the COMPLETE
BEAUTY BIBLE

theCOMPLETE BEAUTY BIBLE

THE ULTIMATE
GUIDE TO
SMART BEAUTY

PAULA BEGOUN

RODALE

Printed in the United States of America
Rodale Inc. makes every effort to use acid-free ∞, recycled paper ♻.

Parts of this book have been published previously as *The Beauty Bible*, 2nd Edition, Copyright © 2002, Paula Begoun and *Don't Go to the Cosmetics Counter Without Me*, 6th Edition, Copyright © 2003, Paula Begoun.
Reprinted with permission from Beginning Press.

Contributing Author: Bryan Barron
Editors: Sigrid Asmus, John Hopper, Jennifer Forbes Provo
Research Assistants: Bryan Barron, Kate Mee
Research for the product reviews
Research Director: Kate Mee
Research Assistants: Shira Druxman, Katherine Siergiej, Lori White

Book design by Erin Smith Bloom and Anthony Serge

Library of Congress Cataloging-in-Publication Data

Begoun, Paula.
    The complete beauty bible : the ultimate guide to smart beauty / Paula Begoun.
        p.   cm.
    "Parts of this book have been published previously as The Beauty Bible, 2nd Edition, Copyright © 2002, Paula Begoun and Don't Go to the Cosmetics Counter Without Me, 6th Edition, Copyright © 2003, Paula Begoun."
    ISBN 1–57954–999–3 hardcover
    1. Skin—Care and hygiene.   2. Beauty, Personal.   3. Consumer education.
I. Begoun, Paula.   The beauty bible.   II. Begoun, Paula.   Don't go to the cosmetics counter without me.   III. Title.
RL87.B3965   2004
646.7'26'082—dc22   2004007915

    4   6   8   10   9   7   5   3   direct mail hardcover

Publisher's Notice

This book is dedicated to women
all over the world
who strive to be the best
they can possibly be.

CONTENTS

part III MORE BEAUTY SOLUTIONS.............289

the COMPLETE
BEAUTY BIBLE

part I

SMART BEAUTY

chapter *1*
COSMETICS COP

WHY YOU NEED TO READ THIS BOOK

Here's the answer, in simple terms: Because reading this book will save you money. Lots of money! Depending on how you spend money on skin care, it can add up to savings of thousands of dollars over the years. More important, it can also help you take better care of your skin. It may literally save your skin if you happen to be using products that are poorly formulated or just plain bad for skin. What you don't know about skin care and makeup can waste money and hurt your skin. The bottom line is simple, too: Getting ripped off isn't pretty.

For those of you who don't know me, let me introduce myself. I am the author and publisher of several best-selling books on the cosmetics industry. My first was *Blue Eyeshadow Should Be Illegal* (which was revised four times and reprinted dozens more); then came *Don't Go to the Cosmetics Counter Without Me* (the sixth edition was published in January 2003); and *Don't Go Shopping for Hair Care Products Without Me*. In addition, I am a syndicated columnist with Knight Ridder News Tribune Service and a consultant to other cosmetics companies, helping them understand the latest research regarding ingredients in relation to skin health.

Over the years my writing has been based strictly on my earnest desire to get beyond the hype and chicanery of the cosmetics industry and to disseminate straightforward information a consumer can really use to look and feel more beautiful.

My expertise, like that of any other consumer reporter who covers such topics as food, cars, or toys, is based on extensive research in the subject area. What makes my situation unique is that I also have over 20 years of personal experience from working as a professional makeup artist and aesthetician and from selling makeup and skin-care products at department stores, salons, and my own stores, and, recently, selling my own product line.

I use my reporting background to continually and extensively research the cosmetics industry. I base all my comments on comprehensive interviews with dermatologists, oncologists, cosmetics chemists, and cosmetic ingredient manufacturers, and on information I've gleaned from both medical journals and cosmetics industry magazines. I am constantly reviewing scientific abstracts and studies. I do not capriciously or abruptly make any conclusions. Everything I report is supported by studies and information from experts in the field, and I document my sources throughout this book. Naturally, there are many who disagree with my assertions, and I do the best I can to present other points of view whenever possible. However, I assure you that a great number of people in the industry agree with my conclusions, even if they can't do so publicly.

In many ways I'm surprised that reviewing, researching, investigating, and questioning the cosmetics industry is what I do for a living. When I started out as a makeup artist back in 1978 it was never my intent to end up writing as a consumer advocate about the cosmetics industry.

At first my quest was personal. I had suffered with acne for many years. I visited over a dozen dermatologists, I tried hundreds of skin-care products from both inexpensive and expensive cosmetics lines, and still I had acne. How could that be? How could all the stuff I diligently applied to my skin—which salesperson after salesperson and doctor after doctor assured me would work—not work? Sometimes one routine worked a little, but not as well as I had hoped and not for very long. And there were always side effects. Most products made my skin so red and irritated I thought it was going to fall off. Slowly but surely I worked my way through the confusion, and after much research and lots more frustration I began to recognize some fundamental problems with the information provided and the products sold by the cosmetics industry. I also found that many of the same difficulties were present in the field of dermatology.

The cosmetics industry's information was little more than marketing mumbo jumbo with exaggerated or misleading claims. In the field of dermatology most doctors don't have time to give their patients the information they need or to explain the limitations and pros and cons of treatment. There is also a great deal of misinformation, not to mention myths that dermatologists generate on their own now that almost 50% of them are selling skin-care products.

In truth, I started out wanting to be an actress, and being a makeup artist was a way to pay the rent. In a very short time it became clear to me that I wasn't going to enjoy much success at acting, or at least I didn't have what it takes to persevere, but I did have what it takes to be a good makeup artist and skin-care consultant. My clientele quickly grew, as did my income. I found I definitely preferred a paycheck to struggling with acting auditions and rejections. Of course, that didn't mean everything was rosy. Along the way, when my freelance makeup business was slow, I supplemented my income with work at department-store makeup counters. But each new job for a different cosmetics line resulted in my being fired.

My first dismissal came after an argument with the line representative of a department-store cosmetics company where I was working. The representative wanted me to say that a toner could close pores and a moisturizer could heal, when I knew it wasn't true. (If a toner could close pores, everyone who used toners would have flawless, poreless skin, and if moisturizers could heal skin, no one would have a pimple or a wrinkle or a scar.) That job lasted about two months.

Several months later, at another department store and for a different cosmetics company, I was involved in a conflict with several of the cosmetics saleswomen working at the other counters. If a customer wanted a particular type of product and I didn't think the product from the line I was selling was right, or if my line didn't offer one, I would walk her over to another counter that I knew had the right product and sell it to her. That caused a nuclear meltdown. I was told to stay behind my counter and not touch another product from any line other than the one I was assigned! (When I recommended that the woman could walk over to the other counter herself, I got in trouble with the sales representatives from my line.) How ludicrous! A great product, five feet away, was out of my reach because it wasn't from the counter I was standing behind.

My final department-store cosmetics counter experience ended when I just couldn't take listening to the distortions and exaggerated claims anymore and decided to go out on my own. I opened my own makeup stores in 1981. I didn't sell blue eyeshadow, wrinkle creams, or toners that claimed to close pores. Along the way, I hooked up with a business partner who was at first thrilled with my ideas and concept, mainly because of the media attention my rather controversial stores attracted.

My stores were generating a lot of attention from the press, and eventually I was asked to make regular appearances on a local TV station in Seattle, KIRO-TV. I also started receiving national and international TV and print exposure.

Eventually my ideas and concept no longer pleased my partner. The department store counters were crowded with women buying blue eyeshadow, wrinkle creams, and toners, so why shouldn't we sell them, too? After all, if you saw women throwing away their money on those sorts of products, at prices ranging from $25 to $250 an ounce for items that cost 75 cents to $4 to produce, you wouldn't want a partner like me, either. I sold my shares back to her in 1984 and stayed at KIRO-TV for the next two years. Sadly, the stores went out of business shortly after I sold them—but I learned a lot about investigative reporting and writing during my time at KIRO-TV in Seattle.

I left the TV station in 1986 after finishing my first book, *Blue Eyeshadow Should Be Illegal*. I decided to self-publish after receiving several rejection letters from major publishing companies telling me that, although they liked my manuscript, I wasn't a celebrity or a model, and no one would be interested in my point of view. I disagreed. I believed lots of women (OK, not all) were tired of hearing useless, and at times incorrect, information from models and celebrities who were born beautiful and knew which makeup artists, photographers, and managers to hire, but very little about the cosmetics they promoted.

I was right, and I sold several hundred thousand copies of my first book! I believed I had given the consumer the more balanced complete information she needed to tackle the cosmetics industry. I was wrong. After I wrote *Blue Eyeshadow*, I received thousands of letters from women asking me, now that they knew how crazy the cosmetics industry was, what they should buy or what I thought of this product or that. It was one thing to have an overview of the cosmetics industry, but quite another to have specific information about a specific product. How could anyone tell if the formulation was effective? How would a person know whether the information about the research done by the doctor or scientist who formulated it was valid? How could someone find out if a company's claims about their impressive study backing up their miracle skin-care product were true? That's when I wrote *Don't Go to the Cosmetics Counter Without Me.*

Meanwhile, the demand to know what works and what doesn't has grown, mainly because the industry has grown. The number of new product lines emerging every day is sheer madness. Between keeping up with infomercials, multilevel direct marketing lines, home shopping network lines, new lines at the department stores and drugstores, and the endless parade of new product launches from existing cosmetic lines, my job was only beginning.

That brings me to today. The cosmetics industry has gone through many changes. In many ways the industry has gotten more complicated, yet as the research into skin and skin-care products has increased it has also become more exciting. My goal in creating this complete beauty bible is to compile and clarify the new data and research to help each woman create the best skin-care routine possible for her specific needs. In addition, I want to help women achieve the best makeup look possible in the fewest steps with the easiest and most effective techniques.

As is true in all the books I write, I also want to separate cosmetics fact from cosmetics fiction and reality from myth, because the fiction and myths spread by the cosmetics industry are nothing less than startling and frustrating. Compared to the information provided by the cosmetics industry, Mother Goose stories sound like the *Encyclopedia Britannica.*

Perhaps the most difficult part of my job is keeping a straight face when I hear the crazy things cosmetics salespeople tell consumers. Combating this endless parade of useless and bizarre information can be maddening. But it's my job and, thankfully, it has been far more rewarding than I ever expected.

EVALUATING PRODUCTS

How I evaluate skin-care formulations deserves some straightforward explanation. Think of the ingredient lists you find on prepared or processed food products, and information on the nutrition content of whole foods. These are the best analogies I can make to ingredient lists on cosmetic products. When it comes to dietary health concerns or awareness, most women start by judging a food on the basis of its ingredient list, or the nutrition content. Information about fat, sodium, preservatives, coloring agents, calories, and many other details is spelled out there. Then the consumer, using various health resources (books, health professionals, research journals, reliable Web sites) can evaluate the Food and Drug Administration (FDA)–mandated ingredient information. Without that information, regardless of how the item tastes (everyone has their own bias), you would never know what you were putting into your body. You could be causing yourself harm by eating more fat than you should, or eating more calories than you should, or skimping on vitamins, antioxidants, fiber, or protein, and on and on, leading to a variety of health problems.

Food labels are incredibly important, and so are the labels on skin-care products. To continue with the food analogy, for example, if one cake mix contains 100 calories per serving but a different cake mix contains 500 calories per serving, that's fundamental information you can use to decide which one you want to buy. Or suppose you are looking for chocolate cake and you find that the mix contains artificial chocolate flavoring—you would probably want to consider another choice. Likewise, if a skin-care product says it is good for sensitive skin but contains ingredients known to cause irritation or breakouts, that is crucial information for making a decision. If a skin-care product sells for $100 but contains the same ingredients as a product that costs $20, that is important information. If a product says it is good for breakouts but contains alcohol and peppermint oil, it would be helpful to know how those ingredients could hurt your face and actually cause more breakouts. That's why the ingredient list is important: It helps you sort through the jungle of choices. Besides, it is a far better starting point for making decisions than are unsubstantiated or one-sided advertising claims.

The fundamental review process for each ingredient or product formulation starts with analyzing the published research about whether or not those ingredients or formulations are capable of providing the asserted benefit.

When it comes to makeup, my team and I actually test a large percentage of the products reviewed. I have purchased over $100,000 worth of cosmetics, and I spend a great deal of time at the cosmetics counters. I use, and test, a lot of makeup, relying on my years of experience along with the feedback I receive from thousands of women.

For makeup application, I make it a point to explain tools and techniques that make sense for everyday use. This isn't the book to use for elaborate or trendy makeup looks. Fashion magazines are replete with those, and you don't need another book to help you paint black smudges all around your eyes or apply glitter from head to toe.

COSMETICS CHEMISTRY—AN ART AND A SCIENCE

I had the opportunity to speak at a meeting of the Society of Cosmetic Chemists, Chicago Chapter, in October 2001. I told this group of accomplished scientists that, despite my anger at the cosmetics industry when it comes to their claims and misleading information, I wanted to affirm that there are wonderful products out there. I know I tend to overemphasize the negative—the crazy claims, high prices, and poor quality—but there are also countless extraordinary products to choose from. This boundless parade of superlative makeup and skin-care products is nothing less than exciting for the consumer.

Every step of the way I am in awe of how beautifully most cosmetics work. Where would we be without the brilliant work of the cosmetics chemists who make the exquisite products we use? Because of their astonishing skill, we have moisturizers that take care of dry skin and help skin heal. They create mascaras that can build thick, lush lashes without flaking or smearing, and foundations that smooth out skin tone, making it look flawless. We have sunscreens that protect skin from sunburn as well as from wrinkles and the potential for skin cancer. There is an endless array of sensuous lipsticks that add relatively long-lasting color and definition to the mouth (and keep it there even longer with the advent of Procter & Gamble's PermaTone lip color—but I'll get into that in the makeup section of this book). Not to mention blushes that softly accent cheekbones and eyeshadows that define eyes, and, well, the list is endless.

I want to sincerely thank all the cosmetics companies who have provided so much of their time and information to me for this book, as well as for my newsletter and my other books. We often don't see eye to eye, but despite our differences, more companies than ever have been generous and forthcoming with information and products.

I also want to thank all the cosmetics chemists everywhere who strive to produce the better and better products that continue to make the beauty industry so incredibly beautiful. I also want to ask cosmetics chemists to do the best they can, whenever they can, to combat the insane marketing departments they have to work with! After interviewing and talking to hundreds of cosmetics chemists over the years, I know most of you don't believe even a fraction of what the advertisements, salespeople, infomercial hucksters, or editorials in fashion magazines say about the products you create. Your work is rooted in science, not hyperbole. I also know this is a risky business. After all, creating products that no one buys is not going to get anyone a promotion, and the marketing department knows all too well what women love to hear, no matter how ridiculous. But try anyway, just to bring a bit of fresh air into an otherwise very cloudy business.

IS BEAUTY EVER NATURAL?

Beauty is definitely in the eye of the beholder, but in our culture, where the cosmetics industry is a $40-billion-a-year industry, beauty takes effort and money. From celebrities to models, and from homemakers to lawyers, hair care, skin care, and makeup are part of a woman's morning ritual. It is probably important for me to make it clear (as the picture of me on the cover of this book shows) that I am hardly anti-makeup, anti-skin care, or anti-hair care—far from it. I do use several skin-care products, I wear makeup (sometimes a lot of makeup), I dye my hair, I have had corrective cosmetic medical procedures (including Botox, breast implants, and nonablative laser resurfacing), I get manicures and pedicures, and I am diligent about wearing sunscreen. Some women may be shocked at the fact that I am not writing about "a return to basics" or making your own cosmetics. My entire perspective throughout every book that I've ever written is to be as nonjudgmental as possible about a woman's personal decisions on what she chooses to do around her own appearance. When it comes to almost all aspects of beauty, I am interested in relating the research in regard to what works and what doesn't. The final decision is always up to the consumer. No matter what that decision is, I want every woman to know what is possible (or impossible) to gain by using a product, so she can purchase what works and not waste money on gimmicks or products that can't possibly live up to their claims.

chapter 2
MIRACLES, FRAUDS, & FACTS: AN A TO Z GUIDE

Whether it's royal bee jelly, yeast extract, vitamins, amino acids, minerals, gems, special water, volcanic mud, DNA, placenta extract, a variety of animal organ extracts, or plants from every corner of the planet, the cosmetics industry wants you to believe that they have a miracle ingredient that can take care of your skin-care woes. To put it simply, every ingredient can't be a miracle. Before you can decide how to take care of your skin, you need to understand what ingredients can and can't do. This chapter focuses on the ingredients that get showcased on a label along with a product's promises of delivering wrinkle-free, acne-free, or just generally flawless skin, as well as the ingredients that have been questioned as being dangerous or a risk to skin. I've included all of the significant ones I am asked about most often. Among the ones listed, there are definitely some genuine, incredibly effective ingredients that can have a positive effect on skin. But there are also many with overblown reputations, or with scant evidence that they are worthwhile for skin when it comes to daily skin care. And, of course, there are those that are just downright silly.

ANTIOXIDANTS AND FREE-RADICAL DAMAGE

An "antioxidant" isn't a type of ingredient. Instead, the name describes the function or action a specific ingredient can have on the skin. Free-radical damage is what antioxidants are supposed to take care of, either by stopping new damage or by reversing earlier damage caused by free radicals. Antioxidants and free-radical damage are considered so vital to our understanding of the origins of cancer, aging, illness, and disease that they have become a profound area of research. Many major universities have an antioxidant or free-radical research department. Dozens of scientific journals are dedicated to these topics alone, including *Free Radical Research, Free Radical Biology and Medicine, Antioxidants and Redox Signaling, Oxidative Stress and Aging, Journal of Anti-Aging Medicine, Mechanisms of Aging and Development, Photochemical & Photobiological Sciences, Photodermatology, Photoimmunology, Photomedicine,* and *Photochemical & Photobiological Sciences.*

Before you can understand the claims being made about many of the skin-care ingredients listed in this section, it is important to have an awareness of what free-radical damage is and what antioxidants can and can't do.

Let's begin by saying that free-radical damage is bad for the skin. It is well-known that oxygen, sunshine (UV rays), and pollution are the main catalysts of free-radical damage. Theoretically, free-radical damage can cause deterioration of the skin's support structures, decreasing elasticity and resilience. What plays a part in slowing down free-radical damage is the presence of antioxidants in the diet, and, possibly, the topical application of antioxidants in skin-care products. Antioxidants are ingredients such as vitamins A, C, and E; superoxide dismutase; flavonoids; beta carotene; glutathione; selenium; and zinc. Technically there are thousands (yes, thousands) of viable antioxidant compounds in the plant world, of which we have so far discovered a mere handful.

Despite the proliferation of skin-care products containing antioxidants, according to many researchers, including Dr. Jeffrey Blumberg, chief of antioxidants research at Tufts University, "There is no conclusive scientific evidence that antioxidants really prevent wrinkles, nor is there any information about how much antioxidant(s) or exactly which one(s) has to be present in a product to have an effect" or if any noticeable effect is even possible.

Even if antioxidants did work on the skin to prevent free-radical damage, the results would hardly be immediate. Free-radical damage in the human body can continue for years and years before any noticeable deterioration can be detected. By the same token, you can't slap the stuff on and expect to immediately notice your wrinkles disappearing.

Despite this lack of hard evidence, fashion magazines and cosmetics companies have heralded the elimination of free-radical damage as the fountain of youth. The excitement about antioxidants is understandable. According to many skin experts (both legitimate experts and those who endorse specific products), all aspects of aging, including wrinkling, are caused by free-radical damage. Vitamin companies and cosmetics companies alike want you to believe their antioxidant products can eliminate it. The evidence is fairly convincing that free-radical damage is an insidious "natural" process that causes the body to break down. What isn't known is whether you can really stop free-radical damage that is taking place on the skin.

Free-Radical Damage

Explaining free-radical damage is like trying to explain how television works. No matter how many times you're told how transmission and reception happen, unless you have a grasp of technology it all sounds like a foreign language. Nevertheless, here's a simplified explanation of free-radical damage.

Free-radical damage takes place on an atomic level. That's really small. To get a sense of an atom's size, imagine that one tablespoonful of water is made up of about 120 billion trillion molecules. Molecules are made of atoms, and a single atom is made up of protons, neutrons, and electrons. Electrons are always found in pairs. However, when oxygen molecules are involved in a chemical reaction, they can lose one of their electrons. This oxygen molecule that now has only one electron is called a free radical. With only one electron, the oxygen molecule must quickly find another electron, and it does this by taking the electron from another molecule. When that molecule in turn loses one of its electrons, it too must seek out another, in a continuing reaction. Molecules attempting to repair themselves in this way trigger a cascading event called "free-radical damage." The action of free-radical damage takes place in a fraction of a second.

How does this affect our skin? Skin cells are formed of numerous parts, including the nucleus, where genetic material in the form of DNA resides; mitochondria, which are responsible for cell respiration and energy production; ribosomes, which are involved in protein synthesis and are composed of RNA, which communicates genetic information; and lysosomes, which are responsible for a cell's enzymatic activity (its chemical actions). These elements are all encased in a plasma membrane (the cell wall). Any of these basic cellular elements—DNA, mitochondria, RNA, and lysosomes—can be broken or impaired by free radicals going about their business of looking for spare electrons.

While we can't see free-radical damage taking place in our skin (at least not without the aid of a skin biopsy and a powerful microscope), we can see it quite clearly in food or even paint. When paint is kept away from air (oxygen) and sunlight in a sealed container, it remains liquid. When it is exposed to air, however, it hardens. What makes this take place? The hardening occurs when an oxygen molecule interacts with the paint and becomes unstable, losing one of its electrons. In searching for another electron, it takes it from the molecule in the paint. This single event happens trillions of times until the paint dries and there are no more electrons available.

What triggers a molecule to let go of one of its electrons, generating free-radical damage? The answer is the presence of oxygen or any compound that contains an oxygen molecule (such as carbon mon**oxide**, hydrogen per**oxide**, and super**oxide**), sunlight, or pollution. Please note that super**oxide** dismutase is an antioxidant enzyme catalase to disarm and destroy the superoxide free radical.

In the human body, free-radical damage is taking place all the time. If you smoke, live in a city, or drive on the highway, that can accelerate the free-radical events taking place in your body at any given moment.

However, to refer to free-radical damage as "damaging" can be misleading. What we call free-radical damage is actually a common life function, in plants and animals as well as in the human body. Immune systems, metabolism, cells communicating with each other, and collagen production (as well as destruction) are all affected both positively *and* negatively by the presence of free-radical damage. This is referred to as the oxygen paradox. We need oxygen for life, but oxygen is also killing us. If you were to breathe pure oxygen for longer than one hour you would die! For all intents and purposes, and in basic terms, oxygen is probably one of the major reasons why, as we grow older, our body's systems start to shut down.

The question that you may be asking at this very moment is this: With all that free-radical damage taking place, and all this oxygen all around us (the air we breathe contains about 20% oxygen), how is it that we are still walking around? Why are we still living? The answer is antioxidants.

Antioxidants

Any substance that impedes or slows down free-radical damage by preventing the oxidative action of molecules is referred to as an "antioxidant." Antioxidants prevent unstable oxygen molecules (made unstable by loss of one electron) from interacting with other molecules (taking one of their electrons) and in turn causing them to become unstable, a process that starts the free-radical chain reaction. Fortunately, a vast assortment of antioxidants are found in both the human body and in the plant world. The full list is beyond the scope of this book. Some of the major categories in the plant world are the carotenoids and flavonoids. Many vitamins have antioxidant properties, including vitamins A, E, and C, as do amino acids such as methionine, L-cysteine, and L-carnitine; enzymes such as superoxide dismutase and catalase; and coenzymes such as lipoic acid and coenzyme Q10. Other antioxidant compounds include glutathione and methylsufonylsulfate.

So what does that have to do with wrinkles? No one is exactly sure, but theoretically when free-radical damage originates from natural environmental factors and fails to be cancelled out by antioxidant protection, then wrinkles appear. If we don't get enough antioxidant protection, either from our own body's production, from dietary sources, or from other sources, including antioxidants we put on our skin, free-radical damage continues unrestrained, causing cells to break down and impairing or destroying their ability to function normally. Instead of helping build collagen or other skin components, free-radical damage destroys them.

There's just one problem with the hope that stopping free-radical damage with antioxidants can protect your skin, and that's the fact that free-radical damage is constant and extensive. How could you ever use enough antioxidants to stop it? How much oxygen, sunlight, or pollution can you really keep away from all skin cells, or even some skin cells? How fast do the antioxidants get used up? Do they last 20 minutes, one hour, two hours, or more on the skin? At this time, no one knows for sure.

Major investigations are now under way in this fascinating area of human aging (intrinsic aging) and sun damage (extrinsic aging), factors that most unquestionably influence wrinkling. However, even though many respected researchers are working on this issue, the research is still in its infancy, and suggesting anything beyond that is sheer fantasy.

Almost every company makes moisturizers that contain antioxidants, so they aren't hard to find. You won't see any difference in your skin, but if free-radical damage, and thus the destruction of the skin's structure, can be slowed or if sun damage can be reduced, then antioxidants should help. Many scientists think that if there is a fountain of youth, antioxidants could be in it. For now, that's only theoretical, and no one can give you any definitive amounts or specific ingredients to look for, despite the cosmetics industry's attempts to do so.

ACETYL GLUCOSAMINE

Acetyl glucosamine is an amino acid sugar, the primary constituent of substances called mucopolysaccharides and hyaluronic acid that are found in all parts of the skin. It has value as a natural moisturizing factor (a natural component of the skin's composition) and is effective (in large concentrations) for wound healing. There is also research showing that chitins (also known as chitosan—which is composed of acetyl glucosamine) can help in the complex process of wound healing (source: *Cellular and Molecular Life Sciences*, February 1997, pages 131–140). As impressive as that sounds, the tiny amount of acetyl glucosamine found in some skin-care products is several orders of magnitude less than the amount of acetyl glucosamine used to heal wounds. Further, it is important to understand that none of this relates to wrinkles. Wrinkles are not wounds. Injuries that cause a breach or tear in the surface of the skin, like those caused by a cut, stab, puncture, or scrape, are unrelated to what causes wrinkles. Something that may help heal a tear in skin is not going to change a wrinkle.

ALGAE

For all intents and purposes algae is little more than pond scum or seaweed (seaweeds are large algae that grow in a saltwater or marine environment). Algae are very simple, chlorophyll-containing organisms, in a family of more than 20,000 different known species. That's a lot of scum and seaweed! A number of these have been used for drugs, where they can work as anticoagulants, antibiotics, antihypertensive agents, blood cholesterol reducers, dilatory agents, and even as insecticides. In cosmetics, algae are used in thickening agents, water-binding agents, and antioxidants. But algae are also potential skin irritants. For example, the phycocyanin found in blue-green algae has been suspected of allergenicity or causing dermatitis on the basis of patch tests (source: *Current Issues in Molecular Biology*, January 2002, pages 1–11). Other forms of algae, such as Irish moss and carrageenan, contain proteins, vitamin A, sugar, starch, vitamin B$_1$, iron, sodium, phosphorus, magnesium, copper, and calcium. For the most part, algae, in their many forms, are probably less of a risk and more of a help to skin when used as antioxidants. But the claims that algae can stop or get rid of wrinkling are completely unsubstantiated.

Names of the algae typically found in cosmetics include *Ulva lactuca, Ascophyllum, Laminaria longicruris, Laminaria saccharine, Laminaria digitata, Alaria esculenta*, various *Porphyra* species, *Chondrus crispus,* and *Mastocarpus stellatus.*

ALPHA LIPOIC ACID

A large quantity of information shows that alpha lipoic acid, when taken *orally* as a dietary supplement, has many potential health benefits. Nevertheless, when it comes to research on what it can do to get rid of wrinkles and make a woman look younger, the information is at best theoretical and (more realistically) inconclusive. While studies of alpha lipoic acid do exist, none have been carried out on people and none have been double-blind or placebo-controlled to evaluate wrinkling (source: *Clinical & Experimental Dermatology*, October 2001, pages 578–582). All of the research has been done on human dermal fibroblasts "in vitro" in cell culture systems. In vitro (test tube) results are always interesting, but it's not known if they translate to human skin. These models do mimic human skin, but something that mimics human skin is still not the same as living skin. It is clear from the research that alpha lipoic acid is a potent antioxidant, but there are many potent antioxidants. Alpha lipoic acid is not the be-all and end-all when it comes to your skin's health.

AYURVEDA

Ayurveda is an alternative health practice developed in India. The term "Ayurveda" is based on two Sanskrit words: ayu, meaning life, and veda, meaning science. Ayurveda is said to be 5,000 years old. That may impress a lot of people, but given that the average human life span prior to the 1900s was less than 50 years, and that the antibiotics developed in the mid-1940s provided health cures previously unknown, the benefits of this ancient science are not necessarily the panacea its adherents would have you believe. Regardless of your belief system, what is absolutely true is that the claims of Ayurveda's effectiveness or lack thereof are primarily anecdotal. That has been changing, however, with some plants proving to be beneficial and others not.

According to an article in the *Indian Journal of Experimental Biology* (May 2000, pages 409–414), the Ayurvedic system of treatments believes that the "living system is made of panch-mahabuta, in the form of vata, pitta and kapha at the physical level and satwa, raja and tama at the mental level. This covers the psychosomatic constitution and [is] commonly known as the Tridosh theory. The imbalance in these body humours [mechanisms] is the basic cause of any type of disease manifestation."

Another interpretation of Ayurvedic theory, in *Alternative Therapies Health Medicine* (March 7, 2001), noted that "The body is composed of 3 body doshas, 3 mental doshas, 7 dhatus, and malas. The harmony among the body doshas of vata (nervous system), pitta (enzymes), and kapha (mucus) and the gunas, or mental doshas (which are human attributes: satogun [godly], rajas [kingly], and tamas [evil]), constitutes health, and their disharmony constitutes disease. The management of illness requires balancing the doshas back into a harmonious state through lifestyle interventions, spiritual nurturing, and treatment with herbo-mineral formulas based on one's mental and bodily constitution."

As you can tell, this is not an easily understood subject. I am not capable of commenting on how or if Ayurvedic principles of any kind can affect skin (though I assure you they do not prevent sun damage—that, at least, is certain). A more complete discussion of Ayurveda would be too complex for the scope of this book and, to say the least, there isn't a shred of research documentation to examine in regard to skin. What I can say is that none of the so-called Ayurveda-based lines I've reviewed have any unique or unusual ingredients. All of the ones I've seen contain the same ingredients that show up in skin-care product after skin-care product, whether they are sold at drugstores, department stores, or health food stores.

BOTANICALS

Is it worthwhile to look for natural ingredients in skin-care products? Leaving aside the fact that the process of removing a plant extract and then stabilizing and preserving it in a cosmetic renders it fairly unnatural, the answer is yes and no. There are bountiful numbers of wonderful plants and plant extracts that have beneficial effects on skin—and there are plenty of plant extracts that present problems for skin, too. Even so, let's say a natural or botanical ingredient is effective as a disinfectant; that doesn't make it better than a synthetically derived disinfectant, it just makes it an alternative. One shortcoming of natural ingredients in skin-care products that the cosmetics industry hasn't addressed is that each natural ingredient has a large range of limitations. These include what happens as a result of the purification process it goes through to get into a product, which part of the plant is effective, bad crops, possible contamination with herbicides, and maintaining consistent concentrations. In many ways synthetic ingredients are often more reliable for the skin.

It is also important to reiterate that just because an ingredient is found growing in nature doesn't mean it's good for the skin. Lots of plants are poisonous if ingested and lots of plants can irritate the skin.

Among the reasons to be wary of natural ingredients (aside from the fact that there is no regulated definition of the word "natural" and cosmetics companies can use it to mean anything, or nothing at all) is that their manufacturers do not make their research available to the Cosmetic Ingredient Review (CIR) panel of the Cosmetic, Toiletry, and Fragrance Association (CTFA). This association is the cosmetics industry's attempt at self-regulation. The efforts of this group are interesting, even though the cosmetics industry doesn't always cooperate. According to an article in *Drug & Cosmetics Industry* magazine (June 1997, page 89), CIR panel members were "frustrated by a lack of specific information to allow them to characterize [natural] ingredients in a manner specific enough to determine safety [or benefit]." The panel further noted that "botanicals are frequently poorly defined, subject to seasonal variations or variations due to different species sources, and varying extraction procedures." Specifically, what is lacking is sufficient information regarding composition, usage concentrations, and possible contaminants, which raises serious doubts about the safety of botanicals and their use.

While plants sound great, pure and natural and all that, and while sesame oil and licorice extract sound far better than capric/caprylic triglyceride and glycyrrhetinic acid, they aren't better or worse. Each has its pros and cons, and it would be a delusion to assume otherwise.

COENZYME Q10—UBIQUINONE

It turns out that despite all the research available on coenzyme Q10 (CoQ10), there are only a handful of studies showing it to have any effect on wrinkles (sources: *Biofactors*, September 1999, pages 371–378; *Zeitschrift für Gerontologie und Geriatrie*, April 1999, pages 83–88). However, neither of these studies was double-blind or placebo-controlled, so there is no way to tell whether or not other formulations could net the same results. What is truly fascinating about CoQ10 has nothing to do with wrinkles. Rather, it is a well-researched nutrient with many studies demonstrating what it can do to improve health. CoQ10 has received particular attention in the prevention and treatment of various forms of cardiovascular disease, strokes, and hypertension. It also has been shown in a small number of studies to increase the metabolism of fat and to increase brain activity. It turns out CoQ10 resides primarily in organs, particularly the heart, with its presence peaking at around age 20 and declining after that. I've seen articles in *Health News* and *International Health News* suggesting CoQ10 should be taken with vitamin E, with a meal containing some fat, or in combination with soy or vegetable oil, which enhances its absorption substantially. "CoQ10 supplements are readily absorbed by the body and no toxic effects have been reported for daily dosages as high as 300 mg though the safety of CoQ10 has not been established in pregnancy and lactation, so caution is advised here until more data becomes available" (source: *International Journal of Alternative and Complementary Medicine*, February 1998, pages 11–12).

Aside from those benefits, there is research showing that sun exposure depletes the presence of CoQ10 in the skin (source: *Journal of Dermatological Science Supplement*, August 2001, pages 1–4). This isn't surprising because lots of the skin's components become diminished upon exposure to the sun. But whether or not taking CoQ10 supplements or applying them to skin stops or alters sun damage is not known.

COLLAGEN AND ELASTIN

Collagen and elastin are best described as the skin's scaffolding. These two proteins create a cross-linked mesh that comprises more than 75% of the skin's structure and shape. They are also responsible for the skin's strength, smoothness, and elasticity. Clearly, collagen and elastin are fundamental to the health and appearance of our skin. One of the more amazing capabilities of collagen and elastin is that they can easily regenerate, which is why our skin is usually able to heal so quickly when wounded. As we age, from both intrinsic factors (chronological aging, health problems) and extrinsic factors (sun damage, pollution, smoking, free-radical damage), collagen and elastin get damaged and depleted. If collagen and elastin are so important and so capable of regeneration, then surely there must be a way to facilitate that process. From the cosmetics industry's perspective, it seems logical to manufacture moisturizers that contain collagen and elastin, and to attempt to convince women that if you apply these substances topically on the skin they will be absorbed and become part of your skin, shoring up and reinforcing your own collagen and elastin. However, the forms of collagen and elastin originally used in moisturizers were good only as water-binding agents because their molecular structure was too large to penetrate skin.

Using newer forms of collagen and elastin ingredients in skin-care products, however, manufacturers were able to break down the collagen and elastin structure, making them soluble and therefore able to penetrate skin. These new substances were referred to as pro-collagen and pro-elastin. Yet even though these newer substances were capable of penetrating skin, there is no research demonstrating that they had any effect on adding to the collagen or elastin content of skin. On the surface, collagen and elastin are nothing more than good water-binding agents (natural moisturizing factors of skin). That's good, but it won't change the shape or resiliency of skin.

Research indicates that it is possible to stimulate your skin to produce more collagen and elastin, but not by putting collagen and elastin on the skin. Rather, tretinoin, AHAs, BHA, and treatments such as laser resurfacing, chemical peels, and microdermabrasion can all provide that benefit. Antioxidants, anti-irritants, and natural moisturizing factors (water-binding agents) contribute to helping skin heal and may possibly help stimulate the production and growth of new collagen and elastin. Growth factors, discussed in this section, also play a role.

COPPER

Copper is an important trace element for human nutrition. The body needs copper to absorb and utilize iron, and copper is also a component of the powerful antioxidant enzyme superoxide dismutase. Copper supplements have been shown to increase superoxide dismutase levels in humans (source: *Healthnotes*—www.healthnotes.com). The synthesis of collagen and elastin is in part related to the presence of copper in the body, and it's important for many other reasons and processes. But is copper important for skin? Some skin-care companies definitely want you to believe this is the answer for your skin. It isn't. However, there is research showing that copper is effective for wound healing (sources: *Journal of Clinical Investigation*, November 1993, pages 2368–2376; *Federation of European Biochemical Sciences Letter*, October 1988, pages 343–346).

As I've mentioned before, wound healing can't be compared to what happens with wrinkles. Wound healing is related to many biophysical processes that have nothing to do with wrinkling. Further, there are lots of substances that repair wounds. Far more research exists on transforming growth factor and epidermal growth factor for wound healing than on copper. And there is also research on the effectiveness of silver sulfadiazine for wound healing (source: *Journal of Vascular Surgery*, August 1992, pages 251–257), tretinoin (source: *Journal of the American Academy of Dermatology*, September 2001, pages 382–386), and curcumin (source: *Journal of Trauma*, November 2001, pages 927–931) to name just a few. Actually there is far more research about tretinoin and the growth factors than there is concerning copper. Copper is still an option, but what, if anything, it may have to do with combating wrinkles is nothing more than conjecture, not fact.

DEAD SEA MINERALS

The Dead Sea in Israel is considered dead because nothing can live in it. Many environmental factors have contributed to making the Dead Sea one of the saltiest lakes in the world. Seawater from the Atlantic and Pacific Oceans has a 3% to 4% salt content; the Dead Sea has a 32% salt content, as well as a large concentration of minerals such as sulfur, magnesium, calcium, bromide, and potassium. If you haven't been to the Dead Sea, I can tell you that the aroma from the sulfur water is overwhelming. It is hard to imagine that anything so noxious would be considered a beauty treatment.

It probably won't come as a shock to you when I tell you that there is no research showing that Dead Sea minerals have any effect on wrinkles. There are, however, several studies demonstrating that these minerals can have a positive effect on psoriatic skin (sources: *Israel Journal of Med-*

ical Sciences, November 2001, pages 828–832; *British Journal of Dermatology*, June 2001, pages 1154–1160; *International Journal of Dermatology*, February 2001, pages 158–159; *Journal of the American Academy of Dermatology*, August 2000, pages 325–326). Psoriasis is a skin condition characterized by rapidly dividing, overactive skin cells. No one is quite sure how the Dead Sea minerals and salts affect psoriasis. One of the more popular theories regarding its benefit is that the mineral content of the water slows down the out-of-control cell division. Some of the research indicates that the benefit is cumulative and the results can last for up to five months.

DEA—DIETHANOLAMINE

In 1999 the National Toxicology Program (NTP) completed a study that found an association between cancer in laboratory animals and the application of diethanolamine (DEA) and certain DEA-related ingredients to their skin (source: Study #TR-478, Toxicology and Carcinogenesis Studies of Diethanolamine (CAS No. 111-42-2) in F344/N Rats and B6C3F1 Mice (Dermal Studies), July 1999—http://ntp-server.niehs.nih.gov/). For the DEA-related ingredients, the NTP study suggested that the carcinogenic response is linked to possible residual levels of DEA. However, the NTP study did not establish a link between DEA and the risk of cancer in humans.

This study "found that repeated skin application to mouse skin of the cosmetic ingredient diethanolamine (DEA), or its fatty acid derivative cocamide-DEA, induced liver and kidney cancer." Besides this "clear evidence of carcinogenicity [only to mouse skin in high concentrations]," the NTP also emphasized that DEA is readily absorbed through the skin and accumulates in organs, such as the brain, where it induces chronic toxic effects. The report went on to explain that high concentrations of DEA-based detergents are commonly used in a wide range of cosmetics and toiletries, including shampoos, hair dyes, hair conditioners, lotions, creams, and bubble baths, plus liquid dishwashing and laundry soaps. "Lifelong use of these products thus clearly poses major avoidable cancer risks to the great majority of U.S. consumers, particularly infants and young children," the report stated.

It is important to note that this conclusion was a stretch. Taking results from high concentrations used on mice and extending them to long-term topical use by humans is not exactly scientific.

According to the FDA (source: *Office of Cosmetics and Colors Fact Sheet*, December 9, 1999), "Although DEA itself is used in very few cosmetics, DEA-related ingredients (e.g., oleamide DEA, lauramide DEA, cocamide DEA) are widely used in a variety of cosmetic products. These ingredients function as emulsifiers or foaming agents and are generally used at levels of 1% to 5%. The FDA takes these NTP findings very seriously and is in the process of carefully evaluating the studies and test data to determine the real risk, if any, to consumers. The Agency believes that at the present time there is no reason for consumers to be alarmed based on the usage of these ingredients in cosmetics. Consumers wishing to avoid cosmetics containing DEA or its conjugates may do so by reviewing the ingredient statement required to appear on the outer container label of cosmetics offered for retail sale to consumers.

"If the FDA's evaluation of the NTP data indicates that a health hazard exists, the FDA will advise the industry and the public and will consider its legal options under the authority of the Food, Drug and Cosmetic Act in protecting the health and welfare of consumers."

I can see why some people may want to avoid DEA in cosmetics, and it is easy enough to do so, but given the specific research data, the entire issue of risk seems rather alarmist. In essence, there is as yet no real evidence demonstrating that people using cosmetics with DEA are any more prone to cancers than those not using them.

DHEA—DEHYDROEPIANDROSTERONE

DHEA (dehydroepiandrosterone) is a male hormone produced in the adrenal glands that contributes to bone density, muscle mass, and skin tone. DHEA production peaks when we are in our 20s and, like all male and female hormones, declines shortly thereafter. Its popularity as an oral supplement comes from its reputation for increasing strength, boosting the immune system, enhancing memory and concentration, reducing depression, preventing weight gain, and heightening libido function. Talk about seductive! A quick search on the Internet for dehydroepiandrosterone brings up over 46,000 Web sites, a good many of which are linked to companies selling DHEA supplements.

The research on DHEA is interesting, albeit controversial. Libido function improvement was shown in research published in the *New England Journal of Medicine* (September 30, 1999) and brain function improvement was discussed in *Brain Research Reviews* (November 2001, pages

287–293). But according to an article in the *Harvard Men's Health Watch* (September 2001), DHEA is not ready for prime time. "In one small trial, 67% of subjects who took DHEA reported an increase in 'well-being,' but objective measurements found no change in body fat or sugar metabolism. In another study, DHEA treatment was associated with an increase in muscle strength and mass at the knee—but only eight men participated in the trial. More recently, doctors in New York administered DHEA in a dose of at least 50 mg a day to 10 men with an average age of 60; after 18 months, there was no change in blood testosterone or prostate specific antigen (PSA) levels." This same article also mentioned a new study from the University of Missouri Medical School that "found no evidence DHEA had any benefits. The [39 men in the study] who took the hormone did not exhibit either a decrease in body fat or an increase in muscle mass; body weight did not change appreciably. Insulin and blood sugar levels were also unchanged. DHEA failed to produce an improvement in sexual function; similarly, there were no changes in overall subjective well-being." Further, Dr. Andrew Weil (at www.drweil.com) warns that DHEA "can increase the risk of breast and prostate cancer, and may elevate the risk of a heart attack."

What does any of this have to do with skin? Aside from the suggested association between DHEA and male hormone levels, and hormone levels having an effect on skin, there is no research showing DHEA has any impact on skin in regard to wrinkling or aging (source: *Clinics in Geriatric Medicine*, November 2001, pages 661–672). Besides, it isn't the male hormones that improve the texture and appearance of female skin. The feel and suppleness of a woman's skin are affected by the levels of her estrogen and progesterone production.

DMAE—DIMETHYLAMINOETHANOL

In regard to dimethylaminoethanol (DMAE), there is no research associating it with the skin in any way. What little research there is about DMAE relates to its effect as an oral supplement, and the findings are mixed. The claims about it being an instant face-lift or an ingredient that can repair skin come primarily, if not exclusively, from Dr. N.V. Perricone's book *The Wrinkle Cure*, but his assertions are not substantiated in any published study or research paper.

DMAE, known chemically as 2-dimethyl-amino-ethanol, has been available in Europe under the product name Deanol for over 30 years.

As an oral supplement it is popularly known for improving mental alertness, much like *Gingko biloba* and coenzyme Q10. However, the research about DMAE does not show the same positive results found with the other two supplements. Because DMAE is chemically similar to choline, DMAE is thought to stimulate production of acetylcholine. And because acetylcholine is a brain neurotransmitter, it's easy to see how it could be associated with brain function. However, only a handful of studies have looked at DMAE for that purpose and they have not been conclusive in the least, and some have shown that DMAE may be problematic or not very effective (sources: *Mechanisms of Aging and Development*, February 1988, pages 129–138; *Neuropharmacology*, June 1989, pages 557–561; *European Neurology*, 1991, pages 423–425).

Aside from what it may do as an oral supplement, the question about DMAE and skin is whether or not a topical application can prevent cell deterioration. Perricone's assertion is that it can, though he doesn't cite a single source that backs up his finding (other than himself and a study where a cream containing DMAE that he sells was applied by seventeen of his own patients).

Despite the lack of evidence supporting DMAE as having any effect on skin, there are hundreds of Web sites claiming that it has. It is possible that DMAE can help protect the cell membrane, and keeping cells intact can have benefit, but so far that appears to be only conjecture and not fact.

EMOLLIENTS

Standard to almost *all* cosmetics, both the so-called natural ones and the not-so-natural ones, are soft, supple, waxlike, emollient, and thickening agents with names that read like a science journal—long and almost indecipherable. These pliable skin-softening agents have many functions. Not only do they have an affinity for skin, effortlessly smoothing over the surface and readily merging with the natural structures of the skin, they also provide the very feel and texture of the cosmetics we use. If a cosmetic has an elegant, smooth feel; or looks like a light, gel-like lotion; or has a soft, translucent appearance; or has a thick, creamy-white texture, it's the mix of these thickening, emollient ingredients that produces those finishes.

The assortment of names these technical-sounding ingredients come in is nothing less than astounding. There are more of them than you can imagine. They range from cetearyl alcohol, to isopropyl myristate, triglycerides, myristic acid, palmitic acid, PEG-60 hydrogenated castor oil, glyceryl linoleate, cyclomethicone, dimethicone, hexyl laurate, isohexadecane, methyl glucose sesquioleate, decyl oleate, stearic acid, octyldodecanol, and thousands more. There are also more understandable or at least familiar "natural" versions such as lanolin, hydrogenated plant oils, shea butter, and cocoa butter.

Together, these unsung heroes of moisturizers, sunscreens, cleansers, foundations, eyeshadows, and blushes are the mainstay of cosmetic formulations the world over. What they all have in common is their molecular resemblance to the natural lipids (sebum or oil) and intercellular substances found in skin. A big issue for dry skin is the very lack of these lipids and intercellular substances. Cosmetics with innumerable formulary recipes are invaluable resources to fill in what the skin lacks. These ingredients are what prevent dry skin, make rough skin feel smooth, soothe irritated skin, and replenish what skin loses from irritation, cleansing products, and sun damage. Although these indispensable substances are relatively indecipherable in the ingredient list, to a cosmetic formulation they are as important as, or even more important than, any natural-sounding ingredient could ever be.

On the other hand, while these thickening and emollient ingredients work great for a wide range of skin types, they may cause problems for someone with oily, combination, or acne-prone skin. Because all of these ingredients to one degree or another mimic the skin's own oil production, they add more to your own naturally abundant oil supply, and that will only make things worse. This is also true for natural-sounding ingredients like jojoba oil, shea butter, cocoa butter, safflower oil, lanolin, olive oil, and so on. This is one of the primary reasons why someone with oily, combination, or acne-prone skin should avoid almost all emollient moisturizers. When you have your own built-in lubrication (the oil produced by the oil glands) flowing freely onto your skin, it makes no sense to apply someone else's fabricated version, too.

EMU OIL

The emu is a large, flightless bird indigenous to Australia, and emu oil has become an important component of the Australian economy. As a result there is research from that part of the world showing it to be a good emollient that can help heal skin. But along with the evidence that emu oil is a good emollient and the companies promoting it for that, there are also companies promoting products containing emu oil for its antiaging, antiwrinkling, and wound-healing properties. So does emu oil live up to these acclaimed properties? Regrettably, none of these promises are supported by research. A study published in the *Australasian Journal of Dermatology* (August 1996, pages 159–161), looked at the "Cosmetic and moisturizing properties of emu oil . . . assessed in a double-blind clinical study. Emu oil in comparison to mineral oil was found overall to be more cosmetically acceptable and had better skin penetration/permeability. Furthermore it appears that emu oil in comparison to mineral oil has better moisturizing properties, superior texture, and lower incidence of comedogenicity, but probably because of the small sample size these differences were not found to be statistically significant. Neither of the oils were found to be irritating to the skin." That's good, but it's hardly a reason to run out and by a product containing emu oil. Further, another study published in *Plastic and Reconstructive Surgery* (December 1998, pages 2404–2407), concluded that applying emu oil on a fresh wound actually delayed wound healing. Emu oil's reputation is driven mostly by cosmetics company claims and not by any real proof that emu oil is an essential requirement for skin.

ENZYMES

Whether in the form of papaya fruit or in a substance such as papain (a proteinase derived from unripe papaya), enzymes have been used for quite some time as exfoliants. They're not as good as AHAs, but they're exfoliants nonetheless. The other new enzymes being put in skin-care potions are supposed to stimulate your skin's own biological processes that have slowed down because of age or sun damage.

Enzymes are proteins that function as biological catalysts. They accelerate chemical reactions in a cell, reactions that would proceed minimally or not at all if enzymes weren't there. Most enzymes—and a lot of different enzymes affect skin cells—are finicky about how they interact. Sometimes it takes several enzymes to produce one chemical reaction. Some enzymes depend on the presence of smaller enzymes, called coenzymes, in order to function. What this boils down to is that it is pretty complicated to stimulate enzyme activity in the skin. One little enzyme in a skin-care product won't turn on your skin's ability to create, say, collagen or elastin. It's a nice idea, but the theory is much more impressive than the effect, if any, on the skin.

Furthermore, even if enzymes were effective in skin-care products, they are an exceedingly unstable ingredient. Enzymes deteriorate quickly, depending on the pH of the product, the presence of other enzymes, and changes in temperature. Most likely, in any enzyme product you buy, the enzyme has deteriorated long before you have a chance to open the product.

GINKGO BILOBA

Research establishing *Ginkgo biloba* as an effective systemic vasodilator (meaning it can increase blood flow and be effective for improving memory and concentration) has increased over the past several years (sources: *Neuropsychobiology*, January 2002, pages 19–26; *International Journal of Neuropsychopharmacology*, June 2001, pages 131–134). When taken internally, there are other benefits (though there is still conflicting evidence) ranging from improvement in overall body circulation to reduced ringing in the ears in the elderly. However, the effects ginkgo may have on brain function and blood flow when taken as a supplement seem to be unrelated to its effects when applied topically on the skin. For skin, ginkgo has components that make it effective as an anti-inflammatory and an aid in collagen production, and it also has antioxidant properties (sources: *Skin Pharmacology and Applied Skin Physiology*, July-August 1997, pages 200–205; *Journal of Pharmacy and Pharmacology*, December 1999, pages 1435–1440).

GLYCERIN

While many cosmetics lines boast all sorts of exotic ingredients, from plant extracts to vitamins, proteins, essential oils, and other exotic and scientific creations, it turns out that plain old glycerin, long known as a humectant, may be a best friend for someone with dry skin. Glycerin is present in all natural lipids, whether animal or vegetable. It can be manufactured by the hydrolysis of fats and by the fermentation of sugars. It can also be synthetically manufactured. For some time it was thought that too much glycerin in a moisturizer could pull water out of the skin instead of drawing it into the skin. That theory now seems to be completely unfounded. What appears to be true is that glycerin shores up the skin's natural protection by filling in the area known as the intercellular matrix and by attracting just the right amount of water to maintain the skin's homeostasis. The intercellular matrix is the mortar that holds layers of skin cells together, creating an intact natural barrier. Keeping the intercellular layer intact keeps bacteria out, moisture in, and the skin's surface smooth. There is also research indicating that the presence of glycerin in the intercellular layer helps other skin lipids do their jobs better (sources: *American Journal of Contact Dermatitis*, September 2000, pages 165–169; *Acta Dermato-Venereologica*, November 1999, pages 418–421).

GRAPE AND GRAPE SEED EXTRACT

A lot of the buzz surrounding grape extracts started with a story in *Consumer Reports* in November 1999 that ranked grape juice just above green tea and blueberries as having strong antioxidant properties. However, the benefits reported both in *Consumer Reports* and in a lead story in *USA Today* (February 2, 2000) had to do with drinking the stuff, not putting it on the skin.

There are no published studies indicating that grapes in any form, applied topically, can affect the wrinkling process (and vineyard workers are hardly wrinkle-free). But when it comes to skin care, there are lots of unpublished studies that "prove" all kinds of things. For example, one cosmetics line points to research by Dr. Stephen Herber of the St. Helena Institute for Plastic Surgery, who conducted a study on the benefits of grape seed, as proof of the efficacy of their products. Not surprisingly, St. Helena is in the heart of California's wine country. This "study," and I use the word loosely, had sixteen volunteers who used pure milled grape seed extract as a topical application to their facial skin twice each day for six weeks. The results? Herber found that most of the volunteers reported improved texture to their facial skin. Others reported effects including an evening-out of complexion pigmentation and excessive oil, a decrease in breakouts, and a decrease in dryness. It only takes a cursory look to notice that this study wasn't done double-blind, that a placebo wasn't used (so we don't know if the results would be the same with a similar or dissimilar type of extract), and that we have no idea of the status of the participants' skin before they started, or what their relation to the product line or researcher was. Even if you buy the results of this study, the study itself used a pure concentration of the substance on the skin, not a product that contained just a small amount of the extract.

Still, none of that would diminish the potential benefit grape extract may have for skin because, aside from the hype, grape seed does contain proanthocyanidin, considered to be a very potent antioxidant (source: *Current Pharmaceutical Biotechnology*, June 2001, pages 187–200). However, there is no research establishing its efficacy on skin.

As I've stated several times throughout this book, and will several times more, antioxidants are a big issue, and there is every reason to believe that there will be great strides in this area. For now, though, it's too early to suggest that we know which antioxidant is the best, how much of it is needed, or whether or not any of them work on the surface of skin to affect wrinkling in a positive way.

HERBAL BREAST ENHANCEMENT?

Most women will do or pay anything to be beautiful, right? That's what a good portion of the cosmetics industry counts on, along with much of the herbal supplement business. While antiaging products are big business, there is also money to be made by convincing women they can take a pill, with all-natural ingredients of course, that will safely enhance the size of their bust. Perhaps images of celebrities with their expansive and overflowing breasts leap to mind along with the hope these products will create the same without surgery. Supplements with names like GroBust, Bust Plus, MiracleBust, Erdic, or Natural Contours abound on the Internet, in vitamin shops, and in mail-order catalogs.

What makes all this unnerving is that by overdosing the body with plant estrogens, these pills can, theoretically, have some effect, although there is no published research indicating that this is the case. Since the female breasts are composed primarily of fat tissue, the only reliable way to increase their size is to gain weight—not something most women want to do. Yet excess estrogen seems to pose that risk, and not only for the breast area. It can also cause bloating and acne. Even more to the point, although plant estrogens (also referred to as phytoestrogens) can have overt health benefits for perimenopausal and menopausal women, there is no research establishing what happens when too much of them are taken, or if there is a negative reaction for younger women who already have sufficient estrogen. But, of course, there are never any downsides to herbal supplements of this kind, at least not any we are likely to hear about from the companies busily selling these products.

The entire issue of breast-enhancement pills is a murky one, saturated with unethical companies doing their best to bilk you out of your money and potentially put your health at risk. For more detailed information about this issue, far more than I can address here, see one of my favorite Web sites, www.dietfraud.com. They have done extensive research on some of the companies selling breast-enhancement pills, including those promoted by some physicians with questionable credentials, and who already have numerous charges of fraud and malpractice lodged against them.

HORMONE CREAMS

The multifaceted and controversial changes a woman experiences, both physiologically and emotionally, during perimenopause and menopause are too complex to cover in this book. However, I would like to provide a bit of insight on the area where perimenopause, menopause, and skin care cross paths, and offer some suggestions and resources so you will be better equipped to make informed decisions.

Thankfully, most cosmetic ingredients are completely benign. I do worry about irritating skin-care products, the lack of sun protection, and how marketing hype about plants and vitamins draws attention away from products that can really help. This last issue has me very concerned about a controversial barrage of skin-care products hitting the market that purportedly contain plant estrogen and/or plant progesterone. Tofu extract is reputedly the source of the plant estrogen, and wild yam extract is the source of the plant progesterone. Skin-care products that contain estrogen and progesterone are aimed directly at female baby boomers who are seeking solutions to the side effects of menopause. When the subject of perimenopause and menopause is on the table, the subsequent discussion usually centers on hormones.

For years, women have relied on oral or vaginally applied hormone replacement therapy (HRT—either estrogen alone or estrogen with progesterone) as their major remedy to ward off perimenopausal and menopausal symptoms such as hot flashes, vaginal dryness, osteoporosis, and changes in skin texture. For many women HRT was nothing short of a blessing. It eliminated hot flashes and vaginal dryness, reduced changes in skin texture, kept osteoporosis at bay, and kept women feeling and looking younger than those women who didn't take HRT.

There is compelling research showing that estrogen loss has a significant impact on skin. The *American Journal of Clinical Dermatology* (2001, volume 2, number 3, pages 143–150) states that "Estrogen appears to aid in the prevention of skin aging in several ways. This reproductive hormone prevents a decrease in skin collagen in postmenopausal women; topical and systemic estrogen therapy can increase the skin collagen content and therefore maintain skin thickness. In addition, estrogen maintains skin moisture by increasing acid mucopolysaccharides and hyaluronic acid in the skin and possibly maintaining stratum corneum barrier function. Sebum levels are higher in postmenopausal women receiving hormone replacement therapy. Skin wrinkling also may benefit from estrogen as a result of the effects of the hormone on the elastic fibers and collagen. Outside of its influence on skin aging, it has been suggested that estrogen increases cutaneous wound healing by regulating the levels of a cytokine. In fact, topical estrogen has been found to accelerate and improve wound healing in elderly men and women."

As beneficial as taking estrogen for skin can be, recent studies have brought to light the serious risks associated with HRT in regard to an increased risk of breast cancer. According to a study conducted by the Fred Hutchinson Cancer Research Center in Seattle, Washington, and a study published in the *Journal of the American Medical Association* (January 26, 2000), and reiterated in another article (August 2001, page 907), there is a correlation between use of ERT [estrogen replacement therapy] and increased risk of heart attack. This is completely opposite from what ERT was originally thought to do, namely, preventing an increase in heart-attack risk that resulted from declining hormone levels. The recent Fred Hutchinson Cancer Research Center study also reported an association between endometrial cancer and ERT, though this is not conclusive due to conflicting research results. (The National Cancer Institute Information Resources, November 1999, released the following statement: "Because reports have shown that estrogen increases the risk of developing endometrial cancer . . . the National Cancer Institute is sponsoring a clinical trial to determine the effects of estrogen in women treated for early stage endometrial cancer.")

A recent follow-up study from Fred Hutchinson Cancer Research Center, Group Health Cooperative, and the University of Washington reported that long-term use of HRT increases the overall risk of breast cancer by about 70%. For one specific type of breast cancer, the risk increases by as much as four times (source: *Seattle Times*, February 13, 2002).

Plant Estrogen

It isn't surprising that alternative, nonprescription sources of estrogen and progesterone would appeal to a wide audience of women enamored with "natural" products, especially given the risks of the medical options available. Plus, there is enticing anecdotal information suggesting that Asian women, who have diets high in soy (an estrogen-laden food), experience low rates of estrogen-positive cancers (particularly breast cancer) and that their menopausal symptoms are reduced (but not eliminated).

According to the research I've seen and the experts I've interviewed, there is indeed reason to believe that a diet consisting of foods high in estrogen, such as tofu, kudzu (a root from Japan but also grown in the United States), dates, pomegranates, and flax seed can prevent some of the side effects of menopause and potentially reduce some risks of estrogen-related cancers. But this is all strictly theory—encouraging, but with simply not enough research to make a definitive statement one way or the other.

The current understanding regarding plant estrogen is that it may work by interfering with the body's own estrogen, preventing it from being out of balance. Plant estrogen may fool the body into thinking it has the right balance of this hormone. If the body has too much estrogen, the plant estrogen may prevent the body from utilizing it (thereby preventing estrogen-related cancers); if the body has too little estrogen (as during the stages of menopause), plant estrogen might make the body think it has more, reducing some of the more uncomfortable side effects. In essence, a woman's estrogen level needs to be in balance for things to go right internally and externally. Too little or too much and you can have problems. It's like any other physical issue. Insulin is a hormone secreted by the pancreas. If too little insulin is present you have diabetes; too much, and you go into insulin shock. The same is true for estrogen: Too much or too little can cause havoc with the body (and the emotions).

As many researchers and gynecologists have pointed out to me, diet may play a significant part in menopausal symptoms. But whether the American diet can duplicate the traditional Asian diet is a good question. There is little information about how many estrogen-laden foods a woman must consume (and for how long) to reduce or eliminate the effects of menopause. In other words, adding estrogen-rich foods or supplements to your diet won't necessarily prevent breast cancer, heart attack, or osteoporosis. (Keep in mind that, unlike the Asian diet, the typical American diet is high in animal protein, which, combined with a low rate of physical activity and exercise, can have an adverse or aggravating effect on menopausal symptoms.)

There are also studies that have shown no improvement or benefit from dietary estrogens (sources: *Journal of Clinical Endocrinology & Metabolism*, January 2002, pages 118–121; *Toxicological Science*, February 2002, pages 228–238), although these were hardly sweeping or conclusive reviews. Clearly this is a health issue that needs to be examined more closely.

But what about estrogen creams? There is no research about plant estrogens showing they provide any benefit when applied topically to skin. But even if there were benefits, how much do you need to rub on your skin to obtain them? When it comes to cosmetics, there is no way to know how much of a plant estrogen extract is being used, or how much may be in a moisturizer. More to the point, because the cosmetics and natural-supplement industries are not regulated, there is no way to really know what you are getting. Until there is, leaving your health up to guesswork and marketing schemes is not a wise choice.

Progesterone in Skin-Care Products

At the forefront of the female hormone battle is a Dr. John Lee, with his books *What Your Doctor May Not Tell You about Menopause: The Breakthrough Book on Natural Progesterone* (Warner Books, 1996) and *What Your Doctor May Not Tell You about Premenopause* [perimenopause]: *Balance Your Hormones and Your Life from Thirty to Fifty* (Warner Books, 1999). Lee's primary thesis is that ERT and HRT were flawed for many reasons. On one level, Lee feels that ERT is problematic because it utilizes synthetic estrogen and/or synthetic progesterone. But a matter of more concern to Lee is that ERT (without progesterone, as it was typically prescribed for years) puts the emphasis on the wrong hormone, namely estrogen, instead of progesterone. Lee's research suggests that too much estrogen, or estrogen dominance as he calls it, is the problem, and that natural progesterone is the only option to combat a woman's hormonal changes.

So what is the difference between progesterone and estrogen? Progesterone is manufactured in the body from the steroid hormone pregnenolone, and is the source or precursor of other steroid hormones, including cortisol, androstenedione, estrogens, and testosterone. For women, progesterone and estrogen work together in a subtle symphonic harmony. This hormonal balance creates the rhythm of the menstrual cycle, and when that harmony gets out of tune, particularly during perimenopausal and menopausal years, the problems for women are significant. Estrogen levels drop by 40% to 60% at menopause, which is just enough to stop the menstrual cycle. But progesterone levels drop, too, and for some women, they may drop to almost nonexistent. According to Lee, "Because progesterone is the precursor to so many other steroid hormones, its use can greatly enhance overall hormone balance after menopause, even for estrogen . . ." although estrogen itself cannot affect progesterone levels.

Menstruation depends on what is taking place in the ovaries and uterus, including the hormones generated by the hypothalamus and pituitary gland in the brain and the corpus luteum in the ovary. During the first half of the menstrual cycle, as an egg follicle grows in the ovary, estrogen is manufactured and released into the blood. As the egg follicle matures in the lining of the ovary, a hormone called luteinizing hormone (LH) causes the egg to be released directly into the ovary. The ovary then starts producing progesterone while estrogen production declines. Progesterone's role is to help the egg to mature even faster, increasing fertility. As you may know, this hormonal fluctuation in estrogen production versus progesterone takes place at midcycle, when a woman is the most fertile. Not surprisingly, the increased progesterone levels correspond to a surge in a woman's sexual drive (after all you can't get pregnant if your libido—brain—doesn't want to have sex). If fertilization does not occur, ovarian production of progesterone falls dramatically. It is this sudden decline in progesterone levels that triggers the shedding of the uterine lining that results in a menstrual cycle. In essence, estrogen encourages the growth of endometrial tissue in the uterus, and progesterone causes this lining to be shed.

In a recent interview with Dr. John Lee, he told me that he "wants people to understand that natural progesterone brings everything back into balance. Around the time when progesterone is low in women, approximately age 45, there is an estrogen dominance occurring in the body, which causes such things as autoimmune disorders, hair loss because there are more androgens [in the body not counterbalanced with progesterone], risk of breast cancer, and a low libido." Lee went on to explain that "natural" progesterone "is the same identical hormone found in women as opposed to the use of synthetic forms of progesterone (progestins) found in prescription-only drugs that merely mimic the effect progesterone has on the body."

So, if Lee is right, why is the research about natural progesterone so controversial? According to Lee it's because "natural progesterone cannot be patented, it is available to everyone and anyone who wants to [can] put it into any lotion or cream they make. Pharmaceutical companies do not fund research that has no likelihood of netting a profit. Therefore, pharmaceutical companies put a lot of money into researching synthetic hormones that . . . can be patented and sold exclusively by the patent holder. It follows that there is a lot of research out there to show that synthetic progesterone and synthetic estrogen work and [explains] why there is little research about the use of natural progesterone [there is simply no profit in the latter]. Pharmaceutical companies do not even broach the issue of natural hormonal options versus synthetic ones with physicians because there is no financial motivation to do so."

There is also controversy among physicians as to whether or not progesterone applied topically can provide the body with the same amounts as synthetic forms of progesterone taken orally. Physicians point out that anecdotal information about positive results from natural progesterone is flawed because in double-blind studies the placebo effect for hot flashes or other physical improvements is about 40% when compared to a test vehicle. Further, when actual blood levels of progesterone are measured, physicians found low levels of natural progesterone, confirming their suspicion that not enough of the natural progesterone is absorbed through the skin. Lee is frustrated by this finding because the medical profession will not accept that "natural" progesterone levels are best tested in saliva and not in blood serum, the way synthetic progesterone is measured. Lee's saliva tests indicate that the natural progesterone creams do produce normal levels of progesterone that can be accurately read.

Is there any risk to applying natural progesterone topically? Lee said he has not seen adverse effects since he began studying it over 20 years ago. This is one aspect of Lee's work that requires more research. Although Lee may not have seen any problems, that doesn't mean they don't exist. After all, Lee would not be the doctor to visit; if problems occurred, women would turn to other doctors for uterine or breast difficulties (he was a family physician). Lee does acknowledge that there is a risk of hyperplasia (an abnormal increase in the number of cells in an organ or a tissue with resulting swelling) and a feeling of lightheadedness and lethargy. However, Lee also points out that "during pregnancy, the placenta produces 300 to 400 milligrams of natural progesterone daily during the last few months of pregnancy, so we know that such levels are safe for the developing baby. But [synthetic progesterones—progestins] even at fractions of this dose, can cause birth defects."

Clearly, more research is needed to settle the issue. But without question this is a growing option for treating the symptoms of hormonal changes. Understanding the options and risks, and being able to separate the truth from what is truly intense hype, both by the "believers" in natural progesterone cream and the "believers" in pharmaceutical or synthetic hormonal therapy, is imperative for women facing this change in their bodies.

And there are lots of formidable believers on both sides of the issue. Typing the term "natural progesterone" into a search engine on the Web brings up over 40,000 hits (and most of those are from companies or doctor's offices selling natural progesterone creams), and searching for "estrogen replacement therapy" brings up just about the same number from medical professionals prescribing ERT. When it comes to natural progesterone products, Lee explained that right now there are about 140 companies marketing natural progesterone creams that come from 20 different labs. And with the baby boomers coming full-fledged into their perimenopausal and menopausal years, there will probably be more and more coming to market. Given that natural progesterone creams are not regulated in any way by the FDA, and that they are, in actuality, merely cosmetics, that means anyone can put them into any product they want to.

According to an associate of Lee's, David Zava, PhD, director of research for ZRT Laboratory in Portland, Oregon, "nearly all of the [natural] progesterone cream products are formulated to deliver about 15 to 30 milligrams of USP-grade progesterone per 1/4 teaspoon of cream." For perimenopausal women, Lee recommends 15 to 24 milligrams applied daily for 14 days before the menstrual cycle is expected to begin and then stopping the day before the menstrual cycle starts. For menopausal and postmenopausal women, he suggests reducing the application to 15 milligrams per day for 25 days and then not using it for 5 days. Lee states that 15 to 20 milligrams "is the same amount the ovaries make naturally."

A study published in the *American Journal of Obstetrics and Gynecology* (June 1999, pages 1504-1511) concurs with Lee's position, stating that "in order to obtain the proper (effective) serum levels with use of a progesterone cream, the cream needs to have an adequate amount of progesterone in it [at least 30 milligrams per gram]. Many over-the-counter creams have little [for example, 5 milligrams per ounce] or none at all. The creams that are made from Mexican yams are not metabolized to progesterone by women. The cream used in the above study (Pro-Gest) contains pure United States Pharmacopoeia [USP] progesterone." Ironically, Pro-Gest was the only cream around at the time Lee started his research.

Lee explains that "the USP progesterone used for hormone replacement comes from plant fats and oils, usually a substance called diosgenin, which is extracted from a very specific type of wild yam that grows in Mexico, or from soybeans. In the laboratory, diosgenin is chemically synthesized into real human progesterone. Some companies are trying to sell . . . 'wild yam extract' [or other plant extracts] . . . claiming that the body will then convert it into hormones as needed. While we know this can be done in the laboratory, there is no evidence that this conversion takes place in the human body." Lee is quick to explain that he doesn't sell any of these products and receives no profit from their sale. He also does NOT recommend the use of natural progesterone creams with any other active hormones or herbs.

So what should you use if you want to give natural progesterone creams a try? Lee recommends creams that contain between 400 and 500 milligrams per ounce of cream. That amount would provide about 20 milligrams per day when applying a quarter teaspoon of the cream. But before you venture out shopping for natural progesterone creams, I strongly encourage you to check out Lee's books (available on www.amazon.com and in most bookstores) and to visit his Web site at www.johnleemd.com. Lee lists the companies that sell products that meet his criteria. There is also a list of products that meet the recommended amount of USP progesterone provided by Aeron LifeCycles Laboratory, San Leandro, California, on their Web site at www.aeron.com.

HUMAN GROWTH FACTOR

It is important to make clear that the topic of human growth factor (HGF) is exceedingly complicated. The physiological intricacies of the varying HGFs and their action challenge a layperson's comprehension.

Nonetheless, because the use of HGF seems to be a direction some skin-care companies are taking, and because there is a large body of research showing its efficacy for wound healing (but not for wrinkles), it does deserve comment. Grasping the full depth of this issue, however, is not within the scope of this book.

HGF is a complex family of hormones that are produced by the body to control cell growth and cell division in skin, blood, bone, and nerve tissue. Most significantly they regulate the division and reproduction of cells. They also can influence the growth rate of some cancers. HGFs occur naturally in the body but they are also synthesized and used in medicine for a range of applications, including wound healing and immune system stimulation. The following are the body's primary HGFs.

> **Epidermal Growth Factor (EGF):** Stimulates cell division of many different cell types.
>
> **Erythropoietin (Epo):** Stimulates the growth of cells that carry oxygen to the body.
>
> **Fibroblast Growth Factor (FGF):** Stimulates growth of the nervous system and bone formation.
>
> **Hepatocyte Growth Factor (HGF):** Stimulates division in cells lining the liver, skin cells, and cells that produce skin color.
>
> **Insulinlike Growth Factor (IGF):** Stimulates fat cells and connective tissue cells.
>
> **Interleukins (IL):** Stimulate growth of white blood cells.
>
> **Nerve Growth Factor (NGF):** Stimulates growth of nerve tissue.
>
> **Platelet Derived Growth Factor: (PDGF):** Promotes the growth of blood clotting factor.
>
> **Transforming Growth Factor (TGF):** Stimulates wound healing and collagen growth.
>
> **Vascular Endothelial Growth Factor (VEGF):** Stimulates the growth of blood vessels.

All of these HGFs are chemical messengers that bind to receptor sites on the cell surface (receptor sites are how cells communicate with any substance to let them know what to do or what not to do). HGFs need to communicate with cells to instruct them to activate the production of new cells or to tell a cell to create new cells that have different functions. Another way to think of HGFs is that they are messengers designed to be received or "heard" by specific receptor sites or "ears" on the cell.

Many HGFs are quite versatile, with the ability to stimulate cellular division in numerous different cell types, while other HGFs are specific to a particular cell type, say blood cells or bone cells.

We are most familiar with HGFs like TGF, in their role in surgical-wound healing. The main task for HGFs is to cause cell division, which is helpful; however, at certain concentrations and lengths of application they can cause cells to overproliferate, which can cause cancer or other health problems.

Skin is an elaborate network of growing tissue that continually regenerates and can usually heal after it is cut, punctured, burnt, or scraped. How skin goes about this process is in many ways a physiological miracle directed by an intricate network of HGFs. "In skin, the most actively regulated growth occurs in the epidermis, the visible, outermost layer. A finely regulated growth factor system maintains homeostasis or biological status quo in the epidermis by adjusting the rates of cell growth versus cell death in response to injury, sunburn, or disease. Failures in this system lead to skin disorders such as psoriasis or even skin cancers" (source: http://www.wound-healing.net/).

But what happens when you put HGFs on skin, particularly TGF and EGF, as some companies claim their products contain? The risk is that they could accelerate the growth of skin cancer by stimulating the overproduction of skin cells. In the case of TGF, which stimulates collagen, that can encourage scarring. Scars are the result of excessive collagen production; if you make too much collagen you get a scar or a knot on the skin such as a keloidal scar. Most of the research on the issue of HGFs for skin has looked primarily at the issue of wound healing, and at short-term use of HGFs. In skin-care products, they would be used repeatedly, possibly over long periods of time.

There is another body of research concerning HGFs, one being touted as the answer for wrinkles. Here is what the research shows: Based on established scientific protocol, you can create "living" skin cells in a petri dish. It is known that normal human skin cells divide a predictable number of times and then die. At first skin cells grow and divide rapidly, and then the division rate slows as we age. Finally the cells cease replicating. In vitro, you can re-create the skin cell's life process and accelerate the effect, so you can watch the growth process of cells in a short period of time (weeks, as opposed to a normal person's life span). If you leave these skin cells alone, they go through a normal life span and eventually stop replicating. However, when you add some forms of HGFs, the skin cells live far longer than they would have on their own. While that sounds like your skin would stay young forever, the other part of the picture is that if you add too much HGF, the skin cells die off sooner than they would have if you hadn't added any! This part of the information is often left out of the impressive data that companies like to publicize in regard to their products.

One other significant shortcoming of HGFs, according to an article by Dr. Donald R. Owen in the March 1999 issue of *Global Cosmetic Industry*, is that "the body produces these [HGFs] in exquisitely small concentrations at just the right location and time. . . . Actual growth factors such as [EGF and TGF-B] are [large] configurations, which do not penetrate the skin. . . . They [also] lose their activity within days in water or even as solids at normal temperatures. . . . [Yet], even after all these complications, the siren's song is too strong. We [the cosmetics chemists] will use them."

The research into HGFs is without question intriguing, but there is much that's not known, especially in terms of long-term risk or stability when they're used in cosmetics and applied to skin. In this arena, if cosmetics companies continue to use HGFs, it's the consumer who will be the guinea pig.

KINETIN

Kinetin is a plant-growth hormone with the technical name N6-furfuryladenine. Several companies, including The Body Shop, Almay, Osmotics, and Kinerase, sell products containing kinetin. (Kinerase is not in any way special just because it is sold through a doctor's office; it contains the exact same kinetin as the less-expensive versions from The Body Shop and Almay, and the more expensive option from Osmotics.)

The unpublished study that created the excitement around kinetin was conducted in part by Dr. Jerry L. McCullough, Professor, University of California, Irvine (UCI). In a letter to me, McCullough stated that in the research done by his team "the UCI study was a double-blind study, which involved subjective assessments of clinical improvement and safety by both the physician and the subject. This is the protocol design used in the pivotal multicenter clinical trials of Renova, which were reviewed by the FDA and led to FDA approval. The above studies focused on the clinical assessment of safety and efficacy as did the kinetin studies. The only objective measures of efficacy in the Renova clinical studies were skin replica analysis and histologic evaluation. The studies at UCI involved over 160 subjects in two studies, each lasting one year. . . . These studies employed objective assessment of the skin-barrier function using measurements of transepidermal water loss (TEWL) in addition to state-of-the-art clinical photography (Canfield Scientific) to document clinical response. I think that the efforts made by Senetek PLC [the company that licenses kinetin to the cosmetics companies] to document the efficacy and safety of this product far exceed those of the numerous antiaging skin products [that] flood the cosmetic counters and Web pages making unsubstantiated claims."

While on the surface it does appear that kinetin can perform like Renova, it is important to recognize that the UCI study does not indicate any results about cellular effects or changes. This study looked at surface improvements. As I've reported in the past, the studies the FDA accepted about Renova's performance for wrinkles were hardly definitive. TEWL tells you about moisturization, not about wrinkles, and while visual assessments may be impressive, they don't tell you if other moisturizers with other ingredients would net you the same improvements. The main interest in kinetin for skin care actually has nothing to do with wrinkles. By contrast, the active ingredient in Renova, tretinoin, has a wealth of established literature regarding its effect in improving abnormal skin-cell production caused by sun damage. That makes Renova (or any other drug containing tretinoin) significant. Kinetin has no such effective data.

What does make kinetin far more interesting are the in vitro and animal studies demonstrating its effect as a growth factor, and how that may affect cellular production. Most of the in vitro or animal-model studies about kinetin were conducted by Dr. Suresh I.S. Rattan, PhD, DSc, Associate Professor of Biogerontology at the University of Aarhus, Denmark, who happens to hold the patent for N6-furfuryladenine for use on aging skin. Rattan discovered this plant growth factor in 1988 and obtained the U.S. patent in 1994. That is, Rattan discovered what happens to skin cells in a petri dish when N6-furfuryladenine is added.

Rattan told me, "Normal cells, as they divide and age, go through a progressive accumulation of changes that are irreversible until they reach a stage where they finally die. This in vitro [meaning in a petri dish as opposed to in humans or animals] form of creating cellular aging, which takes place over one year—consider that it takes our cells more than 70 years to age—is a well-known biochemical phenomenon called the Hayflick Phenomenon, named after the researcher who discovered this method of studying cellular aging in a laboratory setting."

All this relates to N6-furfuryladenine and what it does when added to cells that are aging in a petri dish. Rattan continued, "Normally when we grow cells in culture, as they become older, regardless of sun exposure, they go through over 300 varying changes and alterations. A young cell is plump, round, smooth (and the functions and chemical processes orderly and vigorous). As the cells age, they become irregular, flattened, and large, full of debris—debris meaning they fill up with waste products that they can't get rid of. Further, when you grow normal cells in the lab they have a limited number of times they multiply and divide—termed a cell's replicative life span. But when I added N6-furfuryladenine, the cells did not age as fast: the process slowed down dramatically. In the presence of various concentrations of N6-furfuryladenine, cells act younger, longer."

As exciting as this sounds, and Rattan is indeed excited about his research, he also said, "Topically [applied to the surface of skin] no one knows how or if N6-furfuryladenine is being taken up or used by the cell. There are no studies done on the biochemical action on human skin or animal skin. It has only been observed for in vitro systems. On one level I feel this compound can be a health-preserving molecule. But it would take a lot of money to find out its full potential.

"What will put my mind at rest is knowing what the full up and down side is. We are curious about negative effects; even water is toxic in certain doses. In cell cultures when a concentration of say 250 micromolars [a chemical measure of extremely small sizes] of N6-furfuryladenine was used, we got good results, but when we used 500 micromolars of N6-furfuryladenine the cells started dying."

I suspect that when it's applied topically, kinetin isn't of much use to the skin cell, and even if it could somehow be utilized, there probably isn't enough kinetin in any product to have a negative or positive impact—but that is only a guess, no one knows for sure (source: *Dermatologic Clinics*, October 2000, pages 609–615).

If kinetin isn't a problem for the skin cell, other research does demonstrate quite clearly that it can be a potent free-radical scavenger (antioxidant), which can hypothetically prevent oxidative damage on the skin (oxidative damage is one theory of why skin wrinkles or eventually looks old). But there are many potent antioxidants found in skin-care products these days, from beta glucan to vitamin C, vitamin A, green tea, grape extract, and on and on, that don't have the possible risks and disturbing unknowns associated with kinetin.

LANOLIN

Lanolin has long been burdened with the reputation for being an allergen or sensitizing agent. That has always been a disappointment to formulators because lanolin is such an effective moisturizing agent for skin. A recent study in the *British Journal of Dermatology* (July 2001, pages 28–31) may change all that. This study concluded that "lanolin sensitization has remained at a relatively low and constant rate even in a high-risk population (i.e., patients with recent or active eczema)." Based on a review of 24,449 patients who were tested with varying forms of lanolin, it turned out that "the mean annual rate of sensitivity to this allergen was 1.7%"—and it was lower than that for a 50% concentration of lanolin. It looks like it's time to restore lanolin's good reputation, which is a very good thing for someone with dry skin to know.

MAD COW DISEASE IN COSMETICS?

Mad cow disease and the risk it poses for humans (and, of course, animals) has mostly affected countries outside of the United States, primarily England, and has not been as big a concern here.

Mad cow disease (technically known as bovine spongiform encephalopathy or BSE) is a chronic degenerative disease affecting the central nervous system of cattle. The concern for humans is the risk of eating meat or meat products that contain the BSE pathogen. When the BSE pathogen takes hold in people, it can trigger a variant form of the disease called Creutzfeldt-Jakob disease (after the researchers who identified it). In Europe, over 100 people are now known to have contracted Creutzfeldt-Jakob disease, which leads to dementia and can cause death. The CDC (www.cdc.gov) reports that "in the United Kingdom, this current risk [of Creutzfeldt-Jakob disease] appears to be extremely small, perhaps about 1 case per 10 billion servings [of beef]." It also states that "milk and milk products from cows are not believed to pose any risk for transmitting the BSE agent." While the human toll is infinitesimally small when compared with many other known potentially serious diseases, from malaria to AIDS and even the flu, scientists are concerned that we are on the verge of an epidemic that they want to stop before it gets worse.

While it is important to pay attention to the issue of mad cow disease in relation to eating beef or other meat, the question is whether or not bovine-derived ingredients used in cosmetics can harbor the disease and cause health risks. The answer is that no one knows for sure, but theoretically a remote possible risk does exist. Some researchers feel that there is no evidence BSE can be contracted through the skin (source: *Cosmetic Dermatology*, December 2001, pages 43–47); however, neither cooking, preserving, or any of the other processing most cosmetics go through can eliminate BSE pathogens. That means if animal by-products are used in cosmetics (in particular placenta and spleen bovine extracts), they can pose a risk, albeit remote, to the user. The British BSE Committee in varying reports has mentioned a concern that people could become infected if the creams were used on broken skin. It is important to realize that very few products use those kinds of ingredients.

If you are thinking of buying any cosmetics that contain animal organ extracts of any kind, you may want to reconsider, or discard them if you have already made a purchase. Other than that, at this point, I feel strongly that it isn't necessary to worry about the other ingredients on your cosmetics labels. Aside from the evidence, which does not point to a single case of BSE associated with cosmetics, checking the ingredient label wouldn't be of much help anyway because there is no way to know whether the collagen or ceramide in your product is sourced from animals or plants. I want to stress that from all the research that is out there, this appears to be a negligible issue for your beauty routine.

MINERAL OIL

The notion that mineral oil and petrolatum (Vaseline) are bad for skin has been around for some time, with Aveda being the most visible company to mount a crusade deriding these ingredients. According to many companies that produce "natural" cosmetics, mineral oil and petrolatum are terrible ingredients because they come from crude oil (petroleum) and are used in industry as metal-cutting fluid (among other uses) and, therefore, can harm the skin by forming an oil film and suffocating it.

This foolish, recurring misinformation about mineral oil and petrolatum is maddening. After all, crude oil is as natural as any other earth-derived substance. Moreover, lots of ingredients are derived from awful-sounding sources but are nevertheless benign and totally safe. Salt is a perfect example. Common table salt is sodium chloride, composed of sodium and chloride, but salt doesn't have the caustic properties of chloride (a form of chlorine) or the unstable explosiveness of sodium. In fact, it is a completely different compound with the harmful properties of neither of its components.

Cosmetics-grade mineral oil and petrolatum are considered the safest, most nonirritating moisturizing ingredients ever found (sources: *Cosmetics & Toiletries*, January 2001, page 79; *Cosmetic Dermatology*, September 2000, pages 44–46). Yes, they can keep air off the skin to some extent, but that's what a good antioxidant is supposed to do; they don't suffocate skin! Moreover, petrolatum and mineral oil are known for being efficacious in wound healing, and are also considered to be among the most effective moisturizing ingredients available (source: *Cosmetics & Toiletries*, February 1998, pages 33–40).

NATURAL MOISTURIZING FACTORS AND LIPIDS

One of the primary elements in keeping skin healthy is making sure the structure of the epidermis (outer layer of skin) is intact. That structure is defined and created by skin cells that are held together by something called the intercellular matrix. The intercellular matrix is the "glue" within the skin that keeps skin cells together, helps prevent individual skin cells from losing water, and creates the smooth, nonflaky appearance of skin; these components are called natural moisturizing factors (NMFs). Lipids are the oil and fat components of skin that prevent evaporation and provide lubrication to the surface of skin. It is actually the intercellular matrix along with the skin's lipid content that gives skin a good deal of its surface texture and feel.

When the skin's intercellular matrix and lipid content are impaired, the skin is subject to dryness, an increase in the bacteria that cause blemishes, irritation, flaking, redness, roughness, and a tight, uncomfortable feeling. How do you know if your intercellular matrix and lipid content are intact? A wound or cut is easy to understand because you can see that the skin's intercellular matrix has been impaired and is no longer an intact structure. Damage like that is at one extreme end of the type of problems that can make the skin unhealthy. On the less obvious end are sun damage, irritating skin-care products, dry climates, indoor heat, smoking, and intrinsic aging factors, which all injure the skin's intercellular matrix by depleting the skin's lipid content as well as its content of NMFs. When the lipid content and NMFs are intact they form an adequate barrier that keeps foreign substances out and keeps the appropriate amount of water inside the cells. When the lipid and NMF content of skin is reduced, we experience surface roughness, flaking, small facial wrinkles, and a tight, uncomfortable feeling (source: *Skin Research and Technology*, August 2000, pages 128–134).

It is logical to think that if you replace the components of skin that have been exhausted or destroyed from the varying causes mentioned above, then you can help "repair" skin and keep it intact, allowing it to heal, appear smoother, look healthier, and feel more comfortable. NMFs and lipids make up an expansive group of ingredients that include ceramide, hyaluronic acid, cholesterol, fatty acids, triglycerides, phospholipids, glycosphingolipids, amino acids, linoleic acid, glycosaminoglycans, glycerin, mucopolysaccharide, and sodium PCA (pyrrolidone carboxylic acid). All of these skin-care ingredients are present in the epidermis' intercellular structure between skin cells and in the lipid content on the surface of skin. When any of these ingredients are used in skin-care products, they appear to help stabilize and maintain this complex intercellular-skin matrix. None of these very good NMFs and lipids can permanently affect or change skin, but they are great at temporarily keeping depleted skin from feeling dry and uncomfortable. More important, all of these ingredients, and many more, can help support the intercellular area of the skin by keeping it intact. This support helps prevent surface irritation from penetrating deeper into the skin, helps keep bacteria out, and aids the skin's immune/healing system.

Mimicking the lipid content of skin ingredients are apricot oil, canola oil, coconut oil, corn oil, jojoba oil, jojoba wax, lanolin, lecithin, olive oil, safflower oil, sesame oil, shea butter, soybean oil, squalane, and sweet almond oil, which can be extremely helpful for skin.

Are any one of these ingredients the be-all and end-all for your skin? Hardly! All of them perform similarly. That means that limiting yourself to a single ingredient to answer your skin-care needs, or to a single concept, such as "natural" or "purifying," is the way to do the greatest disservice to your skin.

OLIVE OIL

In the world of skin care, startling antiaging and antiwrinkling proper-ties can be attributed to almost any plant-sourced ingredient. One of the latest ones is olive oil. The concept of olive oil having antiaging proper-ties stems from some evidence that diets high in olive oil may help pre-vent heart disease (sources: *European Journal of Clinical Nutrition*, January 2002, pages 72–81; *Lipids*, November 2001, Supplemental, pages S49–S52; *Lipids*, November 2001, pages 1195–1202). There are also a small number of animal tests showing that topically applied olive oil can protect against UVB damage (sources: *Carcinogenesis*, November 2000, pages 2085–2090; *Journal of Dermatological Science*, March 2000, Supplemental, pages S45–S50).

It does seem that olive oil is a good antioxidant and assuredly it's a good moisturizing ingredient. But research shows similar results for other oils as well. How olive oil's status got elevated so that it's now a show-cased ingredient in expensive skin-care products epitomizes the caprice of the cosmetics industry.

OXYGEN FOR THE SKIN

Here is the most pathetic but clear-cut demonstration of how insane the world of cosmetics truly is. After selling us products to ward off oxygen's effects on the skin (the word antioxidant means anti-oxygen), the beauty industry then turns around and sells us products that claim to provide oxygen *to* the skin. Doesn't the beauty industry have anything better to do? (No, it doesn't, especially if there is an interested consumer willing to make a purchase.)

Many cosmetic products contain antioxidants, ingredients that keep oxygen off the face, such as vitamin C, superoxide dismutase, selenium, curcumin, plant extracts, and vitamin E, among dozens and dozens of others. At the same time, the cosmetics industry also sells products that contain hydrogen peroxide (H_2O_2) or some other oxygen-releasing in-gredient, which supposedly delivers an oxygen molecule when it comes into contact with skin. It makes sense to wonder if the extra oxygen would just trigger free-radical damage and cause more problems for the skin. But if you were also using products that contained antioxidants, wouldn't they "scavenge" up that free-radical oxygen? The answer is that if the product could deliver extra oxygen to the skin it would indeed generate free-radical damage and, based on data from almost every imaginable published study on the subject, that's bad for skin.

So why the concern about supplying oxygen to the skin? Oxygen depletion is one of the things that happens to older skin, regardless of whether it's been affected by sun damage or any other health issue. Why or how that happens is a complete unknown, though it is thought to have something to do with blood flow and a reduction in lung capacity as we age. Nevertheless, delivering extra oxygen to the skin doesn't reverse it. After all, there is plenty of oxygen in our environment. The earth's atmosphere is 21% oxygen; the oceans, lakes, and rivers are about 88% oxygen. Oxygen is a constituent of most rocks and minerals, and 46.7% (by weight) of the solid crust of the earth. Oxygen makes up 60% of the human body, and is in every cell and organ. It is a constituent of all living tissues; almost all plants and animals, including humans, require oxygen to maintain life. However, oxygen is utilized by the body almost exclusively through respiration. Oxygen on the surface may affect the very top layer of skin, but so what? How much extra oxygen does skin need? Again, no one knows. Can it be absorbed? No. Plus, none of this addresses the issue about oxygen generating more free-radical damage, which is one of the reasons the veins and capillaries of the body stop working efficiently.

That brings us to the question, How did this caprice of oxygen booths get started? Oxygen booths (hyperbaric chambers) are used medically to repair skin ulcers and wounds that have difficulty healing. According to the American Diabetes Association's *Diabetes Forecast* (June 1993, page 57), "When you have a stubborn [wound] that won't heal, the white blood cells that fight the infection in the [wound] use 20 times more oxygen when they're killing bacteria. Also, the more oxygen your body has to work with, the more efficiently it lays down wound-repairing connective tissue. Yet just when you need more oxygen, you may have less. If you have neuropathy (diabetic nerve damage), that may cause changes in blood flow, resulting in islands of low oxygen levels in your foot. Less oxygen means slower healing, and a [wound] that doesn't heal could eventually lead to an amputation. So it seems that you should try to get extra oxygen in your blood when you have a foot ulcer, to bring the oxygen levels in the tissues around the ulcer up to normal, or even higher. But sitting in your living room and breathing in 100% oxygen won't do the trick. Under normal circumstances, only so much oxygen will dissolve in your blood." Pressure is needed to allow the oxygen to be used by the body; and sitting in a hyperbaric booth serves that purpose. The article continues, "But it is the inhaled oxygen, which is then absorbed by your blood after you breathe it, that speeds wound healing, not the oxygen drifting past the wound. You may have seen advertisements for devices that encase a person's leg and deliver oxygen to the skin. This is not hyperbaric oxygen therapy, and it's not effective—your skin doesn't absorb oxygen that way. These devices may even reduce the amount of oxygen that gets to your leg."

Moreover, leg ulcers and wounds are a temporary condition, but skin aging is ongoing. The notion that oxygen treatments affect aging, wrinkles, or any other skin malady is a joke. Nary a study exists anywhere to support those ideas, though there is a ton of research showing that the oxidative process generated by oxygen is partly responsible for wrinkles and skin aging in general.

Hydrogen Peroxide

Given what is now known about free-radical damage, I no longer recommend hydrogen peroxide as a topical disinfectant for acne. Oxygen is clearly a problem for skin, and hydrogen peroxide is a significant oxidizing agent. Hydrogen peroxide works by releasing an unstable oxygen molecule onto the skin, and that generates free-radical damage. Hydrogen peroxide is H_2O_2 (water is H_2O). The extra oxygen molecule in hydrogen peroxide is extremely unstable. That's why hydrogen peroxide is packaged in a dark brown, airtight container. On exposure to air or sunlight, hydrogen peroxide's extra oxygen molecule is released and the product becomes just plain water. For skin prone to acne this extra oxygen molecule is capable of killing the bacteria that cause blemishes. Acne bacteria are anaerobic, meaning they don't like oxygen. By giving the skin an extra dose of direct oxygen, hydrogen peroxide can reduce the presence of these problematic bacteria. But because of the cumulative problems that stem from impacting the skin with a substance that is known to generate free-radical damage (which can hurt the healing process, cause cellular destruction, and reduce optimal skin functioning), other options need to be sought. In Chapter 9, Battle Plans for Blemishes, I discuss the different options for combating the bacteria that cause acne.

PROPYLENE GLYCOL

Propylene glycol (along with other glycols and glycerol) is a humectant or humidifying and delivery ingredient used in cosmetics. You can find Web sites and spam e-mails stating that propylene glycol is really industrial antifreeze and the major ingredient in brake and hydraulic fluids. These sites also state that tests show it to be a strong skin irritant. They further point out that the Material Safety Data Sheet (MSDS) on propylene glycol warns users to avoid skin contact because systemically (in the body) it can cause liver abnormalities and kidney damage.

As ominous as this sounds, it is so far from the reality of cosmetic formulations that almost none of it holds any water or poses real concern. It is important to realize that the MSDS sheets are talking about 100% concentrations of a substance. Even water and salt have frightening comments regarding their safety according to the MSDS. It is true that propylene glycol in 100% concentration is used as antifreeze, but—and this is a very big *but*—in cosmetics it is used in only the smallest amounts to keep products from melting in high heat or freezing when it is cold. It also helps active ingredients penetrate the skin. In the minute amounts used in cosmetics, propylene glycol is not a concern in the least. Women are not suffering from liver problems because of propylene glycol in cosmetics.

And finally, according to the U.S. Department of Health and Human Services, within the Public Health Services Agency for Toxic Substances and Disease Registry, "studies have not shown these chemicals [propylene or the other glycols as used in cosmetics] to be carcinogens" (source: http://www.atsdr.cdc.gov).

Polyethylene glycol (PEG) is another ingredient "natural" Web sites have attempted to make notorious. They gain a great deal of attention by attributing horror stories to PEG. For example, several Web sites state the following: "Because of their effectiveness, PEGs are often used in caustic spray-on oven cleaners, yet are also found in many personal care products. Not only are they potentially carcinogenic, but they contribute to stripping the skin's Natural Moisture Factor, leaving the immune system vulnerable." There is no research substantiating any of this. Quite the contrary: PEGs have no known skin toxicity. The only negative research results for this ingredient group indicate that large quantities given orally to rats can cause tumors. How that got related to skin-care products is a mystery to me.

PROTEINS AND AMINO ACIDS

Proteins are fundamental components of all living cells and include a diverse range of biological substances, such as enzymes, hormones, and antibodies that are necessary for the proper functioning of any organism, plant, or animal. There are 20 different amino acids that link together by peptide bonds to form proteins. In skin-care products, proteins and amino acids act as emollients and water-binding agents that help keep the skin's structure intact—they cannot affect, change, or rebuild the structure of skin. Whether the protein in a skin-care product is derived from an animal or a plant, the skin can't tell the difference. There is no research demonstrating that either proteins or amino acids have special properties for skin other than as moisturizing agents.

PYCNOGENOL

There is a great deal of research on pycnogenol, a plant-derived substance found in everything from pine bark to apples, cocoa beans, unripe strawberries, peanut skin, grape seeds, and red wine. However, most of the research dates back to 1990 and earlier (source: U.S. Patent No. 4,698,360 entitled "Plant Extract with a Proanthocyanidins Content as Therapeutic Agent Having Radical Scavenging Effect and Use Thereof"). But a recent study supports the notion that pycnogenol is a potent antioxidant with strong free-radical-scavenging properties (source: *Free Radical Biology and Medicine*, September 1999, pages 704–724). So what about pycnogenol for skin and wrinkles? Like all antioxidants, it can offer benefits for skin, but there isn't a shred of evidence that your wrinkles will melt away or change in any significant manner.

RETINOL

See the section, "Vitamin A: Retinol versus Retin-A and Renova" on page 58.

SODIUM LAURYL SULFATE

Are sodium lauryl sulfate (SLS) and sodium laureth sulfate (SLES) serious problems in cosmetics? I have received more e-mails and letters than I care to count about this concern. I believe that this entire mania was generated by several Neways Web sites, and has been carried over as if it were fact into other so-called "all natural" cosmetics lines.

It seems that most of this issue is based on the incorrect reporting about a study at the Medical College of Georgia. As a reminder, here is what is being quoted: "A study from the Medical College of Georgia indicates that SLS is a systemic, and can penetrate and be retained in the eye, brain, heart, liver, etc., with potentially harmful long-term effects. It could retard healing and cause cataracts in adults, and can keep children's eyes from developing properly." This is supposedly quoted from a report given to the Research to Prevent Blindness conference. While the report on animal models extrapolates concerns about the use of SLS, it draws no hard conclusions, stating that the amount of SLS used was 10% greater than that used in shampoos and that the study was done on animals, not people. The doctor who conducted the study and delivered the final report is Dr. Keith Green, Regents Professor of Ophthalmology at the Medical College of Georgia, who received his doctorate of science from St. Andrews University in Scotland.

I had an opportunity to talk with Dr. Green, who stated that he was completely embarrassed by all this. He told me in a telephone interview back in 1997 that his "work was completely misquoted. There is no part of my study that indicated any [eye] development or cataract problems from SLS or SLES and the body does not retain those ingredients at all. We did not even look at the issue of children, so that conclusion is completely false because it never existed. The Neways people took my research completely out of context and probably never read the study at all." He continued in a perturbed voice, saying, "The statement like 'SLS is a systemic' has no meaning. No ingredient can be a systemic unless you drink the stuff and that's not what we did with it. Another incredible comment was that my study was 'clinical,' meaning I tested the substance on people, [but] these were strictly animal tests. Furthermore, the eyes showed no irritation with the 10-dilution substance used! If anything, the animal studies indicated no risk of irritation whatsoever!" That lack of outcome is in fact why, as of 1987, Green no longer pursued this research. When I asked if anyone has done any follow-up studies looking at SLS and SLES in this regard, Dr. Green said, "No one has done this because the findings were so insignificant."

Resulting mass e-mails continued for some time, carrying on the SLS and SLES myth with a slightly different bent. Yet, according to Health Canada, in a press release, February 12, 1999 (http://www.hc-sc.gc.ca/),

"A letter has been circulating on the Internet which claims that there is a link between cancer and sodium laureth (or lauryl) sulphate (SLS), an ingredient used in [cosmetics]. Health Canada has looked into the matter and has found no scientific evidence to suggest that SLS causes cancer. It has a history of safe use in Canada. Upon further investigation, it was discovered that this e-mail warning is a hoax. The letter is signed by a person at the University of Pennsylvania Health System and includes a phone number. Health Canada contacted the University of Pennsylvania Health System and found that it is not the author of the sodium laureth sulphate warning and does not endorse any link between SLS and cancer. Health Canada considers SLS safe for use in cosmetics. Therefore, you can continue to use cosmetics containing SLS without worry."

Further, according to the American Cancer Society's Web site, "Contrary to popular rumors on the Internet, Sodium Lauryl Sulfate (SLS) and Sodium Laureth Sulfate (SLES) do not cause cancer. E-mails have been flying through cyberspace claiming SLS [and SLES] causes cancer . . . and is proven to cause cancer. . . . [Yet] a search of recognized medical journals yielded no published articles relating this substance to cancer in humans."

That's not to say that sodium lauryl sulfate isn't a potent skin irritant, because it is, and it's considered a standing comparison substance for measuring skin irritancy of other ingredients. In scientific studies when they want to establish whether or not an ingredient is problematic for skin, they compare its effect to the results of SLS. In amounts of 2% to 5% it can cause allergic or sensitizing reactions in lots of people (sources: *European Journal of Dermatology*, September-October 2001, pages 416–419; *American Journal of Contact Dermatitis*, March 2001, pages 28–32). But irritancy is not the same as the other dire, erroneous warnings floating around the Web about this ingredient!

TEA (GREEN, BLACK, AND WHITE)

A significant amount of research has established that tea, including green, black, and white tea, delivers many intriguing health benefits. Dozens of studies point to tea's potent antioxidant as well as anticarcinogenic properties. However, a good deal of this research is on animal models that do not directly relate to human skin (source: *Skin Pharmacology and Applied Skin Physiology*, 2001, pages 69–76). There is only limited information about its effect on skin. The *Journal of Photochemistry and*

Photobiology (December 31, 2001) stated that polyphenols "are the active ingredients in green tea and possess antioxidant, anti-inflammatory and anticarcinogenic properties. Studies conducted by our group on human skin have demonstrated that green tea polyphenols (GTPs) prevent ultraviolet (UV)-B . . . -induced immune suppression and skin cancer induction."

Green tea and the other teas show a good deal of promise for skin but they are not quite the miracle that cosmetics and health food companies make them out to be. As the *Annual Review of Pharmacology and Toxicology* (January 2002, pages 25–54) put it, "Tea has received a great deal of attention because tea polyphenols are strong antioxidants, and tea preparations have inhibitory activity against tumorigenesis. The bioavailability and biotransformation of tea polyphenols, however, are key factors limiting these activities in vivo [in humans]. Epidemiological studies . . . have not yielded clear conclusions concerning the protective effects of tea consumption against cancer formation in humans."

What aren't disputed are the anti-inflammatory properties of tea (green, black, and white). They are also definitely potent antioxidants. All of that is very good for skin but whether or not it has any effect on wrinkles or scars is speculation, not fact.

TEA TREE OIL—MELALEUCA

Tea tree oil has some interesting research demonstrating it to be an effective antimicrobial agent. The *Journal of Applied Microbiology* (January 2000, pages 170–175) stated that "the essential oil of *Melaleuca alternifolia* (tea tree) exhibits broad-spectrum antimicrobial activity. Its mode of action against the Gram-negative bacterium *Escherichia coli* AG100, the Gram-positive bacterium *Staphylococcus aureus* NCTC 8325, and the yeast *Candida albicans* has been investigated using a range of methods. . . . The ability of tea tree oil to disrupt the permeability barrier of cell membrane structures and the accompanying loss of chemiosmotic control is the most likely source of its lethal action at minimum inhibitory levels." In addition, "In a randomized, placebo-controlled pilot study of tea tree oil in the treatment of herpes cold sores, tea tree oil was found to have similar degree of activity as 5% acyclovir" (source: *Journal of Antimicrobial Chemotherapy*, May 2001, page 450). For acne there is also some credible published information showing it to be effective as a topical disinfectant for killing the bacteria that can cause pimples (source: *Letters in Applied Microbiology*, October 1995, pages 242–245).

However, the crux of the matter for tea tree oil is: How much is needed to have an effect? *The Medical Journal of Australia* (October 1990, pages 455–458) compared the efficacy of tea tree oil to the efficacy of benzoyl peroxide for the treatment of acne. A study of 119 patients using 5% tea tree oil in a gel base versus 5% benzoyl peroxide lotion was discussed. There were 61 in the benzoyl peroxide group and 58 in the tea tree oil group. The conclusion was that "both treatments were effective in reducing the number of inflamed lesions throughout the trial, with a significantly better result for benzoyl peroxide when compared to the tea tree oil. Skin oiliness was lessened significantly in the benzoyl peroxide group versus the tea tree oil group." However, while the reduction of breakouts was greater for the benzoyl peroxide group, the side effects of dryness, stinging, and burning were also greater— "79% of the benzoyl peroxide group versus 49% of the tea tree oil group."

Given these results, a 2.5% strength benzoyl peroxide solution would be better to start with to see if it is effective, rather than starting with the more potent and somewhat more irritating 5% or 10% concentrations. However, if you were interested in using a 5% strength tea tree oil solution to see if that would be effective, at this time I know of no products stating the amount of tea tree oil they contain. It appears that almost all of the tea tree oil products on the market contain little more than a 1% concentration, if that, which is probably not enough to be of much help for breakouts.

TOURMALINE

Semiprecious stones and metals have shown up in skin-care products on and off over the years, with silver and gold appearing on the scene periodically. Lately, tourmaline is the gemstone that is showing up in Aveda and Creme de la Mer products (both are owned by the Estée Lauder company), and many women want to know if it has special properties for skin.

Tourmaline is an inert, though complex, mineral. One of its unique properties is that it is piezoelectric, meaning that it generates an electrical charge when under pressure. That's why tourmaline is typically used in pressure gauges. Tourmaline is also pyroelectric, which means that it generates an electrical charge during a temperature change (either increase or decrease). Neither of these actions can take place in a cosmetic, though—and why would you want them to? For example, one of the results of generating an electric charge is that dust particles will become attached to one end of the tourmaline crystal. Who wants that on their skin?

There is a patent for using tourmaline to decrease the need for surfactants, but this patent is for a complicated device and the effect is not generated by the tourmaline itself. Here is a quote from U.S. Patent number 6,308,356, Frederick, et al. October 30, 2001, entitled *Substantially environmental-pollution–free cleaning method and device employing electric energy and surface physical properties*. "The treatment of water by the electrically polar crystalline substance tourmaline requires much longer time to fill up one washing machine tub than the effect lasts. This yields this process of batch treatment before use as impractical as a laundry solution. In the current inventive method the treatment is done simultaneously with the work of cleaning and in the same location as the work of cleaning is being done." In other words, it is a process that uses tourmaline in some way, but the cleaning is not a result of the tourmaline itself (the language is not clear). It doesn't translate to electrifying or illuminating your cosmetics, and especially not in the trace amounts this mineral is found in cosmetics.

After an extensive search, I found no research showing tourmaline has any proven effect on skin whatsoever.

VITAMIN A:
RETINOL VERSUS RETIN-A AND RENOVA

Retinol is the technical name for vitamin A and, despite its recent popularity in skin-care products that proclaim it as an answer for wrinkles, it is hardly new. In fact, it has been around for some time. Retinol gained immense popularity shortly after Retin-A made headlines as a prescription wrinkle cream back in 1987. The active ingredient in Retin-A (and Renova) is tretinoin, which is also referred to as all-trans retinoic acid, an acid form of vitamin A. It wasn't a big stretch for cosmetics companies to take this information and try to convince the consumer that a product containing retinol could produce the same effects as Retin-A. Both are related to vitamin A and they sound almost identical. Headlines everywhere made most people aware of vitamin A, and in no time there was a flurry of knock-off Retin-A soundalike products containing retinol or retinyl palmitate (another vitamin A derivative). It is important to discuss what role, if any, retinol plays in skin care.

There is an abundance of research that shows tretinoin to be effective. Skin does age, whether from sun damage, smoking, or just growing up, and the results are wrinkles, rough skin, sagging, skin discolorations, and thinning of the skin. Changes in the skin are multifold, but one of the primary causes is cellular damage and resulting abnormal growth. An article from *Clinics in Geriatric Medicine* (November 2001, pages 643–659) said "Studies that have elucidated photoaging pathophysiology have produced significant evidence that topical tretinoin (all-trans retinoic acid), the only agent approved so far for the treatment of photoaging, also works to prevent it" (sources: *Cosmetic Dermatology*, December 2001, page 38; Journal of Investigative Dermatology, 2001, volume 111, pages 778–784).

But what about retinol's effect on skin? There is limited evidence demonstrating that retinol can exert the same activity as tretinoin on skin. The problem is that, in the skin, tretinoin (all-trans retinoic acid) is the form of vitamin A that can affect actual cell production by binding to the tretinoin receptor sites on the cell. Retinol needs to *become* tretinoin in the skin if it is to do the same thing. Theoretically, retinol can become tretinoin in the skin, but the process isn't direct. Retinol can be absorbed into the skin and if certain enzymes are present it could then be converted to tretinoin. The question is whether or not, after retinol gets into skin, it is converted into tretinoin, and the research results are conflicting (sources: *Journal of Investigative Dermatology*, 1998, volume 111, pages 478–484; *Journal of Investigative Dermatology*, 1997, volume 109, pages 301–305; *Skin Pharmacology and Applied Skin Physiology*, November-December 2001, pages 363–372).

One more point. Keep in mind that even Retin-A and Renova (the prescription topicals that contain tretinoin) don't produce the kind of results touted by the companies selling retinol products. Ironically, Neutrogena, who sells a retinol product boasting about its antiwrinkle benefits, is owned by Johnson & Johnson, who also happens to own the Retin-A and Renova formulas. If retinol works as well as the label on Neutrogena's product claims, then why would you ever need to use Retin-A or Renova? Perhaps Johnson & Johnson was hoping no one would notice the conflict.

VITAMIN C

Ever since the distinguished Nobel Prize laureate Linus Pauling wrote his now-legendary book *Vitamin C and the Common Cold* back in 1970, vitamin C has become the darling of the alternative healthcare world. The amount of research on vitamin C fills volumes of scientific journals. Vitamin C is essential for collagen formation and helps maintain the viability of the body's lymph system, connective tissue, bone, and cartilage. It is also essential for wound healing and facilitates recovery from burns.

While the information about vitamin C as a dietary supplement abounds, the same cannot be said for what it may do for skin when it comes to wrinkles or aging. In the world of skin care, vitamin C became a cause célèbre after Dr. Sheldon Pinnell from Duke University published a paper in 1992 showing how L-ascorbic acid reduced UVB damage (namely redness and swelling) when applied to the backs of hairless pigs. That was big news and generated product lines based on L-ascorbic acid.

Other doctors, such as N.V. Perricone, M.D. (whose product line bears his name) tout magnesium ascorbyl phosphate as the best form of vitamin C for skin. Still others assert that ascorbic acid is best and can be stabilized. Much of this information is derived from researchers who happen to endorse or are involved in selling products that contain their preferred form of vitamin C. So is there a best form of vitamin C or are any forms of vitamin C the answer for your skin? The answer is a confusing yes and no.

An article in *Plastic and Reconstructive Surgery* (January 2000, pages 464–465) discussed the issue of vitamin C and concluded that the answer is a resounding yes. "Vitamin C is a valuable antioxidant and protectant against photodamage that is created by sunlight in both the UVB and UVA bands. . . . Although oral supplementation may also be useful, topical preparations are able to deliver a higher dosage to the needed area. Topical vitamin C does not absorb or block harmful ultraviolet radiation like a sunscreen. Instead, it augments the skin's ability to neutralize reactive oxygen singlets [free-radical damage] that are created by the ultraviolet radiation, thereby preventing photodamage to the skin. It becomes an integral part of the skin and remains unaffected by bathing, exercise, clothing, or makeup. Used appropriately, topical vitamin C is an important adjunct to the use of sunscreens, an adjunctive treatment to lessen erythema [redness] in skin resurfacing, a helpful adjunct or an alternative to Retin-A in the treatment of fine wrinkles, and a stimulant to wound healing."

If that answer is yes, the answer to the question about which form of vitamin C to choose is not clear. Conflicting research indicates there is no way to know which type of vitamin C is the best. L-ascorbic acid is a good option in terms of its potential bioavailability on skin, but Pinnell's own research shows it is highly sensitive to formulary concerns, including concentration and the pH needed for it to remain stable (source: *Dermatologic Surgery*, February 2001, pages 137–142).

On the other hand, magnesium ascorbyl phosphate is considered stable and there is reliable research showing it to be effective as an antioxidant (sources: *Photochemistry and Photobiology*, June 1998, pages 669–675; *Journal of Pharmaceutical and Biomedical Analysis,* March 1997, pages 795–801). A small number of studies also show that magnesium ascorbyl phosphate can be effective for skin lightening (source: *Journal of the American Academy of Dermatology*, January 1996, pages 29–33). In terms of stability, ascorbyl palmitate may be reliable for skin as well (source: *Biochemical and Biophysical Research Communications,* September 1999, pages 661–665).

Adding to the tangle of information about ascorbic acid, the entire vitamin C molecule has also been shown to be effective as an antioxidant (sources: *Journal of Investigative Dermatology*, February 2002, pages 372–379, and June 2001, pages 853–859). However, you have to balance that with information that ascorbic acid in its pure form is neutralized with water, and given that almost all moisturizing formulations are more than 50% water the chance of ascorbic acid remaining stable (and so available to skin as an antioxidant) is unlikely.

I wish I could point to one clear answer, but there isn't one. Aside from the matter of which form of vitamin C to select, perhaps the fundamental question is whether or not vitamin C is more helpful than any of the other antioxidants described in this chapter. Given the abundance of research on many antioxidants, it is apparent that this vitamin can play a role, but it is hardly the only one to do so, and it is definitely not the "best." What is true for any issue involving skin wrinkling is that aging is more complicated than just the loss or need of vitamin C—or any other vitamin, enzyme, protein, fatty acid, amino acid, or lipid in the skin. We should be concerned about the entire picture, not just one aspect. Besides, there are many other antioxidants that are as good as or even more impressive than vitamin C, including beta-glucan, vitamin E, vitamin A, green tea, grape extract, selenium, curcumin, and superoxide dismutase to name a few; and, according to many researchers dedicated to the study of antioxidants, there are probably thousands of undiscovered antioxidants out there that may be even more significant.

VITAMIN E AND TOCOTRIENOLS

Vitamin E is without question one of the most well-researched vitamins for skin health. It is also, for all intents and purposes, the most well-known antioxidant, both when taken orally as a health supplement and when used in skin-care products. Simply put, vitamin E is an antioxidant superstar. It is a lipid-soluble vitamin (meaning it likes fat better than water) that has eight different forms, of which some are known for being potent antioxidants when applied topically to skin, particularly alpha tocopherol and tocotrienols (sources: *Free Radical Biology and Medicine*, May 1997, pages 761–769; *Journal of Nutrition*, February 2001, pages 369S–373S; *International Journal of Radiation Biology*, June 1999, pages 747–755). However, other studies have indicated the acetate form is also bioavailable and protective for skin (source: *Journal of Cosmetic Science*, January-February 2001, pages 35–50).

Pointing to the significance of vitamin E for skin is an article in the *Journal of Molecular Medicine* (January 1995, pages 7–17), which states: "More than other tissues, the skin is exposed to numerous environmental chemical and physical agents such as ultraviolet light causing oxidative stress [free-radical damage]. In the skin this results in several short- and long-term adverse effects such as erythema [redness], edema [swelling], skin thickening, wrinkling, and an increased incidence of skin cancer. . . . Vitamin E is the major naturally occurring lipid-soluble . . . antioxidant protecting skin from the adverse effects of oxidative stress including photoaging [sun damage]. Many studies document that vitamin E occupies a central position as a highly efficient antioxidant, thereby providing possibilities to decrease the frequency and severity of pathological events in the skin."

In essence, vitamin E functions in the body and on the skin to protect cells against free-radical damage, and an abundant assortment of researchers from diversified medical fields have theorized that this can slow the aging process (sources: *Skin Pharmacology and Applied Skin Physiology*, November-December 2001, pages 363–372; *Free Radical Biology and Medicine*, October 1999, pages 729–737). Theory is not fact, yet the research is definitely compelling for this ingredient. Right now, though, we simply don't know how much is needed or how long it lasts and whether or not any of the benefit shows up as a reduction of wrinkles.

If you thought vitamin E was fascinating, wait until you start hearing about tocotrienols! Tocotrienols are one of vitamin E's eight components and they are fast becoming a popular word in the world of skin care. There is some research showing tocotrienols to be more potent than other forms of vitamin E for antioxidant activity (source: *Journal of Nutrition*, February 2001, pages 369S–373S), but the studies cited in this review were all done on animal models or in vitro. According to the University of California at Berkeley's *Wellness Guide to Dietary Supplements* (October 1999) "[Tocotrienol] research in humans is very limited, and the results conflicting." The research that has been done has centered on large doses of oral tocotrienols, animal studies, or test tubes. Companies that want you to believe tocotrienols are now the answer for your skin are guessing whether or not the laboratory evidence translates to human skin as it exists in the real world (source: *Healthnotes*, http://www.healthnotes.com).

As I have written before about antioxidants, the jury is still out on how much of any topically applied antioxidant is needed to be effective. Full-scale clinical studies on humans to assess the benefits of topical tocotrienols have not yet been performed, so for now (as is true for all antioxidants) choosing it as the "best" one is a leap of faith.

VITAMIN K AND SPIDER VEINS

You may have seen advertisements or heard cosmetics salespeople discussing the effectiveness of vitamin K creams and lotions for reducing or eliminating surfaced spider veins (technically referred to as telangiectasias). These creams can't change spider veins, but let me explain why some people erroneously think they can. Vitamin K in skin-care products is considered a cosmetic ingredient, not a pharmaceutical or drug. As a cosmetic, it is not necessary for companies to prove their claims about what it can do. The only research concerning vitamin K's effectiveness on skin or surfaced spider veins comes from the companies selling these products. One medical source in particular, Dr. Melvin Elson, who sells creams that contain vitamin K, makes a lot of claims about treatment of spider veins. His company, Cosmeceutical Research Institute, is the only source of information suggesting this stuff works. There are no published or peer-reviewed studies that add up to results you can even remotely count on.

According to Dr. Craig Feied, MD, director of the American Vein Institute and Associate Clinical Professor of Emergency Medicine at George Washington University, vitamin K is associated with veins and blood because it is a prominent factor in the blood's ability to clot. If you take too much vitamin K orally, it can cause blood clots (which can lead to death). Blood clots can choke off the blood flow through a vein or capillary and make it atrophy. However, shutting down a vein or a surfaced capillary (spider vein) this way can be risky. Applying vitamin K to the surface of the skin does nothing, and that's good. If vitamin K could penetrate the surface of the skin to affect the blood flow in spider veins, it could also affect the blood flow in healthy veins. If you're already using a vitamin K product, don't worry; for vitamin K to form blood clots to shut down a vein or capillary, you would need to take large doses that would then need to be digested and metabolized in the liver, where proteins are formed. These special proteins are what cause the blood to clot. It isn't the vitamin K that shuts down veins, but a by-product that is created after digestion.

If you are interested in doing something that truly eliminates tiny surfaced spider veins from the face, the Photoderm laser is an option. Photoderm zaps the tiny spider vein and literally makes the blood boil for a moment, which closes down the vein and the surrounding surfaced spider veins. The sensation is about the same as being poked by a tiny needle. It is best for tiny spider veins because it treats only the surface of the skin, where the problem exists. Photoderm can't get deep enough to cause damage or problems for veins you don't want it to affect. Scleratherapy, or salt injections into the surface veins, is another option. (This procedure is discussed further in Chapter 13, Cosmetic Surgery.)

Getting rid of spider veins is one issue, but preventing them is even more important. Sunburn, heat (prolonged exposure to saunas, Jacuzzis, or just cooking for long periods over a hot stove), pressure on the face (from severely blowing your nose, facial exercises, or rough massages), injury, smoking, and repeated local irritation and inflammation from irritating skin-care ingredients can all increase the occurrence of spider veins. Avoid these things and you can reduce the appearance of these veins, as well as their formation.

YEAST

It is a bit odd to think of yeast as a skin-care ingredient worth looking into, yet in many respects it is one of the most paradoxical organisms occasionally found in cosmetics. A simple computer search for brewer's yeast's Latin name, *Saccharomyces cerevisiae*, brings up over 85,000 references. That's amazing! Yeasts are basically fungi that grow as single cells, producing new cells either by budding or fission [splitting]. Because it reproduces well, *Saccharomyces cerevisiae* is the most widely used organism in biotechnology. Nevertheless, some forms of yeast are human pathogens, such as *Cryptococcus* and *Candida albicans*.

In relation to skin there is limited information about how *Saccharomyces cerevisiae* may provide a benefit. Live yeast-cell derivatives have been shown to stimulate wound healing (source: *Archives of Surgery*, May 1990, pages 641–646), but research like this is scant. Most of what is known about yeast is theoretical, and is about yeast's tissue-repair and protective properties (source: *Global Cosmetic Industry*, November 2001, pages 12–13) or yeast's antioxidant properties (source: *Nature Genetics*, December 2001, pages 426–434). As a skin-care ingredient yeast has potential, but what its function may be or how it would affect skin is not understood.

part II

KEEPING SKIN HEALTHY AND RADIANT

chapter 3

SKIN CARE BASICS FOR EVERYONE

SUNSCREEN

Sunscreen, without question, is the most basic and essential part of any skin-care routine—it plays a pivotal role from birth into our old age. No other skin-care product can so greatly and unquestionably influence the health of skin. It may sound simple, but it's a complicated product to understand, thanks to federal Food and Drug Administration (FDA) regulations, formulary considerations, application issues, reapplication concerns, risk of breakouts or irritant reactions, interpreting the SPF number, waterproof claims, and controversial research about ingredients. Because of that complexity, along with the seriousness of sun damage and the vital protection effective sunscreen offers, it deserves a chapter all its own. See Chapter 4, Sun Sense, where it will deservedly receive the attention it merits.

FORGET SKIN TYPE

Some women are quite aware of their skin type; for other women it's a complete mystery, an elusive conundrum of changes that never settles down in one specific direction. What you should know is that regardless of how sophisticated some cosmetics companies are in approaching the issue—whether with computers and questionnaires to help you discover what is going on with your skin, or seemingly knowledgeable salespeople looking at your face and evaluating what you need—their final determination of your skin type is often inaccurate. **That's not to say understanding skin type isn't important, because it is, but not in the way the cosmetics industry approaches it or the way we've been indoctrinated to think about it.**

What I'm really saying is to forget about skin type as the cosmetics industry defines it. The rigid categories you find at cosmetics counters and the information about what your skin needs as analyzed by a salesperson are often wrong or at best incomplete. The concept of skin type, in terms of the standard normal, oily, combination, or dry types, is one of the most misused beauty concepts around. Yet it is usually where making decisions about our skin-care routines begins.

The primary difficulty in understanding your skin type is that, in addition to your skin's condition, you must recognize that outside factors can and do influence what you see and feel on your face. You can't know what skin type you have or what to do about it until you know why skin behaves the way it does. There can be no rational discussion of your skin-care needs until you evaluate what you may be doing that affects your skin's health, such as smoking, subjecting your skin to unprotected sun exposure, or using irritating and drying skin-care products.

What kind of environment you live in absolutely has an impact on skin. Someone living in cool, moist Seattle has radically different skin-care concerns from someone coping with the hot, dry air of Phoenix or Los Angeles. Your skin-care routine also plays a significant factor. Too many of the wrong skin-care products can wreak havoc on your face. For example, overusing moisturizers, scrubs, AHAs, BHA, and masks can all adversely affect skin. Further, health problems such as rosacea or psoriasis or internal health conditions such as a thyroid disorder can affect skin, too.

Those complex, integrated circumstances, combined with your skin's genetic predisposition for certain traits (oily versus dry, prone to breakouts, or sensitive skin), contribute to what takes place on and under your skin. To complicate matters further, skin type is not static. **What you see today may not be what you see tomorrow, next week, month to month, or season to season.** Judging skin type from one moment in time (like when you are shopping at a cosmetics counter and the salesperson says you have dry, oily, or combination skin) doesn't give you enough information to create an effective skin-care routine.

While cosmetics salespeople may ask what skin type you have, their ability to factor in any or even part of this intricate list is at best limited, and may be nonexistent. Nevertheless, aside from genetic traits, environmental factors, hormones, or skin disorders, your present skin-care routine is the pivotal element in the appearance of your skin. The products you use can affect the skin's oiliness, dryness, and sensitivity. The wrong skin-care products can trigger allergies, redness, surfaced capillaries, or changes in skin texture, and can aggravate breakouts. The way your face feels right now can largely (though not solely) be a result of the way you clean your face. Your skin-care routine could be creating the very problems you're trying to eliminate.

For example, if you wash every day with a bar soap (which is drying), followed by a toner (which may also be drying), and several moisturizers (which can be greasy and potentially can block pores), you can create a severe combination skin condition and cause breakouts. Or if you wipe off your makeup with a cold cream (even expensive ones can be greasy) and then follow up with a toner (which might also be greasy or contain irritants), you should not be surprised if you develop breakouts and dull-looking skin. If you have fairly normal skin but you use an alcohol-based AHA toner, plus a scrub, an AHA moisturizer, and a clay mask, your skin may end up looking very dry and irritated, along with showing rashlike pimples.

Typing skin without taking into consideration the products you use relies on the assumption that the skin is the way it is all by itself, regardless of what you do to it, but that is rarely the case. **Before you can know what your skin type really is, you have to start at square one to discover what your skin type is not and find out what is causing the conditions you see on the surface.**

Another problem with what's called skin typing is the assumption that once you've been told your skin type, your skin will be the same forever, or at least until you age. That, too, is rarely the case. Emotions, weather conditions, hormonal levels, menstrual cycles, stress, physical changes, weight fluctuations, and whatever else life brings can directly affect your skin. If your skin-care routine focuses on skin type alone, it can become obsolete the moment the season changes, your work life becomes stressful, or hormonal influences fluctuate (as hormones often do).

To complicate things even more, in any given period of time a woman may have many skin types! Over the years, even when using gentle, irritant-free products, I've experienced irritated skin patches at the same time I had oily skin, or acne flare-ups along with dry skin around my eyes. **It is** not unusual for women to have a little bit of each skin type simultaneously or at different times of the month or week. An overview of how your skin behaves and changes is necessary to assess what your skin needs.

Once skin type is identified, the biggest problem is how the cosmetics industry handles that information. As far as the cosmetics industry is concerned, every woman can and should have normal skin. Yet the very idea of acquiring normal skin is like trying to scale a peak with a slippery, precarious slope. Like the rest of our bodies, skin is in a constant state of change. Even women with perfect complexions go through phases of having oily, dry, or blemish-prone skin. Almost every woman after the age of 40 will have some amount of sun-damaged skin. In reality, no one is likely to have normal skin for very long, no matter what she does. Those of us who struggle with oily skin, breakouts, dry skin, sensitive skin, or sun damage know that normal skin is at best fleeting. **Chasing after normal skin can set you up on an endless skin-care buying spree, running around in circles trying everything and finding nothing that works for very long.**

In any case, identifying skin type is highly subjective. Many women have really wonderful skin but refuse to accept it. The smallest blemish or wrinkle or the slightest sensation of dry skin distresses them. I can't tell you how many women I've met who get one blemish and run to the dermatologist complaining about acne. Or the women who see a line or two around their eyes and immediately buy the most expensive anti-wrinkle creams they can find in the hope of warding off their worst imagined nightmare. Overreacting to what you see in the mirror makes for more mistakes in cosmetics purchases than almost any aspect of skin type. **This is one of those times where being realistic is the most important part of your skin-care routine.**

Identifying your skin type is made even more difficult by the omnipresent combination-skin complaint. Almost everyone at some time or another, if not all the time, has combination skin. This is not out of line—it just happens to be the way the skin functions. The nose, chin, center of the forehead, and the center of the cheek all have more oil glands than other parts of the face. It is not surprising that those areas tend to be oilier and break out more frequently than the other areas. Problems occur when you buy extra products for combination skin because many ingredients that are appropriate for the T-zone (the area along the center of the forehead and down the nose where most of the oil glands on the face are located) won't help the cheek or jaw areas. Some products claim they can regulate themselves over each area of your face, but that's a complete impossibility. The ingredients that can absorb oil can promote dryness and the ingredients that moisturize dry skin can cause breakouts. Mixed together they don't self-regulate, they cancel each other out. **You may need separate products to deal with the different skin types on the face because you should treat different skin types, even on the same face, differently.**

The most frustrating aspect of the skin type idea is the fact that it's often used (by cosmetics salespeople and by the cosmetics industry in its ads) to instill a sense of immediate need. Once your skin is classified as a "type" that isn't normal, or if it stops being normal, then panic can set in. Cosmetics salespeople aim this ploy at the 30-something crowd, with the pitch sounding something like "You had better do what you can do now to make sure your skin doesn't get worse." I've seen it happen a thousand times as I've listened to or been personally subjected to a salesperson's scolding about skin-care mistakes that are destroying my skin. **What destroys skin is unprotected sun exposure, smoking, and using irritating skin-care products. Not using the right skin-care products (other than a good sunscreen) may cause problems, but it does not damage skin in the long run, and that includes not using a moisturizer.**

Determining skin type is not the answer to other skin-care needs that may not be apparent on the skin's surface. For example, sun damage is not evident when you are young, but sun protection is imperative for all skin types. Dry and oily skin that are present at the same time, along with some redness, may be an early sign of rosacea, a condition that cannot be treated with cosmetics and may not be easily diagnosed. Your skin may be breaking out now, but those blemishes on the surface took a few weeks to get there. Breakouts begin in the pores, and may involve sebum (oil), cellular debris (dead skin cells), dead hair shafts, and/or bacteria. It takes consistent, long-term planning to handle each aspect of the blemish problem, and treating only what you see (as in "zapping zits" or "spot treatment") can make matters worse. Large patches of flaky, dry, red skin may be caused by psoriasis, and cosmetics can make this condition worse. Dry patches of rough, abraded skin can be caused by an allergic reaction or by eczema. What you see on the surface of the skin does not always indicate the type of skin-care products you should buy, or even that you need a skin-care product at all.

SKIN TYPE HAS NOTHING TO DO WITH YOUR AGE

Older skin is different from younger skin. That is indisputable. Yet it is a mistake to buy skin-care products based on a nebulous age category. Treating older or younger skin with products supposedly aimed at dealing with specific age ranges is inappropriate because not everyone with "older" or "younger" skin has the same needs. An older person may have acne, blackheads, eczema, rosacea, sensitive skin, or oily skin, while a younger person may have dry, freckled, or obviously sun-damaged skin. Products designed for older skin are almost always too emollient and occlusive, and those designed for younger skin are almost always too drying. Both extremes can cause problems when the key issue becomes your age as opposed to the actual condition of your skin.

Treating older or younger skin with an age-related, unified skin-care routine is a trap lots of women fall into, particularly older women. I understand the anxiety a woman feels when she passes the age of 40 and notices her skin is changing. And when a skin-care routine claims it is best for your age group it is hard not to believe that isn't true. Yet an effective skin-care routine should be based on the current condition of your skin, along with protection from sun damage, regardless of your age. Age is not a skin-care condition! In fact, many of the skin-care concerns associated with age are more often than not shared by women of all ages.

All women, regardless of age, need sun and antioxidant protection, and possibly treatment of skin discolorations (either potential or existing), dry or oily skin, or breakouts. Wrinkles may tend to separate younger from older skin, but the care you give the skin doesn't necessarily differ. Not everyone in their 40s and older has the same skin care needs. In a way it's simple: You need to pay attention to what is taking place on your skin, and that varies from person to person.

DOES SKIN COLOR OR ETHNICITY AFFECT SKIN CARE?

Regardless of skin color or ethnic background, all skin is subject to a range of problems. These skin problems almost always have less to do with color or ethnic background differences than with what they have in common with skin problems in general. Whether it is dry or oily skin, blemishes, scarring, wrinkles, skin discolorations, skin disorders, skin sensitivity, or even risk of sun damage, all men and women share similar struggles. So, while there are some distinctions between varying ethnic groups when it comes to skin problems and skin-care options, overall these differences are minor in comparison to the number of similarities.

According to an article in the *Journal of the American Academy of Dermatology* (February 2002, pages 41–62), "People with skin of color constitute a wide range of racial and ethnic groups—including Africans, African Americans, African Caribbeans, Chinese and Japanese, Native American Navajo [and other] Indians, and certain groups of fair-skinned persons (e.g., Indians, Pakistanis, Arabs), and Hispanics. . . . There is not a wealth of data on racial and ethnic differences in skin and hair structure, physiology, and function. What studies do exist involve small patient populations and often have methodological flaws. Consequently, few definitive conclusions can be made. The literature does support a racial differential in epidermal melanin [pigment] content and melanosome dispersion in people of color compared with fair-skinned persons. Other studies have demonstrated differences in hair structure and fibroblast size and structure between black and fair-skinned persons. These differences could at least in part account for the lower incidence of skin cancer in certain people of color compared with fair-skinned persons; a lower incidence and different presentation of photoaging; pigmentation disorders in people with skin of color; and a higher incidence of certain types of alopecia [loss of hair] in Africans and African Americans compared with those of other ancestry."

One arena where differences do exist was explained in *Contact Dermatitis* (December 2001, pages 346–349). It noted that "there is a widespread, but largely unsubstantiated, view that certain skin types may be more susceptible to the effect of skin irritants than others. One expression of this would be that certain ethnic groups may also be more likely to experience skin irritation. . . . In this study, we have investigated two carefully matched panels of Caucasian and Japanese women volunteers to determine their topical irritant reaction, both acute and cumulative, to a range of materials. The results indicated that the acute irritant response tended to be greater in the Japanese panel and this reached statistical significance with the stronger irritants. Cumulative irritation was investigated only with the weaker irritants and, although again the trend was to a higher response in Japanese compared to Caucasian panelists, this rarely reached significance."

Throughout this book I will point out the special needs, concerns, and treatment options that affect men and women of color when they differ from those of Caucasian skin types. Specifically, I will describe what takes place in keloidal scarring and hyperpigmentation (darkening of the skin).

AVOID IRRITATING YOUR SKIN

I started my career as a cosmetics consumer advocate by warning women about the damage being done to their skin by irritating skin-care ingredients. Over the years my fears about irritation have been confirmed and reinforced by many dermatologists and cosmetics chemists. Indeed, irritation is a bigger problem for the skin than even I had suspected. Irritation can cause an immediate breakout response, it can cause redness, flaky skin (which can clog pores), or rashes, and it can even cause capillaries to surface on the face. More significantly, irritation can destroy the skin's integrity by breaking down the skin's protective barrier, which, over time, damages the skin's structure. Inside the skin, irritation impairs the skin's immune and healing response (source: *Skin Pharmacology and Applied Skin Physiology*, November-December 2000, pages 358–371). Additionally, breaking down the skin's protective barrier can allow the introduction of bacteria, thus raising the risk of more breakouts.

What causes skin irritation? Many elements are responsible for hurting skin including hot water, cold water, sun exposure, pollution, irritating skin-care ingredients, soaps, and drying cleansers, plus just scrubbing the skin. You may think that none of those things bothers your skin. However, it is startling to learn that even if your skin doesn't feel or appear irritated after exposure to those things, it is still being irritated and the skin breakdown is nonetheless taking place. That means if you are out in the sun, sitting in a sauna, or using a skin-care product that contains potentially irritating or sensitizing ingredients, the irritation damage is still taking place even though the skin doesn't show it (source: *Skin Research and Technology*, November 2001, pages 227–237). We can get a clearer idea of how this secret damage takes place by likening it to what happens to skin in response to unprotected sun exposure. Getting tan or sunburned when we are young and throughout our teens seems to be a lot like using a cosmetic coloring because the cumulative damage takes place beneath the skin's outer surface and doesn't show until after many years of exposure.

Avoiding the obvious substances and elements that irritate skin is crucial for healthy skin. This includes not smoking, avoiding unprotected sun exposure at all costs, and not using irritating or harsh skin-care products. Not paying attention to the irritation potential of certain ingredients in skin-care products can be damaging to the health of your skin. What skin-care ingredients irritate skin? That list is presented in the next few pages. Keep in mind that throughout this book when I indicate something is a possible skin irritant, it means it can be irritating to everyone's skin, even if your skin doesn't appear to have a reaction. Some ingredients always create irritation beneath the skin's surface and cause damage, and that is not good for anyone's skin.

Note: Some irritating ingredients can also have positive results for skin, such as AHAs, BHA, Retin-A, Renova, sunscreen ingredients, some antioxidants, and some preservatives [which keep products stabilized]. All of those can be considered essential for many skin types and product formulations, yet they do pose a risk of irritation. In this case, it is simply a tradeoff in which the benefits outweigh the potential negatives. On the other hand, some ingredients are not only irritating but also have no positive impact on skin, meaning they don't help it in any way and are best avoided. Those are the ones I consistently warn about.

LEARNING TO BE GENTLE

Irritation takes a toll on all skin types. Although many things can cause irritation, the skin can respond the same way regardless of the source. While the skin's reaction to irritation is not always visually apparent, when it does react it isn't pretty! Irritation can cause an assortment of problems, from redness to dry patches, blemishes, rashes, cracks along the side of the nose and corners of the mouth and eyes, flakiness, increased skin sensitivity, other skin disorders, and a reduction in the skin's immune/healing response.

Here it's important to say that it is generally believed that irritation is *not* responsible for wrinkles and premature aging of the skin. Some dermatologists suggest, however, that repeatedly using irritating ingredients on the skin can suppress the skin's immune/healing response, making the wrinkling process worse. Many products that are advertised as making skin look instantly younger when placed over the lines on the face contain irritating ingredients (such as alcohol) that swell the skin temporarily. With repeated use, they could actually make the skin more wrinkled.

Take this rule at face value: Thou shalt always treat thy skin gently or it will complain loudly that something is wrong. The skin might react to topical irritation immediately, or it may take some time before signs of irritation show up. Possibly the most ominous aspect of irritation is that your skin doesn't have to exhibit a reaction at all. Your skin can become irritated and you won't necessarily feel or see anything different. If you use irritating skin-care products, your skin may suffer the negative effects whether or not you can see them taking place on your skin (source: *Contact Dermatitis*, November 1998, volume 39, issue 5, pages 231–239).

It logically follows that learning how to be gentle to your face is one of the most important parts of any skin-care routine. There is no way you can ever hope for soft, smooth skin when your face is being irritated every time you take care of it. Irritation-free skin is the goal.

HOW TO BE GENTLE

We do many things to our skin and buy an assortment of skin-care products that can cause serious irritation. Yet it is far easier than you may think to eliminate these skin-"care" culprits. With that in mind, here is a list of typical skin-care procedures and makeup ingredients and specific cosmetics products and tools to avoid or use cautiously. The skin can react negatively to all of the following products, procedures, and ingredients.

Irritating Skin-Care Steps and Products
- Abrasive scrubs
- Astringents containing irritating ingredients
- Toners containing irritating ingredients
- Scrub mitts
- Cold or hot water
- Steaming or icing the skin
- Facial masks containing irritating ingredients
- Loofahs
- Bar soaps and bar cleansers (source: *Dermatology*, March 1997, pages 258–262)

Irritating Ingredients
(These are of greater concern when they appear in the beginning of an ingredient list.)
- Acetone
- Alcohol or SD alcohol followed by a number (Exceptions: Ingredients like cetyl alcohol or stearyl alcohol are standard,

benign, waxlike cosmetic thickening agents and are completely nonirritating and safe to use.)

- Ammonia
- Arnica
- Balm mint
- Balsam
- Bentonite
- Benzalkonium chloride
- Bergamot
- Camphor
- Cinnamon
- Citrus juices and oils
- Clove
- Clover blossom
- Coriander
- Cornstarch
- Eucalyptus
- Eugenol
- Fennel
- Fennel oil
- Fir needle
- Geranium
- Grapefruit
- Horsetail
- Lavender
- Lemon
- Lemongrass
- Lime
- Linalool
- Marjoram
- Melissa (lemon balm)
- Menthol
- Mint
- Oak bark
- Orange
- Papaya
- Peppermint
- Phenol
- Sandalwood oil
- SD alcohol
- Sodium C14-16 olefin sulfate
- Sodium lauryl sulfate
- TEA-lauryl sulfate
- Thyme
- Wintergreen
- Witch hazel
- Ylang-ylang

These ingredients are extremely common; you would be surprised how often they show up in skin-care products for all skin types. Ingredients like camphor, menthol, mint, alcohol, and phenol are sometimes recommended because they are considered anti-itch ingredients. The theory works like this: When your skin itches, the nerve endings are sending messages begging you to scratch. If you place these irritating ingredients over the area that itches, the nerve hears the irritation message louder than it hears the itch message and interprets this as a reason to stop itching. That reasoning is fine if minor, sporadic, occasional itching is your problem. If it is not and those ingredients are present in skin-care products meant for everyday use, they introduce a constantly irritating insult to the skin and cause dryness, rashes, increased oil production, red-ness, and breakouts. None of those side effects are attractive.

Skin doesn't have to hurt, tingle, or be stimulated even a little to be clean. (If the skin tingles, it is being irritated, not cleaned.) The major rule for all skin types is, if a product or procedure irritates the skin, don't use it again.

Exceptions to the rule: When you initially begin to use an AHA or BHA product or Retin-A, Renova, azelaic acid, or Differin, stinging or tingling can occur. You may need to cut back if it is more than a little tin-gling, or stop altogether if these symptoms persist for more than a few weeks or worsen with repeated use.

ANTI-IRRITANTS AND ANTI-INFLAMMATORIES

Avoiding irritating ingredients is important for the health of your skin, but it is also helpful to use skin-care products containing ingredients that mitigate or counter the effects of irritation on skin. Anti-irritants and anti-inflammatories are a group of ingredients known for reducing or re-lieving skin irritation and inflammation. Because irritation and inflam-mation are well-known to be problematic for skin, anti-irritants as well as anti-inflammatories have become popular and necessary terms and components in the cosmetics world and in most medical fields, particu-larly in dermatology. Many ingredients perform as anti-irritants or anti-inflammatories and better ones are being discovered all the time. Interestingly enough, most antioxidants function as anti-irritants, and one of the skin's responses to free-radical damage is irritation and in-flammation. Some of the more popular anti-irritants used in cosmetics are willowherb, willow bark, allantoin, oat extracts, bisabolol, borage, chamomile, comfrey, dogwood, fireweed, *Gingko biloba*, green tea, black tea, grape seed, licorice, coenzyme Q10, and vitamin C, to name a few. These ingredients go a long way toward helping the skin deal with its daily struggle against sun exposure, pollution, skin-care routines (topical disinfectants, sunscreens, and exfoliants can be irritating to skin), makeup, and seasonal environmental extremes.

HEAT IS A PROBLEM

Because irritation is a problem for skin, anything that irritates the skin should be avoided as much as possible. Heat is one of those things that should be avoided. As good as hot water, direct steam, or dry saunas feel on the skin, they end up causing more problems for the health of the skin. For years, I have recommended washing the face with tepid water. This is because hot water burns the skin and cold water shocks it, and both leave it irritated and dry. These two temperature extremes can also injure skin cells, dehydrate the skin, and cause capillaries to surface. Extreme temperatures in any form cause problems for the skin, but heat is the more attractive alternative (most people avoid a cold shower or bath).

Dry heat is clearly dehydrating. Whether the dry heat comes from a dry sauna or an arid desert climate, it pulls water right out of the skin cell. That's bad for any skin type, but especially for someone with dry skin.

Wet heat is a bit more deceptive. We all know how great the skin feels initially when we exit a hot shower, Jacuzzi, or sauna. It feels plump and saturated with water because the skin absolutely loves drinking up all the water it can. After even a short soak in a tub, your skin can swell and become engorged with water. When you leave a bathtub and your fingers are all thick and wrinkly, it isn't because they are dry, but because they are distorted and swollen with water-saturated skin cells. Because the surface layer of skin likes water so much, hot water can enter the skin, stay there, and cause a burnlike reaction. As a general rule, if water feels hot to the touch, it's too hot for the skin, especially the face. Be very skeptical about facial treatments that involve the use of heat or washing your face with hot (or cold) water; down the line, they could cause more trouble for your skin than you want.

DON'T SMOKE

Smoking is, at the very least, equal to the sun in the direct damage it causes to the skin's surface. In actuality, smoking is probably even more insidious than sun exposure when it comes to damaging healthy skin. Not only does smoking cause serious free-radical damage and block the body's ability to utilize oxygen, it also creates necrotic (dead) skin tissue that cannot be repaired. Even more unattractive is the breakdown of the elastic fibers of the skin (elastosis), which gives rise to yellow, irregularly thickened skin (sources: *Journal of the American Academy of Dermatology*, July 1999, "Cigarette Smoking-Associated Elastotic Changes in the Skin," and May 1996, "Cutaneous Manifestations and Consequences of Smoking").

Moreover, smoking causes a progressive cascade of damage inside the body (restricted blood flow, reduced capacity of the blood to take in oxygen, impairment to the body's immune system) that eventually shows up on the surface of skin, making it look haggard and dull. It also creates serious deep wrinkling around the lips and lip area.

While smoking can make skin look prematurely wrinkled and aged, it's unattractive for many other reasons as well, including the permeating smell of smoke on clothing, breath that smells like smoke, and yellow stains on hands, nails, and teeth. Smoking isn't pretty and it can be deadly. Quitting smoking is one of the most healthful things you can do for your skin and body.

EVERYONE HAS SENSITIVE SKIN

Most of us have sensitive and/or irritated skin. Regardless of your primary skin type, ethnic background, or age, minor or major irritating skin conditions can be present, even those you can't feel. The skin can burn, chafe, or crack, and you may have patchy areas of dry, flaky skin related to weather conditions, hormonal changes, the skin-care products you use, or sun exposure. Skin can also break out in small bumps that look like a diaper rash. Skin can itch, swell, blotch, redden, and develop allergic reactions to cosmetics, animals, dust, or pollen.

If that isn't enough to make you itch just a little, then think about the number of cosmetics most women use daily. The average woman uses at least twelve different skin-care, makeup, and hair-care products a day, with each one, on average, containing about 20 different ingredients. That means her skin is exposed to about 240 different cosmetic ingredients on any given day. The fact that any of us have skin left is a testimony to the skin's resiliency and the talent of cosmetics chemists. Whether we like it or not, most of us will react to something along the way, perhaps even daily.

Your skin is the protective armor that keeps the elements and other invaders from entering the body. We protect most of our anatomy with clothing, but our faces are left painfully exposed to everything. It's no wonder the skin on our faces acts up now and then. Sensitive skin is probably the most "normal" type of skin around.

Everyone has the potential to develop sensitive skin, so women of every skin type should heed the precautions for sensitive skin. What are the precautions? There is really only one and it goes for all skin types:

Treat your skin as gently as you possibly can. Whether you think of your face as oily, dry, or mature, you still need to be gentle with your skin and avoid things that cause irritation.

The operative word is gentle. Preventing skin irritation, regardless of your skin type, is the course of action I recommend throughout this book. Of course, some skin types can and should try to tolerate certain potentially irritating ingredients. A topical disinfectant (like 2.5% benzoyl peroxide, for instance) is helpful for someone with acne, while a BHA solution (a salicylic acid exfoliant) is good for someone with blackheads. Likewise, an AHA (an alpha hydroxy acid product used to exfoliate) or Retin-A or Renova (to improve cell formation) are beneficial for someone with sun-damaged skin. But aside from those exceptions to the gentleness rule, if something is irritating, it can be detrimental for all skin types. If it is bad for sensitive skin, it is probably bad for oily skin, acne-prone skin, combination skin, dry skin, or menopausal skin. As you integrate this gentleness philosophy into your skin-care routine, you will slowly solve many of the skin problems you have been experiencing.

FRAGRANCE IN SKIN-CARE PRODUCTS

Hopefully by now you are sensitive (pun intended) to the fact that the cosmetics industry doesn't always tell you the truth about how its products can affect your skin. They are particularly silent on the issue of allergic reactions and unfavorable skin flare-ups that result from ingredients in lots and lots of skin-care products. Allergic reactions and skin sensitivities are not technically the same thing, but they can feel the same on your skin. Regardless of the physiologically precise definition, we have all used some type of cosmetic that causes part of our face or body to burn, tingle, swell, flake, redden, itch, blister, break out, or just feel bad. How could this happen? Given how many products we use and the diversity of ingredients, I'm shocked it doesn't happen more frequently. Interestingly enough, two ingredients almost universally added to cosmetics, fragrance and preservatives, are often thought to be the major culprits when our skin goes a little crazy from a cosmetic (source: *Contact Dermatitis*, June 1999, pages 310–315).

An article in the January 24, 2000 issue of *The Rose Sheet* discussed an advisory report issued by the Scientific Committee on Cosmetic Products and Non-Food Products, a European Commission agency. The report stated that "information regarding fragrance chemicals used in cosmetic products that have the potential to cause allergic reactions should be provided to consumers." According to the article, "It is seen that a significant increase in fragrance allergy has occurred and that fragrance allergy is the most common cause of contact allergy." Concurring with this conclusion is an editorial by Pamela Scheinmann, MD, entitled "The Foul Side of Fragrance-Free Products" (source: *Journal of the American Academy of Dermatology*, December 1999, page 1020). She states that "products designated as fragrance-free should contain no fragrance chemicals, not even those that have dual functions." She continues by saying that the terms "hypoallergenic, dermatologist tested, sensitive skin, or dermatologist recommended are nothing more than meaningless marketing slogans." Further research presented in the *American Journal of Contact Dermatitis* (June 1999, pages 310–315; September 1998, pages 170–175) poses this same concern.

Preservatives are impossible to avoid because without them our skin-care products would become contaminated with mold, fungus, and bacteria and pose a serious problem for our skin in just a short period of time. However, you can and should stay away from cosmetics, particularly skin-care products, that contain fragrance. It smells nice, but fragrance serves no purpose for skin. Even fragrant ingredients that may also offer a positive benefit are easily replaced with ingredients that can perform the same function without the irritation aspect of the fragrant component. It sounds simple enough to avoid products with fragrance, perfume, or parfum by just reading the ingredient list and then not buying those products. But ingredient lists aren't always that easy to decipher.

The cosmetics industry knows that most women emotionally and psychologically prefer cosmetics that smell nice, even if they say they want to avoid fragrance. But if a cosmetics company produces products without fragrance, you will instead get the scent of the ingredients, which are not in the least as appealing as an added sweet, floral, or citrusy fragrance. This is why, in order to kill two marketing birds with one cosmetic stone, companies often list the fragrance components as essential oils or plant extracts rather than listing fragrance or perfume on the label. As lovely as essential oils sound, they are still nothing more than fragrance. **So while you don't see the word "fragrance" on the list, and you may approvingly think wintergreen oil, lemon oil, cardamom oil, ylang-ylang oil, or other oils sound pleasant and healthy, your skin may still respond disapprovingly.**

The next time you admire the fragrant quality of a skin-care product you're about to apply to any part of your body or face, think twice. Similarly, aromatherapy shouldn't be a skin-care treatment, however therapeutic it is for the sense of smell and emotions. Fragrance might be nice for your spirits, but it is a health risk for skin. And it doesn't matter if the source of the fragrance is essential oils or plant extracts; as far as the health of your skin is concerned, they are all the same.

ALLERGIC REACTIONS

An allergic reaction to a substance can look like an irritation or sensitizing reaction but when it comes to what is going on beneath the surface of your skin it is a completely different response. Simply put, an allergic reaction happens when our immune system reacts to a familiar or an unfamiliar substance in a unique way. When our system or skin encounters a particular ingredient or combination of ingredients, the immune system decides whether or not it should accept, reject, or ignore the substance. If the body determines that the substance is unwanted, even when no allergic response existed before, it all of a sudden produces histamines to get rid of it. Allergies can develop immediately or build over time with each additional exposure to the ingredient. That is why many women develop an allergic reaction to a cosmetic that they were able to use for years. What makes identifying the source of the reaction even more difficult is that you can develop an allergic reaction at any time, or even find that you are no longer allergic to a substance you had problems with for years.

In addition to the multiple problems associated with irritation and that cause skin to react negatively, it can be both disconcerting and aggravating to have an allergic reaction to the cosmetics you use. Reactions can be subtle, such as a little itching, minor redness and swelling, or small rashlike pimples. They can also involve a full-blown flare-up that causes intense, but temporary, discomfort and an unsightly appearance or they can trigger a chronic condition requiring medical attention. If you have a tendency toward allergic reactions, your skin's condition can be greatly affected and you will have to pay close attention to what you use. Someone with allergy-prone skin needs to use fewer products with smaller ingredient lists.

I would love to list ingredients that I could guarantee won't cause your skin to have an allergic reaction, but there is no single ingredient or combination of ingredients that can live up to that sweeping claim. Why not? Because everyone is biochemically different. Each of us has a unique chemical makeup, and the endless paradoxical differences in the way our bodies perform is why we can react so differently when exposed to the same thing.

Because of the almost limitless combinations, in all sorts of cosmetic formulations, it is truly impossible to know if, when, or how anyone's skin will react to any cosmetic. Your only recourse, and this is not the best news, is to keep experimenting until you find what works for you. If you do get a reaction, stop using the product immediately. Consult your physician if the reaction is serious or prolonged, return products that are suspect, and keep track of the ingredients included in products to which you seem to be allergic. Also, keep in mind that just because you've used a cosmetic for a long time doesn't mean you won't develop an allergic reaction to it.

Whenever I mention the risks of plants and other potentially sensitizing or allergy-related ingredients throughout this book, remember that the amount of a suspect ingredient can also determine how a product will affect your skin. The less there is of an ingredient—the farther down in the ingredient list it is—the less likely you are to have a reaction to it. Just because the ingredient is suspect or may have a potential for causing skin sensitivities doesn't mean it will always cause problems. Listen to your skin, err on the side of gentleness, and be cautious. **Moreover, be patient. If you do have an allergic reaction, wait until it subsides before you venture out to try something new or different. Pare down to the absolute basics, usually just cleanser and a touch of moisturizer over very dry areas, try a bit of over-the-counter cortisone cream to reduce irritation, and stay out of the sun.**

Reminder: If you have an allergic reaction of any kind to a cosmetic product, stop using it immediately and consult your physician if the problem persists. Also, do not hesitate to return the product to the place where you purchased it and get your money back. It is not your fault that the product caused problems. Also, returning the product gives the cosmetics company essential information about how their formulas are working.

Is there one line of cosmetics that's best for sensitive or allergy-prone skin? It would be great if there were, but it just doesn't exist. Allergic skin reactions are amazingly random and dissimilar. What you're sensitive to often has little to do with what someone else reacts to, and beyond that there's the intricate interaction of ingredients being combined on the face. The culprit may not be the product you think caused the problem. You may think a new moisturizer made your eyes swell, but it could be the resins from that reliable nail polish you were wearing in combination with the new moisturizer that triggered the problem.

BATTLE PLAN FOR ALLERGY-PRONE OR SENSITIZING SKIN REACTIONS

Whether or not you have sensitive or allergy-prone skin, chances are that at some point you've had a sensitizing or allergic reaction to a cosmetic you've applied somewhere on your face or body. For some, simply identifying which product caused the problem and stopping its use is enough to improve the appearance of skin almost immediately, or at the very least in a day or two. For others, even after you've stopped using the offending item or items, your skin can remain rashy, reddened, flaky, dry, swollen, and irritated for days—and for some, even months. There is no known medical reason why some skin types can't shake a sensitizing or allergic reaction, but there are a few relatively simple things you can do to wage a successful battle against your skin's response to a product or products it doesn't like.

1. **Be certain you are dealing with an allergy or sensitizing reaction to a product and not with a skin disorder.** Many skin conditions such as psoriasis, rosacea, eczema, folliculitis (an inflammation of the hair follicle), and reactions to food can account for the skin becoming irritated, swollen, red, itchy, flaky, or rashy. A great resource for identifying whether or not what is occurring on your face is a skin disorder is the *Primary Care Dermatology Atlas* at http://www.medscape.com/px/dermatlas?src=search, where you can search over 2,600 images of skin problems. (You will need to create a user name and password, but otherwise this amazing source is a free online service of Medscape.) This gives you a way to identify whether or not your skin is similar in appearance to the images found for a particular skin disorder.

2. **Find what product(s) or ingredient(s) is causing the problem and stop using it.** Sometimes that is a simple enough procedure. If you started using a new concealer and within a few hours that area became red, itchy, and swollen, it would be clear that the concealer is the problem and you would stop using it. Unfortunately, it isn't always that easy.

This discovery process can be very difficult because many skin reactions don't happen all that quickly. It may be several weeks or even months or years of using a product before your skin has a negative reaction to it. For some unknown reason your skin can develop allergic or sensitizing reactions over time. Further, given the number of cosmetic products women use daily, each one containing a disparate range of ingredients, it is no wonder that pinning down exactly which one caused the problem can be a challenge. To make matters even more complicated, it may not be a single product but the combination of products worn one over the other that caused the problem (maybe the concealer isn't the problem, but the mix of concealer, foundation, and moisturizer together that sparked the reaction). The key is to be patient and diligent, experimenting with the item or items you suspect and then watching how your skin responds when you discontinue using them.

3. **Whether or not you've been able to identify the problem product, an over-the-counter cortisone cream can be your skin's best friend.** Lanacort or Cortaid are excellent over-the-counter cortisone creams that function as anti-inflammatories. When either of these are applied to irritated, inflamed skin they can turn off the reaction that is causing the problem. It is essential to be conscientious about using these on a regular, methodical, though short-term, basis while your skin is having problems. For example, once the skin irritation shows up, keep applying the cortisone cream over the affected area for several days, even a day or two after everything seems back to normal. Remember that the skin can hold on to a sensitizing or allergic reaction for a long period of time, even after you've stopped using the offending product. And don't be afraid about the short-term use of an over-the-counter cortisone cream. It is the long-term, consistent use (for more than two or three months) of cortisone creams that can damage collagen and elastin in the skin, not short-term use.

4. **While you are combating the allergic or sensitizing reaction, do not use any other skin irritants of any kind over the affected area.** Fragrances, scrubs, washcloths, AHAs, Retin-A, Renova, benzoyl peroxide, skin lighteners, or other skin-care products with active or abrasive ingredients can trigger skin irritation and will only add to the problem.

5. **Avoid saunas, steam, sweating (if possible), or rubbing the affected area, all of which can help retrigger the reaction.**

6. Finally, if matters don't improve after four to six weeks, or if the re-action is severe from the beginning, you should see your dermatolo-gist for an evaluation.

7. If you suspect that you are having a serious allergic reaction (in the form of hives, extremely swollen skin and eyes, or red patches over the skin that feel warm or tingle), consult your physician to discuss varying options. Prescription-strength topical cortisone, oral cortisone, or oral antihistamines may be necessary.

WHAT ABOUT MOISTURIZER?

Not everyone needs or should use a moisturizer, especially women with oily, combination, or acne-prone skin. That sums it up. I can't think of any other skin-care product that is more misunderstood, misused, and abused than moisturizer. How did things get so out of hand? The only answer is that things tend to get out of hand in the world of cosmetics!

Ironically, from a formulary point of view, I like more moisturizers than I dislike (putting aside the nasty debates over cost versus perfor-mance or exaggerated claims). Yet I've found that because most women overuse moisturizers, these products can cause some surprising skin problems. A lot of women (maybe most) still cling to the erroneous be-lief that moisturizers somehow prevent wrinkles. Not just moisturizers with a high SPF, which do stop further skin damage if they contain tita-nium dioxide, zinc oxide, or avobenzone, but all moisturizers. The mis-taken notion that dry skin is more prone to wrinkles than oily skin remains firmly implanted in the mind of the consumer, and that's on top of all those claims about firming, toning, repairing, and lifting the skin made by companies that sell all sorts of other creams, gels, and lotions.

The only reason to use a moisturizer is if you have dry skin or wrin-kled skin and you want it to look smoother (moisturizers can smooth over, not change, wrinkles). If you don't have dry skin, there is no reason to use a moisturizer. If you have oily skin or skin that breaks out, the worst thing you can do is use a moisturizer of any kind. It really is that simple. What happens when you overuse a moisturizer? Pores get clogged and blackheads can develop; dead skin cells get trapped and have a harder time naturally sloughing off, which can leave the skin looking dull; and you run a higher risk of getting patches of dermatitis, increasing the number of breakouts, and creating your own combination-skin predicament. Additionally, oversaturating the skin can turn off the skin's own immune/healing response. Overdoing it with moisturizers can actually prevent the skin from repairing itself.

Recognizing that a moisturizer isn't for everyone doesn't mean that your skin doesn't need the benefit of sunscreen ingredients, anti-irritants, antioxidants, or water-binding agents. It just means you need to reconsider the type of products you use that contain these kinds of ingredients. Many toners use no thickening agents that can clog pores or occlude skin but do contain antioxidants, anti-irritants, and water-binding agents. Further, many foundations now contain effective sunscreens, so that you don't have to load up your skin with layers of unnecessary products.

DO YOU NEED A MOISTURIZER?

Dry skin is technically a condition caused by a lack of moisture in the skin's top layers, combined with a breakdown of the skin's intercellular matrix (the components that fill the area between skin cells) and an inadequate supply of lipids and oils from the oil glands. If the oil glands aren't doing their job of forming a protective barrier composed of lipids and other substances that prevent evaporation, you can have dry skin. In addition, anything that depletes or damages the skin's intercellular matrix, such as sun damage, environmental factors, or drying skin-care products, can create the need for a moisturizer.

Generally, you can assume that if you are using a gentle skin cleanser and no other irritating skin-care products and your skin still feels dry several minutes after you wash your face, you should use a moisturizer. (**This assumes you are not using a drying or irritating cleanser. It is critical to make sure the dryness of your skin isn't caused by your cleansing products.**) If your skin feels tight, dehydrated, taut, or uncomfortable from dryness by midday or at the end of the day, it is essential to use a moisturizer. Fine lines that improve with the application of a moisturizer, especially around the eyes, are a great reason to use a moisturizer. Just keep in mind that it is best to use the most lightweight moisturizer possible that makes a difference. If none of these problems are present, you don't have dry skin, so don't use a moisturizer. (Obviously, sunscreen is another story, but I'll delve into that in the next section.)

I know giving up a traditional moisturizer may be hard to do, but think about it the next time you reach for one. Ask yourself if your skin really needs this or if it would be better off with an AHA product or a lightweight moisturizer for just around the eyes instead. Or perhaps a well-formulated toner with antioxidants, anti-irritants, and natural moisturizing factors (also called water-binding agents) may be all your skin needs. You can even try a simple experiment to see if your skin does better by using moisturizer only on the dry spots or wrinkled areas rather than applying it all over. (Again, this presumes your skin-care routine is not drying out your skin.)

It's important to note that several skin conditions can look like dry skin but are not, and that they may be exacerbated by the use of moisturizers. Eczema, seborrhea, rosacea, early signs of skin cancer (called actinic keratosis), psoriasis, sun-damaged skin, and even overuse of heavy moisturizers can all resemble dryness but are not helped by using moisturizer. Eczema requires a cortisone cream; seborrhea, rosacea, and psoriasis require topical prescription medications to control the condition; skin cancer or actinic keratosis demands immediate medical attention; and sun-damaged skin is better off with an alpha hydroxy acid product to help exfoliate skin. Overusing moisturizers can not only mask these problems, but also can cause breakouts, make the skin appear dull and thick (by holding down skin cells and preventing exfoliation), and inhibit the skin's natural immune/healing response.

WHAT MAKES A GREAT MOISTURIZER?

As any cosmetics chemist will tell you, there are countless formulary possibilities for moisturizers, far too many to narrow them down to any one ingredient or even to a handful of ingredients. There are truly myriad possible ingredient combinations that can be used to create a great moisturizer. There simply isn't a single best one, which explains why a company like Estée Lauder can sell over 300 antiaging products when you count the varying cosmetics companies under their banner. The cosmetics industry–induced hype that one ingredient holds the answer for skin is a complete fabrication. Whether it is vitamin C, green tea, grape extract, seaweed, beta glucan, alpha hydroxy acid, or some rare mushroom extract, to name just a few, none of them can deliver on the promise for wrinkle-free skin. Instead, each one has a specific benefit to consider, and there is no research establishing any one of them as being preferred over the other (source: *Cosmetic Dermatology*, December 2001, pages 37–39).

So what does constitute a great moisturizer? For daytime, the crucial aspect of any moisturizer is that it must be a well-formulated sunscreen.

Besides protecting your skin from the sun, an excellent moisturizer will contain emollients, water-binding agents (ingredients that attract water to the skin and help keep it there), anti-irritants, and antioxidants.

Emollients

Emollients are lubricating ingredients that are critical for making dry skin not feel dry. These provide dry skin with the one thing it's missing—lubrication—in the form of substances that resemble those the skin produces for itself. Emollients are ingredients like plant oils, mineral oil, shea butter, cocoa butter, petrolatum, cholesterol, and animal oils (including emu, mink, and lanolin, the latter probably the one ingredient that is most like our own skin's oil). All of these are exceptionally beneficial for skin and are easily recognizable on an ingredient list. Far less easy to comprehend on the label are a wide range of ingredients like triglycerides, palmitates, myristates, and stearates. These substances are generally waxy in texture and appearance but are what give most moisturizers their elegant texture and feel. Overall, emollients create the fundamental base and texture of a moisturizer and impart a creamy, smooth feel on the skin. Silicones are another interesting group of lubricants for skin. These have the most exquisite silky texture and an incredible ability to prevent dehydration without suffocating skin. All of these ingredients, in endless variations, spread over the skin to create a thin, imperceptible layer, re-creating the benefits of our own oil production, preventing evaporation, and giving the skin the lubrication it is missing.

Natural Moisturizing Factors (NMFs) or Water-Binding Agents

Natural moisturizing factors (NMFs) or water-binding agents work great for dry skin, and most are suitable for all skin types. "Water-binding agent" and NMF are general terms that refer to ingredients that can keep water in the skin or repair the skin's intercellular matrix (fundamental external structure). There are many ingredients that have these functions. Humectants, for example, attract water to skin and are one vital component of a moisturizer. But what good is getting water to the skin if the structure isn't there to keep the water from leaving? It turns out skin cells usually have plenty of water if they don't become degraded or damaged. Once skin is irritated, overcleansed, exposed to the sun, dehydrated from air conditioning or heaters, and so on and so on, the integrity of the skin is compromised. That means the substances that keep the skin cells bound together to create the surface structure we see as skin (the intercellular matrix) are depleted. This intercellular structure is made up of many different components, ranging from ceramides to lecithin, glycerin, polysaccharides, hyaluronic acid, sodium hyaluronate, sodium PCA, collagen, elastin, proteins, amino acids (of which there are dozens), cholesterol, glucose, sucrose, fructose, glycogen, phospholipids, glycosphingolipids, and glycosaminoglycans, to name just a few. All of these give the skin what it needs to keep skin cells intact. Just adding water is meaningless if the skin doesn't have the wherewithal to keep the water inside, or if the intercellular matrix is damaged. When a moisturizer does contain a combination of these NMFs and water-binding ingredients, it reinforces the skin's natural ability to function normally and that temporarily reduces the presence of dry skin.

Anti-Irritants

Anti-irritants are another vital component of any skin-care formulation. Regardless of the source, irritation is a problem for all skin types, and is ubiquitous and almost impossible to avoid. Whether it is from the sun, the environment, or from the skin-care products a person uses, irritation is a constant assault on the skin. Ironically, for skin-care products, even such necessary ingredients as sunscreen agents, preservatives, exfoliants, and cleansing agents can cause irritation. And other ingredients are irritating or have no real benefit for skin care, such as fragrance and sensitizing plant extracts. Further, oxidative damage from pollution, sun exposure, and air can cause irritation and damage to skin. Anti-irritants thus are a growing addition to many skin-care products to help skin handle the impact or to reduce the irritation skin is subjected to on a daily basis. Anti-irritants are incredibly helpful because they allow the skin healing time and can reduce the problems oxidative damage causes. Anti-irritants include substances with names like bisabolol, allantoin, burdock root, aloe, licorice root, grape extract, glycyrrhetinic acid, green tea, vitamin C, chamomile extract, willowherb, white willow, willow bark, and many, many more.

Antioxidants

Antioxidants are a fascinating part of a moisturizing formula. There's now a growing body of research that shows antioxidants to be a potential panacea for skin's ills and it's nothing less than impressive. What makes antioxidants so intriguing is that they seem to have the ability to reduce or prevent some of the oxidative damage that destroys and depletes the skin's function and structure, while also preventing some solar degeneration of skin (sources: *Cosmetic Dermatology*, December 2001, pages 37–40; *Current Problems in Dermatology*, 2001, volume 29, pages 26–42, "The Antioxidant Network of the Stratum Corneum"). All of that is incredibly beneficial for cell turnover, healing, and reducing dehydration. I suspect that antioxidant research for skin will become even more fascinating over the years. Meanwhile, lots of antioxidants are showing up in skin care these days, such as selenium, superoxide dismutase, vitamin A (retinyl palmitate and retinol), vitamin C (ascorbyl palmitate and magnesium ascorbyl palmitate), beta glucan, vitamin E (a-tocopherol, tocotrienol), curcumin, coenzyme Q10, alpha lipoic acid, green tea, grape extract, and forms of rosemary and lemon bioflavonoids.

All of these, combined in more permutations than you can imagine, create the moisturizers I consider "best" for skin. There is no one mixture or best ingredient though, just like there isn't just one best chocolate cake. I wish there were, but the brilliance of cosmetics chemists lies in their ability to put these ingredients together in many ways to create wonderful products. There are just too many options to sum it up in any one formula. (Antioxidants have been discussed in more detail in Chapter 2, Miracles, Frauds, & Facts: An A to Z Guide.)

ARE SERUMS NECESSARY?

Hearing the word "serum" evokes a sense of a medical fluid of some kind, something more technically advanced for your skin. It may make you think of blood serum, the fluid, colorless part of the blood. It may even trigger memories of being given a shot of specially prepared serum to protect you from an illness. But in cosmetics serums are not an authentic or distinctive formulation. Cosmetic products labeled as serums are using a term with no real meaning or specific definition of any kind. Rather it is just a clever marketing ploy used to make a standard product sound like something impressive and different from a moisturizer. This way the cosmetics industry can lead women to believe that they are purchasing a unique product that is worth the extra money and is a necessary addition to their skin-care routine.

Technically, serum is defined as any watery animal fluid, and surely that doesn't sound appealing! Yes, the name "serum" may give you the sense that these are something medical or therapeutic, but that is nothing more than a psychological impression, not a tested formulary attribution. In the cosmetics world a serum is just a lightweight, gel-like moisturizer with a consistency that is less viscous or emollient than the average lotion or creamy moisturizer. These serums also tend to contain more silicone than other moisturizers, as opposed to thickening agents, so it's very likely that the silky feel you experience is from the silicone they contain. Serums may moisturize, but the name is nothing more than a marketing term. They are not a uniquely formulated product that provides an uncommon benefit for skin.

EXFOLIATING SKIN

The issues around skin exfoliation are complicated, but exfoliation itself is essential for skin health, and most skin types can benefit from exfoliation. Despite the risks of irritation, removing the damaged outer layer of skin is an essential skin-care need of many different skin types. If you have dry skin, oily skin, blackheads, acne, sun-damaged skin, flaky skin (not caused by a skin disease or a skin disorder), or a rough surface texture, those problems are best handled by products that exfoliate and help dead skin cells slough off from the surface of the skin. (Disinfectants, which can also be irritating, are essential for treating acne; see Chapter 9, Battle Plans for Blemishes, for more information about the pros and cons of disinfectants.) The goal is to use the most effective, least irritating products for exfoliating skin. The only skin types that need to be very cautious about using exfoliating products are those with extremely sensitive skin or older skin, and those with skin diseases or disorders such as rosacea, eczema, dermatitis, or seborrhea.

EXFOLIATING OILY SKIN

Let's start with oily skin or skin with clogged pores. Blackheads or blemishes can occur if the oil gland produces too much sebum. Sebum is a soft wax that should liquefy when it reaches the surface of the pore, spreading a thin, imperceptible protective layer over the skin. But when too much sebum is produced, the liquefying process can get backed up. Add to that problem a tendency for skin cells that should be naturally sloughing off to instead fall inside the pore and get stuck. The more skin cells that build up in the oil gland, the more oil will be held back from flowing easily out of the pore (the pore is the exit path for oil), and the result can be a blackhead or a blemish.

Often with oily skin, cells that should be shedding on a regular, daily basis are being held back. One thing that keeps cells from sloughing off is that self-same oil (sebum). The oil works as an adhesive, preventing the shedding skin cells from going where they are supposed to go—off the face. One way to keep pores from getting clogged is to help skin cells shed as freely as possible so they don't get trapped inside the pore. The more you keep skin cells exfoliating in a normal manner, the less cell debris can fill up the pore.

Another issue for oily skin with clogged pores is that the oil gland itself has a skin lining (epithelial lining). For some reason, this lining inside the pore can become thickened or misshapen and choke off and block the flow of oil out of the pore. Using exfoliants that can exfoliate the lining of the pore, thus restoring a more natural shape, can encourage a normal flow of oil and eliminate clogged pores.

EXFOLIATING DRY SKIN

The reasons for exfoliating dry skin are different from the ones for treating oily, blemish-prone skin, though the objective is the same: removing dead skin cells that are not shedding normally. Skin can be dry for many reasons, including lack of moisture, a buildup of dead skin cells that don't easily shed, and abnormal skin cells that adhere together in a way that prevents normal exfoliation and normal moisture retention. (Dry-looking skin can also be caused by moisturizers that are too emollient and hold dead skin cells in place, preventing healthy shedding. When this happens, the surface of the skin feels "greasy" or moist, and the underlying layer feels dry.) When you help dry skin shed dried-up, dead skin cells, it can make room for plumper (moisture-filled), less-dry skin cells to come to the surface, which can lend a fresher look to the skin. This also allows moisturizers (the least amount and lighter texture, the better) to more easily penetrate the skin because there are fewer dried-up skin cells in the way to block absorption. Exfoliating helps the dead surface-skin cells shed at a more normal rate, making room for the lower layers of newer skin cells. And for dry skin it is also helpful to efficiently remove dead skin cells to reduce the chance of pores becoming clogged and creating blackheads and whiteheads.

EXFOLIATING SUN-DAMAGED SKIN

One of the primary manifestations of sun-damaged skin is that the outer layer of skin becomes thickened, similar to a callous. This thickened layer is your skin's response to the damage caused by unprotected exposure to ultraviolet (UV) radiation from the sun. While this thickened layer provides a minimal amount of sun protection (it is thought to protect with the equivalent of an SPF of 2), it ends up creating far more problems than advantages. As you will learn in Chapter 4, Sun Sense, on sun protection, an SPF of 2 is truly meaningless and useless for skin. This thickened outer layer of the skin produced by sun damage causes skin to look dull and more wrinkled than it really is; it also adds a yellowish or gray tint to skin and reduces the ability of good skin-care ingredients to penetrate. Using effective topical exfoliants to remove this thickened, unattractive outer layer of skin can help skin feel smoother; look less wrinkled; have a healthier, more normal skin color; and reduce the chance of clogged pores. (Removing this layer of unhealthy skin does make the skin more sun sensitive, the way it was before it became sun damaged. Though it is always imperative to use a sunscreen, it is even more so if you are regularly using an exfoliant of any kind.)

WHICH EXFOLIANTS TO USE?

For many skin types, the issue is not whether to exfoliate, but which type you should use and how often. There are a lot of exfoliating products out there waiting to peel the money from your pocketbook as well as skin cells from your face. Scrubs, soaps with exfoliating ingredients, toners, facial masks, facial peels, abrasive sponges, washcloths, and facial brushes are all designed to exfoliate. Overkill (as in doing too much to the skin) becomes an issue when your skin-care routine includes more than one exfoliating product or if the one you are using is too strong. In the world of consumerism, if a little is good, a lot must be better, and the cosmetics industry is right there with a host of products. Ignore them; it only takes one product to do the job, and your task is to choose the best product for your skin type.

I do not recommend exfoliating facial masks because often, in addition to the exfoliating ingredient, they also contain a number of other irritating ingredients. Also, exfoliation works best when done consistently, while facial masks tend to be used irregularly and infrequently.

Facial brushes and washcloths are options, but I find they are both almost impossible to keep clean, they tend to exfoliate unevenly, they exfoliate only on the very surface of the skin, and they are not as effective or as gentle as other alternatives. Abrasive sponges, such as loofahs, are way too irritating from the neck up, and are also very difficult to keep clean, meaning they could cause problems by harboring bacteria that can cause infection.

Cosmetic scrubs can be a good way to remove the dead surface layer of skin, but there are difficulties with these types of exfoliants, too. Many of them contain gritty abrasives that can be unnecessarily irritating. These abrasive fragments are not uniform in shape and can literally cut the skin. In addition, cosmetic scrubs often contain thick waxes and creams so you can smooth them more easily over your skin, yet these waxes can clog pores and leave a film over the face, which reduces exfoliation. Some scrub products also contain harsh ingredients such as peppermint, menthol, eucalyptus, alcohol, and roughly ground scrub particles that are simply unnecessary and overly irritating. The problems with all mechanical scrubs—even the one I recommend, namely plain baking soda or baking soda mixed with Cetaphil Cleanser—are that the scrubbing action is mostly on the surface, and the mechanical action against the skin can cause too much irritation. You need to exfoliate, but how to do that gently is the question.

AHAS AND BHA

There are two primary topical ways to exfoliate skin, either with a product containing alpha hydroxy acids (AHAs) or one with beta hydroxy acid (BHA). AHAs have lost much of the popularity they enjoyed since they were first introduced when Avon launched its Anew line with AHAs in 1992, but nevertheless their effectiveness for skin remains a convincing option.

There is only one BHA (beta hydroxy acid, or salicylic acid), but there are a variety of AHAs. The five major types of AHAs that show up in skin-care products are glycolic, lactic, malic, citric, and tartaric acids. Of these, the most commonly used AHAs are glycolic and lactic acids because of their special ability to penetrate the skin, plus they have the most accumulated research on their functionality for skin. A search of the published literature for glycolic and lactic acids lists over 200 varying studies, while there are only a handful for the other three AHAs put together. A similar search for salicylic acid (BHA) reveals over 450 different published studies evaluating its effectiveness.

What glycolic, lactic, and salicylic acids can do is "unglue" the outer layer of dead skin cells, helping increase cell turnover by removing the built-up top layers of skin, allowing healthier cells to come to the surface. Removing this dead layer can improve skin texture and color, unclog pores, and allow moisturizers to be better absorbed by the skin. Both AHAs and BHA affect the top layers of skin, and they help to improve the appearance of sun-damaged skin, dry skin, and thickened skin caused by a variety of factors, including abnormal cell growth, smoking, and heavy moisturizers. Reminder: Sun damage in particular causes the top layer of skin to thicken, creating a dull, rough texture and appearance on the surface of skin; AHAs nicely remove this thickened layer, revealing the more normal-appearing skin cells underneath (sources: *Archives of Dermatologic Research*, June 1997, pages 404–409; *Dermatologic Surgery*, May 1998, pages 573–577).

There is even a good deal of research showing that the use of glycolic acid can improve the appearance of skin discolorations, increase collagen production, and reinforce the barrier function of skin (source: *Dermatologic Surgery*, May 2001, pages 429–433).

Because AHAs and BHA work through a chemical rather than a mechanical process, they can produce better results than cosmetic scrubs, which work only on the exposed surface of the skin. And because AHAs and BHA work just on the top layers of skin (or, in the case of BHA, inside the pore), there is no risk that you will lose too much skin. That is, they don't keep on exfoliating away layers of skin without stopping, as can happen with a scrub. Technically, there is a drop-off rate, meaning the AHA and BHA will exfoliate just the dead or damaged skin and leave the healthy skin alone.

The fundamental difference between AHAs and BHA is that AHAs are water-soluble, while BHA is lipid-soluble (oil-soluble). This unique property of BHA allows it to penetrate the oil in the pores and exfoliate the built-up skin cells inside the oil gland. AHAs are much less able to do this because they can't get through the fat content of the oil (sebum). Therefore, BHA is indicated for use where blackheads and blemishes are the issue, and AHAs are more suitable for sun-damaged, thickened, dry skin where breakouts are not a problem (source: *Global Cosmetic Industry*, November 2000, pages 56–57).

I wish the discussion of AHAs and BHA could end here. I wish you could find a good AHA product by looking for glycolic or lactic acid on the ingredient list if you have sun-damaged, thickened, dry skin. Or that if you tend to have blackheads or blemishes and wanted to find a good BHA product, you would only need to look for a product that contains salicylic acid. But, alas, it isn't that simple. AHAs and BHA are effective as exfoliants only at certain concentrations (the quantity of the ingredient present in the product) and at very specific pHs (referring to the acidity or alkalinity of a product).

PH-SENSITIVE AHAS AND BHA

When it comes to AHAs and BHA, the crucial information comes in two parts: One is the type of ingredient and its concentration in the product, and the other is the pH of the product. AHAs work best at concentrations of 5% to 8% and at a pH of 3 to 4 (this is more acid than alkaline or neutral), and their effectiveness diminishes as you go past a pH of 4.5. BHA works best at concentrations of between 1% and 2%, and at an optimal pH of 3, diminishing in effectiveness as you go past a pH of 4. Both AHAs and BHA lose their effectiveness as a product's pH goes up and the concentration of the ingredient goes down. This is so central to the whole subject of exfoliation and cell turnover that it bears repeating: **AHAs work best in a 5% to 8% concentration, in a product with a pH of 3 to 4; BHA works best in a 1% to 2% concentration, in a product with a pH of 3 to 4** (source: *Cosmetic Dermatology*, October 2001, pages 15–18).

If the cosmetics industry isn't forthcoming about the necessary percentages and pH for a BHA or AHA product (and most companies aren't), how can you tell if it provides decent or effective exfoliation? Consumers can't, not unless they are shopping with pH measuring paper in hand, which is exactly how I go about rating exfoliant products. As a general rule, it is best if the AHA ingredient is either second or third on the ingredient list, making it likely that the product contains a 5% or higher concentration of AHAs. For salicylic acid, because such a small amount is required, it is fine if the ingredient is located toward the middle or end of the ingredient list. (To establish the pH of a product you can always do what I do, test each product with a pH strip, but that is hardly practical for most women.)

Aside from the way they can exfoliate the skin when the concentration and pH level are right, AHAs can also have water-binding properties. They can provide an added benefit by helping to keep water in the skin at the same time that exfoliation is taking place. They also have water-binding properties at any pH, so even if the product can't exfoliate skin it still can aid in moisturizing the skin.

BHA, though it provides more penetrating exfoliation into the pore, ends up being less irritating than AHAs. This is due to BHA's relation to aspirin. BHA, as salicylic acid, is derived from acetylsalicylic acid, which is the technical name for aspirin, and aspirin has anti-inflammatory properties. On the skin, BHA retains many of these anti-inflammatory effects.

Keep in mind that none of these AHA or BHA products, regardless of concentration, pH, or type, can prevent aging or change a wrinkle. Researchers theorize that AHAs, and possibly BHA, can increase collagen and elastin, much as Retin-A and Renova can. But this is only theory, and there is no research to prove it. Meanwhile, AHA and BHA products can definitely smooth the skin, improve texture, unclog pores, and give the appearance of plumper, firmer skin (because more healthy skin cells are now on the surface). And when you stop using them the skin goes back to the condition it was in before you started.

AHA CONFUSION

Estée Lauder was one of the first department-store lines to launch an AHA product, Fruition. It was an overnight success, but not because of its AHA content: Fruition contained less than 2% AHA. At that percentage, AHAs are little more than good water-binding agents. That isn't bad; it just isn't what makes AHAs and BHA such fascinating ingredients. Consumers must have complained, because shortly thereafter Lauder launched Fruition Extra, which contains a decent amount of AHA and has a good pH. It's absurdly expensive for what you get, and of course the company never bothered to explain why you now needed Fruition Extra if the original Fruition was supposed to be so amazing and wondrous for the skin.

Another example: Clinique's Turnaround and Total Turnaround products, all of which contain about a 1% concentration of BHA, and have a pH of around 5. That high pH makes them ineffective as exfoliants. In reality, TurnAround can't turn around even one skin cell.

Then there are AHA soundalikes, including sugarcane extract, mixed fruit acids, fruit extracts, milk extract, and citrus extract, and BHA soundalikes such as wintergreen extract. You may think these are better, more natural AHAs or BHA products when you see these less technical, more familiar names, but that absolutely isn't the case. Without knowing exactly what type of AHA or BHA ingredient you are buying, there is no way to know for sure what you are putting on your skin or how effective it really is. Although glycolic acid is derived from sugarcane and lactic acid is derived from milk, that doesn't mean sugarcane extract or milk extract are the same as glycolic or lactic acid. Just because a product contains sugarcane extract doesn't mean that the acid has been extracted from the sugarcane. And even if the acid has been extracted, you can't tell how concentrated it is, and what about the pH? It's all too vague and meaningless, making it impossible to determine what you are really buying. My advice is to be very suspicious of any product that claims an association with AHAs or BHA but contains some variety of soundalike ingredients.

BHA CONFUSION

Products boasting that they contain a natural source of salicylic acid (BHA) usually add willow bark. Willow bark contains salicin, a substance that when taken orally is converted by the digestive process into salicylic acid. That means the process of converting willow bark to salicylic acid requires the presence of certain enzymes to turn the salicin into salicylic acid. The digestive conversion processes can turn salicin into saligenin, and then into salicylic acid, but this is complicated. Further, salicin, much like salicylic acid, is stable only under acidic conditions. The likelihood that willow bark in the tiny amount used in cosmetics can mimic the effectiveness of salicylic acid is at best problematic, and in all likelihood impossible. However, willow bark may indeed have some anti-inflammatory benefits for skin because, in this form, it appears to retain more of its aspirin-like composition.

WHAT ABOUT HIGHER CONCENTRATIONS OF AHAS?

I am very concerned about the introduction of products with higher percentages of AHAs, as is the FDA (source: FDA *Consumer Magazine*, March-April 1998, revised May 1999). Various cosmetics lines have introduced products like this, including one called M.D. Formulations, sold by doctors and salons. M.D. Formulations sells AHA products at 10%, 15%, and 20% concentrations in appropriate pHs of 3 to 4.

Removing the outer layer of skin can be taken too far, however, and many cosmetic dermatologists and researchers worry that increased irritation and exfoliation caused by such high concentrations of AHAs can actually hurt skin. Without more evidence showing a genuine benefit from higher concentrations (none exists at this time), I am not willing to recommend that anyone put their skin at risk in that way. Most likely the positive results women and men may perceive with higher concentrations of AHAs come from the swelling and edema they cause. That may diminish the appearance of wrinkles and make the skin feel smoother, but it is most likely not best for the long-term health of the skin due to the increased amount of constant irritation.

If you use a well-formulated AHA product (5% to 8% concentration, with a pH of 3 to 4) or BHA product (1% to 2% concentration with a pH of 3 to 4) but you don't "feel" it working on your skin, that doesn't mean it isn't working. Quite the contrary, it is indeed working—without causing your skin any discomfort or irritation.

POLYHYDROXY ACIDS

It's no secret that alpha hydroxy acids (AHAs) may be irritating. In fact, for them to be effective they need to produce a little bit of irritation. Yet for some skin types that little bit can be too much. The search for an effective form of AHA (as mentioned above, glycolic acid and lactic acid are considered the most functional forms) or an extra ingredient that can enhance performance and reduce irritation has been a popular topic of discussion among cosmetics formulators. Gluconolactone and lactobionic acid are types of polyhydroxy acid that NeoStrata believes serves both ends: They are supposed to be just as effective as AHAs but also less irritating. (NeoStrata is the company that holds the patent on glycolic acid as an antiwrinkle agent, as well as a patent for gluconolactone for reducing the appearance of wrinkles.)

Gluconolactone and lactobionic acid are chemically and functionally similar to AHAs. The significant difference between them is that gluconolactone and lactobionic acid have a larger molecular structure, which limits their penetration into the skin, resulting in a reduction of irritating side effects. This more controlled release into the skin supposedly doesn't hamper effectiveness. So are gluconolactone and lactobionic acid better for your skin than AHAs in the form of glycolic acid or lactic acid? There is a small amount of research indicating this to be the case but it is hardly conclusive (Cutis, February 2003, pages 14–17). Rather, if you have had trouble using AHAs in the past due to irritation, polyhydroxy acids may be the best for your skin type.

HOW DO YOU USE AHAS OR BHA?

Strictly based on your skin type and skin-care needs, you can apply an AHA or BHA product once or twice a day. Also, depending on your skin's sensitivity you can apply either of these around the eye area, making sure to keep them off the eyelid and away from the eye itself. Apply the AHA or BHA product after the face is cleansed and after your toner has dried (if you are using one). Once the AHA or BHA has been absorbed, you can apply any other product, such as additional moisturizer, eye cream, sunscreen, or foundation. It is not essential to wear moisturizer over an AHA or BHA product. That totally depends on what type of skin you have, how it reacts to the AHA or BHA product, and what kind of base the AHA or BHA is in. Some AHAs and BHA come in moisturizing bases, and most skin types do not require another moisturizer.

I generally recommend using an AHA or BHA in a gel or liquid form so you don't have to apply a moisturizing base where you don't need it. That way the AHA or BHA goes on first and the moisturizer goes over it only where the skin is dry or taut. Never purchase an AHA or BHA product that includes other irritating ingredients such as alcohol, menthol, camphor, eucalyptus, mint, or citrus. AHAs and BHA can be irritating enough by themselves (removing dead, damaged skin cells is not a gentle process), and there is never a reason to add more irritation, especially when it provides no benefit for the skin. The only reason possible irritation from AHAs and BHA is allowable is because their ability to exfoliate is useful for solving many skin-care problems.

I never recommend cleansers that contain AHAs or BHA, for several reasons. First, if they are in a water-soluble cleanser, you run the risk of possible contact with the eyes, which can cause irritation. Second, AHAs and BHA work on the skin or the pores when they have been absorbed. When they are in a cleanser, they get rinsed down the drain before they can work. (Some companies shockingly recommend leaving the cleanser on the face for several minutes so the AHAs or BHA can be absorbed into the skin, but that means the detergent cleansing agents would be left on the skin for longer than necessary, and that absolutely can cause unwanted irritation.) Finally, the skin needs only one good exfoliant, and that's it. Overexfoliating will further irritate the skin, and the long-term effects of that are unknown.

In terms of sunscreens, it would be great if an AHA or BHA product had a good SPF rating (at least SPF 15, with FDA-approved UVA protection). That way, if you wanted to use an AHA or BHA product during the day along with a sunscreen, you would only have to apply one product instead of two. **With the exception of Exuvience by NeoStrata, there are no sunscreens currently on the market that contain an effective concentration of AHAs or BHA with a proper pH level as well as an effective SPF formulation (effective meaning an SPF 15 with one or more of these active ingredients: avobenzone, titanium dioxide, or zinc oxide). Why? Because to be stable, sunscreen formulations usually require a pH higher than what is acceptable for an effective AHA or BHA product. As a result, sunscreen needs to be a separate step from the application of AHAs or BHA (or Retin-A and Renova, for that matter).**

As you search for an AHA or BHA product, cosmetics salespeople will tell you to use theirs along with their complete program, including two or three other moisturizers, toners, cleansers, eye creams, throat creams, and anything else they can sell you. Be prepared for the hard sell when it comes to AHA or BHA products! Many cosmetics companies treat them like the fountain of youth, and they are not. They do not stop wrinkling, they merely smooth the surface skin for as long as you continue to use them. Some companies deal in specialty AHA products that contain higher percentages (from 8% to 15%). However, higher percentages may guarantee higher irritation, and there is little research indicating what kind of risk or harm that might pose over time. Be aware that many, many AHA and BHA products are poorly formulated, with ineffective concentrations and pH levels. The purpose of AHAs and BHA is to exfoliate the skin. They can do that only at the appropriate concentration and pH. An AHA or BHA product that has a low concentration and a high pH may feel good on the skin, but it is good only as a moisturizer. That isn't bad, but it won't exfoliate the skin.

By the way, many AHA or BHA products designed for oily skin contain alcohol. I do not recommend these because of the risk of increased irritation and sensitization they pose. Likewise, someone with oily skin or breakouts will have problems with an AHA or BHA that comes in a moisturizing base because the ingredients may make the skin feel slick and can clog pores. Those with oily skin types need to look for AHA or BHA products in a gel or liquid form that are irritant-free (meaning no alcohol, plants, fruit extracts, or witch hazel) and as lightweight as possible. More of these are becoming available, but the pickings are still relatively slim if you're looking for a good, reasonably priced AHA or BHA product that won't adversely affect oily skin types.

As a general rule (though there are definitely exceptions and personal preferences that alter this rule), if you are using one good AHA or BHA product, you should not use additional exfoliating products such as cosmetic scrubs, washcloths, and facial masks (clay or drying masks). Also, stay away from overdoing exfoliation. Lots of cosmetics companies put AHAs and BHA in everything they make. Remember, the skin can handle only so much irritation; one effective exfoliant is all that is necessary for anyone's skin.

Most people experience a tingling or slight stinging sensation when they use AHA or BHA products with appropriate concentrations and pH. Some people have had minor to severe flaking and redness. Minor reactions are to be expected, given the nature of AHAs and BHA. However, long-term irritation, redness, flaking, or patches of dermatitis are not healthy for the skin, and if any of these symptoms occur, you should reduce the frequency of application or consider a gentler (less concentrated) product. Listen to your skin. If it gets very dry and flaky, use an additional moisturizer for a period of time until the skin calms down and gets used to the new level of exfoliation. If it gets red and irritated, use the product less frequently, though still regularly (perhaps once a day, or two or three times a week). If it still gets very dry and irritated, consider stopping altogether. Severe irritation is not the goal or the desired result.

One more key point. As you probably already know, it is imperative that you wear a sunscreen every day, one with an SPF of at least 15 that includes avobenzone (trade name Parsol 1789), titanium dioxide, or zinc oxide to protect skin from UVA damage. Exfoliating the skin leaves it more vulnerable to sun damage and that means you need mandatory, maximum sunscreen protection every day.

The FDA has confirmed that there is a risk of UVB sun sensitivity (sunburn) following the use of AHAs. That makes sense, given that

AHAs work to remove sun-damaged skin, and that leaves the skin some-what more vulnerable. Of course this sensitivity is easily preventable with the diligent use of lower concentrations of AHA (10% or less) and a sunscreen. Research does show AHAs to be safe in 4% to 8% concentrations with a pH of 3 to 4 (source: *Journal of Cosmetic Science*, November/December 2000, pages 343–349).

TRETINOIN (RETIN-A, RENOVA, ETC.)

Even after discussing AHAs and BHA at length, I do not want to play down the considerable importance of tretinoins for skin because they are major players when it comes to changing the way skin behaves. If you have sun-damaged, dry, wrinkled, or acne-prone skin, you should become familiar with the names Retin-A and Renova and their active ingredient tretinoin.

Let me make it perfectly clear from the beginning that **Retin-A and Renova are not exfoliants**, though many people think that's what they do. It is also vital to clarify how important it is to consider these products (or any topical prescription medication containing tretinoin) as elements of basic skin-care treatment. This is because tretinoin affects and improves actual cell production deep in the dermis, far away from the surface of skin (sources: *Clinical and Experimental Dermatology*, October 2001, pages 613–618; *Clinical Geriatric Medicine*, November 2001, pages 643–659; *Photochemistry and Photobiology*, February 1999, pages 154–157).

Tretinoin can help skin look and feel smoother and function more normally, but the process is subtle and very different from the action of removing surface layers of skin to create a smoother texture and appearance. AHAs and BHA affect the *surface* of the skin (epidermis) or the lining of the pore by actually ungluing or dissolving layers of skin cells. In contrast, tretinoin affects the *dermis*, where new skin cells are produced. Why the confusion about the effect tretinoin can have on the skin? Primarily it's due to the fact that using products containing the drug tretinoin can cause irritation and inflammation, resulting in the skin becoming flaky and dry. This flaking and dryness is not exfoliation, nor is it a desirable or advantageous result. If tretinoin causes your skin to be consistently dry and flaky it is a problem, and you should probably avoid the products that contain it.

For a bit of history, the original patent for the use of tretinoin to treat acne and sun-damaged skin was held by a division of Johnson & Johnson. The only prescription products that contained tretinoin were varying forms of Retin-A and Renova. Johnson & Johnson's patent for tretinoin expired in the mid-1990s. Now there are a handful of other topical prescription drugs containing tretinoin that are also an option for skin, including Tazorac, Avita, and generic tretinoin.

The FDA approved Renova for use as a wrinkle cream in December 1995. That makes Renova the only medication ever approved by the FDA for the treatment of sun-damaged skin and wrinkles. Yet the research concerning Renova in regard to "wrinkles" was not exactly exciting. According to the FDA, "Studies on Renova showed that after 24 weeks approximately 30 percent of people who used the product for fine wrinkles or spotty discoloration had moderate improvement, 35 percent had minimal improvement and 35 percent had no improvement. Among individuals who used the product, about 16 percent had moderate improvement in skin roughness, 35 percent saw minimal improvement and 49 percent had no improvement. Renova does not eliminate wrinkles or repair the sun-damaged skin that leads to cancer. Nor is there evidence that Renova treats coarse skin, deep wrinkles, skin yellowing or other skin problems" (source: *FDA Talk Paper*, January 2, 1996).

While Renova and other tretinoin products won't erase wrinkles, they can do remarkable things for the health of the skin. Tretinoin has the ability to locate receptor sites on the skin cell that accept certain specific components of vitamin A. The tretinoin attaches to this receptor site, which provides information to the cell, telling it to behave in a healthier manner. In this way, tretinoin can play a vital role in changing the way skin cells are formed and shaped. This is different from exfoliating. If a skin cell has a healthier form and shape, it can do its job of natural exfoliation and look the way it did (to some extent) before it was sun damaged.

Regardless of these positive effects, tretinoin products will be useless if you do not wear a sunscreen as well. Not a wrinkle cream in the world, even one approved by the FDA, can have positive results if you don't use an effective sunscreen; without that, you are just putting back more of the damage you don't want.

Tretinoin products aren't cheap. Renova costs about $60 for a 40-gram tube (a one- to two-month supply), and that doesn't include the cost of a visit to your doctor. But Tazorac and Avita or generic tretinoins are half that price and just as effective.

Many physicians recommend applying both tretinoin and AHAs, using AHA in the morning and tretinoin at night or one over the other. How BHA figures into use for different skin types is not clear. Because people react differently to skin-care products, I would suggest experimenting to see which item or items work best for you. There is no reason in the world not to judiciously try out such a combination, always remembering sunscreen, to see what has the most benefit for your skin.

Again, what tretinoin, AHA, and BHA products have in common is that once you stop using them, your skin will revert to the way it was before. These products will not produce permanent change. The smooth exterior lasts only as long as you use them. This is one of the major reasons that researchers don't believe AHAs, BHA, Retin-A, or Renova really change the deeper layers of the skin.

Tretinoin Care

If you do choose to get a topical prescription tretinoin product, it is important to be careful when using it, as with AHA and BHA products. Review and remember the following list of cautions.

* It is always dangerous to tan, but it is especially problematic after you start using topical tretinoins (because they can be irritating and cause peeling) or an AHA or BHA product. As the surface skin peels and the callous of damaged skin is removed to reveal healthier skin, the skin becomes more sensitive to sunlight and is, therefore, even more subject to serious sunburn and sun damage. Also, tanning will negate any positive effects you hope to gain from using these products. You should already be using an effective sunscreen every day, but if you are using any of the above-mentioned products, it is vital to wear a sunscreen rated at least SPF 15, with the UVA-protecting ingredients of avobenzone (Parsol 1789), titanium dioxide, or zinc oxide, whenever you venture outside. The idea is to keep your sun exposure to a minimum.
* Tretinoin, as well as AHA and BHA products, can irritate the skin. If you use any other irritant on the skin at the same time you will exacerbate the initial negative side effects of the product. You must eliminate all of the following from your skin-care routine during your first months of using these products: all astringents, toners, fresheners, clar-

ifying lotions, refining lotions, and the like that contain irritating ingredients. Also avoid scrubs, clay and peel-off facial masks, bar soaps, and skin-care products that contain fragrances. Finally, it is best to avoid saunas and steam rooms (used on a regular basis, saunas and steam rooms can surface tiny capillaries, causing a spider web of tiny red lines on the face.

• If you want products with tretinoin, AHAs, or BHA to work, you must use them regularly. To sustain the results, you must continue using them on a regular, patterned cycle for the rest of your life. The changes they allow to take place on the skin are not permanent. Once you stop using the product, the skin slowly reverts to its original condition. Using something forever is a tremendous commitment. But according to the majority of women I've interviewed and who have written to me, the difference is positive enough to warrant a long-term relationship.

EXFOLIATING TREATMENTS

While we are on the subject of exfoliation, you should know there are deeper forms of exfoliating than products that contain a 5% to 8% concentration of AHAs or 1% to 2% concentration of BHA. The deeper options are treatments you can receive from a salon or spa or at a doctor's office. These include AHA or BHA peels, microdermabrasion, nonablative laser resurfacing, and ablative laser resurfacing. All of these are valid options for dealing with wrinkles and some kinds of scarring. You may also be pleased to hear that in many ways the decision to go with one of these is less baffling than you think. That's because it isn't about which method is effective (they are all effective in their own way for removing surface layers of skin); rather, it is a question of money, tolerance, how comfortable you are about the risks (if any), and, finally, what results you hope to achieve. When considering any of these skin-resurfacing methods, the questions you need to answer are how much risk you can tolerate, what your budget is, how long you want the results to last, what the condition of your skin is, and what your skin color is. Once you understand how the answers to those questions affect your choice you can start shopping for what you want as opposed to being sold a service by a convincing doctor or aesthetician.

Note: I discuss each of the following procedures further in Chapter 13, Cosmetic Surgery.

Superficial Microdermabrasion

Facialists typically perform this type of procedure but it is also available from some dermatologists and plastic surgeons. It is little more than a deep surface scrub done with a machine that shoots finely ground mineral crystals onto the skin and then vacuums them back up. This involves superficial abrasion of the skin's surface (removing the nonliving skin cells that occupy the top three to five layers of skin only). This surface layer has no capillaries and is nonpigmented, which is why its removal causes no bleeding, crusting, or skin discoloration. Left on its own, sun-damaged skin takes on a dull or thick appearance and fine lines seem more apparent because the surface skin cells slough off unevenly. Regular superficial microdermabrasion treatments with an appropriate system can temporarily improve the appearance of skin, but that's about it.

Microdermabrasion presents minimal to moderate risk, but that has little to do with your skin type or color and more to do with your reaction to the procedure and the skill of the technician. For some skin types, the irritation is too much; also, some aestheticians get carried away and go over and over an area, causing wounds and oozing. To obtain lasting or noticeable results, microdermabrasion needs to be constantly repeated because once (and even three or four times) is not enough.

The most typical result is a noticeable reduction in the appearance of some wrinkling and red skin discolorations (superficial scarring). However, this takes repeated sessions, and it is believed that the outcome is most likely a reaction to the skin being irritated and not from a change in the lower layers of skin. But that conclusion is open to debate, with most studies substantiating the concern (source: *Dermatologic Surgery*, November 2001).

There is no downtime associated with superficial microdermabrasion, although the skin of some women does get red, dry, and flaky. The price varies widely, but generally the procedure can be pricey—and to get the smooth skin you are looking for, the repeated treatments can go on forever. The results also vary depending on the skill of the technician.

Risk: Minimal. Some women can experience redness, flaking, dryness, and irritation, but this usually diminishes within a few days. If you are prone to cold sores (*Herpes simplex*) around your mouth or on your face, this can trigger an outbreak.

Cost: Moderate to expensive. A series of microdermabrasion treatments can range from $300 to $600 for three treatments. That's pricey, considering the short-term nature of the results, and over a few years the amount can add up.

Results: After two to three treatments a noticeably smoother surface, with wrinkles and redness from surface acne scars reduced but not eliminated. Has no effect on ice-pick or dented scars from acne or chicken pox.

Duration: Improved appearance can last for one to three months, but treatments must be repeated for improvements to stick around.

Deep Microdermabrasion

Deep microdermabrasion is (or should be) performed only by physicians and involves disruption of part of or the entire epidermis. The skin cells of the epidermis have capillaries and varying degrees of melanin; therefore, their disruption can cause bleeding, crusting, and skin discolorations, particularly in darker-skinned individuals. It was believed, when microdermabrasion technology was new, that this deeper disruption of the skin would cause dermal remodeling of collagen and should, therefore, reduce the appearance of acne scars, pits, and deeper wrinkles. Histologic confirmation of this has yet to be established and clinical correlation remains controversial (source: *Cosmetic Dermatology*, March 2001).

Deeper microdermabrasion shares risks that are similar to AHA peels, which are reviewed in the following section. Last, it should be mentioned that both superficial and deep microdermabrasion may in fact be safer than some glycolic or salicylic acid chemical peels in darker-skinned individuals because acid peels may alter pigmented cells in the epidermis.

AHA peels ranging between 20% and 40% concentrations in a pH of 2 to 3

AHA peels using concentrations of over 50% are done strictly by physicians. There are no BHA peels in any concentration available as a nonmedical treatment. AHA peels in concentrations of 40% or less are done by both physicians and facialists. There is a vast difference between results and risks at these varying concentrations (see the next section). At lower concentrations, AHA peels are similar in efficacy and results to microdermabrasion, with AHAs having a slight to moderate edge in creating a smoother appearance and less noticeable wrinkles and scars with only one to three applications. However, to obtain more significant, lasting results, takes subsequent treatments—up to three or six over the period of a year. Both microdermabrasion and low-concentration AHA peels require repeated treatments.

While microdermabrasion may not produce the same quality of noticeable results, there are far fewer risks associated with it. Even low-concentration AHAs can result in extreme redness, flaking, a burning sensation on the skin, and even some oozing and scabs.

Several cosmetics companies sell products claiming to be at-home peels. Thankfully, none of these are effective. These types of products may have a high AHA content, but none of them have a pH low enough to exfoliate skin. That's good news. The risks to skin of using a truly effective at-home peel include possible burns from leaving it on too long or not treating the skin appropriately afterward.

Risk: Minimal to moderate. Some women can experience extreme redness, flaking skin that can last for a week, irritation, and dryness, although this usually diminishes in a week or two. If you are prone to cold sores (*Herpes simplex*) around your mouth or on your face, this process can trigger an outbreak.

Cost: Moderate to expensive. A series of AHA treatments can range from $300 to $600 for three treatments, and the treatments need to be repeated to maintain the effect.

Results: After two to three treatments a noticeably smoother surface, with less-noticeable wrinkles and less obvious redness from surface acne scars. Has no effect on ice-pick or dented scars from acne or chicken pox.

Duration: Improved appearance can last from two to three months.

AHA peels ranging between 50% and 70% concentrations in a pH of 2 to 3, or BHA peels at 8% to 13% concentrations in a pH of 3

These high-concentration peels are performed strictly by physicians—and with good reason: The risk to skin is far higher, with many concerns about hypo- or hyperpigmentation, severe irritation, and risk of infection. As you may suspect, the higher risk goes hand-in-hand with more impressive, longer-lasting results. These kinds of medical peels can make a significant difference in the appearance of skin. They can fundamentally change the appearance of wrinkles and surface scarring; however, they still won't have an effect on ice-pick or dented scars from acne or chicken pox. Peels like this also have a far longer duration, with the effects lasting between two and three, and up to five years.

Risk: Moderate. Most women will experience severe redness, flaking, and oozing skin, and that can last for one to four weeks. The risk for these effects is reportedly somewhat less with a BHA peel because BHA's relation to aspirin may provide an anti-inflammatory effect along with the peeling action. There is also the possibility of a minimal risk of skin discoloration (either darkened areas of skin or lighter areas of skin). However, when this does occur it more often than not doesn't last, and fades with minimal treatment of prescribed skin lighteners. This risk of discoloration is more significant for those with darker skin tones. If you are prone to cold sores (*Herpes simplex*) around your mouth or on your face, this can trigger an outbreak.

Cost: Expensive. A high-concentration AHA or BHA peel can range from $1,000 to $2,500.

Results: After healing is completed the skin will have a markedly smoother appearance, with facial lines and surface scarring greatly reduced. High-concentration AHA and BHA peels have no effect on ice-pick or dented scars from acne or chicken pox.

Duration: Improved appearance can last from two to five years.

Nonablative Laser Resurfacing

In the world of making skin look younger there are many paths to take, and a number of nonablative laser treatments ("nonablative" meaning noninjurious or without damaging or burning skin tissue) are available options. Nonablative lasers include the N-lite laser, Nd:YAG laser, Flash-lamp laser, Pulsed Light laser, and Cool-Touch laser. All of these are options for minimizing the appearance of wrinkles and skin discolorations. But what are nonablative laser treatments, and how do they compare to other forms of laser resurfacing?

Nonablative (or coblative) laser resurfacing is very different from ablative laser resurfacing treatments, which became popular over the past several years and involved a machine that would "ablate" skin tissue with extreme heat generated by laser pulses. (The most well-known types of ablative lasers are the CO_2 Pulse Laser and the Er:YAG laser.) Ablative laser resurfacing procedures absolutely made a remarkable difference in the appearance of skin, particularly in terms of long-lasting improvement in the appearance of deep wrinkles, surface wrinkles, and skin discolorations. But as wonderful as that sounds, there are risks with ablative laser resurfacing, which include swelling, scabbing, oozing, bleeding, flaking, redness, and irritation that could last for an extended period of time. There is also a definite risk in terms of even longer-term skin discoloration and scarring.

The laser procedure being performed by plastic surgeons and dermatologists alike is termed nonablative laser resurfacing or dermal remodeling because it does not injure skin tissue. That means little downtime and few to none of the risks associated with ablative laser resurfacing. However, nonablative resurfacing doesn't produce the same dramatic results as ablative resurfacing can. According to an article by Dr. David Goldberg in *LaserNews* (July 2000), "Nonablative dermal remodeling leads to improvement in photodamaged skin and rhytids (wrinkles) without any obvious wound. . . . However, at the present time, the clinical improvement seen with such techniques is less than that following the inelegant ablative laser resurfacing techniques."

Risk: Minimal. Some women can experience redness, flaking, dryness, and irritation, but this usually diminishes within a few days. If you are prone to cold sores (*Herpes simplex*) around your mouth or on your face, this can trigger an outbreak.

Cost: Moderate to expensive. $300 to $1,000 per treatment. Typically, two to five treatments are needed.

Results: After a series of treatments, noticeable improvement is visible on areas of skin discoloration, rough surface texture (sun damage), and reduction of postinflammatory hyperpigmentation. The impact on wrinkles is not as impressive as with ablative laser treatments but an improved appearance is still possible.

Duration: Improved appearance can last from two to four years, but varies depending on how many treatments you have had.

Nonablative laser resurfacing does require multiple treatments to maintain or achieve better results, but the smaller risk and minimal to no downtime to let the skin heal (relative to that of ablative techniques) is a huge benefit. This method is indeed a consideration, but it is not a panacea for getting rid of wrinkles and skin discolorations—it's just one of the many options to consider.

Ablative Laser Resurfacing

This is the prince of all peels. Other than a face-lift, this is the last of the effective surface treatments to help reduce the appearance of wrinkles. Because the process is so involved, including a discussion of the different laser options, I provide a more in-depth analysis in Chapter 13, Cosmetic Surgery, examining the options for this complicated, though highly effective and long-lasting, resurfacing cosmetic-surgery procedure. Put simply, and aside from questions about the types of machines available, this procedure is both extremely effective and most risky. The results can be astounding, but when it's overdone or done with poor pre- and postoperative procedures, it can give the skin a plastic look. When done right, it can smooth out a good deal of wrinkling, uneven skin texture, skin discoloration, and acne scarring. It can't undo deep folds or heavily sagging skin, but it can retract some sagging. It cannot eliminate dented or ice-pick scars.

Preoperative care, including the use of skin lightener (to reduce the risk of skin discoloration), Renova or Retin-A to improve the skin's healing ability and the general health of the skin, and the use of effective sunscreens is important, and it can help achieve positive results. It is also essential that the patient stop smoking, if not permanently, for at least as long as possible before treatment (smoking not only causes wrinkles but it can also weaken the skin's immune system enough to put the patient in a higher risk category). Postoperative care varies, but silicone bandages are considered one of the best options, along with antibiotic creams and oral antibiotics. There should be minimal exposure to sun and irritating skin-care products of any kind.

Risk: Moderate to severe. Most women will experience severe redness, flaking, and oozing skin that can last for two to five weeks. There is also a possible risk of skin discoloration (either darkened areas of skin or lighter areas of skin). This risk of discoloration is more significant for those with darker skin tones. If you are prone to cold sores (*Herpes simplex*) around your mouth or on your face, this can trigger an outbreak.

Cost: Expensive. Prices range from $2,500 to $5,000.

Results: After healing is completed the skin will have a markedly smoother appearance, with facial lines and surface scarring greatly reduced and some eliminated altogether. Deep, furrowed lines will not be affected much. Laser resurfacing can greatly improve and eliminate some acne scarring. It cannot eliminate sagging skin but some retraction will be visible.

Duration: Improved appearance can last from three to seven years.

chapter 4
SUN SENSE

UNDERSTANDING UV

Before you can understand how to protect skin from the sun it is helpful to know what exactly you need protection from. Sun feels great, especially when you're outdoors and it's shining. But even on a cloudy day, when you can't see the sun, the sun's rays are ever-present and ever attacking the skin. Basically, the sun's infrared rays (IR) keep us warm and the visible rays provide daylight. But while the sun's ultraviolet radiation (UVR) is also important, its effects are serious for skin and eyes.

UVR is divided into three different bands: UVA, UVB, and UVC. Virtually all UVC radiation is filtered out by the atmosphere so that none actually reaches the earth's surface (although ozone depletion has some researchers worried about this one, too). In direct contrast to UVC, UVB and UVA rays both reach the earth in significant amounts.

UVB radiation, the rays of the sun that burn, is much stronger in some ways than UVA radiation, and it has a considerable capacity to cause instant skin damage in the form of blistering sunburns. However, the earth is bombarded with about 100 times as much UVA as UVB, so while it may be weaker, UVA radiation still has a potent impact on the skin.

All UVR is strongest between 10 A.M. and 2 P.M. Clouds filter some, but not most, of the UVR, which is why you are still likely to get burned on an overcast day. Different surfaces, such as water, cement, sand, snow, and even grass, can reflect UVR, causing a double whammy for the skin.

Altitude is also a sun enhancer because for every 1,000-foot increase in altitude the UVR potency increases by 4%.

Pollution's effect on the ozone layer, located many miles above the earth's surface, is serious business for many reasons, but this discussion is about what that means for skin. When intact, the ozone layer filters out much of the sun's UVB radiation, but it has relatively little effect on UVA. It is the sunburning UVB rays that increase when the ozone layer is eroded, which means more serious burns for those who dare to go outside without protection.

By the way, UVB rays can't get through glass, so there's no risk of sunburn when you sit in a car or next to a window, but that's the good news. The bad news is that UVA rays *can* get through windows. Normal glass doesn't protect skin from UVA damage, so sitting in a car or next to a window that lets daylight through offers no UVA protection whatsoever. (Sunglasses are very important, but I discuss that later in this chapter.)

TO TAN OR NOT TO TAN? NOT!

FACT: There is no such thing as a safe tan. ALL tanning is a problem. Actually, any and all unprotected sun exposure is damaging to skin. Most of us think sun damage occurs from baking in the sun and getting a deep, dark tan. That is only part of the picture. Sun damage begins the moment you walk out of the house, anytime during the day, whether it is sunny or cloudy (at least 40% to 50% of the sun's rays penetrate cloud cover). It may take 20 minutes for some of us to get burned, or an hour or two for some of us to start tanning, but the damage associated with wrinkling and skin cancer begins the moment your skin is exposed to sunshine. It is the repeated sun exposure, just several minutes a day, 365 days a year, *even when sitting near a sunny window*, that adds up to a great deal of damage, both aesthetically and physically.

But back to tanning. Turning any shade that is darker than your own natural skin color, whether you have very light or very dark skin, is the skin's defensive response to sun damage. It may look nice, but it isn't nice for the skin. Melanocytes are skin cells that contain the brown-colored protein called melanin. These brown skin cells determine a person's natural skin tone. Surprisingly, the difference between the lightest skin color and the darkest is only a very small amount of melanin. With exposure to sun, the melanocytes produce more melanin, and tanned skin is the result. But here's another shock: Despite the fact that tanning is a protective response, it isn't all that helpful. By some estimates, a tan provides an SPF of only about 2. Sorry, there just isn't any way a tan of any kind can be considered healthy. As one dermatologist described it, a tan is the same as a callus on your foot. Yes, it protects the foot, but who wants that kind of protection and why continue doing what caused the callus in the first place?

Because melanin isn't a very reliable sunscreen, dark-skinned people still suffer negative effects from sun exposure. Ashen skin color, mottled skin, wrinkles, and even skin cancer can happen to those with dark skin. Skin cancer is less likely, but the risk of skin damage and wrinkling is certain.

The most damning result of sun exposure is that it does serious damage to the entire system, beyond the problems that eventually take place on the skin's surface. The skin contains components that are central to the body's immune system. The Langerhans cells in the epidermis prevent bacteria from attacking the system and prevent cell mutation, making these cells indispensable to good health (source: *Journal of Investigative Dermatology*, January 2002, pages 117–125). Yet a few minutes of unprotected sun exposure can damage the Langerhans cells in ways that can last for weeks.

In addition to damaging the immune system, the sun also directly attacks the collagen structure of the skin, changing it from a cohesive network of support into a disorderly, weakened mass. While the sun is busy destroying collagen underneath the surface of the skin and the Langerhans cells throughout, it also thickens the exterior of the skin, chokes off the skin's blood supply, and reduces the skin's elasticity (sources: *Clinical Experimental Dermatology*, October 2001, pages 573–577; *Journal of the American Academy of Dermatology*, July 2001, pages 610–618). Sun tanning is not pretty.

Dear Paula,

With summertime just around the corner, I thought that I might share the knowledge I have learned over the years about self-tanning products. I have used self-tanning products since they were first introduced on the market. I am a 49-year-old female and enjoy being "tan." My best advice is to get just a little bit of a real tan. I live in the Houston/Galveston area and usually in late spring (late April, early May) I will lay out in the early part of the day (10 A.M. to 12:30 P.M.) and then apply the self-tanner. This helps achieve a real bronze-colored tan. If you like being tanned it's worth your time and effort, because it sure beats the alternative, namely skin cancer.

Wanda, Houston, TX

Dear Wanda,

I am sharing your letter because I am afraid that there are women who may share your belief that a little bit of tanning is safe, but that is absolutely not the case! The skin turning color is a danger sign of damage and abnormal cell production. It is not safe or healthy. Any amount of tanning puts the skin at high risk for cancer, not to mention wrinkles. I cannot advocate your routine and would suggest you reconsider what you are doing. Your belief that you are preventing problems for yourself by tanning in the morning and getting just a "little" color is dangerous thinking and you are putting your health and skin in jeopardy. One more point: In reality you are exposing your skin to sun at the worst time—right in the middle of the day (given that the sun is strongest between 10 A.M. and 2 P.M.) when UVA and UVB rays are at their most potent.

SUN STRATEGY

If you take to heart only one section of this book, make it this one. What makes the following information so vital is not only the prevention of wrinkles, but also the prevention of many forms of skin damage. We're talking serious skin care.

Perhaps the most important fact about sun protection is that the Food and Drug Administration (FDA) stringently regulates sunscreens as over-the-counter drugs, not as cosmetics. While cosmetics don't have to prove their claims, or their efficacy for that matter, over-the-counter drugs have to prove both efficacy and safety and their formulations are tightly controlled. The FDA also allows only specific claims to be made for specific ingredients. That means if a product is labeled SPF 15, whether it's Chanel or Coppertone, it must utilize one or more of the limited number of approved sunscreen ingredients, in very specific concentrations, that are allowed to receive such a rating (source: FDA *Cosmetics and Colors Fact Sheet*, June 27, 2000).

SPF stands for "sun protection factor." But the SPF number tells you only about how long a product will protect you from getting a sunburn, protecting your skin from the sun's UVB rays. Surprisingly, it doesn't provide any information about the sun's UVA rays. The sun's UVA rays have no apparent, immediate impact on skin, but they are thought to be the cause of wrinkles, hyperpigmentation, and skin cancer (source: *Photodermatology, Photoimmunology & Photomedicine*, February 2001, pages 2–10). So, while SPF is important it does not tell you everything you need to know in order to purchase an effective sunscreen.

It turns out that the difference in UVA versus UVB protection is incredibly significant for the health of the skin. Until as recently as 1997, in the United States, the typical SPF 15 formulation provided protection only from UVB radiation, which unquestionably prevented sunburn and deep tanning. Anyone who applied a sunscreen correctly knew they wouldn't get burned and could stay in the sun with no painful side effects. Yet despite this remarkable protection, as well as the notably increased use of sunscreens, skin-cancer rates did not decline. If anything, they increased. So why weren't sunscreens doing their part to reduce the problem?

To the dismay of dermatologists, oncologists, and researchers, it eventually became clear that UVB radiation is not the culprit in many types of skin cancers. Rather, UVA radiation is the primary cause of skin cancer. **In addition, because sunscreens were so successful at preventing sunburn (protecting against UVB radiation), they allowed people to stay out in the sun for even longer periods of time, absorbing more cancer-causing UVA radiation.** It was found that while the typical SPF 15 sunscreen formulation protected against about 97% of UVB radiation, it kept out only a limited amount of UVA radiation. Keeping a large percentage of the UVB rays off the skin felt great, but evidently that wasn't enough for the long-term health of the skin. It is easy to see why cancer rates were going up, not down (source: *Journal of Investigative Dermatology*, November 2001, pages 1186–1192).

So how do you know if your sunscreen is protecting your skin from the sun's UVA rays? There is only one way to tell. You must look at the *active* ingredient list on the sunscreen you own or are thinking of buying, looking for one of the following ingredients: avobenzone, titanium dioxide, zinc oxide, and (outside of the United States) Mexoryl SX (source: *Photodermatology, Photoimmunology & Photomedicine*, December 2000, pages 250–255). If one of these three ingredients isn't present it is a product you should throw out and absolutely should not purchase.

If you are looking for a sunscreen—and everyone must wear a sunscreen 365 days a year—you now need to pay attention to more than just the SPF. The SPF is still important, but it's only part of the story. What counts, and regardless of what sunscreen products you buy—whether tints, foundations, oil-free sunscreens, sprays, or lotions—they must be rated at least SPF 15 or greater and they must have the UVA-protecting ingredients avobenzone (Parsol 1789), titanium dioxide, zinc oxide, or Mexoryl SX on the active ingredient list. It is acceptable to have titanium dioxide and zinc oxide as the only sunscreen ingredients present, while Mexoryl SX and avobenzone can be used in conjunction with other sunscreen ingredients. (Avobenzone may also be listed as butyl methoxy-dibenzoylmethane.)

WHAT ABOUT SPF?

A sunscreen's SPF rating is incredibly important, but it is no longer the only guide when buying sunscreens. All the SPF number lets you know is how long you can stay in the sun without burning while wearing that product. For example, let's say you're like me and you can stay in the sun for about fifteen minutes before your skin starts to turn pink. Applying a sunscreen rated SPF 15 (both the new formulations with avobenzone, titanium dioxide, or zinc oxide or without) will allow you to stay in the sun fifteen times longer (three and three-quarters hours: 15 times 15 minutes) without getting pink. In other words, the SPF number, 15 in this case, multiplied by the amount of time you can normally stay in the sun without getting pink, is how long you can stay in the sun after you've applied the sunscreen. If you normally can stay in the sun 25 minutes without getting pink, applying an SPF 15 sunscreen would let you stay in the sun six and one-quarter hours (15 times 25 equals 375 minutes) without burning.

However, as we now know, the SPF rating refers only to protection from UVB radiation. It gives you no information about protection from UVA radiation, which can cause skin cancer and wrinkles. If that SPF 15 or SPF 30 doesn't contain avobenzone, titanium dioxide, or zinc oxide you are receiving minimal protection from UVA radiation and it is a dangerous product to consider using.

APPLYING SUNSCREEN

Now that so many products contain sunscreen (foundation, concealers, moisturizers, and even face powders), the next question is, What about application? That's a great question! The major issue for the use of any well-formulated sunscreen (SPF 15 or greater with UVA protecting ingredients) is liberal application. Protection is determined not only by the SPF number and the UVA ingredients the product contains but also by how thickly and evenly it is applied, and when, where, and how often the sunscreen is reapplied. There is often a mismatch between the expectation versus the reality of actual use (source: *Journal of Photochemistry and Photobiology*, November 2001, pages 105–108).

Keep in mind that everyday liberal application, applied 20 minutes before you step outside (not once you get to the car, or get to the beach, or do anything—but before you leave the house) is the key element of getting the best protection possible. But within your skin-care routine, exactly when does sunscreen get applied? If you are applying several skin-care products, ranging from toners to acne medications to moisturizers, **the rule is that the last item you apply during the day is your sunscreen.** If you apply sunscreen and then apply, say, your moisturizer or an acne product, you could inadvertently be diluting or breaking down the effectiveness of the sunscreen you've just applied.

Any skin-care product, or even just water (and almost all moisturizers are more than 50% water), applied over a sunscreen reduces its effectiveness. This is why you have to reapply sunscreen after swimming or perspiring. If you use moisturizers, which are always lipid soluble, over your sunscreen you are breaking the sunscreen down via dilution or removal, and that is a serious problem. I have seen information in some fashion magazines suggesting that you should apply sunscreen first because putting it on over other skin-care products would block its absorption and that absorption is necessary for a sunscreen to be effective. This is dangerous information. If anything, research indicates that sunscreen can readily be absorbed through other cosmetic ingredients. An article in the *Journal of Investigative Dermatology* (2001, volume 117, pages 147–150) stated that "in contrast, when applied [in light amounts], thickening agents promote penetration, most likely through greater stratum corneum diffusivity arising from an enhanced hydration by the thicker formulations . . ." and suggests people " . . . recognize that thicker formulations may sometimes enhance the penetration of other topical agents when applied 'in use.' "

What about applying foundation (one that doesn't contain sunscreen) over the sunscreen you've just applied? If the foundation is a thin, watery-type foundation or you're using a tinted, lotion-type moisturizer (which doesn't contain sunscreen) you would in all likelihood reduce the potency of the sunscreen underneath. However, if you are applying a standard liquid foundation, a cream-to-powder or stick foundation, a cream foundation, or a pressed-powder foundation, and as long as you are smoothing it over the skin and not wiping it off or rubbing it too heavily into the skin, there is minimal risk that you are affecting the sunscreen underneath. However, if there is even a small risk that you are diluting the effectiveness of your sunscreen with foundation, you should consider wearing a foundation that contains sunscreen, too.

If you are using more than one product containing sunscreen, such as an SPF 15 moisturizer and an SPF 8 foundation, it is important to understand that does not add up to an SPF of 23. You would get some increased SPF value for protection, but there is no way to know what amount of increased protection that would be. If you want to get the protection of SPF 30, then that is the SPF number you should look for. If you are mixing SPF products, both must contain the UVA-protecting ingredients of avobenzone, titanium dioxide, zinc oxide, or Mexoryl SX.

What if your foundation is the product you've chosen for sun protection? **Then the trick is to be sure you've applied it evenly and liberally.** If you apply it too thinly or blend most of it off instead of using it full-depth, you would not get the amount of protection listed on the label.

I am concerned about the new pressed powders with SPF ratings. While I don't doubt the validity of the SPF number, I worry that most women do not apply pressed-powder foundations liberally enough to get the amount of protection indicated on the label. **If you lightly dust the powder over the skin there is no way you will get the SPF protection indicated on the label.** You must be sure you apply the pressed powder in a manner that completely and evenly covers the face. I believe that pressed powders are an iffy way to get sun protection for the face, but they *are* a great way to touch up your makeup during the day and reapply sunscreen at the same time.

SUN-BELIEVABLE—AN OVERVIEW

While the world of skin care is definitely providing better and better sunscreen products, and although most of my readers already know the basics and even a lot of the more detailed sunscreen information, it never hurts to go over the salient points one more time. It will also help you handle the new myths that companies generate as they try to defend their products as being the best when they aren't.

- **There is no such thing as a safe tan,** at least not from the sun or tanning beds. Even if you tan slowly without burning, the damage to skin is still hazardous to the health of your skin.
- **UVB** rays are the sun's burning rays, which have an immediate harmful impact on skin.
- **UVA** rays are the sun's silent killers. You don't feel them, but they are the primary cause of skin cancer and wrinkles! (UVA rays also penetrate through clear glass windows.)
- Skin damage from the sun begins within the first minutes your skin is exposed to sunlight.
- Even on a cloudy day the sun's rays are ever-present and ever attacking the skin.
- Sitting in the shade or wearing a hat protects only from a small portion of the sun's rays. Plus, other surrounding surfaces such as water, cement, and grass reflect the rays from the ground to your skin, giving you a double whammy of damage.
- Altitude is a sun enhancer; for every 1,000-foot increase in altitude, the sun's potency increases by 4%.
- According to the FDA, a product's SPF (sun protection factor) number tells you how long you can stay in the sun while wearing it without getting burned. Here's how it works: If it normally takes you 20 minutes in the sun before you start turning pink, an SPF 15 product will let you stay in the sun for five hours without burning. The formula is 20 (minutes) $\times$ (SPF number) 15 = 300 (minutes), or five hours. But that five hours applies only if you aren't swimming or perspiring. If you are active or if you get wet, you need to reapply the sunscreen after 60 to 90 minutes.
- SPF numbers are crucial, but they are a measurement that only pertains to sunburn (UVB rays). **There are no numbers to tell you about protection from UVA radiation.** For that protection you have to check the active ingredient list. Make sure that either **avobenzone** (which may also be listed as Parsol 1789 or butyl methoxydibenzoylmethane), **titanium dioxide,** or **zinc oxide** or, outside of the United States, **Mexoryl SX** is one of the active ingredients. If one of these doesn't appear in the

active ingredient list (it doesn't count if it is just part of the regular ingredients) you will not get adequate UVA protection.

- Several sunscreen ingredients are approved for use in the United States for sunburn protection, and they have a wide variety of technical names. Two of these are benzophone and oxybenzone, and while they sound like avobenzone and they do offer some UVA protection, they are not as effective in protecting from the entire range of UVA radiation as are avobenzone, titanium dioxide, zinc oxide, or Mexoryl SX (source: *Photodermatology, Photoimmunology & Photomedicine*, December 2000, pages 250–255).

- For more technical specifics about the issue of UVA versus UVB protection, refer to the *Skin Therapy Letter* published by the Division of Dermatology at the University of British Columbia (1997, volume 2, number 5, "Update on Sunscreens"). This informative article states that the "UVA [range is] 315 [through] 400 nanometers" [according to the FDA the UVB range is from 280 to 315]. The range of protection for the following sunscreen ingredients is listed as: "padimate O, 290–315 nanometers; benzophenones, 250–350 nanometers; octyl methoxycinnamate, 290–320 nanometers; avobenzone, 320–400 nanometers; titanium dioxide, 290–700 nanometers; and zinc oxide, 290–700 nanometers." Skin receives the best protection when a sunscreen uses ingredients that screen the entire range of UVA and UVB.

- **Waterproof sunscreens are actually not waterproof,** and the FDA is ordering manufacturers to eliminate such a claim from sunscreen labels. Sunscreens can be water resistant, but they are never waterproof. Water-resistant sunscreens must be reapplied every 40 to 80 minutes if you are sweating or swimming.

- A product with an SPF 2 blocks only about 50% of the UVB rays; an SPF 10 filters out about 85% of the UVB rays; an SPF 15 stops about 95%, and an SPF 30 through SPF 50 stops about 97%. So even if the SPF number on the label of your sunscreens is an ultrahigh SPF 50, it still has limitations. (Note that new FDA regulations state that no sunscreens will be allowed to have ratings over an SPF 30+.) These percentages explain why you still might get some color after prolonged exposure to the sun despite slathering sunscreen on your skin.

Another reason you may get color despite using generous amounts of a good sunscreen is because of the following. Along with the change that eliminates SPF ratings over 30, the FDA is going to crack down on all "unsupported, absolute, and/or misleading and confusing terms such as 'sunblock,' 'all-day protection,' and 'visible and/or infrared light protection.' " Why the concern about "sunblock" as a term? Because all sunscreen agents, even zinc oxide and titanium dioxide (which are often thought of as "blocking" UV rays), work the same way. All sunscreen agents work because they disperse and break up UV radiation, not because they "block" the sun's rays.

- **Always apply sunscreen at least 15 to 20 minutes before going outside.** This gives the sunscreen time to be absorbed and to spread over and into the skin.

- **You must apply sunscreen liberally.** According to a press release from the American Academy of Dermatology (May 21, 1999), "sunscreen users are only applying 50 percent of the recommended amount, so they are only receiving 50 percent of the SPF protection." Is anyone out there really applying the right amount? This is an important issue because liberal application is essential, and skimping on it just because your sunscreen is expensive can be dangerous to your skin's health. After all, how likely are you to liberally apply an expensive sunscreen that would be gone in a few days if you were using it correctly? Not applying sunscreen liberally can negate any benefit you may assume you are getting from the SPF number on the label.

- If you are using AHAs, BHA, Retin-A, Renova, Differin, or any other topical, pharmaceutical tretinoin (Tazorac, Avita, generic tretinoin), they can make your skin more vulnerable to sun damage. This information isn't news for those of you who are already diligent about using sunscreen, but if you are not being diligent then remember that these ingredients expose healthy layers of skin and make it even more at risk for sun damage and sunburn with even minimal sun exposure.

- Getting sunburned is bad enough, but what you may not know is that **sunburn continues to develop for 12 to 24 hours after the initial burn takes place!** For detailed information on how to handle a sunburn, please see "Sunburn" on page 133.

- If you have **babies or small children,** the sunscreen protection issue should absolutely be of primary concern, as their delicate skin is even more sensitive to the sun's damaging rays. Here, you need to know that all sunscreen formulations that have an SPF are regulated closely by the FDA; and the formulations don't differ in any way because of the age of the intended user. Although kids' products often come in very cute packaging, the formulation you choose should be of greater concern and must contain one of the UVA-protecting ingredients mentioned on page 125, either avobenzone, titanium dioxide, or zinc oxide.

• If you are looking for a less-irritating sunscreen for your kids or yourself, choose one that contains only pure titanium dioxide or zinc oxide as the active ingredient; these are definitely less irritating than products made with other types of sunscreen agents.

• If you're determined to tan, the only safe way to do it is with the self-tanning products sold by countless cosmetics lines.

IS SUNSCREEN IN FOUNDATION RELIABLE?

An article published in the *Journal of the American Academy of Dermatology* (October 2001, entitled "Degradation and Migration of Facial Foundations") concluded that foundations with sunscreen are not reliable for sun protection. Dr. Zoe Diana Draeolos, the author, is a dermatologist who really and truly does test products, and her work is impressive and considered dependable. However, I wouldn't conclude from her study that foundations with sunscreen are completely unreliable and therefore unusable for sun protection.

The summary of this study was that you would need to reapply a foundation with sunscreen at least every two hours (or apply a sunscreen over it) for continued protection. However, looked at more closely, this conclusion was not based on any sunscreen testing as such. Rather the results were based on examining twelve participants who applied the following foundations: Clinique Pore Minimizer (no longer made), Neutrogena Healthy Skin SPF 20, Revlon ColorStay SPF 6, L'Oréal Visuelle (no longer made), Cover Girl Ultimate Finish, and Estée Lauder Impeccable SPF 20. Over an eight-hour period "the migration of the iron oxide pigment [the coloring agent] over the skin surface was monitored in 12 white female subjects with dry (4 subjects), normal (4 subjects), and oily (4 subjects) skin." Following application, each participant was photographed with a specialized video that magnified the skin. The pictures revealed that after two hours the foundation began to travel into facial lines and eventually, by the end of the day, it also had moved into the hair follicles. About the movement, the study commented that "this was particularly true for those participants who had oily skin and for those who used the cream-to-powder foundations." Cream-to-powder foundations are often the greasiest types of formulations (especially in the case of Lauder's Impeccable).

I agree that this study poses concerns that require further investigation, but please realize that the study did *not* test whether or not sun protection was still present, it just noted that the pigment colors of the foundation migrated into lines and hair follicles. There was no UV skin testing done at any point, which would be the only way to know how much sun protection (if any) was still present. In other words, did the sunscreen protection degrade because of migration with the foundation's color? Yet sunscreen testing would have been pointless for this study because three of the foundations didn't even have sun protection (and one only had an SPF 6). More precisely, the conclusions were based on the *assumption* that the sunscreen efficacy dissipated in relation to the pigment movement of a foundation. That means the conclusions about what happens to sunscreen protection when foundations with sunscreen are used were not based on actual testing or proof. Instead, an educated guess was offered, based on the opinion that if the iron oxide pigments in the foundation migrate, the migration must take the active sunscreen agents away with it. A guess is not scientific nor a final determination of any kind.

Another issue here was the unrealistic expectation that you're going to reapply your foundation with SPF (or apply a sunscreen over your previously applied foundation) every two hours! That is impractical in every respect because for most women it would mean redoing almost every other part of your makeup, from concealer to blush, eyeshadow, and eyebrows as well. Instead, it would be far more helpful to touch up your foundation during the day with a pressed powder that has an SPF 15 or higher and that also has UVA protection.

On an anecdotal, personal note, as someone who is diligent about wearing foundation with sunscreen and a moisturizer with sunscreen on my body (both containing titanium dioxide), I found that after two months in Florida last year the only part of my body to *not* get a drop of color was my face. There was a decidedly noticeable change of color on my arms and hands.

More important, application and wear are issues for *all* sunscreens. Another study went so far as to suggest that reapplying your sunscreen "liberally to exposed sites 15 to 30 minutes before going out into the sun, followed by reapplication of sunscreen to exposed sites 15 to 30 minutes after sun exposure begins" is the optimal way to ensure the best protection (source: *Journal of the American Academy of Dermatology*, December 2001, pages 882–885). Liberal application as well as even, smooth application is critical. From there, you should monitor how your sunscreen wears so you know you're not sweating it off, rubbing it off, washing it off (particularly for the hands), or degrading it by virtue of your own oil production. I know this is a lot to pay attention to, but it is our first line of defense against photodamage, which is truly what causes the skin to wrinkle.

WATER RESISTANT, NOT WATERPROOF

The FDA's 2002 regulations regarding sunscreen require companies to eliminate the use of the word "waterproof" as a valid claim. In truth, no sunscreen can be waterproof because it must be reapplied if you have been sweating or immersed in water for a period of time. The only approved terms for use on sunscreens, reflecting studies that prove they have limited ability to stay in place when people are in water or sweating, are "water-resistant" or "very water-resistant." A product that is water-resistant means the label's SPF value has been measured after application and 40 minutes of water immersion; it must keep the same SPF value to use the term water-resistant. A very water-resistant product means the SPF value on the label must remain intact after 80 minutes of water immersion.

If you are swimming or sweating, you absolutely should use a sunscreen that's labeled water resistant or very water-resistant. Water-resistant sunscreens are formulated quite differently from regular sunscreens. Water-resistant sunscreens use acrylate technology in their formulations, which helps them hold up remarkably well under water. Acrylate-type ingredients are, like hairspray, holding agents. These plasticizing ingredients form a film over the skin and can take a great deal of wear and tear in contact with water before the sunscreen protection is rinsed away.

For normal wear, I do not recommend daily application of water-resistant sunscreens. The acrylate-type ingredients that help keep sunscreens on when swimming or sweating also make them somewhat tacky or sticky under makeup. For regular application, when you aren't exercising outside or taking a dip, a regular sunscreen with SPF and good UVA protection is the best choice.

TITANIUM DIOXIDE AND ZINC OXIDE

Titanium dioxide and zinc oxide are often referred to as "nonchemical" sunscreen ingredients, but this is misleading at best. In every aspect and by every definition titanium dioxide and zinc oxide are chemicals. What these two substances do have in common is that they are inert minerals used as sunscreen ingredients. They also have minimal to no risk of causing an allergic reaction and are considered benign and safe for skin. Along with their safety they have a superior ability to protect skin from the sun's UVA radiation (sources: *British Journal of Dermatology*, November 2001, pages 789–794; *Lasers in Surgery and Medicine*, September 2001, pages 252–259). One drawback that these two ingredients also share is that, when they are present in large enough concentrations to impart optimal UVA protection, they tend to leave a white cast on the skin. Ingredient manufacturers are working to make better, microfine versions of titanium dioxide and zinc oxide to help reduce or eliminate this problem. In the meantime it is a shortcoming of two otherwise outstanding options for sun protection.

Some media attention has been given to research that compares microfine zinc oxide to microfine titanium dioxide. This study concluded that "microfine zinc oxide is superior to microfine titanium dioxide as a sunscreen ingredient" (source: *Dermatologic Surgery*, April 2000, pages 309–314). However, this study was about a commercially available form of zinc oxide and no other study has supported the results. Nonetheless, if you feel that zinc oxide is a preferred sunscreen ingredient it only takes a quick review of the active ingredient label to see if the product you are using contains it.

One misconception that often comes up about titanium dioxide and zinc oxide is the notion that they are "sunblocks" and, therefore, better than traditional sunscreens. However, titanium dioxide and zinc oxide function fine as sunscreens. In fact, the FDA is disallowing the term "sunblock" on all products that have an SPF. The *Federal Register* (May 21, 1999, volume 64, number 98) Final Sunscreen Monograph states: "While micronized titanium dioxide does not meet the proposed definition of a sunscreen opaque sunblock, the agency has not included the use of this term in the final monograph (see section II.L, comment 52 of this document). . . . In addition, the proposed definition of 'sunscreen opaque sunblock' in Sec. 352.3(d) applied only to titanium dioxide and is inconsistent with how micronized titanium dioxide functions as [a] sunscreen active ingredient (Ref. 44)"; and " . . . micronized titanium dioxide absorbs short wavelength UV radiation and reflects and scatters long wavelengths, thereby functioning similarly to chemical UVB radiation sunscreens." This is a very technical way of saying that titanium dioxide and zinc oxide need to be applied in the same manner as any sunscreen: liberally, and 20 minutes before going outside.

AVOBENZONE UNDER FIRE

A story that appeared in the May/June 1998 issue of *Health* magazine raised concerns about the stability of avobenzone in sunscreen formulations. According to the article, recent research conducted by Robert Sayre, a physicist in photobiology at the University of Memphis, suggests that avobenzone may break down in as little as 30 minutes when exposed to sunlight.

That published study has created quite a stir in the cosmetics industry and among dermatologists, oncologists, and scientists in the biomedical arena. "Stir" is actually an understatement; shock and confusion may be more accurate. If Sayre is right, a lot of sunscreen products should be thrown in the garbage. But so far the primary response is confusion because no one understands how Sayre came up with his findings, given how incredibly well-researched and scrutinized avobenzone is as a sunscreen ingredient. There are no other studies substantiating Sayre's results anyplace in the cosmetics or medical world.

Avobenzone is not some untested or untried sunscreen agent. It has been around since 1981 and is the most-used sunscreen ingredient in the world. It is the number-one sunscreen agent used in Canadian, Australian, and European sunscreen formulations. In the United States, the FDA approved avobenzone's use as a sunscreen agent only after more than seven years of study. Avobenzone had to meet scrupulous performance standards when Hoffman LaRoche applied for it to receive new drug status from the FDA. New drug status is the most stringent FDA classification possible and requires more safety studies and efficacy substantiation than you can imagine. Avobenzone held up under all of the FDA's safety and potency protocols, or it wouldn't have been approved.

Even more significant, the June 1996 issue of *Journal of Chromatography Biomedical Applications* (pages 137–145) contained a study that examined the issue of sunscreens degrading when exposed to sunlight.

The conclusion for avobenzone was as follows: "After 72 hours Parsol 1789 [avobenzone] in the sample exposed to the sun was decreased by up to 25% of the initial concentration." That 25% decrease was after 72 hours (far longer than anyone is supposed to rely on a sunscreen) and is a far cry from the 50% decrease reported by Sayre after only 30 minutes.

In particular, one must ask the author of a study like this whether his research has been peer reviewed and published in a scientific publication, and whether the results have been validated. To the best of our knowledge, none of the above has taken place. (There have also been no other studies supporting Sayre's work.)

For many reasons I find Sayre's research and conclusions incredibly suspect. Sayre looked at the issue of stability in vitro only, he did no studies in vivo. In vitro (meaning in a petri dish) photostability measurements cannot be substituted for in vivo (meaning on a live person) determinations of UVB and UVA photoprotective efficacy. Plus, he did not use the required application amount and smaller amounts mean less protection, something the American Academy of Dermatology and I have been warning about for some time. Avobenzone is extremely reliable and a safe source for UVA sun protection.

SUNBURN

Most of us know about sunburn. Spending even a short time in the sun can be all it takes to get a serious, painful burn. As I stated earlier, sunburn continues to develop for 12 to 24 hours after the initial burn takes place. It goes without saying that it would be best if we all knew enough to take care of our skin and never get a sunburn, or tan for that matter, but that isn't realistic. So knowing how to take care of sunburn is essential, both to keep from making the problem worse and to help skin heal.

Essentially, treating sunburn is the same as treating any other burn. Do not cover it with thick salves (butter is the worst). That will trap the heat and cause more damage. Get the skin in contact with cool compresses immediately (do not put ice directly on the skin—that's too cold and can cause a different kind of burn on the skin). Then keep applying cool compresses on and off for several hours. Do not soak the skin with water; too much water in the skin can inhibit the skin's healing response (source: *Contact Dermatitis*, December 1999, pages 311–314).

SUN RISK FROM USING AHAS, BHA, OR TRETINOIN?

As I've already described in the previous chapter one of the major signs of sun-damaged skin is that the outer layer of skin becomes browned, thickened, and wrinkled. To some extent that does serve as protection, but it isn't very good protection (it barely rates an SPF 2), nor is it very attractive! AHAs and BHA (because they exfoliate the built-up damaged surface layer of skin) and tretinoin or products containing it (because they change abnormal cell production back to some level of normalcy) can help remove some of that thickened exterior. That change to the exterior of the skin does leave it more vulnerable to the effects of sun exposure. Yet it is far better to improve the appearance of damaged skin by removing that layer than it is to leave it in place for inadequate, coarse, and defective sun protection. After all, it isn't the AHAs or the tretinoin that cause the skin to be more sensitive to sunlight. All they do is remove the old, sun-damaged skin. Sunscreen is always important, *always*, but it becomes even more essential to protect the fresh skin cells you get if you are using AHAs or tretinoin on a regular basis.

CAN SUNSCREEN CAUSE CANCER?

Media headlines sometimes have a way of creating news sensations where none exist, or making something sound new and eye-popping when the information is really well-established and even dated. You may have seen stories in the media regarding a study claiming that sunscreens do not help protect a person from skin cancer. According to an epidemiological review of ten previously published studies, presented at an American Association for the Advancement of Science meeting in Philadelphia, February 1998, by Dr. Marianne Berwick, an epidemiologist at Memorial Sloan-Kettering Cancer Center in New York, "Based on the evidence, we conclude that sunburn itself probably does not cause melanoma, but that it is an important sign of excessive sun exposure, particularly among those who are genetically susceptible because of their skin type." Well, of course!

Dermatologists have debated for some time whether or not sun exposure is related to skin melanomas, so there is conflicting information for this deadly form of skin cancer. However, basal cell and squamous cell carcinoma are directly linked to sun exposure. Further, the fact that sunburn has *not* been implicated in the occurrence of some skin cancers has long been concluded in Europe and Australia, and recently here in the United States (due to the research about the effect of UVAs on skin). But that's about UVA protection versus UVB protection. The importance of protecting skin from UVA rays (skin-cancer and wrinkle-causing rays) as well as UVB rays (sunburning rays) has now been demonstrated. I'm not sure how Berwick missed this one, but she did. Her study did look at sunscreen use over the past ten years. However, she should have checked into the formulations that were used during that period. It is only recently that cosmetics chemists have started formulating sunscreens with ingredients that can protect equally from both UVB and UVA damage. People who used traditional sunscreens over that ten-year period were putting their skin at risk because they were getting sunburn protection only, while still being exposed to harmful UVA rays. At the time, UVB sunburn-preventing products were so effective that people stayed out longer than they might ever have before, thus exposing their skin to the sun's more damaging UVA rays for longer periods of time.

Others have raised questions about how Berwick's study was conducted and the conclusions her team reached. Dr. Roger Ceilley, former president of the American Academy of Dermatology, refuted the suggestion that long-term sunscreen users derived no benefit from sunscreen. "The study looked at patients who were using sunscreens before 1980, well before broad-spectrum, Sun Protection Factor (SPF) 15 became widely available in 1984. There is a period of at least 10 to 20 years from sun exposure to the clinical appearance of skin cancer. Sunscreens would have had little impact on the patients studied. Many well-documented studies from notable organizations such as the U.S. Department of Health and Human Services (Food and Drug Administration), the American Academy of Pediatrics, the American Cancer Society, and the American Society of Plastic and Reconstructive Surgeons join the American Academy of Dermatology in saying that the use of sunscreen products is an important tool in the prevention of skin cancer" (source: *American Society for Photobiology Online Newsletter*, Summer 1998, volume 27, issue 2).

Studies also abound regarding the appearance of thickened, yellowed, mottled, sun-damaged skin versus the smooth, even, wrinkle-free appearance of someone who has stayed out of the sun; the contrast is a classic in dermatological annals. Staying completely out of the sun isn't possible (nor would it be healthy). However, good sun protection is, at the very least, essential for reducing or stopping the damage that causes most of the wrinkles we see on our skin, basal cell carcinoma, squamous cell carcinoma, and very likely melanoma (source: *American Journal of Clinical Dermatology*, 2001, volume 2, issue 3, pages 131–134).

CAN SUNSCREEN AFFECT SKIN NEGATIVELY?

A paper presented at the March 2001 meeting of the American Physical Society by Johannes Norrell et al., Department of Physics at the University of Alabama at Birmingham, created quite a stir regarding the safety of sunscreen ingredients. Because his paper is titled "The Sunscreen Octyl Methoxycinnamate Binds to DNA," it is easy to see why someone might be concerned. The abstract from this presentation stated the following: "Sunscreens are designed to prevent skin cancer by absorbing ultraviolet radiation from the sun before it gets to the DNA in skin cells. The purpose of this work is to determine whether or not octyl methoxycinnamate, an active ingredient in many sunscreens, will bind to DNA. If so, the sunscreen could transfer the energy it absorbed from the sun to the DNA and cause damage. To determine this, we prepared samples with varying concentrations of cinnamate added to herring sperm DNA, sonicating the mixture to disperse the hydrophobic sunscreen into solution. We conclude that the octyl methoxycinnamate can indeed bind to DNA in aqueous solution."

Before you go checking your bottles of sunscreen for this very popular sunscreen ingredient, let me add a bit of fuel to the fire and inform you that many sunscreen ingredients, from oxybenzone to titanium dioxide, zinc oxide, padimate-O, homosalate, benzophenone-3, phenylbenzimidazole sulphonic acid, and 2-phenylbenzimidazole, just to name a few, all have some intimidating negative research about their potential effects on skin. These aren't junk science articles, either—they are all from very notable publications, including such well-respected journals as *The Lancet*, *Journal of Investigative Dermatology*, and *Mutation Research*. Rather than elaborate on each specific paper (which would take pages and pages), let me sum up the major issues.

Despite the limited amount of research being conducted on the harmful effects of sunscreen ingredients, the majority of the research on these ingredients has been done in vitro (in test tubes) and not in vivo (on human skin). In other words, how does octyl methoxycinnamate's effect on herring sperm relate to its effect when used on human skin? None of the papers described research conducted on humans and, therefore, the results are not conclusive in the least. Plus, there is much debate among researchers themselves about what any of this research means. For example, an article in *The Lancet* (February 14, 1998) stated that the concerns in regard to using oxybenzone "for large surface area application for extended and repeated periods . . . are not warranted." Further, an article in *Science News* (June 6, 1998), which compared the handful of research papers on this issue, concluded that hundreds "of experiments have shown that sunscreen-protected skin seems to suffer less DNA damage than unscreened skin."

Going beyond possible DNA damage, the whole arena of sun protection becomes even murkier, given the way sunscreens interact with the very light they are meant to direct away from skin cells. Several published studies show oxidative damage in vitro from varying sunscreen ingredients. Science News (in the same article) mentioned that " 'the sunscreen [ingredient] actually forms oxygen radicals that we would like to protect the skin against, but sunscreen also reacts with and traps them,' mitigating harmful effects. . . . Some scientists argue that it is by trapping radicals that sunscreen blends offer their protection."

Some in vitro studies have indicated that there is a possibility that certain sunscreen ingredients can be absorbed into skin. However, there are still many researchers who believe that most sunscreen ingredients stay on the surface of skin (where skin cells are dead) and do not penetrate into lower layers of skin, where the real damage occurs. If that's the case, it means the negative effects seen for surface skin in test tubes may be irrelevant.

Another concern about sunscreen is whether the ingredients may possibly exert estrogenic effects. This was examined in a study published in *Environmental Health Perspective* (March 2001). The research was done on rats that were *fed* sunscreen ingredients, not on topical application to rat skin or anyone else's skin. Eating pure sunscreen ingredients is not the same thing as applying them to the skin, any more than applying chocolate to the skin is the same as eating it! There is concern that sunscreen ingredients found in lakes, particularly 4-methyl-benzylidene camphor (4-MBC), may be associated with estrogenic effects on fish, but again this is about consumption, not application, and unless you are living in lake water, the issue appears to be unrelated to humans.

All these issues are significant and deserve more research, but none of the findings indicate that anyone should give up using sunscreen. Besides, it is important to realize that no one sunscreen ingredient stands out as more of a problem than any other in these studies. Also, none of the research demonstrates that there are actual, in vivo human risks related to the topical application of the sunscreen ingredients currently being used in products. Finally, it is imperative to note what a massive amount of research does show: That *not* wearing sunscreen is related to lots of serious skin problems.

WHY YOU MAY STILL GET TAN WHEN USING SUNSCREEN

There are many reasons why you may still be getting some tan despite diligent use of sunscreen. One likely cause is the fact that even the best of sunscreens still let some sun rays through. A high SPF number is not about better or deeper protection, but just longer protection—an SPF 30 means you can stay in the sun 30 times longer than it would normally take you to get a slight burn. For most skin types that would provide over eighteen hours of sun exposure without getting sunburned. It's impressive, but it is also only about the length of time the protection lasts.

High SPF numbers give the false impression of providing enhanced protection when that is not the case (that's why the FDA no longer allows products to be labeled as having SPFs over 30). A well-formulated sunscreen with an SPF 30 still only protects your skin from about 97% to 98% of the sun's rays. That means 2% to 3% of the sun's rays are still getting through, and that can trigger melanin production (the skin's tanning response). This is especially true for those with darker skin tones or for those who have a lot of previous sun damage, because for them hypermelanin production is more likely to take place.

Further, most people misunderstand or have poor information about how to get the best sun protection. Please review the "Applying Sunscreen" and "Sun Strategy" sections in this chapter. It is essential to apply sunscreen liberally and to be sure that the active ingredients include the UVA-protecting ingredients of avobenzone, titanium dioxide, or zinc oxide.

Keep in mind that you must:

• Apply sunscreen every day of your life, not just when you think you will be spending extended time in the sun.
• Apply sunscreen liberally.

- Apply sunscreen 20 minutes before going outside.
- Reapply water-resistant or very water-resistant sunscreen every 40 to 80 minutes if you are spending extensive time in the sun and are swimming, exercising, or perspiring heavily.
- Reapply sunscreen on your hands every time after you wash them.
- Avoid direct sun exposure as much as possible. It also helps to wear a broad-brimmed hat, sunglasses, and long sleeves when you're outside or at the beach.
- Try to avoid spending more than a few minutes out in the sun when it's most intense (between 10 A.M. and 2 P.M.).
- Seek shade whenever possible for "sun breaks" on long days outdoors.

SPF-RATED CLOTHING

After you've dressed in the morning and because you take great care of your skin, you apply a well-formulated sunscreen to the areas of your body that will be exposed to the sun. You are confident that the parts of your body covered by clothing are protected from the sun and therefore don't need sunscreen. Think again. Just because some of your body is under wraps doesn't mean it is protected from sun damage. While clothing can be an excellent form of sun protection, if the fabric is sheer, lightweight, or has any transparency (meaning it lets daylight through) it also lets the sun's damaging rays through. "The most important determinant is tightness of the weave. Fabric type is less important. Thickness is also less important than regular weave. Protection drops significantly when the fabric becomes wet. Color plays a minor role with dark colors protecting [slightly] better than light colors. A crude test of clothing is to hold it up to visible light and observe penetration. The FDA defines clothing with an SPF rating as a medical device. One approved line of clothing with an SPF 30 or greater rating is Solumbra" (1-800-882-7860) (source: *eMedicine Journal*, July 31 2001, volume 2, number 7, and http://www.fda.gov).

Sun damage is not to be taken lightly, and lightweight clothing can be a problem. When in doubt, apply sunscreen all over and then get dressed.

HOW LONG DO SUNSCREENS LAST?

How long does sunscreen last in the container? Should you throw it away after a year or two if you haven't used it up? Sunscreens don't last forever, on your skin or in the bottle. The FDA considers sunscreens over-the-counter (OTC) drugs, meaning they are subject to much more stringent guidelines and regulations than cosmetics. According to the FDA's OTC regulations, sunscreens should be stamped with an expiration date if they have less than three years of acceptable stability testing. If they do have three years' worth of acceptable stability testing they do not need to be stamped with an expiration date. That confusing bit of legislation is almost impossible for the consumer to understand. In the long run you are best off looking for a sunscreen product that is stamped with an expiration date so you know how long it has been on the shelf, but those without expiration dates are not a problem in terms of meeting FDA guidelines.

SHOPPING FOR SUNSCREENS

To recap, it is no longer good enough (or safe enough) to buy a sunscreen based only on its SPF rating. It is now essential to buy sunscreens that are not only at least SPF 15 but also contain avobenzone, titanium dioxide, or zinc oxide as one of the active ingredients. When those ingredients are present, either alone or with other sunscreen agents, you are guaranteed of getting equal protection from UVA and UVB radiation. UVB radiation causes sunburn, but UVA radiation is far more insidious and causes skin cancer and skin damage.

Please understand that labeling on sunscreens can be misleading. If the label says "protects from UVA and UVB radiation" but you don't see avobenzone, titanium dioxide, or zinc oxide listed in the active ingredients, the sunscreen will not provide adequate protection from skin cancer and wrinkle-causing rays, despite the claim. The reason products can say this even when they don't contain the pertinent ingredients I've mentioned is because of a technicality. Sunscreen formulations without UVA-protecting ingredients do block a small portion of the sun's UVA rays, it's just insufficient. Yes, you do get some UVA protection with most sunscreen formulations, but not enough to really protect you from skin damage, cancer, and wrinkles. So when the product states you'll be "protected from UVA and UVB rays," it isn't exactly lying even though it doesn't contain avobenzone, titanium dioxide, or zinc oxide. But it isn't telling the whole truth, either. The FDA has not established any guideline or measurement when it comes to UVA protection; the only way the consumer can obtain any information is to check the active ingredients for the UVA-protecting ingredients of avobenzone, titanium dioxide, and zinc oxide.

SUN PROTECTION FOR DIFFERENT SKIN TYPES

Perhaps one of the most irresponsible, reckless, and unethical marketing positions the cosmetics industry takes is selling skin-care routines that don't include sunscreen. Many cosmetic lines sell an endless array of cleansers, toners, antiwrinkle treatments, eye creams, throat creams, face creams, and facial masks yet never mention the indispensable need for regular, consistent use of a sunscreen. Almost every line does have "sun-care" products, but they are often promoted separately from the "daily-care" routines. I've personally spoken to hundreds and hundreds of cosmetics salespeople about their products and repeatedly found a gross lack of information about sun protection. I'm always told how important moisturizers, eye creams, serums, toners, cleansers, and eye-makeup removers are, but almost never do I hear about the value of daily sunscreen use.

There are indeed many ways to get good sun protection, regardless of your other skin-care needs. This is so important that I consider it unconscionable to discuss any skin-care routines, skin-care problems, or skin-care concerns without also including a discussion of sun protection. If you've been intrigued by a new miracle skin-care line, but a sunscreen is not mentioned, that company clearly does not take skin care seriously or ethically. You should not be wasting your money and hurting your skin by considering a company that would ignore such a vital component of healthy skin care.

Now that you understand the importance of using sunscreen on a daily basis, finding the right product is not easy. Perhaps the trickiest part of sunscreen use is finding one that doesn't cause problems, particularly if you have normal to oily skin, acne-prone skin, or sensitive skin. Active sunscreen agents including avobenzone, benzophone, octyl methoxycinnamate, oxybenzone, padimate O, and many others can cause irritation on the skin, creating patches of dryness, itching, rashlike breakouts, redness, and swelling. Because these particular sunscreen agents can be potentially irritating, many dermatologists feel that titanium dioxide and zinc oxide are the best sunscreen ingredients, since they are almost benign on the skin and are excellent screens for both UVA and UVB radiation. I wish the subject could end here and I could unequivocally recommend titanium dioxide and zinc oxide as the only sunscreen ingredients to look for, but that isn't the case. As safe and effective as titanium dioxide and zinc oxide are they can be occlusive, meaning they can block and clog pores.

The issue for any ingredient that can cause breakouts is threefold: how occlusive it is (meaning blocking oil flow out of the pores), how irritating it is on the skin (perhaps causing rashlike breakouts), and how much the ingredient duplicates what the pore already produces, adding more fuel to the fire. Titanium dioxide and zinc oxide pose the first problem for skin. Are you guaranteed to break out if you use a sunscreen with titanium dioxide? Absolutely not, but it is a possibility. Everyone's skin reacts differently to any and all cosmetic ingredients. One other issue with a sunscreen that uses only titanium dioxide and/or zinc oxide as the active ingredient is a cosmetic one, as these products tend to leave a white appearance and can feel somewhat heavy on the skin. That can be a problem for all skin types. In response to that shortcoming, many sunscreen products combine titanium dioxide with other sunscreen agents, which reduce the amount of potentially irritating ingredients while also decreasing some of titanium dioxide's occlusive tendency.

SUNSCREENS FOR OILY SKIN

The search for a sunscreen that is appropriate for oily skin can be a frustrating, lifelong pursuit. Even those I've created for my line can have problems for some people. There are difficulties of several kinds. First, the types of ingredients that can be used to suspend sunscreen agents are not exactly the best for oily skin. Regardless of the claim on the label, there are risks that the base formulation can clog pores or feel slippery or greasy on the skin. There's also the problem that the sunscreen ingredients themselves can cause an irritated breakout reaction, a response to the synthetically derived sunscreen agents. (Regrettably, that is the nature of almost all active ingredients used in cosmetics—"active" meaning they actually do something on the skin. Whether they are AHAs, Renova, benzoyl peroxide, hydroquinone, or sunscreen ingredients, if they work, they can be irritating.) In the case of titanium dioxide and zinc oxide, even though they are relatively innocuous and have minimal to no risk of irritation on skin, they can still clog pores, being the thick creamy ingredients that they are. Finally, given the wide variety in formulations, there is no way to quantify which ingredients are more problematic than others. What's my advice? The only true answer is to experiment. I wish there was a slam-dunk solution I could offer, but there are no product lines that can legitimately make the claim that their sunscreen won't cause breakouts (and those of you with this problem already know that).

For oily skin, or any skin type for that matter, wearing a foundation with a high SPF is an excellent idea, particularly for women with oily skin who don't want to wear layers of skin-care products. This is also an option for women who are just tired of wearing layers and layers of skin-care products and makeup. Luckily, there are now many well-formulated foundations and tinted moisturizers with good SPF numbers containing avobenzone, titanium dioxide, or zinc oxide. **The one negative about using a foundation with sunscreen is that you need to apply it generously; thin, sheer applications don't work. Plus, as the foundation shifts during the day it is essential to touch it up with a pressed powder containing an SPF 15 and including UVA-protecting ingredients of avobenzone, titanium dioxide, or zinc oxide.**

If you wear a foundation with a good SPF you might forget to use a sunscreen on your hands, neck, throat, chest, or any other area of your body that is exposed to the sun on a daily basis. Those brown "age spots" and crepey skin textures are related to sun damage. Like wrinkling on the face, wrinkling on the rest of the body can't be mitigated without daily use of sunscreen, and that means reapplying your sunscreen every time you wash your hands and taking care to put sunscreen on any exposed parts of your body day in and day out.

FOR THE LITTLE ONES

If you have babies or small children, the issue of sunscreen protection should certainly be of primary concern. Their delicate skin is even more sensitive to the sun's damaging energy. Whether or not you are diligent about staying out of the sun or using sunscreen for yourself, you must be diligent when it comes to the health of your children.

An article in the *Archives of Pediatrics & Adolescent Medicine* (August 2001, pages 891–896) stated that "the regular practice of sun protection for children rarely takes place and primarily consists of applying sunscreen rather than methods that reduce sun exposure. This flies in the face of definitive knowledge that skin cancer, both melanoma and nonmelanoma, has reached epidemic proportions, that excessive sun exposure is associated with the subsequent development of most types of skin cancer, and that as much as 80% of lifetime sun exposure takes place during child-hood. . . . [S]un protection should take its place among topics like car seats, smoke alarms, safe water temperature, and bicycle helmets."

When should you start using sunscreen for children? It's generally thought to be safe when they are six months old or older. But according to an August 1999 press release from the American Academy of Pediatrics, "The issue of whether sunscreen is safe for infants under the age of 6 months remains controversial. Concerns have been raised that human skin under 6 months may have different absorptive characteristics; biologic systems that metabolize and excrete drugs may not be fully developed in children [younger than] 6 months."

Despite these concerns, the Australian Cancer Society in a Position Paper entitled, "Sun Protection and Babies," August 2000, supported by the Australasian College of Dermatologists, concluded: "There is no evidence that using sunscreen on infants is harmful. Although premature babies may have increased skin permeability consistent with incomplete development of the skin, the structure of the stratum corneum (the skin layer principally determining permeability) in full term babies is indistinguishable from that of adults [thus] providing an effective barrier. If infants are kept out of the sun or well-protected from UVR by clothing, hats and shade, then sunscreen need only be used occasionally on very small areas of a baby's skin. When used according to these guidelines, it is unlikely that the small amount of organic sunscreen components absorbed would exceed the metabolic capacities of the liver. In this position statement, the term 'infant' refers to babies from birth to 12 months of age." Before you make a decision for your child, check with your physician for his or her recommendation.

When choosing a sunscreen for your child it's easy to be attracted to the sunscreen products with pictures of cute babies on the label. However, despite these marketing tactics, formulations of products aimed at children are no different from the formulations of products for adults. All sunscreen formulations that have an SPF are regulated closely by the FDA; the formulations do not differ in any way between those intended for adult use and those meant for infants and children. The only difference I've ever noted in baby products is the use of fragrance. Certain fragrances may make you think of little ones, but fragrance can be irritating for all skin types, and baby formulas tend to contain more than many adult products do.

Of greater concern is that many sunscreens claiming to be for children do not contain the UVA-protecting ingredients of avobenzone, titanium dioxide, or zinc oxide. If one of these ingredients is not present in the active ingredient list on the label, do not buy it, or if you already own one, now that you know better, do not use it again, but throw it out immediately.

If you are looking for a less irritating sunscreen for your kids, choose one that contains only pure titanium dioxide or zinc oxide as the active ingredient, which are definitely less irritating than products with other inorganic sunscreen agents.

VITAMIN D AND SUN

Exposure to sunlight allows the human body to produce vitamin D, and vitamin D deficiencies can be a serious health problem. Some people worry that if they use sunscreen it will cancel out their body's ability to absorb vitamin D from the sun. Regarding this issue, a June 1999 article in *Cosmetic Dermatology* (page 43) discussed a presentation given by Mark Naylor, MD, assistant professor in the Department of Dermatology at the University of Oklahoma, which described some of "the latest studies proving that ultraviolet exposure is neither required for vitamin D sufficiency nor [that vitamin D is] a scientifically proven cancer fighter. Prospective sunscreen trials examining whether sunscreen contributes to vitamin D deficiency found that regular sunscreen users were not vitamin D deficient."

THE ART OF SELF-TANNING

Self-tanners are the only way to get a tan that is safe for the skin. All self-tanners are virtually equal in that they use the same ingredient, dihydroxyacetone (DHA), to chemically turn the skin brown. Some products contain a greater concentration of DHA than others, and the higher the concentration the faster the skin will turn color. The key to a good result is the application, which is always tricky. It takes experimentation to figure out how much to use, how dark to go, what areas to go over lightly (like knees and elbows), what areas to avoid (like palms of hands and armpits), and where to start and stop the application (do you stop at your ankles or continue down to your toes?). All of these are questions you need to answer for yourself, depending on your own personal preferences and blending techniques.

Note: If you choose to buy a self-tanner, whether it contains a sunscreen or not, please be aware that self-tanned brown skin does not offer any protection from the sun. All of the rules for wearing sunscreens still apply when you are using these products.

During the summer months, fashion magazines are replete with advertisements and stories about the best self-tanners and the optimal application for obtaining the best results. Varying products proclaim they are streak-free, won't turn orange, dry in five minutes, tan in under an hour, or have special color indicators. Those claims are often unreliable or misleading. Essentially, any self-tanner can be streak-free if you apply it evenly. A product that has "color indicators" simply refers to one with a temporary color that helps you see where you've applied it. That is helpful, but still not foolproof, because the tint can dissipate quickly in some areas, leaving you wondering where it was applied. (However, products that aren't transparent are definitely a great place to start, helping improve your odds of putting it on right.)

As far as the color of the tan you get, there are basically no color differences between products. As stated earlier, this is because all self-tanners contain the same ingredient, dihydroxyacetone, which turns skin brown. DHA is a simple sugar involved in plant and animal carbohydrate metabolism, so you can even think of it as being all natural. How fast your skin turns color also has to do with how much DHA the product contains and how your skin reacts to this ingredient. DHA browns the skin through its interaction with the amino acid arginine, which is found in surface skin cells (source: *Chemical Engineering News*, June 2000). Drying time is irrelevant because the tanning effect really depends on the chemical changes taking place in your skin cells. That's why, if you aren't patient and your skin rubs against your clothes (whether the self-tanner is completely dry or not), it will cause smudging or an uneven appearance.

Products that claim to turn your skin tan in less than an hour may actually be a problem because if you make a mistake in application (which is almost inevitable at first) it will also be almost instantaneously noticeable. A self-tanner that takes a few applications to achieve the color you want may be a better option as you learn how your skin reacts and hone your technique.

Regardless of the claims made about any self-tanner, it turns out that which product you choose isn't anywhere near as important as your technique and diligence. The following list will help you get the absolute best results with minimum problems. Just let me warn you, trying to do this fast will make your skin look more strange than tan.

1. It takes time, so apply self-tanner in the evening, allowing yourself at least a half hour, although an hour would be best. (For those who think the time it takes to apply self-tanner is inconvenient, remember how many hours it used to take in the sun to get the same amount of color? And with self-tanners there's no risk of wrinkles or skin cancer.)

2. Self-tanners grab on to surface skin cells, and you may have more in some areas than others. To help achieve a uniform appearance, take a shower or bath and exfoliate your skin, either with a washcloth or some baking soda, or both. Don't overscrub, but do pay extra attention to your knees, ankles, feet, elbows, and neck.

3. After showering and completely drying off, apply a minimal thin layer of moisturizer over the areas where you will be applying self-tanner. This will help the self-tanner glide on more easily and not stick over dry patches. A little extra moisturizer over ankles, knees, and elbows can prevent those areas from looking patchy. I have seen some recommendations that suggest mixing self-tanner with your moisturizer, but don't do it because that will encourage streaking (unless you can precisely mix the two together), and it will take longer for the self-tanner to absorb and dry.

   Body Sense: *Perspiration can make self-tanners streak, so take a cool shower or bath to keep yourself from sweating. Your skin must be completely dry to get the best results. Do not apply self-tanner in a steamy, hot bathroom.*

4. It is best to apply the self-tanner while naked, but wearing an old bathing suit (one you don't plan to wear outside) can help you determine where you want your tan to be. Either way, have a game plan of where you want to stop and start the color. (Do you want tan armpits, the entire arm tan? What about the heels of your feet, your ears, or the palms of your hands?) Remember that self-tanners will stain clothing until they completely absorb into the skin and take effect in the skin cell.

   Body Sense: *Applying self-tanner on your back requires a friend with a helping hand, although you can use a long-handled paintbrush. I vote for the friend (or significant other) as the paintbrush poses some issues of dripping and uneven application.*

5. Apply self-tanner to one section of your body at a time. Be more con-

cerned about even application than rubbing it all the way in. Avoid areas of your body where you do not want to have color.

6. To prevent tan palms you can try using surgical or plastic gloves to apply the self-tanner. This can work well, but can also make application trickier. Another option is to wash your hands after you've applied the self-tanner to a section of your body, or just to wash them every few minutes. If you wait too long you will have strange-looking palms. It helps to have a nail brush handy to be sure you get the self tanner off your cuticles and the area between your fingers.

7. Different parts of your body "pick up" self-tanner more easily than others. For example, some people find that their legs turn brown more easily than their arms or torso, while others find that their faces and necks change color fastest. Experience will help you determine which is true for you. Be careful around your nose, eyes, ears, hairline, and lips. A cotton swab can help blend a thin, even amount smoothly over those areas. To keep your hair from turning color, apply a layer of conditioner or Vaseline over the hairline.

8. Wait at least fifteen minutes before getting dressed. Do not exercise or swim for at least three hours.

9. If you make a mistake and end up with streaky or dark areas of skin, consider using my 2% Beta Hydroxy Acid Solution or Neutrogena's Clear Pore Clarifying Gel (with 2% BHA) over those spots. Then, in the morning, manually exfoliate those areas with a wet washcloth, and voilà! Bye-bye streaks!

10. Problem Areas. As an option for your hands (which can be particularly tricky to get looking natural) apply self-tanner as you would a moisturizer, but then quickly wipe your palms off on a slightly soapy washcloth. Then take a Q-tip dipped in cleanser, eye-makeup remover (one that is not greasy so it doesn't spread or smear), or nail polish remover and carefully use it to wipe around the nails and cuticle area and between your fingers. Another option is to use a makeup sponge to apply self-tanner to the back of your hands, tops of your feet, temples, and hairline. By holding the sponge deftly between two fingers, you only need to worry about preventing this small area from becoming the wrong color.

Body Sense: *Skin-care products such as AHAs, BHA, topical scrubs, Retin-A, and topical disinfectants can affect the self-tanner's action on your skin or even eliminate the color by exfoliating the surface skin cells (self-tanners only interact on the surface of skin). It is best not to* *apply these products the evening you apply a self-tanner. However, if you must do so, wait at least two to three hours before you do.*

11. Reapply self-tanner as you feel the need. Generally it will start wearing away in about three to four days as the surface layers of skin shed.

All of these are valid application techniques, but none offers a guarantee, which is why it takes experimenting and going slow to get the best results.

SUN-TANNING MACHINES

According to the FDA, the FCC (Federal Communications Commission), the American Academy of Dermatology, and the Skin Cancer Foundation, sun-tanning machines are nothing more than skin cancer machines and should be made illegal. The research for this is startling. Sun-tanning machines radiate the most damaging effects of the sun only inches away from your body, and, worse, they are available day after day, month after month, in areas of the country where you would not normally see the sun on a daily basis. In addition, they allow exposure of body parts that are usually covered. They pose the same serious risk of skin cancer that unprotected exposure to the sun allows (source: *Journal of the American Academy of Dermatology*, May 2001, pages 775–780).

Shockingly, I have received pamphlets and brochures from tanning-machine companies and from salon managers who own these machines explaining how safe these machines really are because of the type of radiation they emit. It makes me want to scream, or cry, or both. None of it is true or substantiated by anyone other than those who market the use of tanning machines. Please, if you heed no other information this book provides, protect your skin from sun damage, both artificial and natural. There are lots of ways to look and feel beautiful, but this isn't one of them.

TANNING PILLS?

Tanning pills come in two forms: those that contain tyrosine and those that contain concentrated doses of beta-carotene. Let's start with tyrosine. The FDA has debunked tyrosine as a tanning accelerator. The marketing pitch is that tyrosine is needed by your body to produce melanin, which is a true statement. Tyrosine is an amino acid that is a precursor for the production of melanin. Ergo, the logic (albeit flawed) follows: Taking pills with tyrosine will increase melanin production. It just isn't true—only exposure to UVA or UVB sun rays can activate tyrosine and other elements in skin to initiate (or trigger) melanin production, the pigment we see as a tan.

Here's what the FDA says about tyrosine in the *Office of Cosmetics and Colors Fact Sheet* (June 27, 2000): "Lotions and pills marketed as "tanning accelerators" generally contain tyrosine (an amino acid), often in combination with other substances. Tanning accelerators are marketed with the claim that they enhance tanning by stimulating and increasing melanin formation. The FDA has concluded that these 'tanning accelerators' are actually unapproved drugs, and the agency has issued warning letters to several manufacturers of these products. There are no scientific data showing that they work; in fact, at least one study has found them ineffective." No research supports the oral consumption of tyrosine as having any effect on the color of skin. In another report the FDA stated "In fact, an animal study reported a few years ago demonstrated that ingestion or topical application of tyrosine has no effect on [melanin production] (source: FDA Web site, http://www.fda.gov/ora/inspect_ref/igs/cosmet.html).

A self-tanning pill, called Elusun, shows up on many Internet sites. Elusun's claims are at best misleading and, at worst, potentially dangerous. Elusun claims that it can prevent the skin from aging during sun exposure; that's not only completely false information, but also a truly harmful statement. Without sunscreen that contains UVA-protecting ingredients, *all* sun exposure is damaging, and no oral vitamin or supplement can change that.

Does Elusun color the skin? Yes, by giving the skin high doses of beta-carotene (an FDA-approved vitamin supplement and food-coloring agent). Beta-carotene is the stuff that makes carrots orange and, if you consume enough of it, it can alter the skin's color. However, according to the FDA, megadoses of beta-carotene "enter the blood stream and are partially deposited in skin tissue, giving the skin a tanlike color . . . [but they are not] approved for [tanning] use, and products containing them are considered adulterated. Some reports of adverse reactions associated with 'tanning pills' have mentioned stomach cramps, hepatitis, nausea, diarrhea, and deposition of the color in the retina of the eye."

Megadoses of beta-carotene can be harmful (source: FDA Web site, http://www.fda.gov/ora/inspect_ref/igs/cosmet.html).

Aside from pills that contain beta-carotene, there are others that contain another food-coloring substance called canthaxanthin. This ingredient works much like beta-carotene, but, according to the FDA "At least one company submitted an application for the approval of canthaxanthin-containing pills as a tanning agent, but withdrew the application when side effects, such as the [formation] of crystals in the eye, were discovered."

The FDA also states on its Web site that "In recent years, 'suntan accelerators' have appeared on the market. They claim to enhance tanning by stimulating and increasing melanin formation. . . . One type of suntan accelerator is based on bergapten (5-methoxypsoralen) which is found in bergamot oil and is a well-known phototoxic substance (responsible for Berloque dermatitis). Bergapten increases the skin's sensitivity to ultraviolet light, intensifies erythema formation, and stimulates melanocytes to produce melanin. It has also been reported to be photo-carcinogenic in animals" (source: FDA Web site, http://www.fda.gov/ora/inspect_ref/igs/cosmet.html).

SKIN CANCER AND SUN DAMAGE

According to the Centers for Disease Control and Prevention (CDC) and the American Academy of Dermatology (AAD), one million new cases of skin cancer are diagnosed each year. That gives skin cancer the unfavorable distinction of being the most common form of cancer in the United States. As reported by Dr. Darrell S. Rigel from the New York University School of Medicine, the chance for an American to develop melanoma in their lifetime is 1 in 84. Those aren't the kinds of odds you want to gamble on, at least not when it comes to losing portions of your skin, or your life.

Most skin cancers fall into three categories: basal cell carcinomas, squamous cell carcinomas, and melanomas. Basal cell carcinomas and squamous cell carcinomas are caused by repeated, unprotected sun exposure (source: *American Journal of Clinical Dermatology*, May-June 2000, pages 167–179).

However, there is some controversy as to whether or not melanomas are caused by unprotected sun exposure. Despite the disagreement, many, if not all, dermatologists feel that the best available evidence suggests counseling patients to lower their exposure to sunlight and advising them that the use of a broad-spectrum sunscreen with a high protection factor decreases the risk of developing melanoma (sources: *Archives of Dermatology*, December 2000, pages 1447–1449; *Journal of the American Medical Association*, June 2000, pages 2955–2960).

As a general theory, scientists believe that exposure to UVA and some UVB radiation triggers mutations in replicating skin cells, causing their genetic coding to go haywire. The cells forget how to maintain the normal cell turnover process because of the radiation damage. Fortunately, nonmelanoma skin cancers are relatively easy to treat if detected in time, and are rarely fatal. Melanomas are a much more dangerous and life-threatening form of cancer.

An article in the *Journal of Epidemiology* (December 1999, Supplement, pages 7–13) summed up the issue quite nicely, "Skin cancer is the most commonly occurring cancer in humans. . . . Descriptive studies show that incidence rates of the main types of skin cancer, basal cell carcinoma, squamous cell carcinoma and melanoma are [highest] in populations in which ambient sun exposure is high and skin transmission of solar radiation is high, suggesting strong associations with sun exposure. Analytic epidemiological studies confirm that exposure to the UV component of sunlight is the major environmental determinant of skin cancers and associated skin conditions and evidence of a causal association between cumulative sun exposure and SCC, solar keratoses and photodamage is relatively straightforward. . . . Complementary to [population and research] data is the molecular evidence of ultraviolet (UV) mechanisms of carcinogenesis [cancer] such as UV-specific mutations in the DNA of tumor suppressor genes in skin tumors. With increased UV irradiation resulting from thinning of the ozone layer, skin cancer incidence rates have been predicted to increase in the future—unless, as is hoped, human behavior to reduce sun exposure can offset these predicted rises."

In addition to sun protection, you should be aware of some early, telltale signs of skin cancer. Early detection of skin cancer can save your skin and your life. If you perceive a change in your skin that you are not sure about, talk to your doctor; even a minor difference in a mole or a freckle, or a blemish that doesn't look normal, can be an indication of skin cancer.

The five most typical characteristics of skin cancer are:

1. An open sore, any size, that bleeds, oozes, or crusts and remains open for three or more weeks. A persistent, nonhealing sore is one of the most common signs of early skin cancer.
2. A reddish patch or irritated area that doesn't go away and doesn't respond to cortisone creams or moisturizers. Sometimes these patches crust over or flake off, but they never go away completely.
3. A smooth growth with a distinct rolled border and an indented center. It can look like a small blemish or wound, but tends to grow and doesn't heal.
4. A shiny bump or nodule with a slick, smooth surface that can be pink, red, white, black, brown, or purple in color. It can look like a mole, but the texture and shine are what make it different.
5. A white patch of skin that has a smooth, scarlike texture. The area of white skin can have a taut, clear appearance that stands out from the appearance of the surrounding skin.

The American Academy of Dermatology has a list of the "A, B, C, Ds" of identifying skin cancer, as follows:

Asymmetry: One half of the lesion or suspect area is unlike the other half.

Border: There is an irregular, scalloped, or poorly circumscribed border around a suspected skin lesion or mole.

Color: Color varies from one area to another, with shades of tan, brown, black, white, red, or blue.

Diameter: The area is generally larger than 6mm (the diameter of a pencil eraser).

ACTINIC KERATOSIS

If you have had any amount of unprotected sun exposure and you are between the ages of 30 and 80 you might have noticed uneven, rough-feeling, slightly raised, occasionally crusty, and generally light brown or light pink patches on your chest, hands, arms, or neck. These discolorations are called actinic keratosis or solar keratosis, and are distinct from other types of brown discolorations that show up on skin. According to the Skin Cancer Foundation, "One in six people will develop an actinic keratosis in the course of a lifetime." The more typical brown spots that appear on skin due to sun exposure are called melasmas. Melasmas look more like brown freckling and are not raised, rough, or crusted, and are considered benign. Actinic keratosis lesions, though not cancerous, are problematic because they are considered indicative of a precancerous skin condition and require evaluation by a dermatologist. If you are in doubt as to whether or not a brown patch on your skin is a melasma or an actinic keratosis, it is best to ask your doctor.

Prevention is the best method of averting the occurrence of these types of brown patches (meaning daily and liberal use of effective sunscreens). Unfortunately, because most of us were not aware of appropriate sun protection for much of our lives, many of us have a pretty good chance of seeing one of these patches crop up somewhere on our bodies.

There are a number of ways to deal with removing actinic keratosis. The primary techniques are curettage, cryosurgery, and photodynamic therapy, plus topical chemotherapy options (source: *American Journal of Clinical Dermatology*, May-June 2000, pages 167–179).

Deciding what to do depends primarily on the status of the lesion and how much the appearance bothers you. This requires a discussion with your dermatologist to evaluate your various options.

A typical method of removal is to scrape or cut the lesion off with procedures called **curettage, electrodesiccation,** or even simple scraping with a surgical razor. Curettage refers to cutting out the lesion with a curette, a spoon-shaped implement that has a sharp edge. Electrodesiccation uses an electric current to remove the skin tissue while it simultaneously controls bleeding. In both instances a biopsy is done to check on the status of the lesion. Both of these methods can cause scarring, and recurrence of the lesions is a problem.

Cryosurgery uses extreme cold, in the form of liquid nitrogen, to get rid of the unwanted tissue. This method doesn't cause bleeding or scarring but it can leave behind a white mark that often doesn't regain normal skin color. There is also a strong likelihood of recurrence.

When there are numerous actinic keratosis lesions present, two topical medications are sometimes used. The first, **5-fluorouracil** (brand name Efudex), a chemotherapy agent for some cancers, is applied to the spots twice a day for three to five weeks. The side effects of this treatment can be significant, though temporary. Inflammation, burning, stinging, crusting, and some discomfort or pain are typical, but healing takes place one to two weeks after treatment is discontinued. It is considered a highly effective treatment.

Another chemotherapy agent used topically, **masoprocol** cream, 10% (brand name Actinex), is similar to 5-fluorouracil in terms of application and results, although there is a far higher risk of contact dermatitis with masoprocol than with 5-fluorouracil.

Immune response modulators are capable of selectively destroying abnormal skin cells. In a small study group "six men with actinic keratosis were treated with imiquimod 5% cream (trade name Aldara) three times a week for 6–8 weeks. In the event of a local skin reaction treatment was modified to two times per week. Results: All the AK [actinic keratosis] lesions were successfully cleared. . . . Histologically [under the skin], no apparent signs of persisting AK could be detected, and no recurrences were reported during follow up" (source: *British Journal of Dermatology*, May 2001, pages 1050–1053). Aldara is a potential option to discuss with your physician.

Chemical peeling uses trichloroacetic acid (TCA), which is applied under light sedation. Much like any other cosmetic chemical peel, this causes the top layers of the skin to slough off, to be replaced within a few weeks by growth of new skin. A TCA peel is used when deeper penetration is needed to remove the lesion. The downsides to this method are the need for sedation, which makes it rather inconvenient, and the prolonged healing time; the upside is that the eventual results are considered quite good.

The newest treatment recently approved by the FDA is called **photodynamic therapy**. This is an interesting procedure that involves the topical application by a physician of a prescription-only cream containing aminolevulinic acid (brand name Levulan Kerastick). About 14 to 18 hours after the cream has been applied the area is exposed to a particular light source, called BLU-U or Blue Light, for approximately 15 to 20 minutes. This is considered a very successful treatment with little risk to skin. However, after the aminolevulinic acid has been applied, the skin becomes abnormally sensitive to daylight or bright indoor lighting until the treatment is completed. It is critical to wear sunlight-protective clothing and to avoid any exposure to the sun because sunscreens will not protect you. It is also important to avoid sitting close to any light source. Side effects during treatment usually include burning, a crawling feeling, itching, numbness, and stinging sensations, darkening or lightening of treated skin, crusting, scabs, and red itchy bumps. However, once treatment is discontinued the reaction and brown spots are gone and tend not to return.

AFTER-SUN CARE

I worry about the concept of "after-sun care." It sounds as if you can undo all the sun damage you incurred during the day. I admit it's a great marketing concept, but it is risky business for someone to buy into the notion that skin can be repaired following unprotected sun exposure. If you leave your skin defenseless and exposed to the sun's rays, and then slather some lotion, toner, or serum on afterward, you cannot miraculously or even in a minor way heal, eliminate, correct, or cancel the devastating injury to your skin (and all sun exposure over time is devastating).

Slathering too much moisturizer on after a long day outside, or just in general, can prevent the skin from doing what it does on its own naturally, namely healing. This is because too much moisturizer can turn off the skin's natural ability to heal. Most skin is best left alone or, at most, given a lightweight, thin layer of moisturizer, especially after sun exposure.

What about taking care of sunburn? Well, why are you getting sunburned in the first place? Why would you ever leave your house any time of the day or year without a good sunscreen on (one rated at least SPF 15 that contains either avobenzone, titanium dioxide, or zinc oxide as the active ingredients)? OK, that's enough guilt, just don't do it again, and now take care of your burn wisely.

It is essential to treat sunburns the same way you would treat a burn injury from any heat source. Unquestionably, whenever the skin is burned you first need to cool it off to prevent the skin tissue from either retaining the heat or continuing to react negatively. Trapping the heat in the skin by covering it with a thick, waxy, or heavy lotion or cream will literally let the skin continue to fry, even after the heat source has been removed. Likewise, it promotes swelling, redness, and pain.

Some of you may remember the days when you got burned in the kitchen and your grandmother or mother would slather butter on it. Absolutely nothing could have been worse for the skin. Butter, like any emollient moisturizer, places a relatively occlusive layer over the skin, encapsulating the heat and preventing it from leaving the skin. It does nothing to reduce the swelling or redness.

All burns need to be cooled to dissipate the heat simmering in the lower layers of skin and to reduce the resulting inflammation. If you have sunburn over most of your body, a cool to slightly cold bath (not ice-cold; ice or icy water applied directly on the skin is too severe and can burn the skin in other ways). If you do want to use a moisturizer or soothing agent, I recommend a light layer of aloe vera, but not for the reasons the cosmetics industry tells you to use the stuff. Using aloe vera helps cool the skin and prevents trapping the heat the way creams and emollient moisturizers do.

If your burn is serious or extremely painful, do not hesitate to find the nearest hospital emergency room. Heat trauma from sunburn can be a serious threat to your health.

WHY ALOE VERA MAY WORK ON SUNBURNS

We are now learning that moisturizers can be overdone and can hamper the skin's healing process. Lots of people attribute miraculous benefits to the aloe plant for helping the skin heal. Yet there is no real evidence that aloe vera helps the skin in any significant way. An article in the *British Journal of General Practice* (October 1999, pages 823–828) stated that "topical application of aloe vera is not an effective preventative for radiation-induced injuries. . . . Whether it promotes wound healing is unclear. . . . Even though there are some promising results, clinical effectiveness of oral or topical aloe vera is not sufficiently defined at present." There is also research that has isolated certain components of aloe vera and demonstrated it has some effectiveness for wound healing and as an anti-irritant (sources: *Journal of Ethnopharmacology*, December 1999, pages 3–37; *Free-Radical Biology and Medicine*, January 2000, pages 261–265).

Regardless of the disparate information, there is enough anecdotal evidence about aloe vera to make its reputation hard to ignore. It turns out that aloe's reputation may have less to do with what it does for the skin than with the things it helps you keep off the skin. In other words, if you apply pure aloe to sunburn or some other injury site, you won't apply anything else. In essence, you are just cooling off the skin and leaving it alone to do its own thing. Once the aloe juice dries—and because it is mostly water that happens fairly quickly—the skin can heal quite nicely on its own.

BUYING SUNGLASSES

Wearing sunglasses on a regular basis is critical for the health of your eyes. The lens of the eye turns out to be a pretty good absorber of UVA rays, but, unlike the skin, the lens cannot slough off damaged cells. That means there is no way for the lens to ever repair itself. Protecting the eyes isn't just a cosmetic issue, it is about keeping your sight undiminished for as long as possible. Your eyes need protection from ultraviolet radiation, and whether you buy inexpensive or expensive sunglasses, it is a waste of money if they don't supply it.

Eyes exposed to sunlight are at risk for cataracts, sunburn (the eyeball itself can get sunburned), irritation, skin cancer of the eyelid, and dry eyes. Fortunately, most sunglasses do protect us well from the sun, but there is no easy way to know which ones do and which ones don't. Some sunglasses come with labels indicating they offer UV radiation protection, but there are no regulations or standards in this field. It doesn't hurt to buy sunglasses with a UV protection label, but there are some things you need to check out to make sure you purchase a pair that does more than just look good.

I strongly recommend buying sunglasses that hug the face and have wide rims and sidepieces. This way, you shield the eyes from any sunlight coming in from above, below, or around the sides, as well as protect more of the delicate skin around the eyes from sun damage.

The American Academy of Ophthalmology (http://www.aao.org/) offers a few extremely helpful guidelines for finding the best protection.

1. Select sunglasses that block ultraviolet rays. Don't be deceived by color or cost. The ability to block UV light is not dependent on the darkness of the lens or the price tag. You should always buy sunglasses with this feature. Shop for sunglasses that block 99 or 100% of all UV light. Some manufacturers' labels say "UV absorption up to 400nm." This is the same thing as 100% UV absorption.
2. Ideally, your sunglasses should wrap all the way around to your temples, so the sun's rays can't enter from the side.

3. Even if you wear contacts with UV protection, remember your sunglasses.

4. Be sure that the lens tint is uniform, not darker in one area than another.

Another test to be sure the glasses are well made is to hold them out from you at arm's length. Look through them from this distance at a straight line such as the edge of a bookcase or wall. Then slowly move the glasses across the straight line. If the straight edge distorts, sways, curves, or moves, the lenses have imperfections and you should not buy them.

Tinted sunglasses have an impact on what kind of sun exposure you get, aside from their impact on the face. Red- and yellow-tinted lenses can cut haze, but may not adequately protect from sun exposure, though if they had a UV coating they would work to protect against sun damage. Check them in daylight or consult an ophthalmologist. Gray, green, and brown tints are known for providing good viewing as well as good sun protection. Black and blue tints can be too dark, impairing good vision.

chapter 5

SKIN-CARE PLANNING

WHY DOES IT HAVE TO BE SO COMPLICATED?

As I look over the material and research I've accumulated, from magazine articles and books on botanicals and herbs to medical and scientific journals, as well as from interviews with dermatologists, oncologists, and cosmetics chemists, I am amazed at the depth of information available on skin and skin care. It is also mind-boggling to realize how many thousands of products you can choose from when it comes to everything from cleaning the face to protecting skin from the sun, moisturizing, fighting blemishes, or treating a large number of skin problems. You wouldn't think that taking care of your skin could be so complicated or shrouded in such controversy, but the truth is, it *is* very complicated.

Despite being such a small part of the whole body, the face has the lion's share of topical problems, far more than what takes place from the neck down. Acne, wrinkles, sagging, sunburn, blackheads, dryness, rosacea, eczema, psoriasis, seborrhea, dry patches, swelling, and allergies, not to mention our concepts of beauty, are most evident on the face. There is a lot of money to be made if a cosmetics company can get a consumer to believe that their product(s) will make her more beautiful and do something to tackle one or more of those facial dilemmas. If a company can make the stuff sound utterly unique for the skin, even when it isn't, the sales figures rise astronomically. No wonder the claims are so hard to decipher!

As complicated and emotional as skin care can be, the actual skin-care routines can really and truly be streamlined and concise. By now you have an overview of what works and what doesn't when it comes to cosmetics claims and various skin-care ingredients. You are also aware of how the cosmetics industry may be damaging your skin and what current research is revealing about optimal skin care. The next step is to arrange all these data in a way that helps you find an effective skin-care routine so you can stop wasting money on useless products that may be hurting your skin.

CLEANING THE SKIN

No other aspect of skin care is quite as basic as this one. Cleaning the face sets the stage for everything else that will take place on the skin. More so than any other part of your skin-care routine, it is essential that the cleansing products you use be gentle. **Overcleaning or using cleansers that are too drying is a major cause of irritation, dry patches, and redness. Not cleaning the skin well enough can clog pores or leave a residue on the face that can prevent skin cells from sloughing off. Using a cleanser that leaves a greasy film on the face can clog pores and prevent moisturizers from being absorbed and doing their job. It is essential to get this step right, and that means thoroughly, but gently, cleaning the face** (source: *Cutis*, December 2001, pages 12–19. Note: "cutis" is Latin for skin).

EYE-MAKEUP REMOVERS

In the past I have been hesitant to recommend wiping off makeup. Repeated pulling at the skin can be problematic because it stretches skin and damages the skin's elastin fibers. Elastin is a stretchable elastic protein found in skin tissue that is responsible for the flexible, resilient nature of healthy skin. When skin is being pulled and yanked, elastin's orderly arrangement can change. Regardless of the direction you pull—up, down, or sideways—if you see the skin move, you are tugging on the skin's elastic fibers and helping the skin to sag sooner than it would otherwise. No matter how gently it's done, this pulling distends the tissue more than enough to stretch it. Watch closely in the mirror the next time you start wiping off your makeup, particularly eye makeup. Notice that even when you are trying to be gentle the skin is shifting around, movement that inevitably causes wrinkles and sagging.

So how do you get your makeup off? If your makeup is water soluble, the process is pretty straightforward. Because so many water-soluble cleansers use mild ingredients that don't affect the eyes any differently than makeup removers do, they can easily remove all of your makeup, including eye makeup. Using water with a water-soluble cleanser that slips over the face and is easily rinsed off decreases friction and minimizes pulling. If you are used to wiping off makeup, it can take a while to get used to washing it off, but it is the most effective and least damaging way to remove eye makeup.

The exception to this rule is when you are using waterproof or water-resistant makeup, waterproof mascara, heavy or thick foundations, or ultra-matte or transfer-resistant foundations such as Revlon's ColorStay foundations. In those instances, it is necessary to use a gentle, wipe-off makeup remover to help get all your makeup off, and to be as delicate as possible in doing that.

If you do use a water-soluble cleanser to remove your makeup, you may find some residual eye makeup gets left behind. In those circumstances, when you are done cleaning your face, dip a cotton swab in the eye-makeup remover to get the last remnants of your eye makeup; you can also use your toner (assuming it is gentle) to gently remove whatever makeup was left behind on your face.

WASHCLOTHS

Using a washcloth can prove irritating for some skin types and should probably be avoided. However, if you are using ultra-matte foundations, heavy or thick foundations, or layers of makeup, you may find that most gentle, water-soluble cleansers, no matter how effective the cleansing agents are, will have a difficult time cutting through them. To be sure you are cleaning these off thoroughly, especially to help prevent breakouts, it is extremely helpful to use a washcloth in conjunction with a water-soluble cleanser. The goal is to always remove your makeup thoroughly every night (leaving any amount of makeup on all night long can cause irritation, breakouts, or dryness). Be prepared for ultra-matte foundations or heavy makeup to pose a tricky twist to the proceedings.

THE WATER

It's important to pay attention to the right type of cleanser, but it is also important to pay attention to the temperature of the water you use. For the most part, water is one of the most nonirritating things you can use on your skin (though on rare occasions there are people with serious atopic dermatitis who find water irritating to the skin). Although water is the most gentle part of cleaning the face, it is gentle only when it is tepid. Hot water can burn and irritate the skin, and cold water will shock and irritate it. Because the goal is to always be gentle to reduce irritation, redness, and swelling, and to prevent any negative impact on the skin's immune response, using tepid water is essential (sources: *Advances in Skin & Wound Care*, 2000, volume 13, pages 127–128; *Acta Dermato-Venereologica*, July 1996, pages 274–276).

Water is also frictionless, a beneficial quality that is another very important reason to use it. When you splash your face with tepid water, your hands glide over the face, letting you avoid pulling and tugging at the skin. That means you can remove makeup without stretching the skin tissue, making it overall a better way to treat skin.

HARD VERSUS SOFT WATER

Hard water is a common problem found in many homes. If you live in a hard-water area, the use of a water softener can make a difference in how your hair and skin feel. What is hard water? The term "hardness" simply describes the total concentration of calcium and magnesium ions present in the water. Why is hard water a problem? Hard water is an issue when it comes to any type of washing because with hard water it can take twice as much cleanser, shampoo, or laundry detergent to achieve the same level of cleanliness as it does when using soft water. That's the efficiency side of it. The other issue with hard water is that cleansing agents of any kind combine with the calcium and magnesium ions in the water to form a film that doesn't easily (or even completely) rinse off. That film attaches to all kinds of surfaces, including almost imperceptibly to clothes, and it can be seen on dishes, bathtubs, and, yes, on skin and hair. In fact, the squeaky sound you hear after washing your face or hair is from the presence of calcium, not the effect of having clean skin. That means there really is no such thing as "squeaky-clean." And yes, the film remains on your skin even after rinsing, and that clogs pores and coats hair. Moreover, the calcium and magnesium are drying in and of themselves (as are most minerals) when found in high concentrations. According to an article in *Contact Dermatitis* (December 1996, pages 337–343) even "using the more mild wash procedure, skin sites treated under conditions of hard [water] were significantly drier, had more [redness], and were less hydrated than corresponding sites treated with [soft] water. All [three] surfactant cleansers behaved similarly. We also found the hardness of the rinse water to be the more significant factor versus that of the wash water."

According to several water-softening companies I called, the most economical way for you to soften household water is with an ion-exchange water softener. These units exchange the hard calcium and magnesium minerals for sodium, which has softening properties on skin. This can be a far less costly process than trying to find hair-care products that make your hair feel softer and fuller, when the issue is really the quality of your water supply.

What to expect: If you do choose to try a water softener in your home, you will find, when the "hard" minerals are removed from the water, that cleansers will no longer form a film and you won't get much of a bathtub ring. You are also likely to experience a slippery feel on the skin and hair, almost too much "softness," and that can take a while to get used to. Soft water can also tend to make hair more flyaway, which would call for different hair-care products than you would have used when your hair was being rinsed with hard water.

CHOOSING THE BEST CLEANSER

Using the right cleanser makes all the difference in the world because it determines how your skin is going to react to everything else you put on it. Overcleaning your face and drying it out causes problems a moisturizer can't correct. Greasing up your skin with a wipe-off, cold cream–type cleanser can clog pores and leave a film on the skin, which means all the other products you put on will be sitting on top of that instead of being easily absorbed. Trying to degrease the skin with a drying toner after using this kind of greasy makeup remover can cause irritation and a range of other problems. Using a gentle, water-soluble cleanser is the best option for the entire face, and this is true for all skin types.

Most of us are familiar with the three primary categories of cleansers available: wipe-off cleansers (including cold creams and milky makeup removers), soaps of all kinds (including bar cleansers, which technically are not soap), and water-soluble cleansers (creamy, lotion, or shampoo-type cleansers that rinse off).

A good water-soluble cleanser is a terrific invention. It is a cross between a shampoo and a cold cream, and it is not a soap. What differentiates a good water-soluble cleanser from a poor one? Three basic qualities: (1) It washes off makeup without leaving the face dry (like soaps) or greasy (like cold cream), (2) it contains no fragrance (fragrance is an irritant, though water-soluble cleansers without fragrance are hard to find) or abrasive, scrublike particles (scrubs should be used carefully and judiciously not as part of cleaning skin), and (3) most important of all, it is gentle to the skin. Some cleansers on the market are labeled "water soluble," but in actuality they need to be wiped off with a wet washcloth. If the cleanser must be wiped off with a tissue or washcloth, it is anything but water-soluble. These types of cleansers may still be an option for someone with dry skin but only a very soft, nonabrasive washcloth will be gentle to skin.

Water-soluble cleansers are not only the gentlest way to clean the face, they are also the most efficient. Everything is done at the sink. Using a water-soluble cleanser eliminates the need for a separate eye-makeup remover or for boxes of tissues to wipe the face with. Imagine splashing your face generously with (tepid) water, then massaging a water-soluble cleanser on evenly over your face, including the eyes, and then rinsing it off with more water, preferably with your hands. Once the face is rinsed, it shouldn't feel greasy or dry.

I'm not referring to needing to use a washcloth with water to remove your cleanser when I say a product is water soluble. Water-soluble cleansers should splash off without the aid of a washcloth; if you prefer to use something besides your hands, use the softest washcloth you can find. Many people use smoother cloths on their kitchen counter than they do on their face!

Not all water-soluble cleansers are created equal, and finding a good one can be tricky. Just because a cleanser is labeled water-soluble doesn't mean it comes off with water or is gentle. Plenty of cleansers have names that sound great, with words like "Milky" or "Creamy" or "Foaming" or "Gel." But many of them leave the face feeling greasy and need to be wiped off, or they rinse off too well, leaving the face feeling dry and irritated.

I also recommend that you avoid water-soluble cleansers that contain AHAs, BHA, or disinfectants. These may be well-formulated products but they can all be irritating to the eye area, and because they are rinsed, the active ingredients are washed away before they have a chance to have their intended full, positive impact on the skin.

When I first began recommending water-soluble cleansers years ago, there was really only one available. That was Cetaphil Gentle Skin Cleanser, which is still available and is excellent for someone with dry, sensitive skin. Today, there are more water-soluble cleansers to choose from than I ever thought possible. Not all of them are really water soluble and many are too drying, but many are very gentle on the skin, remove all the makeup without causing irritation or dryness, do not burn the eyes, and leave no greasy residue.

One thing most water-soluble cleansers have in common, regardless of price, is the same basic ingredient list. You'll find they have water and one or more detergent cleansing agents such as sodium laureth sulfate, ammonium laureth sulfate, cocamidopropyl betaine, or sodium cocoamphopropionate, among others. Cleansers designed for dry skin often contain oils and leave a greasy residue. When someone with dry skin uses a cleanser supposedly designed for her skin type, and then follows that with a rich, creamy moisturizer, too many emollients can build up, causing the skin to look dull and preventing cell turnover. On the other hand, cleansers designed for normal to oily skin can contain one or more standard detergent agents that can be overly drying and irritating for skin, such as sodium lauryl sulfate, TEA lauryl sulfate, and sodium olefin sulfate (when listed as one of the first ingredients on the label). Drying out the skin is always a problem and often creates the artificial need for a moisturizer, which just greases things back up. This cycle of greasing up dry skin or drying out oily or combination skin causes more skin problems than almost any other facet of skin care.

The following information from an article in *Cutis* (December 2001, Supplemental, pages 12–19) nicely sums up the need for mild cleansing products: "The choice of a mild cleansing agent is important in the adjunctive management of various skin conditions, such as atopic dermatitis, acne vulgaris, rosacea, photoaging, retinoid-induced irritant dermatitis, and sensitive skin. There are three major categories of cleansing agents: soaps, synthetic detergents, and lipid-free cleansing agents. The irritancy potential of cleansing agents is a function of a number of factors, including the pH, type of surfactants, and amount of skin residue. Furthermore, the presence of humectants and emollients also can influence the overall mildness of a cleansing agent. Agents with slightly acidic or neutral pH, nonionic surfactants, and minimal skin residue may be preferable for people who are at increased risk for irritancy reactions."

In Part V, Navigating the Cosmetics Counter, I review some popular water-soluble cleansers.

Summary: Use only water-soluble cleansers that rinse off completely when water is splashed on the face, leaving the face with a clean, soft feeling that is neither dry nor greasy. Creamy, water-soluble cleansers can be an option for dry skin as long as they are used with an extremely gentle washcloth.

Basic directions: Wash your hands first and then splash the face generously, including the eyes, with tepid water (not hot or cold). Once the face is soaking wet, take your cleanser and massage it generously all over the face, including the eyelids. Rinse very well. If traces of makeup are left behind, or if you have very oily skin, you may need to repeat this step. Another option is to first cleanse the eye area and rinse, then do the rest of the face separately and rinse again. Do this step twice a day or whenever you need to clean the face, whether or not you are wearing makeup. Use a gentle washcloth if you are wearing heavy makeup, ultra-matte foundation, or other hard-to-remove makeup.

WHAT ABOUT BAR SOAP?

For many reasons it is best to avoid bar soap, especially from the neck up, but it can also be helpful to avoid it from the neck down. This is particularly true if you have problems with dry skin or breakouts. Just be aware that there are issues with using most bar soaps or bar cleansers no matter what type of skin you have.

Many women believe that the tight sensation they feel after washing with soap means that the face is clean. You know the feeling I'm talking about, where if you open your mouth it pulls the skin around your eyes? The thinking is that the more squeaky-clean your face feels, the better off you are. But that feeling you associate with being clean is nothing more than irritated, dried-out skin. The difficulty with asking someone to break a soap habit is that soap really does clean the skin thoroughly. Unfortunately, it cleans too thoroughly, and that can be irritating! If your skin feels tight for more than two minutes after you wash, you have to run to your moisturizer to prevent it from feeling pulled or taut; if you have oily skin, the oil resurfaces in seconds no matter how clean you felt initially; and if you have combination skin, you reinforce that dual condition.

The major issue with bar soap is its high alkaline content (meaning it has a high pH). "The increase of the skin pH irritates the physiological protective 'acid mantle' and changes the composition of the cutaneous bacterial flora and the activity of enzymes in the upper epidermis, which have an acid pH optimum" (source: *Dermatology*, March 1997, pages 258–262). That technical description basically explains that skin's normal pH is about 5.5, while most bar soaps have a pH of around 9 to 10, which negatively impacts the surface of skin by causing irritation and increasing the presence of bacteria in the skin. There is definitely research showing that washing with a cleanser that has a pH of 7 or higher, which is true for many bar soaps and bar cleansers, increases the presence of bacteria significantly when compared to using a cleanser with a pH of 5.5. (sources: *Clinics in Dermatology*, January-February 1996, pages 23–27; *Dermatology*, 1995, volume 191, issue 4, pages 276–280).

What about specialty soaps that come in clear bars, have nonsoap-sounding names, or contain creams and emollients that appear to have none of the properties of regular soap? Bar cleansers (which are technically not soap) often have a lower pH and are therefore far less irritating to skin. However, the ingredients that keep the bar cleanser in its bar form can theoretically absorb into skin and clog pores. There is also no way for a consumer to test each particular bar to be sure the pH is compatible with skin. Further, many of the so-called gentle bar cleansers I've reviewed contain fairly drying, irritating, and potentially pore-clogging ingredients. So much for specialty soaps being different. Even worse, the soaps designed for oily or acned skin contain even harsher ingredients. Soaps designed for dry and sensitive skin often contain beneficial ingredients such as glycerin, petrolatum (mineral oil), or vegetable oil, and while they might make the face feel somewhat less stiff after you rinse, they won't prevent the irritation caused by the other ingredients.

Here's a rundown of some basic categories of soaps. Remember, just because a product is advertised as gentle doesn't mean it is.

Castile soaps use olive oil instead of animal fat, but the cleansing agent, sodium hydroxide, is still fairly irritating to the skin.

Transparent soaps look milder or less drying because of their unclouded, clear appearance, but many contain harsh cleansing ingredients, and the ingredients that give the bar its shape can clog pores.

Deodorant soaps are always irritating for the face and should be used only on other parts of the body, if at all. The ingredients used to reduce bacteria are too harsh for the delicate skin of the face and they don't stay on the skin long enough to have any real disinfecting effect.

Acne soaps often contain very irritating ingredients in addition to harsh cleansers that, especially when combined with other acne treatments, can super-irritate the skin. There is no reason to overclean the skin. Breakouts have nothing to do with how clean your skin is! A study in *Infection* (March-April 1995, pages 89–93) demonstrated that "in the group using soap the mean number of inflammatory [acne] lesions increased. . . . Symptoms or signs of irritation were seen in 40.4% of individuals." Furthermore, if the acne cleanser contains antibacterial agents, the benefit would be washed down the drain.

Cosmetic soaps or bar cleansers are sold at the cosmetics counters for more money than they are worth. Although these are advertised as being gentle or specially formulated, they are no better than or different from what you can buy at the drugstore. The irritating and pore-clogging ingredients are still included regardless of the price or claim.

Superfatted soaps contain extra oils and fats that supposedly make them more gentle for the face. Basis Soap is one of the most popular superfatted specialty soaps. However, the extra glycerin, petrolatum, or beeswax in these soaps won't prevent irritation and can cause breakouts.

Oatmeal soaps are supposed to be better at absorbing oil and soothing sensitive skin than other soaps or bar cleansers. There are studies demonstrating that oatmeal can have anti-irritant properties. How that translates into a bar cleanser is unknown, but the benefits are probably nonexistent given the amount of time the oatmeal is actually on the skin and the presence of other irritating ingredients. Plus, the oatmeal particles are fairly large and end up usually being abrasive on skin, and that isn't gentle in the least.

"Natural" soaps are those that contain vitamins, fruits, vegetables, plants, flowers, herbs, aloe, and specialty oils; these ingredients are gimmicks and serve no purpose on the face. They don't nourish the skin or provide any other health benefit; that is sheer marketing whimsy and nothing more. Plus, the cleansing agents and the ingredients that keep the soap in bar form are the same as in any other bar cleanser.

Beauty bars such as Dove are about 50% sodium cocoyl isethionate (a form of coconut oil) and, although it is not as irritating as other cleansing agents found in soaps, it is still potentially irritating and drying, especially in such a high concentration. Dove claims to be moisturizing, and it does contain emollients to help soften the effect of the cleansing agent. If the manufacturers left out the drying and irritating ingredients altogether, they wouldn't need to add emollients to counteract them. Also, the ingredients that help the bar keep its shape can clog pores.

WHAT DO TONERS TONE?

In reality, toners—also referred to as astringents, clarifiers, refiners, fresheners, and tonics—don't tone anything. At least not by the dictionary definition of "tone," which refers to the "normal firmness of a tissue or an organ." The term "toner" is a caprice invented by the cosmetics industry and, therefore, it can mean anything they want it to. I have heard that toners do everything from balance the skin and close pores to deep-clean and prepare the skin for other products. They do none of that. In fact, toners of any kind do not close pores; they do not deep-clean pores; and they do not reduce oil production. If toners could do any of that, given the repeated daily use of these items by most women, who would have a pore left?

There are no ingredients in toners that can firm skin and return it to its normal state. What well-formulated toners can do is help reduce inflammation, add water-binding agents and natural moisturizing factors to skin, help remove the last traces of makeup, and impart some lightweight moisturizing ingredients to skin. However, not all toners are created equal, and many are poorly formulated, meaning they have a real capacity to cause irritation, redness, and dryness. No matter what toners may be called (astringent, freshener, pore cleanser, clarifying lotion, witch hazel, and so on) and whether or not they are inexpensive or expensive—if they contain irritants they are bad for skin. The only toners you should ever consider using are those that are as irritant-free as possible.

In the past, the primary ingredient in most toners—even many of those designed for dry skin—was usually SD alcohol with a number following it. This is one of the kinds of alcohol that burn like crazy when you put them on a cut or wound, and it's extremely drying and irritating for all skin types.

Fortunately, the use of alcohol in toners has definitely decreased over the past several years. However, it still shows up in astringents and toners aimed at those with oily or acne-prone skin. If you were under the impression that alcohol is somehow helpful for acne you would be mistaken. For alcohol to be an effective disinfectant, it needs to be 60% to

SKIN-CARE PLANNING   *171*

70% pure alcohol. Most astringents are in the 20% range. Even at a 40% level, you would not get an effective disinfectant, although you would get an effective irritant that kills skin cells and destroys the skin's intercellular layer. Further, irritation and dryness deplete the skin's intercellular matrix and protective outer barrier, and that damages the skin's ability to heal at the same time it increases the presence of bacteria in the skin. All of that can only make breakouts worse in the long run (source: *Archives of Dermatological Research*, 1995, volume 287, issue 2, pages 214–218).

Note: Do not be confused by cosmetics that contain ingredients that sound like alcohol but are not. For example, cetyl alcohol, stearyl, or other alcohol esters are not the type of alcohol I'm warning you about. Remember the ingredient list will say "SD alcohol" followed by a number, or use the term "ethanol" or "isopropyl alcohol" on the label. Those are the kinds to avoid.

Aside from alcohol, other irritating ingredients found in toner-type products include acetone (that's nail polish remover), citrus (lemon, grapefruit, and orange juice are incredibly irritating to the skin because of their high acid content), camphor, mint, peppermint, menthol, volatile plant extracts, fragrance (or essential oils, which are nothing more than fragrance additives), and witch hazel. All of these ingredients can hurt the skin because of irritation or skin sensitivity, and should be avoided.

If a toner does contain irritants, all that irritation does to a pore is temporarily cause it to swell, which can make the pore look smaller for maybe a few minutes. Toners that contain alcohol can remove the surface oil from the skin, but if you've cleansed the skin properly there should be no excess surface oil left. You can't get inside the pore with a toner to deep-clean it without causing damage (if you could, we would all have spotless, empty pores), so toners surely don't work in that capacity. Most of all, toners do not reduce oil production. Oil production is controlled primarily by hormonal activity (source: *Medical Electron Microscopy*, March 2001, pages 29–40). There is nothing you can put topically on skin to stop the oil production triggered by hormones.

Irritant-free toners are an excellent skin-care option for all skin types. They are fine as an extra cleansing step after removing the cleanser. Toners can also soothe skin, lightly moisturize it, and provide some antioxidant and anti-irritant protection. For some skin types, a toner can be the only moisturizer needed. That makes irritant-free toners a wonderful cleansing, lightweight moisturizing aid. What is in these products that makes them beneficial to the skin? Well-formulated toners usually are a blend of water-binding agents, natural moisturizing factors, anti-irritants, antioxidants, lightweight emollients, and gentle cleansing agents. There are great toners in all price ranges.

It is best if the toner is fragrance-free, but those are hard to find. In Part V, I review some popular toners.

Summary: Many irritant-free toners are a fine alternative as an extra cleansing step after cleaning the skin with a water-soluble cleanser. Toners won't close pores and they won't deep-clean, but depending on the formulation they can leave the face feeling soft and smooth, remove the last traces of makeup or oil, reduce or eliminate irritation, provide antioxidant protection, soothe the skin, and lightly moisturize skin. For some skin types, a toner can be the only moisturizer you need to use.

Basic directions: After cleansing the face, soak a large cotton ball with the toner and gently stroke it over the face and neck.

EXFOLIATING THE SKIN

As I explained in Chapter 3, exfoliating skin or removing excess or built-up dead skin cells on the surface of skin or in the pore can be helpful for almost all skin types. During the 1970s the only way to exfoliate the skin was to use toners that contained alcohol, which literally burned skin cells off, leaving dry and irritated skin in their wake. In the 1980s, the main choices were mechanical scrubs with ingredients such as honey and al-mond pits, cleansers with scrub particles, facial masks, more irritating toners, and loofahs. Most of these worked, but they took a toll on the face and irritation was a typical problem. When it comes to mechanical scrubs, my favorite recommendation was and still is mixing Cetaphil Cleanser with baking soda to create an effective, gentle, and extraordi-narily inexpensive scrub. Other mechanical scrubs, with their detergent cleansing agents and wax bases, just can't compare.

However, with the advent of alpha hydroxy acids (AHAs) and beta hy-droxy acid (BHA), mechanical scrubs are now a supplement for exfolia-tion, not the primary choice. AHAs and BHA chemically exfoliate the skin instead of physically abrading it. Chemical exfoliation provides even exfoliation with less physical damage to the skin.

Remember that AHAs exfoliate the surface skin (they do not penetrate into the pore) and, therefore, are the best option for normal to dry skin or sun-damaged skin that doesn't break out. BHA can exfoliate the surface of skin as well as skin within the pore (BHA is lipid soluble) and is, therefore, preferred for those with normal to oily skin that is prone to breakouts or clogged pores.

I review some popular exfoliants in Part V, Navigating the Cosmetics Counter.

Summary: For oily skin, one of the ways to keep pores from getting clogged is to help skin cells shed as freely as possible so they don't get trapped inside the pore. The more you keep skin cells exfoliating in a normal manner, both on the surface of the skin and inside the pore, the less cell debris can fill up the pore and obstruct oil flow out of the pore (source: *Journal of the European Academy of Dermatology and Venereology*, 2001, volume 15, Supplement 3, pages 43–49).

When you help dry skin shed excess dried-up skin cells, it can make room for plumper, moisture-filled skin cells to come to the surface, which can lend a fresher look to the skin. It also allows moisturizers (the fewer and lighter, the better) to more easily penetrate the skin because there are fewer dried-up skin cells in the way to block absorption. Exfoliating helps the dead surface-skin cells to slough off evenly and at a more normal rate, making room for the lower layers of newer skin cells to arrive.

If you decide to use a reliable AHA product for dry or sun-damaged skin, or a BHA product for normal to oily skin or skin prone to breakouts, the question is: Do you still need to use a physical scrub? There is no definitive answer, so you will have to judge for yourself. Most women with normal to dry skin that is sensitive, allergic, or mature should use one, and only one, exfoliant and no other. Someone with normal to oily skin with breakouts can use a BHA product and may find benefit from a gentle physical exfoliant as well. Stick with Cetaphil Cleanser and baking soda for the gentlest results and listen closely to your skin; irritation is never the goal.

Note: The only skin types that may need to stay away from exfoliating are those with extremely sensitive skin, thin skin, and skin diseases or disorders such as rosacea, eczema, dermatitis, or seborrhea, unless approved by a dermatologist.

Basic directions: After cleansing and toning, when the skin is dry, place a small amount of AHA or BHA on your fingertips and smooth it over the entire face, avoiding direct contact with the eyes. First-time users who have sensitive skin should apply it once a day (preferably at night). Depending on your skin's tolerance, you may even want to apply it every other day. If the exfoliant you choose isn't in an emollient base or isn't emollient enough, apply a moisturizer over dry areas. In the morning, apply sunscreen after applying the exfoliant.

If you start out using the chemical exfoliant once a day or every other day, after four weeks you can start increasing usage to twice a day.

If you are using an alkaline cleanser such as bar soap (which you shouldn't be, but just in case you are), wait fifteen minutes before applying any chemical exfoliant because the high pH of the cleanser can affect the acidity of the exfoliant. Nearly all other skin-care products are formulated with a pH of 7 or less (pH 7 is neutral, like water), with the majority around a pH of 5.5, and will not affect the efficacy of the AHA or BHA.

SUNSCREEN

Regardless of the time of year, where you live, the color of your skin, or the amount of time you spend in the sun, sunscreen should be an essential part of your morning skin-care routine. It takes only a few minutes in the sun—the time it takes to walk to your car or to your office—for sun damage to begin. Over time this can cause serious wrinkling, even if you don't tan on a regular basis.

There are several ways to fit this vital skin-care step into your daily routine. Most sunscreens come in a moisturizing base, which means you most likely do not need any additional moisturizer if you have dry skin. As long as one of your daytime products (either a moisturizer or foundation) is an SPF 15 or greater that includes the UVA-protecting ingredients of avobenzone, titanium dioxide, or zinc oxide, it is a fine choice.

Basic directions: During the day, sunscreen is the last thing you apply to the skin because applying anything else over it could dilute its effectiveness. Sunscreen is applied after you have finished cleansing, applying toner, disinfectant, chemical exfoliant (AHA or BHA), topical prescription medications such as Retin-A, Renova, Tazorac, generic tretinoin, or Differin, and skin-lightening products. If you have very dry skin and feel the moisturizer in your sunscreen is not enough, you can apply a moisturizer over the drier areas and then apply sunscreen over that.

MOISTURIZING

If you have dry skin, dry, wrinkled skin, or dry areas (like on the cheeks or around the eyes), you need a moisturizer; otherwise you don't. It's that simple. If you don't have dry skin or you have normal to oily skin, you can obtain many of the benefits moisturizers contain (antioxidants, anti-irritants, water-binding agents, natural moisturizing factors) in a well-formulated toner. Avoiding using a cream-, lotion-, or serum-style moisturizer when you don't have dry skin can help prevent breakouts and feeling greasy and shiny through your makeup by midday, and encourage your skin to do its own natural exfoliation.

Always use the lightest moisturizer capable of making your skin feel soft without feeling greasy or layered. There are more wonderful moisturizers available than bad ones. They contain a vast array of emollients, water-binding ingredients, natural moisturizing factors, soothing agents, anti-irritants, and antioxidants in a dizzying range of permutations with an equally dizzying range of prices. Unfortunately, there is no one formula I can point to as the single best one, so don't let the cosmetics industry convince you such a thing exists. It turns out there are hundreds and hundreds of great moisturizers with great ingredients and very few poor ones.

The worst thing about moisturizers is they are often overpriced and erroneously labeled as wrinkle creams, firming and lifting lotions, and serums to make them seem more exotic and miraculous than they really are. While women the world over search for the best wrinkle creams, you can be ahead of the game, and take better care of your skin, either by leaving this step out altogether (because you now know that overmoisturizing the skin is bad) or by using a great but inexpensive moisturizer that can do the job as well as, if not better than, the expensive stuff. Strangely enough, the expensive stuff almost always has too much fragrance (which can cause allergic reactions or irritation), too many plants (and, therefore, a higher risk of skin reactions), and coloring agents (products sell better if they look pretty, even if the result isn't better for the skin), and all of these can be problematic for skin.

The only thing that distinguishes a daytime moisturizer from a nighttime moisturizer is that the ones for daytime should include sunscreen. All the other claims and descriptions explaining why daytime products are different from nighttime products are bogus. Make sure your daytime moisturizer is rated SPF 15 or greater and contains one or more of the UVA-protecting ingredients avobenzone, titanium dioxide, and zinc oxide. There are great, state-of-the-art moisturizers with sunscreen available, and more are being created all the time.

At night almost any moisturizer will do, depending on your skin type.

Always use the lightest formula possible and only over dry areas. There is no reason to apply moisturizer where the skin isn't dry. And don't expect any moisturizer you apply at night to work by somehow "banking" or "depositing" the right ingredients in the skin so it would build up interest for the next day's wear and tear.

Many excellent moisturizers are reviewed in Part V, Navigating the Cosmetics Counter, and on my Web site, www.cosmeticscop.com.

Basic directions: During the day, follow the guidelines for applying the sunscreen. If you have dry skin, that's your daytime moisturizer. At night, over clean, dry, or slightly damp skin, sparingly apply the moisturizer over dry areas. Dab it on and let it be absorbed; don't rub it in (rubbing isn't good for the skin). At night, moisturizer is the last thing you apply. If you are using an AHA or BHA product in an emollient base, or using Renova, which comes in a moisturizing base, azelaic acid in a cream base, or Differin in a cream form, that is the last thing you apply and probably the only moisturizer your skin needs. If you feel some areas of your face need a little more moisturizer, apply that to the drier areas of the face after you've applied the AHA, BHA, Renova, Retin-A, azelaic acid, or Differin.

WHAT ABOUT EYE CREAMS?

Most women believe that eye creams are specially formulated for the skin around the eye area. Although the eye area does tend to be more prone to allergic or sensitizing reactions and often shows wrinkles before other areas of the face, it turns out that product formulations for eye creams don't differ from those for face products. There is no evidence, research, or documentation validating the claim that eye creams have special formulations setting them apart from other facial moisturizers. It only takes a quick look at the ingredient labels of any moisturizer or eye moisturizer to see that they don't differ except for the price and the tiny containers the eye creams come in. Eye creams are a whim of the cosmetics industry designed to evoke the sale of two products when only one is needed.

The only time you might want to use a different product around the eyes is if the skin there happens to indeed be different from the skin on the rest of the face. For example, if your face is normal to oily and doesn't require a moisturizer except occasionally on the cheeks or around the eyes, then an emollient, well-formulated moisturizer of any kind will work beautifully.

Ironically, one of the drawbacks of many so-called eye creams is that they rarely contain sunscreen. For daytime, that makes most eye creams a serious problem for the health of skin. You could believe that you were doing something special for your eyes, but you would actually be putting them at risk of sun damage and wrinkling by using an eye cream without sunscreen. This is another example of the way cosmetics marketing and misleading information can waste your money and hurt your skin.

DRY PATCHES OF SKIN

There are many reasons why skin can develop dry patches. Makeup left on overnight can cause irritant or allergic reactions; then there are drying skin-care products, dermatitis, eczema, and heavy moisturizers that can cause a buildup of dead skin cells. Any and all of these can contribute to dry patches of skin. The best advice is to avoid drying skin-care products and use only the lightest-weight moisturizer for dry skin areas.

If the dry patches are chronic or itchy, they are probably a form of topical dermatitis or eczema and may require treatment by a dermatologist. If you've done your best to eliminate the cause of the problem and the problem persists, one of the best ways to calm down the appearance of dry patches is with an over-the-counter cortisone cream. Lanacort and Cortaid are 1% hydrocortisone creams meant for dry patches of skin, for short-term use only. It is amazing how effective they can be. If the problem lingers, consult a dermatologist, but for many people this is all it takes.

DRY UNDERNEATH AND OILY ON TOP

Several things can cause the combination of a layer of dry, flaky skin combined with oily skin. Often using the wrong combination of skin-care products causes this condition. An emollient, wipe-off cleanser, followed by a toner that is too emollient for your skin type, and then an unnecessarily emollient moisturizer can prevent the lower layer of skin from exfoliating, creating a thick, dry, flaky lower layer and a greasy layer on top. Conversely, if you have oily skin, using a drying face cleanser followed by a toner with irritating or drying ingredients, and then an emollient moisturizer can create the same condition. The drying toner and cleanser can cause the skin to be dry and flaky, while the emollient moisturizer adds to your own excess oil production, aggravating it and making the skin look both oily and dehydrated. The condition of dry skin underneath and oily skin on top rarely requires additional skin-care products. Instead, taking a completely different approach and eliminating overly drying or overly emollient products can help a great deal.

It is also possible that the dry layer covered by an oily layer could be a result of psoriasis, rosacea, seborrhea, or eczema. Chapter 11, Common Skin Disorders, deals with these skin problems at length.

SKIN LIGHTENING

Brown spots on skin are called chloasma or melasma and can happen for several reasons. One repercussion of sun damage is areas of skin discoloration known as solar lentigenes, more popularly called liver spots, sun spots, or age spots. They are definitely not associated with the liver, but they often have everything to do with unprotected sun exposure. On lighter skin types, solar lentigenes emerge as small brown patches of freckling that grow over time. On women with darker skin tones, they appear as small patches of ashen-gray skin that tend to enlarge over time.

Brown or ashen patches of skin can also occur due to birth control pills, pregnancy, or estrogen replacement therapy. In those instances, the discoloration is referred to as pregnancy masking or hormone masking.

Regardless of the source, the issue is the same: site-specific, increased melanin production, or hyperpigmentation. Melanin is the pigment or coloring agent of skin. It is created by melanin synthesis, a complex process controlled partly by an enzyme called tyrosinase.

When it comes to selecting treatment for these areas, one important factor to consider is the depth of the discolored pigment within the skin. In most situations the discoloration is superficial. In a few cases, the discoloration lies deep in the dermis. If the pigment is in the epidermis, it can be helped with skin-lightening products, both over-the-counter and prescription types. If the pigment is deeper, laser treatments are a consideration. For topical treatments, according to an article in the American Journal of Clinical Dermatology (September-October 2000, pages 261–268), "Topical hydroquinone 2% to 4% alone or in combination with tretinoin 0.05% to 0.1% is an established treatment. Topical azelaic acid 15% to 20% can be as efficacious as hydroquinone.... Tretinoin is especially useful in treating hyperpigmentation of photoaged skin. Kojic acid, alone or in combination with glycolic acid or hydroquinone, has shown good results, due to its inhibitory action on tyrosinase. Chemical peels are [also] useful to treat melasma."

Sunscreen

Diligent use of a sunscreen alone allows some repair as well as protection from further photodamage (source: *British Journal of Dermatology*, December 1996, pages 867–875). No other aspect of controlling or reducing skin discolorations is as important as the use of sunscreen, SPF 15 or greater with the UVA-protecting ingredients avobenzone, titanium dioxide, or zinc oxide. Using skin-lightening products or laser treatments without also using a sunscreen is a waste of time. Sun exposure is one of the primary, fundamental causes of hypermelanin production. Before you consider any other treatment for skin discolorations, this is unconditionally the first and most practical step.

Laser Treatments

Pigment deep in the dermis does not respond well to topical agents. Resurfacing procedures such as chemical peels and laser treatments may significantly help some of these problems, but the results are not consistent, problems can occasionally occur, and without strict use of a sunscreen with UVA-protecting ingredients the discolorations almost always come back. Moreover, laser treatments of this kind are often a problem for those with darker skin tones. However, after taking all of the risks into consideration, when laser treatments do work they can make a marked difference in the appearance of the face, arms, hands, and chest, which are the areas of the body most prone to hypermelanin production. The results can be startling and completely eliminate any appearance of the problem.

Hydroquinone

Over-the-counter skin-lightening products often contain 2% hydroquinone, while 4% concentrations are available only from a physician. Hydroquinone is a strong inhibitor of melanin production (source: *Journal of Dermatological Science*, August 2001, Supplemental, pages S68–S75), meaning that it lightens skin color. Hydroquinone does not bleach the skin (calling it a bleaching agent is a misnomer); it only disrupts the synthesis of melanin hyperpigmentation.

Hydroquinone in the medical literature is considered the primary topical ingredient for inhibiting melanin production. Using it in combination with other options listed here can make a marked difference in the appearance of skin discolorations (sources: *Journal of Cosmetic Science*, May-June 1998, pages 208–290; *Dermatological Surgery*, May 1996, pages 443–447).

Some concerns about hydroquinone's safety on skin have been mentioned, but research indicates that reactions are minor or a result of using extremely high concentrations (source: *Critical Reviews in Toxicology*, May 1999, pages 283–330).

According to Howard I. Maibach, MD, Professor of Dermatology at the University of California School of Medicine, San Francisco, "Overall, adverse events reported with the use of hydroquinone . . . have been relatively few and minor in nature. . . . To date there is no evidence of adverse systemic reactions following the use of hydroquinone"—and it has been around for over 30 years in skin-care products. Maibach also stated that "hydroquinone is undoubtedly the most active and safest skin-depigmenting substance." Research supporting Maibach's contentions was published in the *Journal of Toxicology and Environmental Health* (1998, pages 301–317).

Hydroquinone can be an unstable ingredient in cosmetic formulations. Upon exposure to air or sunlight it can turn a strange shade of brown. It is thus essential, when you are considering a hydroquinone product, to be sure it is packaged in a nontransparent container that doesn't let light in and that minimizes the amount of air exposure. Hydroquinone products packaged in jars are not recommended because once opened they quickly become ineffective.

Tretinoin

A great deal of research shows that the use of tretinoin (all-trans retinoic acid) is effective in treating skin discolorations (sources: *Acta Dermato-Venereologica*, July 1999, pages 305–310; *International Journal of Dermatology*, April 1998, pages 286–292; *Journal of the American Academy of Dermatology*, March 1997, pages S27–S36). However, the response to treatment is less marked than with hydroquinone or azelaic acid. Results can also take far longer with tretinoin than with other treatments, requiring at least six months or more before improvement is seen. As such, tretinoin is generally not recommended as the only treatment option for skin discoloration, but is used in combination with other effective topicals (source: *eMedicine Journal*, www.emedicine.com, November 15, 2001, volume 2, number 11). Even though tretinoin can be disappointing for skin lightening, that should in no way diminish the critical role it plays in the overall improvement in skin from the standpoint of cell production, collagen production, elasticity, skin texture, and dermal thickness. Tretinoin in combination with more effective skin-lightening treatments is a powerful alliance in the battle against sun-damaged and aged skin.

Alpha Hydroxy Acids

Alpha hydroxy acid products, in and of themselves, in concentrations of 4% to 10% are not effective for inhibiting melanin production and thereby won't lighten skin discolorations. However, there is evidence that in combination with other treatments such as kojic acid, hydroquinone, azelaic acid, and laser resurfacing they can be very effective for improving the overall appearance of sun-damaged skin and possibly help the other ingredients penetrate the skin better.

Much as laser treatments do, AHA peels (using 50% concentrations) have impressive results for removing skin discolorations (source: *Dermatological Surgery*, June 1999, pages 450–454). Only a physician should perform these types of facial peels.

Kojic Acid

Kojic acid is a by-product in the fermentation process of malting rice for use in the manufacture of sake, the Japanese rice wine. There is definitely convincing research, both in vitro and in vivo, and also in animal studies, showing kojic acid to be effective for inhibiting melanin production (source: *Archives of Pharmacal Research*, August 2001, pages 307–311). Both glycolic acid and kojic acid or glycolic acid with hydroquinone are highly effective in reducing the pigment in melasma patients (source: Dermatological Surgery, May 1996, pages 443–447). So why aren't there more products available containing kojic acid? Kojic acid is an extremely unstable ingredient in cosmetics formulations. Upon exposure to air or sunlight it can turn a strange shade of brown and lose its efficacy. Many cosmetics companies use kojic dipalmitate as an alternative because it is far more stable in formulations. However, there is no research showing that kojic dipalmitate is as effective as kojic acid, though it is a good antioxidant.

Azelaic Acid

Azelaic acid is a component of grains such as wheat, rye, and barley. It is effective for a number of skin conditions when applied topically in a cream formulation at a 20% concentration. For the most part, azelaic acid is recommended as an option for acne treatment, but there is also some research showing it to be effective for the treatment of skin discolorations. For example, "The efficacy of 20% azelaic acid cream and 4% hydroquinone cream, both used in conjunction with a broad-spectrum sunscreen, against melasma was investigated in a 24-week, double-blind study with 329 women. Over the treatment period the azelaic acid cream yielded 65% good or excellent results; no significant treatment differences were observed with regard to overall rating, reduction in lesion size, and pigmentary intensity. Severe side effects such as allergic sensitization or exogenous ochronosis were not observed with azelaic acid" (source: *International Journal of Dermatology*, December 1991, pages 893–895). However, other research suggests that azelaic acid is more irritating than hydroquinone mixed with glycolic acid or kojic acid (source: *eMedicine Journal*, www.emedicine.com, November 5, 2001, volume 2, number 11). Azelaic acid is a consideration for skin lightening if you have had problems using hydroquinone along with tretinoin.

Arbutin

Plant-derived skin-care ingredients send a definite siren call to consumers. Anyone developing "natural" alternatives to hydroquinone has an eager audience ready and willing to give it a try. To that end, arbutin, a hydroquinone derivative isolated from the leaves of the bearberry shrub, cranberry, blueberry, and most types of pears, serves that purpose.

Because of arbutin's hydroquinone content it can have melanin-inhibiting properties (source: *Journal of Pharmacology and Experimental Therapeutics*, February 1996, pages 765–769). Although the research describing arbutin's effectiveness is persuasive (even if most of the research has been done on animals or in vitro), concentration protocols have not been established. That means we just don't know how much arbutin it takes to have an effect in lightening the skin. Moreover, most cosmetics companies don't use "arbutin" in their products because there are patents controlling its use in skin-care products for skin lightening. To get around this problem many cosmetics companies use plant extracts that contain arbutin, such as bearberry. No research exists showing that the plant-sourced arbutin has any impact on skin and especially not in the tiny amounts it is used in cosmetics. The only product I've seen with a pure and rather high concentration of arbutin (about 5%) is Shiseido's Whitess Intensive Skin Brightener *($120 for 1.4 ounces)*. I doubt if it's really worth the price just to see if this amount of arbutin can have an effect on skin as an alternative to hydroquinone, given that arbutin doesn't work any better than hydroquinone. Plus this product contains alcohol and menthol, which would make it potentially as irritating to skin as hydroquinone.

Magnesium Ascorbyl Phosphate

This form of vitamin C is considered stable and an effective antioxidant for skin. For skin lightening there is only a single study showing it to be effective for inhibiting melanin production (source: *Journal of the American Academy of Dermatology*, January 1996, pages 29–33). The study concluded that a moisturizer with a 10% concentration of magnesium ascorbyl phosphate "suppressed melanin formation. . . . The lightening effect was significant in 19 of 34 patients with chloasma or senile freckles and in 3 of 25 patients with normal skin." One study is not exactly anything to write home about, not to mention that at present there are no products on the market containing 10% magnesium ascorbyl phosphate. Most skin-care products containing magnesium ascorbyl phosphate have less than a 1% concentration.

Combination Treatments

Diligent and consistent use of sunscreen with the UVA-protecting ingredients of avobenzone, titanium dioxide, or zinc oxide is the first line of defense when tackling skin discolorations. Many researchers feel that 2% to 4% hydroquinone lotions can be more effective when combined with Retin-A or Renova and AHAs. Higher strengths of hydroquinone (over 2%) are available only from a physician and can possibly help deeper sources of pigment discoloration, although they can be a problem for darker skin tones. It is also extremely helpful to consider chemical peels or laser treatments to remove or lighten skin discolorations and then use topicals to maintain the improvement (source: *Cosmetic Dermatology*, August 2001, pages 13–16).

FACIAL MASKS

If there is one truly optional step in skin care, masks are it. Whatever miraculous properties are attributed to masks, no research supports the assertions of benefit attributed to the special muds, minerals, vitamins, or plant life these products contain. These exotic components range from seaweed to volcanic earth, unusual muds, enzymes, vitamins, and just about anything else you can think of, all associated with a fantastic jumble of characteristics to make the products seem life-altering for your skin. Cellulite is smoothed, wrinkles are eliminated, and acne is cured, all with the application of a facial mask! I would offer to sell you a bridge if you believe any of this, but there aren't enough bridges in the world to accommodate the number of women taken in by these claims.

A recent example of the insanity regarding facial masks or mud mask spa treatments are the preposterous claims that revolve around moor mud. Depending on the Web site, the multitude of claims made for this substance range from curing vaginitis to healing arthritis, acne, and wrinkles. Based on the fact that it was used by the Romans in 120 B.C. (at least that was the information proffered by several spas offering moor mud treatments), the association with ancient medicine must have value. (Though I doubt any of the people proposing these claims would want to get sick in ancient Rome.) Here are the qualities another spa attributed to their moor mud: "As biological beings, the atoms in the human body have an intrinsic affinity for like atoms in nature, so whether moor products are taken internally or externally, the body automatically extracts the substance it needs to reestablish order and harmony." First, if that were accurate then there would be no risk of poisonous substances in nature, and that simply is not true. Moor mud refers to wet earth with a limited ability to grow plant life because of the acidic nature of the land.

Other claims for masks say they offer the benefit of detoxifying properties. Again, there is no research showing this to be the case, but the world of cosmetics or spa treatments is all about outlandish claims, not proof. To begin with, what exactly are these toxins that need to be eliminated from our bodies, and that supposedly cause so many skin problems? Where is the information or data indicating exactly what toxins need to be removed from the body and how is this taking place? If it is possible to "detox" by the application of a facial mask, what biological or physiological process is taking place to allow that to happen? Are the toxins being leached through skin? Drained out of the body in some fashion? This all adds up to magic along with some murky smoke and mirrors. It isn't based on a shred of reality.

Despite the litany of bogus claims ascribed to facial masks, they still can have a benefit for some skin types. Someone with dry skin may find an emollient facial mask soothing and relaxing. Someone with oily skin may find a facial mask with oil-absorbing properties beneficial. It is that uncomplicated.

Facial masks, by their very design, are meant to be used occasionally. But they are much like dieting or exercising—when it is done occasionally, little gain can be derived. The skin's need for antioxidants or anti-irritant protection, skin barrier repair, or (for someone with breakouts) the need for disinfecting or oil absorption is a daily one, not solved by a once-a-week fix.

SHOULD YOU GET A FACIAL?

I suspect there is more pressure lately to spend money on facials than ever before. The rapid proliferation of day spas, which seem to be showing up in every hair salon and mall from Manhattan to Los Angeles, probably brought this form of beauty treatment back into the spotlight. While there are reasons to consider having a facial, it is very important to keep in mind that there is very little a licensed aesthetician can provide that regular use of good skin-care products can't duplicate—and do better.

(Let me emphasize the need to consult only a licensed aesthetician. Although "licensed" doesn't tell you anything about the capability of the aesthetician, it does mean the person has been trained in sanitation and application techniques and, more to the point, has been tested on those procedures and is certified to be able to accomplish those tasks. Of course, while that is just the beginning of what you should expect in the care of your skin, it is essential to know that your skin will be handled in as safe and hygienic a manner as possible.)

Given the popularity and effectiveness of high-concentration alpha hydroxy acid peels and the occasional or regular need to remove stubborn blackheads and deep-rooted blemishes, facials can indeed play an important role in a person's skin-care needs. AHA peels at concentrations of 20% to 35% with a pH of 3.5 are extremely effective at providing a temporarily smooth appearance to the skin. That is within the ability of a good facialist, and the results can be very satisfying. But be extremely cautious. This is, at best, a controversial salon treatment. Many cosmetic surgeons and dermatologists (and the FDA) consider AHA peels unsafe when done by someone without medical training. That is an extremely rational concern, especially considering the wide disparity in training and licensing, even though there are plenty of doctors who charge exorbitant prices for AHA peels but have an assistant or an aesthetician in their office perform the service instead.

When it comes to acne, a reliable aesthetician can definitely soften the skin and safely remove blackheads and blemishes without scarring. In cases like these, there is every reason in the world to get a facial every six weeks to every other month. But please don't expect any of this to permanently stop breakouts. If anything, facialists can get carried away with applying creams and masks, and rubbing and wiping at the skin, which can cause blemishes and irritation. **Keep in mind that the skin-care products sold by facialists and spas are not any more effective or better formulated than those sold anywhere else.**

Along with the viable and relaxing facial treatments out there, a host of facial masks and procedures that pass as premium skin care are really nothing more than a waste of time and money. Lymph drainage treatments are one of the many spa services that are claimed to rid the body of toxins, cellulite, wrinkles, and on and on. Lymph massage does have validity for those with lymphedema, a consequence of diseases such as cancer that require the removal of lymph nodes. However, the massage associated with lymphedema is not about "draining" lymph or removing toxins. Rather it is about preventing the pooling of lymph into the extremities when the lymph system has been compromised in a given area.

The concept of draining lymph glands from the outside in to remove toxins makes as much sense as the idea of draining your hormonal system or blood system from the outside in. The lymph system carries our body's immune defenses. Lymph runs through the body like blood does, in veins and capillaries. You wouldn't want someone draining your blood or hormones (without lots of proof that it was safe and worthwhile), and the same goes for the lymph.

chapter 6

SKIN-CARE BATTLE PLANS

GETTING STARTED

The following list is a fairly comprehensive compilation of the most effective skin-care routines for different skin types. Remember, before you choose a routine for your specific skin type, you must determine if what you are seeing or feeling on your skin is being caused by the skin-care products you are presently using.

Whatever is happening to your skin indicates the direction you should follow, which may indicate treating several different needs at the same time. If your cheeks are dry, your forehead is breaking out, and you have some brown discolorations and patches of rosacea, it will take a combination of products used on different parts of the face to address each issue.

Moreover, your skin-care needs may change depending on the time of year or the climate you find yourself in. **Respond to what you see or feel on your face and change what you are doing based on what your skin is telling you.** (This always assumes that you are using gentle, nonirritating, and nondrying products on your skin.) For example, the cleanser you are using may be fine in a humid, temperate environment, but it may be too drying for an arid, hot climate. It will take some experimentation to find what feels best for your skin in different situations, paying attention to what works and what doesn't.

Exception to the rule: Although it is best to only treat what is happening with your skin now, some skin-care problems require consistency

187

even when the problem is not present on the face. If you tend to break out or have psoriasis, rosacea, or seborrhea, a consistent program is essential. For breakouts you must use an exfoliant and disinfectant daily in order to see a continued difference. I explain in Chapter 9, Battle Plans for Blemishes, why you can't spot-treat blemishes. For psoriasis, rosacea, or seborrhea, consistent treatment is also paramount even when the problem isn't present.

The chapters following this elaborate on some of the more challenging skin-care dilemmas women face. Here I list some basic skin-care steps for all skin types.

Normal Skin with no signs of wrinkles or sun damage

A.M.

Water-soluble cleanser
Toner
Sunscreen in a lightweight or matte base (SPF 15 or greater with avobenzone, titanium dioxide, and/or zinc oxide)

P.M.

Water-soluble cleanser
Toner (optional)
Lightweight moisturizer (only over dry patches and around the eyes)

Normal Skin with signs of wrinkles or sun damage

A.M.

Water-soluble cleanser
Toner (optional)
Sunscreen (SPF 15 or greater with avobenzone, titanium dioxide, and/or zinc oxide in a lightweight moisturizing base)

P.M.

Water-soluble cleanser
Toner (optional)
AHA in a lightweight lotion (can be used in the A.M. as well)
Tretinoin product
Skin-lightening product
Moisturizer for dry areas, including the eyes

Oily Skin with no signs of wrinkles or sun damage

A.M.

Water-soluble cleanser
Toner (optional)
BHA product in a gel or liquid base
Sunscreen (preferably in a foundation or a very lightweight lotion base with SPF 15 or greater containing avobenzone, titanium dioxide, and/or zinc oxide)

P.M.

Water-soluble cleanser
Toner (optional)
BHA product in a gel base
Moisturizer (for dry areas only, including the eyes)
Absorbent facial mask

Oily Skin with signs of wrinkles or sun damage

A.M.

Water-soluble cleanser
Toner (optional)
Moisturizer (for dry areas only, including the eyes)
Sunscreen (preferably in a foundation or a very lightweight lotion base with SPF 15 or greater containing avobenzone, titanium dioxide, and/or zinc oxide)

P.M.

Water-soluble cleanser
Toner (optional)
BHA product in a gel base
Skin-lightening product (optional)
Tretinoin product (optional)
Moisturizer (for dry areas only, including the eyes)
AVOID absorbent facial masks

Combination Skin

A.M.

Water-soluble cleanser
Toner (optional)

BHA product in a gel or liquid base
Moisturizer (for dry areas only, including the eyes)
Sunscreen (preferably in a foundation rated SPF 15 or greater with avobenzone, titanium dioxide, and/or zinc oxide)

P.M.

Water-soluble cleanser
Toner (optional)
BHA product in a gel or liquid base
Tretinoin product
Moisturizer (for dry areas only, including the eyes)
Absorbent facial mask over oily areas only

Combination Skin prone to breakouts

A.M.

Water-soluble cleanser
Toner (optional)
Topical disinfectant (only over areas with breakouts)
BHA product in a gel or liquid base
Moisturizer (for dry areas only, including the eyes)
Sunscreen (preferably in a foundation rated SPF 15 or greater with avobenzone, titanium dioxide, and/or zinc oxide)

P.M.

Water-soluble cleanser
Toner (optional)
Topical disinfectant (only over areas with breakouts—but not benzoyl peroxide if you are using Retin-A, Renova, Avita, Tazorac, or generic tretinoin)
BHA product in a gel or liquid base
Tretinoin product
Moisturizer (for dry areas only, including the eyes)
Absorbent facial mask over oily areas only

Combination Skin with signs of wrinkles or sun damage and prone to breakouts

A.M.

Water-soluble cleanser
Toner (optional)

Topical disinfectant (only over areas with breakouts—but not benzoyl peroxide if you are using Retin-A, Differin, Avita, Tazorac, or generic tretinoin)
BHA product in a gel or liquid base
Moisturizer (for dry areas only, including the eyes)
Sunscreen (preferably in a foundation rated SPF 15 or greater with avobenzone, titanium dioxide, and/or zinc oxide)

P.M.

Water-soluble cleanser
Toner (optional)
BHA product in a gel or liquid base
Topical disinfectant (only over areas with breakouts—but not benzoyl peroxide if you are using Retin-A, Differin, Avita, Tazorac, or generic tretinoin)
Tretinoin product
Skin-lightening product
Moisturizer (for dry areas only, including the eyes)
Absorbent facial mask over oily areas only

Dry Skin with no signs of wrinkles or sun damage

A.M.

Water-soluble cleanser
Toner (optional)
Moisturizer
Sunscreen in a moisturizing base (rated SPF 15 with avobenzone, titanium dioxide, and/or zinc oxide)

P.M.

Water-soluble cleanser
Toner (optional)
AHA product in a moisturizing base
Moisturizer (over dry areas)

Dry Skin with signs of wrinkles or sun damage

A.M.

Water-soluble cleanser
Toner (optional)
Moisturizer

Sunscreen in a moisturizing base (rated SPF 15 or greater with avobenzone, titanium dioxide, and/or zinc oxide)

P.M.

Water-soluble cleanser
Toner (optional)
AHA product in a moisturizing base
Tretinoin product
Skin-lightening product
Moisturizer (over extremely dry areas)

Very Dry Skin and Fragile Dry Skin

Follow Dry Skin routine above, only at night the last thing to apply is
plain olive oil, or another nonvolatile plant oil such as sweet almond
or evening primrose, over excessively dry areas

Sensitive/Allergy-Prone Oily Skin

A.M.

Water-soluble cleanser
Toner (optional)
Over-the-counter cortisone cream (only when irritation or skin reactions occur—if skin reactions are persistent seek medical advice)
Sunscreen (preferably in a foundation rated SPF 15 or greater with titanium dioxide and/or zinc oxide as the only actives, and no other
sunscreen agent)

P.M.

Water-soluble cleanser
Toner (optional)
Over-the-counter cortisone cream (only when irritation or skin reac-
tions occur—if skin reactions are persistent seek medical advice)
BHA in a gel or liquid solution
Lightweight moisturizer (over dry patches or around the eyes)

Sensitive/Allergy-Prone Dry Skin

A.M.

Water-soluble cleanser
Toner (optional)

Over-the-counter cortisone cream (only when irritation or skin re-actions occur—if skin reactions are persistent seek medical advice)
Sunscreen in an emollient moisturizing base, SPF 15 or greater, with titanium dioxide and/or zinc oxide as the only actives, and no other sunscreen agent

P.M.

Water-soluble cleanser
Toner (optional)
Over-the-counter cortisone cream (only when irritation or skin reac-tions occur—if skin reactions are persistent seek medical advice)
BHA in a moisturizing base
Moisturizer

Rosacea with oily, flaky skin

A.M.

Water-soluble cleanser
MetroGel, MetroLotion, or azelaic acid 20% (prescription-only top-ical medications)
Sunscreen (preferably in a foundation rated SPF 15 or greater with titanium dioxide and/or zinc oxide as the only actives, and no other sunscreen agent)

P.M.

Water-soluble cleanser
MetroGel, MetroLotion, or azelaic acid 20% (prescription-only top-ical medications)
BHA product in a gel or lotion base

Rosacea with dry, flaky skin

A.M.

Water-soluble cleanser
MetroLotion, MetroCream, or azelaic acid 20% (prescription-only topical medications)
Sunscreen in a moisturizing base, SPF 15 or greater with titanium dioxide and/or zinc oxide as the only actives, and no other sunscreen agent

P.M.

Water-soluble cleanser
MetroLotion, MetroCream, or azelaic acid 20% (prescription-only topical medications)
BHA in a moisturizing or lotion base
Emollient moisturizer (for dry areas)
For other prescription options for rosacea refer to Chapter 11, Common Skin Disorders.

Seborrhea

A.M.

Water-soluble cleanser
BHA product and/or prescription steroids and coal-tar lotions
Sunscreen in a moisturizing base, SPF 15 or greater with titanium dioxide and/or zinc oxide as the only actives, and no other sunscreen agent

P.M.

Water-soluble cleanser
BHA product and/or prescription steroids and coal-tar lotions
Emollient moisturizer (for dry areas)
For associated prescription options for seborrhea refer to Chapter 11, Common Skin Disorders.

Psoriasis

A.M.

Water-soluble cleanser
BHA product
Sunscreen in a moisturizing base, SPF 15 or greater with titanium dioxide and/or zinc oxide as the only actives, and no other sunscreen agent

P.M.

Water-soluble cleanser
BHA product
Emollient moisturizer (for dry areas)
For associated prescription options for psoriasis refer to Chapter 11, Common Skin Disorders.

Any skin type with patches of dermatitis, eczema, or rashlike areas

A.M. & P.M.

Follow the skin-care regime for your skin type. Before applying the appropriate sunscreen, apply an over-the-counter cortisone cream over inflamed areas only and only intermittently. (Lanacort® and Cortaid® are over-the-counter cortisone creams found at the drugstore.) Repeated use of topical cortisones can thin skin. If your skin condition persists seek medical advice.

All Skin Types prone to blemishes or blackheads:
see Chapter 9, Battle Plans for Blemishes.

chapter 7

BATTLE PLANS
FOR WRINKLES

Note: Cosmetic medical procedures such as Botox and face-lifts as well as some spa procedures such as microdermabrasion and low-concentration chemical peels are discussed in Chapter 13, Cosmetic Surgery.

HOW SKIN AGES AND WRINKLES

How the skin ages and wrinkles is a very complicated process that involves an almost limitless range of physiological occurrences. There isn't any one cause that can be addressed with a cosmetic to erase or minimize the inevitable, because the "aging" process itself is so complex and intricate. Skin, all by itself, ages in many identifiable ways. Adding one plant extract or a vitamin to the skin won't address what is needed to deal with the myriad issues for slowing down the aging process. A series of extrinsic factors (sun damage, pollution, free-radical damage, smoking) and intrinsic factors (genetically predetermined cell cessation, chronological aging, hormone depletion, immune suppression) all culminate in what we define as aged skin.

It isn't just oxygen depletion, free-radical damage, collagen destruction, reduced cell turnover, abnormal cell formation, decreased fat content, intercellular deficiency, genetically predetermined cell shutdown, hormone loss, and so on, that affect the way skin ages—it is a combination of all these things and more taking place.

Looking at the issue objectively can help us better understand what is happening to our skin and what can and can't be done for it. Gaining insight into why wrinkle products make the claims they do and why it is most unlikely that they can actually live up to those claims will ultimately benefit our skin and our budget, too. For example, while we know that collagen and elastin, the support structures of the skin, break down and flatten as a result of repeated sun exposure, they also become less pliant and more hardened with age, so the skin becomes less elastic. Some products claim to only build collagen or only improve elastin. That is much like building a house with only cross beams and no support beams. One without the other is useless because the house won't stay erect without both of them.

It would take an entire book to evaluate every element of the skin affected by intrinsic (genetically induced) and extrinsic (environmentally induced) age factors, but it is important to get a basic sense of what is taking place to better understand why most antiaging or antiwrinkle creams can't possibly live up to their claims.

For example, one notable characteristic of older skin versus younger skin is that younger skin has more fat cells in the dermis than older skin. That is one reason older skin looks more transparent and thinner than younger skin and why someone 30 pounds or more overweight tends to have fewer wrinkles. Furthermore, for some unknown reason, the skin keeps growing and expanding as we age, despite the fact that the supporting fat tissues of the lower layers of skin are decreasing. That is why the skin begins to sag: Too much skin is being produced, but there aren't enough bones (remember, bone also deteriorates with age) and fat to shore it up. Simultaneously, the facial muscles lose their shape and firmness, giving the face a drooping appearance.

Certain components of the skin also become depleted with age. The water-retaining and texture-enhancing elements in the intercellular structure such as ceramides, hyaluronic acids, polysaccharides, glycerin, and many others are exhausted and not replenished. The skin's support structures, collagen and elastin, deteriorate or are damaged. Older skin is also more subject to allergic reactions, sensitivities, and irritation than younger skin due to a weakening immune system.

On a deeper molecular level, the DNA and RNA genetic messages to the skin cell for reproduction slow down and the cells stop reproducing as abundantly or in the same way as they did when we were younger. This preprogrammed change makes cells become abnormally shaped, which further changes the texture of the skin and prevents the cells from retaining water. This is why older skin tends to be drier than younger skin. This change in the skin's DNA and RNA seems to happen for a variety of reasons: It is genetically predetermined, a result of sun damage, and a result of an inflammatory response from free-radical damage built up in the skin cells over a period of time (source: *Annals of the New York Academy of Sciences*, April 2001, pages 327–335).

You have probably connected the dots and noticed that many of these factors of aging are targeted by corresponding cosmetic ingredients that claim to counteract the effect of their naturally occurring depletion. Collagen, elastin, ceramide, hyaluronic acid, polysaccharide, DNA, RNA, and other skin components are popular additions to wrinkle creams. (DNA and RNA are the biggest jokes in this group of ingredients because not only don't you want to mess around with the cell's genetic coding, you can't. If you could, you would have the cure for cancer!)

Putting collagen and elastin in a skin-care product may sound convincing, but they can't bond to the collagen and elastin in your skin, although they can work as moisturizing ingredients. Ingredients like ceramides and hyaluronic acids do work to help support the intercellular structure of the skin, but there is no research demonstrating that they prevent its continuing depletion.

Good old glycerin is also abundant in the layers between the skin cells, and it's just as reliable in helping the skin to feel better, but the cosmetics industry doesn't talk much about glycerin because it is too commonplace to sound distinctive. Unfortunately, the cosmetics industry loves to use phrases such as "replaces what skin has lost" that lead you to believe these kinds of ingredients can affect skin structure in some permanent way. They can't. The point of all of this is that growing old cannot be reversed, much less with a skin-care routine or a handful of specific skin ingredients.

DRY SKIN DOESN'T CAUSE WRINKLES

I understand how difficult it must be to overcome the bombardment of moisturizers claiming to take care of wrinkles and dry skin, yet it is completely false that dry skin and wrinkles are related. **How do we know dry skin and wrinkles are not associated? Because after slathering on tons of moisturizers and wrinkle creams and lotions over the years, women still get lots of wrinkles regardless of their skin type.** Even women who use expensive products still get wrinkles and make appointments with plastic surgeons. Moreover, kids with dry skin don't have wrinkles, and women with oily, sun-damaged skin do have wrinkles. Scientifically, we know dry skin and wrinkles are not associated because when you look at the skin under a microscope there is no physical evidence that the two are linked. Dry skin may look more wrinkly, but that doesn't mean those wrinkles are permanent.

The dilemma is that, in fact, dry skin does look more wrinkled and—here's the crux of the confusion—wrinkled skin looks better with a good moisturizer on it. That's how we get sucked into this myth about wrinkles and dry skin. A woman with oily skin has her own built-in moisturizer (that's basically what moisturizers are: oils or oil-like ingredients and water), which helps her skin look smoother without the aid of a moisturizer.

The truth is, moisturizing the skin does not have any long-term effect on wrinkles. That doesn't mean moisturizers can't make wrinkles less apparent, because they absolutely do, but the notion that these soothing creams, lotions, gels, and serums do anything to prevent or stop wrinkling in its tracks is wishful thinking fostered by constant reinforcement from the cosmetics industry. We know the cosmetics industry tells us lots of things that aren't true. This myth just seems more believable as we become more worried about wrinkles.

Another important distinction between dry skin and wrinkles is that when the outer layer of skin becomes dry or irritated the surface can literally crack, and something referred to as fine lines can appear. These fine lines are not the same as permanent lines caused by intrinsic (genetic aging) or extrinsic (sun damage) factors. This type of dry-skin damage can look wrinkled, which is why the elusive term "fine lines" is used. That also explains why the cosmetics industry uses the term fine lines, because those are just what moisturizers can easily correct. Fine lines (better described as nonpermanent lines) nicely disappear with almost all moisturizers; on the other hand, permanent lines don't go away no matter how much moisturizer you put on them. Extremely dry skin can crack and chafe if it isn't moisturized, causing a parched appearance and a tight, irritated feeling, which is why dry skin is so uncomfortable.

Keep in mind that part of what makes the skin feel parched and dry is that the skin's intercellular matrix is deteriorating. The intercellular matrix is the glue within the skin that keeps skin cells together and helps prevent individual skin cells from losing water. It is actually the intercellular matrix that gives skin a good deal of its surface texture and feel. This matrix is composed of such substances as glycerin, cholesterol, sodium PCAs (NaPCA), and mucopolysaccharides, among many others referred to throughout this book as water-binding agents and natural moisturizing factors (NMFs). Water (as in moisture) doesn't help that part of the skin's health at all. Emollients, lipids, and NMFs do.

THE BACKSIDE TEST OF AGING

A great many of the wrinkles and signs of aging we see on our face, hands, arms, and chest are a result of sun damage. The amount of evidence supporting this is overwhelming (source: *Journal of Photochemistry and Photobiology,* October 2001, pages 41–51). However, you can prove this for yourself with something I call the backside test of aging. I've talked before about this indisputable, clear-cut evidence of wrinkling's direct relationship to sun damage, and it is as valid today as it was years ago when Dr. Kligman, the inventor of Retin-A, first described the phenomenon.

Here's how it works. If you are over the age of 40, preferably not more than 20 pounds overweight (fat helps plump up skin and smooth out wrinkles), you need only compare the skin on your face, hands, or the other parts of your body that are consistently exposed to the sun, with the skin on your backside. (If you don't meet the qualifications for this test, you can sneak a peek at women in the locker room at your exercise club and do the test surreptitiously.) Most people who have never, or rarely, exposed their bare backside to the sun will find a radical difference between it and those parts of the body that have been exposed to the sun. What you will notice is crepey skin on the face and hands, some loss of elasticity, lines, furrows, some skin discoloration (usually darkening, redness, or ashiness), and signs of new freckling. However, the skin on your bottom will be smooth, evenly toned (no freckling or discoloration), and elastic (unless there has been a fluctuation in weight, in which case the backside may be out of shape and saggy), without lines, crow's feet, crepiness, or any sign of wrinkles. These differences become more prominent the older you are and the more sun exposure you've experienced.

How does the cosmetics industry account for this difference in skin texture and appearance when it comes to wrinkle products? Or why doesn't your backside or tummy area need wrinkle creams like the face does? The cosmetics industry doesn't have an explanation; they just ignore this fact and so does the consumer. I imagine that if you don't see the contradiction right there in front of you on a daily basis, you might not notice this clear evidence about what causes skin wrinkling.

CELLULAR RENEWAL AND REPAIR

Cellular renewal and repair are well-established marketing terms used by the cosmetics industry to sell skin-care products. The ability to generate healthy cell growth (in other words, the way that younger skin cells reproduce) is a claim many antiwrinkle and antiaging moisturizers make.

This idea of stimulating healthy cell growth definitely has some basis in scientific research, as I point out throughout this book. But the cosmetics industry distorts the concept of cellular renewal into a great deal of misinformation represented by overpriced products. Here are the facts about what it is possible to do for skin, regardless of the price tag on the product you are buying.

Essentially anything that protects skin can help encourage healthy cell production. This is particularly true for sunscreen and, theoretically, for products that contain antioxidants and anti-irritants. As described in the sections on tretinoin and alpha hydroxy acids in Chapter 5, you can even effect some repair and generation of collagen and elastin.

Skin cell production slows down with age or sun damage. That can leave older, dried-up cells on the skin's surface longer than is normal. Skin cells can become misshapen, sticking together unevenly, causing problems with moisture content, and producing a dry, dull, and extremely flaky layer of surface skin. All of this builds a very good case for exfoliation. Removing dead skin cells helps pave the way for plumper, healthier skin cells to surface, which can make a huge difference in the appearance of the skin. When this takes place, underlying skin density improves, moisture content goes up, and skin functions better (oil flows more easily out of the pores, and blackheads and blemishes decrease now that the dead skin cells that were in the way are gone). All of that can be termed cellular renewal and repair, but it doesn't take an expensive product to gain this kind of benefit. And, as you might expect, many of the other claims circling around cellular renewal make it sound like you can expect 20-year-old skin again, and that is not the case.

For most of our lives cellular renewal and repair is an inherent process all skin goes through. New skin cells are generated in the deepest structures of the skin, then migrate up to the skin's surface, changing their shape and size as they go. At the end of their life cycle, at the surface, the flattened and dried-up cells are shed. Healthy, newly produced skin cells make this trek to the surface over a period of about 28 to 45 days. As we age, due to both extrinsic and intrinsic aging factors, that process can become impaired, negatively affecting the skin's appearance.

What can go wrong with skin cells as they are born, work, die, and shed? Depending on your age and genetic predisposition, a lot. In most women under the age of 40 with normal skin, new skin cells are generated and move upward through the layers of the epidermis, with a complete turnover taking place every 28 to 45 days. But for some women, particularly older women and women affected by the sun damage, smoking, genetic abnormality, or pollution that causes free-radical damage, the process is not always smooth, and problems occur along the way that can affect the appearance of the skin. When skin cell turnover is sluggish, the turnover process can take much longer, leaving dead skin cells on the surface longer. These dead skin cells that hang around longer than they should have a dull, flat, thickened appearance and a grainy, coarse texture. Doing things to improve this process can also be termed cellular renewal or cellular repair.

Aside from helping skin improve cell production and cell turnover, cellular repair and renewal can also refer to anything that helps reinforce or fortify the skin's intercellular matrix—the substance between the cells that forms the skin's protective barrier. Ingredients in skin-care products such as glycerin, hyaluronic acid, ceramides, glycosaminoglycans, vitamins, amino acids, and phospholipids can help this part of the skin. That's a benefit because keeping the intercellular matrix intact is the skin's first line of defense against many elements that can harm healthy skin.

Inasmuch as many things can help skin with cellular renewal and repair, it is still not the panacea the cosmetics industry makes it out to be. Even if women could use every product recommended for antiaging, there is still a genetically preprogrammed turnoff point where all skin cells stop reproducing the way they did when they were young. Remember, all cells are regenerated again and again. For a good deal of our lives we continue producing new cells, but as genetic aging (over our natural life span) takes place, the process simply slows down, almost to the point of shutting down completely. There are some who would suggest that growth factors can prevent the cells from shutting down, but this research is in its infancy and no one yet knows the consequences of attempting to affect or change genetic aging. After all, having skin cells that don't know when to die is the very definition of cancer.

FACIAL EXERCISES

I am completely bewildered by the enthusiasm and passion the practice of facial exercises seems to generate. The number of questions I receive asking me if these work to get rid of wrinkles is just astounding. I also get swarms of letters from women telling me that I have my nonexercised head screwed on wrong when I suggest that facial exercises don't work. Banners on infomercials and advertisements that claim facial exercises can achieve something akin to a nonsurgical face-lift with only five minutes of effort a day keep a lot of women making strange faces in the mirror. But is there any information or research that would somehow explain the mania surrounding all this stretching and toning of the face muscles?

For the most part, facial exercises of any kind are more likely a problem for skin than a help. The reason why facial exercises can have little to no benefit is because loss of muscle tone is not a major cause of wrinkles or sagging skin. In fact, muscle tone is barely involved in these at all. The skin's sagging and drooping—and most every facial wrinkle—are caused by four major factors.

1. Deteriorated collagen and elastin (due primarily to sun damage)
2. Depletion of the skin's fat layer (a factor of genetic aging and gravity)
3. Repetitive facial movement (particularly true for the forehead frown lines and for smile lines from the nose to the mouth)
4. Muscle sagging due to the loosening of facial ligaments that hold the muscles in place

It turns out that facial exercise is not helpful for worn-out collagen, elastin, or the skin's fat layer because none of that is about the muscles, it's strictly about layers of skin and fat tissue. It is especially not helpful for the lines caused by facial movement! Rather, facial exercises would only make those areas appear more lined. The reason Botox injections into the muscles of the forehead, laugh lines, and lines by the temple and eye area work at smoothing out lines in those places is because Botox *prevents* the muscles from moving! It actually prevents muscle movement of any kind, including movements like squinting and raising the eyebrows that create wrinkles in those areas.

Facial exercises also won't reattach facial ligaments; that is only possible via surgery. One step involved in a surgical face-lift is to actually re-drape the muscle of the cheek and the jaw, drawing it back and then literally stitching it back in place where it used to be. So if facial exercise could positively impact the muscle tone of the cheek and jaw it would cause a bulge in the wrong place. This is because exercise doesn't reattach the ligaments, it would just tone the sagged muscle, making it appear fuller lower down, and that would only make skin look more droopy in that area.

The ads for facial exercises often tout the fact that the facial muscles are the only muscles in the body that insert (or attach) into skin rather than into bone. They then use this fact to explain why, if you tone facial muscles, they directly affect the appearance of the skin. What this reasoning leaves out is that skin movement itself is one of the elements that causes the skin to sag and that helps the elastin in skin to become exhausted. If you are doing facial exercises and can see your skin move or frown lines and laugh lines look more apparent, that will only make matters worse.

While every dermatologist and plastic surgeon I've ever interviewed found facial exercises either silly or detrimental, there was one exception. As I was researching this I found the name of one dermatologist who wasn't part of the crowd and who was repeatedly quoted on Web sites selling facial exercise programs. Dr. Wilma Bergfeld, Head of Clinical Research, Department of Dermatology at The Cleveland Clinic, and the first woman president of the American Academy of Dermatology (1992) was being quoted as someone who thought facial exercise was worthwhile. I had to hear this for myself. I spoke with Dr. Bergfeld and it turns out she isn't quite a supporter of facial exercises. "While there is no research or studies demonstrating facial exercises as being helpful, it is a reasonable assumption that it may be useful," she said. "Though I don't recommend them I do believe they could work in some controlled situations. However, you would never want to do anything that moves the facial skin, especially as it ages, or overmanipulate the skin," Bergfeld added, "because it would create more wrinkling [and] increase the loss of elasticity in the skin."

If facial exercise that moves the skin is problematic, what about electrical stimulation for the facial muscles? Wouldn't that form of involuntary stimulation tone the muscles without causing movement of the skin? The answer to that question is a resounding yes. It would exercise the muscle without moving skin. But there is no research demonstrating that this wouldn't make matters worse by creating surfaced capillaries (after all, electrical shocks to the muscles would zap capillaries, too, and that can be a problem), and it doesn't address the issue of the muscle being toned in the wrong area (given that most women start this treatment only after the muscles have already sagged and stretched). And finally, it won't affect the ligaments that have caused most of the sagging and drooping in the first place.

FACIAL MASKS FOR WRINKLES

Lots of facial masks, if not the majority, are little more than clay, mud, or earth minerals. Although there is much ado about the quality of clay from various parts of the world, conjuring images of volcanic ash or minerals derived from exotic waters, the truth is that clay is clay, and its value for the skin is negligible. Clay has some ability to absorb oil, and when the mask is removed it takes a layer of skin with it, which can make your face feel smoother—temporarily. But that doesn't compare in the least with regular use of AHAs, BHA, or tretinoin.

When facial masks don't contain clay, they often contain a plastic-like hairspray ingredient that places a Saran Wrap-like layer over the face. These peel-off masks, when they don't contain other irritants, can be fun. Like the clay masks, they take off a layer of skin when they are removed but, as with the clay masks, the benefit is at best insignificant and very short-term. Some facial masks contain AHAs or BHA. Although these ingredients definitely benefit the skin, they work best when used daily, not once a week or once a month.

You might be thinking, "But facial masks feel so good." As long as facial masks don't contain irritants, they do feel good, and your face can feel nice and temporarily smoother after they are removed because they take off the top layer of skin. You can mimic this effect by placing a layer of glue on the back of your hand, letting it dry, and then peeling it off. The back of your hand will feel incredibly smooth, at least for a short period of time. That's fine, but there is no long- or short-term benefit. There may even be a problem if peeling off these masks also removes some of your skin's intercellular protection.

If you are going to use a facial mask, and you have normal to dry skin, I suggest using only those that are lightweight and soothing—no peeling agents or clay needed.

SUNSCREEN, TRETINOIN, AND AHAS— A VERY GOOD PLACE TO START

One of the fundamental characteristics of sun-damaged skin is that the outer layer becomes thickened and yellow and the underlying layer, where new skin cells are produced, becomes damaged, generating abnormal cell growth and hypermelanin production. The abnormal cell growth also results in malformed elastin, collagen deterioration, and distorted circulation of the blood and lymph systems. Regular use of sunscreen can slow this damage, allow for some improvement, and prevent further destruction. But topical tretinoin has been shown to partially reverse the clinical and histological (structural) changes induced by the combination of sunlight exposure and chronological aging. A formulation of tretinoin in an emollient cream (as in Renova, Avita, Tazorac, or generic tretinoin) has been extensively investigated in multicenter double-blind trials and has been shown to produce significant improvement within four to six months of daily use, compared with the vehicle alone, as part of a regimen including sun protection and moisturizer use.

Histological (structural) changes in the epidermis and dermis that were noted after twelve months suggest that tretinoin repairs photodamage by reconstitution of something called the rete pegs (the anchoring structure of skin that binds the outer layer of skin to the lower layer), repair of keratinocyte ultrastructural damage (surface-skin-cell damage), more even distribution of melanocytes and melanin pigment, deposition of new papillary dermal collagen, and improvements in vasculature (arrangement of blood vessels).

Alpha-hydroxy acids (AHAs) have also been widely used for therapy of photodamaged skin, and these compounds have been reported to normalize hyperkeratinization (overthickened skin) and to increase viable epidermal thickness and dermal glycosaminoglycans content. To sum this all up, recent work has substantially described how the aging process affects the skin and has demonstrated that many of the unwanted changes can be improved by topical therapy (sources: *Cutis*, August 2001, pages

135–142; *Journal of the European Academy of Dermatology and Venereology*, July 2000, pages 280–284; *American Journal of Clinical Dermatology*, March-April 2000, pages 81–88; *Skin Pharmacology and Applied Skin Physiology*, May-June 1999, pages 111–119; *Journal of Cell Physiology*, October 1999, pages 14–23; *British Journal of Dermatology*, December 1996, pages 867–875).

There is every reason to consider using the combination of sunscreen (SPF 15 or greater with the UVA-protecting ingredients of avobenzone, titanium dioxide, and/or zinc oxide), topical tretinoin, and an AHA lotion, gel, or moisturizer as an effective approach for combating wrinkles. A litany of research points to these as being as basic as it gets for your skin when it comes to battling wrinkles.

HORMONES FOR WRINKLES

A great deal of research has affirmed the notion that hormone loss contributes to wrinkles and changes in the skin associated with aging. An article in the *American Journal of Clinical Dermatology* (2001, volume 2, issue 3, pages 143–150, "Estrogen and Skin. An Overview") stated that "estrogen appears to aid in the prevention of skin aging in several ways. This reproductive hormone prevents a decrease in skin collagen in postmenopausal women; topical and systemic estrogen therapy can increase the skin collagen content and therefore maintain skin thickness. In addition, estrogen maintains skin moisture by increasing acid mucopolysaccharides and hyaluronic acid in the skin and possibly maintaining stratum corneum barrier function. Sebum levels are higher in postmenopausal women receiving hormone replacement therapy. Skin wrinkling also may benefit from estrogen as a result of the effects of the hormone on the elastic fibers and collagen. Outside of its influence on skin aging, it has been suggested that estrogen increases cutaneous wound healing by regulating the levels of a cytokine [proteins that generate an immune response]. In fact, topical estrogen has been found to accelerate and improve wound healing in elderly men and women." Similar research in *Maturitas*, the official journal of the European Menopause and Andropause Society (July 2001, pages 43–55), concluded that "HRT . . . regimes significantly improved parameters of skin aging."

There are compelling reasons to consider hormonal treatment as part of a battle plan for wrinkles. It is a multifaceted as well as a controversial issue. The following information will provide an overview to help you create a dialogue with your physician to evaluate all the options available to you.

SKIN CARE FOR PERIMENOPAUSE AND MENOPAUSE?

It has been said that menopause starts the day you get your first menstrual cycle. I don't know if that's a hopeful comment or a depressing one, but any way you slice it, a woman will have periods for about 40 years after they first begin, and then they'll stop. Though there is still a great deal of research that needs to be done on all the issues surrounding perimenopause (referring to the symptoms in the years before the onset of menopause), menopause (the actual cessation of the menstrual cycle), and postmenopause, there is a lot that is known regarding the health and appearance of skin, hair, the body, and other physical as well as psychological aspects of this challenging and intricate life event.

Perimenopause and menopause are brought about by the body's changes in hormone production. The irksome side effects of menopause are caused primarily by the imbalance between a woman's female hormones (estrogen and progesterone, which become depleted) and her male hormones (like androgens such as testosterone). Because the male hormones decline more slowly, there are proportionately more of them, so they have a stronger impact. This imbalance, for example, can affect hair growth. When estrogen levels decrease, many women experience an increase in androgen production, resulting in varying amounts of dark hair growth on the face—particularly around the chin and moustache area above the lip. Ironically, while the hair on your face may get darker, the hair on your head will have reduced growth and you may experience some balding; even the individual hairs actually become smaller in diameter.

The lessening and eventual loss of estrogen and progesterone also affect skin negatively. Aside from problems caused by sun damage, perimenopausal and menopausal women experience thinner, looser and less elastic skin, reduced production of collagen, cessation of oil gland function, and dry skin. Other parts of the body are also influenced by the diminishing amount of female hormones; the vaginal lining becomes thin and can burn and itch, and the breasts' mammary tissue is replaced with more fat tissue, which can cause sagging.

To make matters even more frustrating, perimenopause and menopause can also bring hot flashes, flushes, night sweats and/or cold flashes, a clammy feeling, intermittent rapid heartbeat, irritability, mood swings, trouble sleeping, heavier periods, flooding, loss of libido, itchy skin, and more brittle nails, among other symptoms.

As complex and multifaceted as this all sounds, there are actually some fairly exciting options for addressing the side effects of perimenopause and menopause, and these include both alternative herbal options and conventional Western medical choices. For the purpose of this section I'm going to highlight a few of the current options, but I cannot encourage my readers strongly enough to seek out as much information as they can, or to find a doctor who is an expert in this arena.

Warning: Please avoid the Web sites, companies, or physicians who do not offer a balanced approach to this issue. Medical options are not evil or dangerous, as many alternative-based supplement companies assert, and herbal alternatives are not as ineffective (or as unproven) as many medical doctors assert. Both approaches play a role in mitigating some of the more annoying (as well as intolerable) symptoms of perimenopause and menopause.

Hormone Replacement Therapy (HRT) or Estrogen Replacement Therapy (ERT). There are many prescription-only hormone replacement options to consider. HRT, taken in pills or skin patches, has been shown to restore some amount of the skin's support tissue and elastic quality. A number of studies have demonstrated that ERT and HRT can increase the thickness and elasticity of skin as well as lessen the appearance of skin's aging (sources: *Skin Research and Technology*, May 2001, page 95; *Maturitas*, May 29, 2000, pages 107–117). *The American Journal of Clinical Dermatology* (2001, volume 2, issue 3, pages 143–150) summed up what all of these reports concluded by stating, "Estrogen appears to aid in the prevention of skin aging in several ways. This reproductive hormone prevents a decrease in skin collagen in postmenopausal women; topical and systemic estrogen therapy can increase the skin collagen content and therefore maintain skin thickness. In addition, estrogen maintains . . . stratum corneum [skin] barrier function. . . . Skin wrinkling also may benefit from estrogen as a result of the effects of the hormone on the elastic fibers and collagen. . . . It has been suggested that estrogen increases cutaneous wound healing."

There are risks associated with ERT and HRT and there are controversies regarding their effects on heart disease, osteoporosis, and breast cancer. But there seems to be little opposition to the notion that they ease hot flashes, night sweats, mood swings, and vaginal thinning. It is essential to weigh the pros and cons of ERT and HRT to decide if they are the right direction for you.

Herbal alternatives (phytoestrogens, also called plant estrogens). As someone who has been drinking eight ounces of soy milk per day and eating lots of tofu for the past six years, as well as applying an over-the-counter progesterone cream for the past several months, I can attest to the benefit of both. But that is only anecdotal, and I would never want you to rely on anecdotal information for any health matter. However, there is a great deal of research pointing to phytoestrogens and natural progesterones as valid options for perimenopausal and menopausal symptoms. Research on Dr. Andrew Weil's Web site (http://www.drweil.com) offers a very balanced approach between herbal and medical choices, and includes the medical options of HRT and ERT and herbal alternatives such as soy, black cohosh, dong quai, damiana, evening primrose oil, and borage oil.

Further, a paper on this issue published in the journal *Endocrine-Related Cancer* (June 2001, pages 129–134) stated that "current descriptive epidemiology data in Asian women and the absence of any obvious harmful effects of soy-rich diets constitute arguments which encourage Western women to adopt a diet low in saturated fats and . . . soy supplement." However, this same study discussed the need for more studies to establish the safety of consuming plant estrogens, especially given the American woman's propensity for believing that if a little is good then a lot must be even better. When you add to this the fact that there is no way to measure how much soy to eat or how much progesterone to rub on your body, you find that the alternative supplement world is one of personal experimentation. That isn't bad, but whether or not there are risks is just now being studied.

It is probably wise for women to get a baseline estrogen count around the age of 40 and then again at 45 to determine what normal is for you. That way you can monitor the changes and balancing effect that varying combinations of supplements are having on your body.

There are a lot of believers in natural progesterone and it definitely has helped change some of the problematic bleeding I've been experiencing over the past several years. However, it's important to point out that while natural progesterone is absolutely an option, you should be aware that natural progesterone creams are not regulated in any way by the FDA, and so they are, in actuality, merely cosmetics. That means any cosmetics company can put progesterone into whatever product they want to.

Skin care options. I would love to say that there are skin-care products out there that positively affect the changes that occur in peri-menopausal and menopausal skin, but there aren't. There is simply no information suggesting that applying soy extract, black cohosh, or evening primrose oil to the skin can mitigate any of the changes taking place in the epidermis and dermis, and definitely not in comparison to taking those substances orally. None of those substances are a problem if they show up in skin-care products, but their benefits are most likely not any different from those of other anti-inflammatory and antioxidant cosmetic ingredients.

The truth is the real basics for skin care continue to apply to peri-menopausal and menopausal women alike: sun protection, treating the skin type you have (not all menopausal women have dry skin), considering using Retin-A or Renova, and using gentle skin-care products. If you have dry skin, use an emollient moisturizer with antioxidants and anti-inflammatory agents (which most products these days contain). The use of hydroquinone or arbutin-based skin-lightening products is another important option. But there is nothing you can apply to skin (other than over-the-counter products containing USP progesterone or prescription-only estrogen creams) that can alter the actual condition of your skin caused by the depletion of hormones.

Note: What about the use of effective AHAs and BHA for menopausal women? This depends more on the condition of your skin than anything else. For some women (usually those over 70—well after menopause) the skin can become so thin it can literally tear when gently scratched or rubbed. This thinning is a result of many factors but primarily it is brought about by a combination of estrogen loss, genetic aging, and sun damage. All of these things cause the skin cells to produce less skin and less healthy skin. In terms of genetic aging, skin cells seem to have a pre-programmed mechanism that slows down skin-cell turnover, causing a buildup of dead skin cells on the surface of skin. It would be helpful if there were a way to tell skin cells not to slow down production, stay healthy (produce normally), and not build up on the surface of skin.

Renova is the only real option we have for producing healthy cells. As for AHAs and BHA, they indeed help the outer layer of skin to shed by removing built-up dead skin cells. For some women in their 70s, 80s, and 90s with extremely fragile skin that may be problematic (they may indeed need the dead skin cells to stick around on the surface for as long as possible). However, for many women who don't have that kind of fragile skin the benefit of removing surface dead skin cells is that it absolutely helps improve the appearance of skin and allows healthier skin cells to come to the surface. It is also thought that AHAs and BHA can stimulate the production of collagen, which also has benefit.

chapter 8

BATTLE PLANS
FOR DRY SKIN

UNDERSTANDING DRY SKIN

Before I go about creating a battle plan for dry skin it is essential for you to have a fundamental understanding of what dry skin is all about so you know exactly what kind of problems you are dealing with. Ironically, dry skin does not seem to be about a lack of moisture. The studies that have compared the water content of dry skin to normal or oily skin don't seem to find a statistically significant difference in moisture content between them (source: *Journal of Cosmetic Chemistry*, September/October 1993, page 249). As mentioned in the earlier discussion of moisturizers, too much water can be a problem because it can disrupt the skin's intercellular matrix, the substances that keep skin cells bonded to each other, ensuring that the outer layer of skin is intact and smooth.

What is thought to be taking place in dry skin is that the intercellular matrix has somehow become impaired or damaged and that creates water loss. It's not that the skin doesn't have enough water, but rather it doesn't have the ability to prevent water loss, or to keep the right amount of water in the skin cell. When the intercellular matrix is disrupted, it impairs the integrity or health of the skin and the skin inevitably becomes dry, literally torn and ruptured.

There are some genetic factors that create this weakened or ineffective outer layer of skin but some of the things we do to our skin cause dryness as well. Perhaps the biggest offense is the use of drying skin-care products such as soaps, harsh cleansers, or products with drying or irritating ingredients. All of these disrupt the outer layer of the skin, destroying the intercellular matrix and causing dry skin. In skin-care products, the ingredients that are the worst culprits are alcohol, witch hazel, fragrance, camphor, menthol, citrus, and peppermint.

Weather and the way we heat and cool our homes, cars, and workplaces are also problematic for creating or worsening dry skin. Constant exposure to arid environments, as well as to air blasting from dry heaters or air conditioners, also destroys or impairs the skin's outer layer and intercellular matrix. Adding a humidifier to your home can make a world of difference to prevent external factors like this from causing dry skin to occur in the first place.

Unprotected sun exposure is another factor that damages the outer layer of skin. Sun damage causes abnormal cell production, resulting in a malformed outer layer of skin. In this situation skin cells adhere poorly to each other and the result is that the surface of new skin being formed is continually unhealthy and unable to provide reliable protection. Removing the damaged outer layer of skin can also make a world of difference in the health and appearance of the skin's surface. AHAs, BHA, and cosmetic skin-resurfacing procedures handle this problem beautifully. Tretinoin is also helpful for its role in improving cell production.

Perimenopause and menopause also factor into the causes of dry skin. Estrogen helps maintain skin's moisture content by increasing mucopolysaccharides and hyaluronic acid in the skin, helping to maintain the function of the skin's outer layer. Loss of estrogen also reduces the lipid content of skin, which eliminates the skin's natural protection against dryness.

TOO MUCH WATER CAN BE A PROBLEM

While companies love touting how much water their products can put in your skin it turns out that may not be a good thing because too much water is particularly hard on dry skin. Overhydration can indeed be a problem, and products that brag about increasing water content in skin cells by 180% can be doing more harm than good. Supporting this contention was a recent article in the May 2000 issue of *Cosmetics & Toi-*

letries magazine. The article on page 18 reviewed a book by Loden and Maibach called *Dry Skin and Moisturizers, Chemistry and Function.* One of the points in this book that impressed the reviewer was the fact that "prolonged water contact is not innocuous. Intense dermatitis can occur simply by prolonged water exposure. . . . Water alone also disrupts the SC [stratum corneum—the outer, surface layer of skin]. . . . Their studies show that water can directly disrupt the barrier lipids [protecting skin covering] and are consistent with surfactant-induced intercellular lamellar bilayer disruption." That means water can break down the stuff that binds skin cells together, actually degrading skin in the same way that strong cleansing agents can. (**Note:** *Cosmetics & Toiletries* magazine is a cosmetics industry journal read by cosmetics executives, formulators, and packaging companies.)

Another article, in *Contact Dermatitis* (December 1999, pages 311–314), stated that "Water is a skin irritant, which deserves attention because of its [pervasiveness]. . . . In occupational dermatology, the importance of water as a skin irritant is especially appreciated. The irritancy of water has been demonstrated by occlusion experiments; occlusion with either closed chambers or water-soaked patches has been shown to produce clinical and histopathological inflammation. Functional damage, as revealed by increased transepidermal water loss, has also been shown. . . . However, much remains to be done to clarify the risk factors and mechanisms of water-induced irritation."

What this means is that those with dry skin should avoid soaking in a tub or taking long showers. Water is great, but it can be overdone and end up causing more problems than it helps.

DRINKING WATER

Wouldn't it be great for those with dry skin if just drinking eight or more glasses of water a day could prevent or change dry skin? Drinking water is definitely important for the health of the body but that doesn't translate to getting rid of dry skin. If all it took to eliminate dry skin would be to drink water no one would have dry skin! Attempting to overdrink is always accompanied by an almost immediate need to go to the bathroom, where the excess water is quickly eliminated. So even if the extra water could be delivered to skin cells it would never have the chance to get there.

BATTLE PLAN FOR DRY SKIN

To prevent or eliminate dry skin, the goal is to maintain the health of the skin's intercellular matrix. Moisture loss is definitely a symptom of dry skin, but simply giving the skin moisture won't repair the intercellular matrix because it has no water content to begin with. Rather the intercellular matrix is made up of substances like glycerin, lecithin, cholesterol, hyaluronic acid, and on and on, but not water.

Without question, moisturizers play a significant role for dry skin, and the number of products aimed at this problem is staggering. Fortunately, almost all moisturizers are wonderfully able to take care of most dry skin conditions. Yet for a number of men and women even a well-formulated moisturizer can't take care of the type of dryness they have and special management must be practiced.

Dry skin does show improvement and feels vastly better when emollients and lipids are used and dry air is kept off the skin. Here are some practical recommendations for winning this battle:

- If you can add a humidifier in your home, bedroom, or workplace, do so. This can make a huge difference in the feel of your skin.
- Use gentle cleansers from head to toe. Harsh or drying soaps or cleansers of any kind will either create dry skin or make matters worse.
- Avoid immersing your skin in water for long periods of time.
- **At night, apply an effective AHA or BHA product.** This is great for dry feet, legs, and arms, as well as the face. You may have to experiment to find out how frequently to apply these types of products, but it is essential to exfoliate the outer layer to get rid of the unhealthy buildup of dry, sun-damaged skin.
- In the morning it is essential to apply an emollient moisturizer with an SPF 15 or greater that has the UVA-protecting ingredients avobenzone, titanium dioxide, or zinc oxide.
- At night an emollient moisturizer that's made with lipids (plant oils), natural moisturizing factors (ceramides, hyaluronic acid, vitamins, polysaccharides), and water-binding agents (glycerin) can help a great deal.
- For very dry skin, apply a layer of olive oil or safflower, almond, or canola, over your nighttime moisturizer as an extra treatment.
- Medical hormone replacement therapy or alternative sources of hormones can also reduce or eliminate dry skin.

chapter 9

BATTLE PLANS
FOR BLEMISHES

UNDERSTANDING WHAT CAUSES A BLEMISH

There's no way around it: One of the most worrisome and prevalent skin-care problems many women suffer through at some time in their lives is some degree of acne. Whether it's blackheads, whiteheads (milia—hard white bumps that do not contain pus and are not swollen or red), papules (inflamed, red, raised bumps that do not contain pus), or pustules (inflamed, red, raised bumps that contain pus), blemishes are commonplace skin imperfections. The language may not be pretty, but "acne affects approximately 95% of the population at some point during their lifetime." This common disorder can range from mild to severe forms, can sometimes cause extensive scarring, and can occur somewhere between the ages of 11 and 50 (source: *Journal of Cutaneous Medical Surgery*, June 2000, Supplemental, pages 2–13).

Regardless of your age, gender, skin color, or ethnicity, what causes acne is the same across the board (source: *British Journal of Dermatology*, May 2000, pages 885–892). As a result there are certain basics for fighting breakouts that are essential if you are going to have any chance of winning the battle. To create a plan of action—and it does take an organized plan of action—it is essential to let go of the inaccurate but persistent and pervasive information concerning blemishes and instead learn what really can help your skin. You can't choose wisely if you don't know what you're fighting against. If you don't understand all your options and don't focus on what can work and what can't, you will end up making the condition worse than it was to begin with, or find temporary relief, only to have the problems show up time and time again.

First and foremost, you need to get over three myths about treating breakouts—because not only will they fail to prevent or eliminate a blemish, but they can also cause a whole range of additional skin problems.

The first myth is the notion that you can dry up a blemish. Water is the only thing you can dry up and a blemish has nothing to do with being wet. Skin cells, however, do contain water, and when you dry up the skin you are really drying up the water in the skin cell. Drying up skin impairs the intercellular matrix (skin's protective barrier), which can increase the presence of bacteria in the pore and cause flaking and a tight, dry feeling. None of that stops breakouts but it can lead to irritation and add another predicament to your skin-care woes. What's true is that blemishes can be aggravated by oil production, which needs to be reduced and/or absorbed. Absorbing oil on the skin or in the pore is a radically different process from drying up skin.

The second myth is that blemishes are caused by dirty skin. Unfortunately, this mistaken belief causes harsh overcleaning of the face with soaps and strong detergent cleansers. That only increases the risk of irritation and dryness, and doesn't do anything to prevent blemishes. Not only that, the ingredients in bar cleansers and soaps that keep them in a hard bar form can clog pores and actually cause breakouts. The truth is that gentle cleansing and overall gentle skin care are critical to getting breakouts under control (source: *Cutis*, December 2001, Supplemental, pages 12–19).

The third myth is that you can spot-treat blemishes. Sadly, lots of products are based on this concept. However, once you see a blemish, you can't just zap it into oblivion in the hope of changing anything. For most types of blemishes (other than those created by an immediate reaction to a cosmetic or some other topical irritant or sensitizing reaction), by the time it shows up on the surface of the skin, it has been at least two to three weeks in the making. The truth is, it takes time for conditions in the pore to create a blemish. If you don't understand and you don't learn how to deal with that somewhat lengthy process, you can't successfully tackle recurring breakouts. Dealing with only the blemishes you see means that the blemishes that are forming won't be stopped.

Remember, you can't dry up a blemish because it isn't wet, and irritating ingredients not only may make matters worse by creating more redness and swelling, but also hurt the skin's ability to heal. The best course of action is to work on the cause of the blemish, not the aftermath.

WHAT CAUSES BLEMISHES?

What truly causes breakouts? There are four major factors and one minor one that contribute to the formation of blemishes.

1. Hormonal activity
2. Overproduction of oil by the oil gland
3. Irregular or excessive shedding of dead skin cells, both on the surface of skin and inside the pore
4. Buildup of bacteria in the pore

Less likely to cause problems but still a problem for some is:

5. Irritation or sensitizing reactions to cosmetics, specific foods (rarely), or medicines

Fundamentally, this is how a blemish occurs. Inside an oil gland a type of bacteria called *Propionibacterium acnes* (or *P. acnes*) finds a perfect environment for growth. Dead skin cells and excess oil in the oil gland provide just the kind of conditions that *P. acnes* needs to thrive. As *P. acnes* reproduces, irritation and inflammation occur, which is why most blemishes are red and swollen (source: *Seminars in Cutaneous Medicine and Surgery*, September 2001, pages 139–143).

Each hair follicle grows from a sebaceous (oil) gland that secretes an oily, firm wax called sebum. The structure that the oil gland and hair follicle share is called the pilosebaceous duct or unit, more popularly referred to as a pore. When things are going well, the sebum smoothly leaves the pore and imperceptibly melts on the skin's surface, helping to keep the skin surface moist and smooth. When things aren't going well, as when the pore becomes plugged with sebum and dead skin cells and bacteria run amok, a blemish is the outcome. Surplus sebum is generated primarily by hormonal activity (source: *Journal of the American Academy of Dermatology*, December 2001, pages 957–960). When too much oil is produced, it can become mixed with dead skin cells from the skin's surface, with poorly sloughed skin cells from the pore's lining, and with small pieces of hair debris from the follicle. This combination of sebum, dead skin cells, and small pieces of hair can clog the pathway out of the hair follicle/oil gland, creating quite a backup. Now you've got problems.

When your body produces too much oil, and dead skin cells on the surface of skin or inside the pore aren't shed normally, they can join together in blocking the exit from a pore. All this excess oil and dead skin cells solidify as a soft, white substance that plugs the pore. If the surface of the pore is covered by skin, it is called a whitehead (milia). If the pore is open, without any skin covering, the top of the plug is exposed to air and darkens, causing a blackhead.

Whiteheads and blackheads become pimples when *P. acnes* begins growing inside the plug, causing irritation and inflammation. This inflammation and excess oil causes the wall of the oil gland to rupture, spilling the contents (oil, cell debris, bacteria, and all) into the surrounding skin tissue. The body's immune system then responds, sending lymph to the inflamed area to help with repair (and causing swelling), and you now have a pimple.

This still leaves some pretty important questions unanswered. What causes the hormones to increase oil production, and can you slow it down? How do the skin cells build up and clog the pore, and how do you stop that from happening? How do you stop the bacteria that cause the inflammation and redness? And who can break out or get acne, and why?

WHY ME?

Why my skin? Why another blemish or blackhead? Why can't I have smooth, poreless skin? Why me? Believe me, I know this feeling.

Why do you suddenly, at the age of 28 or 48, have blemishes? Why haven't you outgrown the blemishes and oily skin that have plagued you since you were 14, and that at 35 are worse than ever? Why, at 40, do you have incessant blackheads and breakouts that won't go away no matter what you do, and you've done everything? Why do you still have acne when you're 18 and have tried oral antibiotics, Retin-A, sulfur masks, topical antibiotics, and every cosmetic skin-care routine imaginable? These are great questions and I understand them well.

Regardless of how old you are, breakouts and oily skin are upsetting, and anyone can be a victim. The main culprits in all these scenarios are hormones, because hormones are what affect oil production, and because their levels fluctuate at different times of life.

Breaking out is definitely most prevalent during adolescence. Statistics suggest that three out of four teenagers have problems with breakouts and various forms of acne. That isn't surprising when you consider that adolescence is a time of colossal hormonal changes that stimulate sebaceous (oil) glands and increase sebum production, which in turn increases the chances for breakouts. But acne can happen at any age. More than 40% of all women will experience some form of acne (source: *Journal of European Dermatology and Venereology*, November 2001, pages 541–545).

Anything that can raise hormone levels—stress, the menstrual cycle, pregnancy, birth control pills, or certain medications such as corticosteroids and lithium—can act as a trigger. Specific foods are not responsible for breakouts, but an individual can have allergies to specific foods. There is also speculation that foods with hormone additives (specifically poultry and beef), iodine in food (shellfish), or fluoride in toothpaste may aggravate blemishes.

There's no question that hormone activity is the main thing responsible for oily skin and breakouts. When hormones gush, blemishes can flare, but hormones alone are not enough to create this annoying skin malady. For some unknown reason(s), something goes wrong in the oil gland, blocking the natural flow of oil. Theories about what causes acne generally focus on a genetic predisposition that creates either a defective oil gland, a malfunctioning pore lining that doesn't shed properly, or oil (sebum) that itself is in some way abnormal (too thick or irritating to the skin). In real life, you have to address most, if not all, of these issues if you want to reduce the chances of breakouts.

There are many theories why some people have more severe cases of acne than others. Some suggest that it's increased levels of male hormones, while others say that a genetic abnormality of the oil gland is the culprit. Hypersensitivity to *P. acnes* may also account for the great variation in the severity of acne (source: *Dermatology*, 1998, volume 196, issue 1, pages 80–81). There is even research showing that the actual fatty acid components of the oil gland may be responsible. Most likely it's a combination of all these that cause the differences between those with mild or severe breakouts.

YOU CAN'T ZAP ZITS

Most of us have sought relief from the emotional pain and humiliation that often accompany acne, whether it is one blemish or many, by going to drugstores or cosmetics counters where acne products and skin-care regimes line the shelves. Myriad products promise clear skin, and several pledge to zap zits, dry up blemishes, and drink up oil. The commercials and ads sound convincing, but a closer look reveals that many of these products really can't zap zits or dry up oil (you can never really dry up oil). Spot-treating only the blemish you see doesn't prevent other blemishes from forming. It takes consistency (regularly exfoliating, disinfecting, absorbing oil, hormonal balance) to stop breakouts. Further, many of these products that assure you they can zap zits contain drying, irritating, or sensitizing ingredients that actually make matters worse.

If you just pay attention to what you see on the surface without taking into consideration what is occurring underneath, you can't help heal the skin, reduce breakouts, or prevent scarring. Finding solutions that address each problem—hormonal activity, oil production, exfoliating the skin (and the pore), and killing the bacteria that cause the infection—is the only course of action that makes sense. Focusing on that single lesion without keeping the entire picture in mind can result in more breakouts, increased risk of scarring, and additional skin problems such as redness, surfaced capillaries, irritation, and dry skin.

WHAT YOU CAN DO

Effective blemish treatment works by reducing oil production, eliminating skin-cell buildup on the surface of skin and in the pore, and killing the bacteria, *P. acnes*, that caused the inflammation in the first place. That's why the best course of action for blemishes is twofold: topical (what you put on the skin, whether it's an over-the-counter or a prescription option) and systemic (prescription oral medication that addresses the issue of oil production and bacterial growth).

Topical Options

Clean the skin gently with a water-soluble cleanser that doesn't contain ingredients that can clog pores or irritate the skin. This helps reduce further irritation and redness, which would make matters worse. **Remove dead skin cells and encourage healthy skin-cell turnover** from both the skin's surface and inside the pore to help skin shed more normally.

Absorb or reduce excess oil to reduce the main cause of clogged and enlarged pores.

Kill the bacteria (*P. acnes*) that is causing the eruption, inflammation, redness, and swelling.

Systemic Options

Take oral antibiotics to eliminate bacterial growth.

Use birth control pills and hormone blockers to control oil production.

Apply topical retinoids (Retin-A, Tazorac, Avita, generic tretinoin, Differin) to normalize cell function, allowing the pore to function normally.

Take Accutane, the only prescription medication capable of curing acne.

You need to experiment to discover exactly how to put these various steps together in a combination that works for you. Unfortunately, there isn't one absolutely right way. It is essential to try different options until you find what suits your skin type and your specific condition. If you are consistent and avoid veering from your special battle plan, you stand a pretty good chance of winning a good part of the war against blemishes and blackheads. But the battle plan must deal with all of a blemish's causes.

WHAT YOU SHOULDN'T DO

Don't use harsh or irritating skin-care products. Throughout this book I discuss the need for gentle cleansing for all skin types. This concept is particularly difficult for someone with oily or blemished skin to believe, despite the research backing it up, because the desire to *really* clean the skin is almost irresistible. Yet, a paper published in the *Proceedings of the Fourth International Symposium on Cosmetic Efficacy* (May 10–12, 1999, entitled "The Effects of Cleansing in an Acne Treatment Regimen") concluded that 52% of the time a hydrating face wash gave better results in reducing comedones, papules, and pustules when used with benzoyl peroxide. **By comparison, this type of gentle cleanser was more effective than either soap or a benzoyl peroxide cleanser alone.**

What is most frustrating is that many of the blemish products on the market actually make breakouts worse or cause more skin problems than you started out with. Products designed to tackle acne often contain ingredients like harsh surfactants and overly abrasive scrub particles, as well as alcohol, menthol, peppermint, camphor, and eucalyptus, lemon, or grapefruit oils. All of these ingredients are extremely irritating, and the resulting irritation can impair the skin's ability to heal or to fight bacteria.

What makes all these standard, harmful "blemish fighting" ingredients worse is that they don't reduce any of the factors causing breakouts. They can't disinfect, reduce oil production, affect hormonal activity, or help exfoliation. Instead, they kill more skin cells than necessary, which can further clog pores, produce dry skin, cause irritation, and make skin redder. **A blemish by definition is already irritated, red, and swollen, so it doesn't make any sense to use ingredients that will make it even more irritated, red, and swollen.**

Skin-care products with irritating ingredients, such as facial masks, astringents, toners, and facial scrubs (which also contain waxes), are a big no-no. These can all hurt the skin, and that can aggravate acne. If a product irritates the skin, if it tingles or burns, it is not helping. And not only does irritation stimulate oil production, promote redness, increase swelling, and dry out the skin, it can also add small rashlike pimples to the breakouts you're already trying to deal with.

Bar soaps and bar cleansers are often recommended for acne, yet all of them contain ingredients that can clog pores. Soaps contain tallow and bar cleansers contain other heavy, wax-based thickening agents that can clog pores. Shockingly, high-pH soaps and cleansers (those with a pH of 8 or higher) can actually increase the presence of bacteria in the pore! All this makes matters much worse inside the pore, again greatly increasing the risk of breakouts.

Oversqueezing, picking, digging, scraping, or poking at pimples may be hard to resist, and you may think it speeds healing, but in fact it sets you up for more problems. Creating scabs and constantly reinjuring the lesion just increases the chances of scarring. There is nothing wrong with gentle squeezing to remove a blemish's contents, but unless you are extremely careful you will create more problems than you started with.

Many women think they can use hot compresses to bring pimples to a head. Actually, hot compresses severely damage skin by burning it; the heat causes more redness and swelling; and the whole process can also rupture the pore, increasing the possibility of more breakouts. The same is true of steaming the face or using hot water. Hot water burns the skin, impairing the skin's ability to heal and fight bacteria. Tepid water is what you need to help soothe the skin and calm things down. Use tepid water and a gentle, water-soluble cleanser on the face, and do not wipe off makeup. Wiping and rubbing will make the irritation worse, and can also make the skin sag and cause wrinkles.

Be careful that the breakouts you're struggling with aren't a result of hair products getting on the face. Hairspray, mousse, hair gel, and other styling products contain polymers (plastic-like, film-forming ingredients) that can clog pores and cause pimples.

Don't smoke. A study in the *British Journal of Dermatology* (July 2001, pages 100–104) concluded, "According to multiple logistic regression analyses acne prevalence was significantly higher in active smokers (40.8% . . .) as compared with nonsmokers (25.2%). A significant linear relationship between acne prevalence and number of cigarettes smoked daily was obtained. . . . In addition, a significant dose-dependent relationship between acne severity and daily cigarette consumption was shown by linear regression analysis. . . . Smoking is a clinically important contributory factor to acne prevalence and severity."

WHEN TO SEE A DERMATOLOGIST

Some women run to see a dermatologist the second they see a blemish. Others put it off well past the time when over-the-counter options have stopped working even though their breakouts are still rampant. Though there are many options for dealing successfully with breakouts outside the realm of prescription medications, if your acne is severe or chronic it may indeed be best to seek medical attention. Dermatologists have a host of options in their arsenal that can be more effective than over-the-counter products in reducing sebum production, creating healthy skin-cell turnover, and fighting bacterial infection.

Most prescription-only options such as tretinoins (Retin-A, Tazorac, Avita, generic tretinoin), Differin (technically adapelene), and azelaic acid (trade name Azelex), plus topical antibiotics, oral antibiotics, and hormone blockers have no nonprescription counterparts. Dermatologists also have one option that can be an absolute cure for acne and breakouts. That option is Accutane, the only medication that has a chance of curing acne as opposed to just keeping it under control. All of these options are discussed in this chapter.

Nonetheless, it is completely acceptable to start with the options avail-able over the counter or from some cosmetics lines. Some of these are similar to what a doctor would prescribe, such as salicylic acid products to exfoliate and benzoyl peroxide products to disinfect. If you select this course of action, it is essential to use only what works and to use it con-sistently. If after a period of time you find those options don't work or aren't working as well as you would like, you can always make an ap-pointment with a dermatologist.

WHAT ABOUT DIET?

There is little, if any, scientific evidence that diet affects acne, although specific food allergies certainly can be a contributing factor—but that de-pends on what you personally are allergic to. Not everyone has the same food allergies. Likewise, drinking soda pop, not exercising, popping vi-tamins, and eating healthy or unhealthy foods will neither help nor hurt acne. Lots of Olympic-caliber athletes have acne-prone skin, and lots of people who don't exercise and are overweight have a flawless com-plexion. However, if certain foods—such as nuts, shellfish (because of their iodine content), milk products, or wheat—seem to make your acne worse, it is best to avoid them (try omitting them one by one) to see if it makes a long-term difference in your skin.

Incidentally, fluoride in toothpaste may be the source of breakouts around the mouth. The research for this is very old, with a couple of studies published in the 1970s and 1950s. That is not exactly current in-formation, but if you tend to have acne just around your mouth, it is simple enough to try nonfluoride toothpaste for a while and see if things improve. If your acne is indeed triggered by fluoride, consult your den-tist about alternative cavity-prevention treatments.

OIL-FREE IS A BAD JOKE

The joke is on us, because while "oil-free" is a meaningless claim it may mislead consumers into buying products that can actually clog pores. There are plenty of ingredients that don't sound like oils but that can ab-solutely aggravate breakouts. On the other hand, not all oils clog pores. **Yet, many cosmetics (anything that isn't in a liquid form) contain wax-like thickening agents that may clog pores.** Simple, standard moisturizing ingredients that are great for dry skin can cause problems for someone with oily skin or breakouts. When any product looks like a cream or a lotion (as opposed to a fluid), the ingredients that give it that consistency may clog pores. Despite the problems these ingredients can cause, they show up in lots and lots of so-called oil-free products.

Above and beyond the products that claim to be oil-free, label after label promises that the product is "noncomedogenic" or "nonacnegenic." Most of us have bought products with this assurance, only to find that they did cause breakouts. I wish I could say otherwise, but the truth is you can't trust any product that makes the claim that it's not comedogenic because there is no approved or regulated standard for that assertion. Aside from the regulatory aspect of this bogus claim, I'm certain all of us have used products that promised not to cause breakouts and yet we still broke out. What many women already know from experience is that trying to guess how their skin will react based on a product's promises, especially when it comes to blemishes, is truly a lost cause—or at the very least a difficult problem with no easy, slam-dunk answers.

WILL IT MAKE ME BREAK OUT?

So if you can't trust the terms "oil-free," "noncomedogenic," or "nonacnegenic," how do you know if a product will cause problems? Why does it seem so impossible to find products that won't cause breakouts? It's because *most* ingredients used in cosmetics can cause breakouts, depending on your skin type.

There is evidence that some specific ingredients can trigger breakouts, but there are no absolutes. I wish there were, but there aren't. Several Web sites that showcase lists of comedogenic ingredients have caused quite a stir for many women. The major source of information for these data appears to be *Dr. Fulton's Step by Step Guide to Acne*, published in 1983 by Harper & Row (though credit is not given on any Web site, it is the exact same information presented in the book). At the time (and 1983 is a long time ago), Fulton's research on the causes of breakouts was unprecedented. Fulton applied cosmetics ingredients to rabbits' ears and waited to see what happened. As promising as this research was, it has never been repeated, and is rarely cited in later research (except when it suits a company's marketing agenda). There are many reasons why lists of this kind are unreliable.

First, the methodology involved pure concentrations of the ingredient, not the concentrations that are used in actual cosmetic formulations, which are usually only a fractional percentage. It also didn't address the issue of usage and application. For example, the exposure risks of specific ingredients are very different for a cleanser, which is left on the skin for a few seconds, and a lotion or liquid, which is left on the skin for hours. Beyond this, the research didn't look at the host of plant extracts or sunscreens in cosmetics that were introduced during the early 1980s. To call this list out of date and inconclusive would be an understatement.

I have to admit that I'm also to blame for some of the confusion. In my books I have included a list of ingredients that may cause breakouts. I based this list on the emollient or waxlike characteristics of the ingredients and on findings in more contemporary research when it was available. I warned against products that contain ingredient groups such as triglycerides, myristates, palmitates, and stearates, but it was probably not wise to include such a list because in some ways it is misleading information. For example, isopropyl palmitate is a waxy thickening agent used to bind other ingredients together, has an emollient feel on skin, and is used most frequently in moisturizers for dry skin. On the other hand, ascorbyl palmitate is a stable form of vitamin C that is used in small amounts in skin-care products, and is not a problem for skin. So much for following the rule about palmitates. Further, depending on the ingredient, just because it is present in a formulation means nothing if it is toward the end of the ingredient list—while if it's the second, third, or fourth ingredient it may be problematic. But that may not be true if there are many of these kinds of ingredients strewn across a label and, therefore, present in small amounts. Also, keep in mind that even the most notorious ingredients (such as isopropyl myristate) won't cause problems for everyone. Just because an ingredient *may* cause breakouts doesn't mean that it will.

Another point these kinds of lists can't account for is that there are thousands and thousands of cosmetic ingredients being used in skin-care and makeup products today. A lot of them are emollients, waxy thickening agents, or irritants that can cause skin problems. Whether they do or not, however, is completely dependent on the amount used and the nature of the individual ingredient (some ingredients cause problems in far smaller amounts than other ingredients, while others cause problems in various combinations). A comprehensive list would not only be impossible, but also would be nothing more than guesswork.

There are no easy answers for this one, but you can understand that trying to research, categorize, classify, and make absolute conclusions about 50,000 ingredients with an infinite number of possible combinations is just not humanly possible. So, what's a woman to do when trying to fend off blemishes and still use skin-care and makeup products? While I still think some ingredients are more problematic than others, the easiest and most reliable quality for a consumer to consider is consistency of the product. The thicker the product (meaning those with a high, thick, or creamy viscosity), the more likely it is to cause problems. That means you can feel safer with a gel or serum (because these have a low or watery viscosity).

What about greasiness? It is safe to assume that a product with plant or mineral oils of any kind listed high up on the ingredient list might make the skin feel greasy. But greasiness doesn't necessarily trigger breakouts.

Finally, it makes more sense to watch out for irritating ingredients than so-called pore-clogging ingredients. It doesn't take much alcohol, menthol, peppermint, balm mint, eucalyptus, camphor, lemon, grapefruit, or lime to cause a negative skin reaction that can impede the skin's healing process by stimulating bacteria production—and that won't help heal blemishes.

BLEMISH FIGHTING BASICS

Each of the following products and product categories reflects state-of-the-art treatments for blemishes, acne, and blackheads. How to put them all together is addressed in the "Battle Plans for Fighting Blemishes" section on page 252.

All of the products starting on page 231 address each of the factors that cause pimples. These are the best options for reducing oil production, for disinfecting the skin, for improving exfoliation, and for controlling hormonal activity, and are a potential cure for blemishes. Finding the combination that works for you is the first goal, and then you must focus on hitting all the steps and carrying them out consistently.

Gentle cleansing is the first place to start. I've already elaborated on the need for gentle cleansing, but let me say it one more time for added emphasis. Using a water-soluble cleanser gently cleans your skin without stimulating the oil glands, increasing redness, or creating dryness. This step is standard for any skin-care routine because it makes an instant difference in the appearance and feel of the skin, and it is essential for reducing breakouts. Once you stop using drying, irritating, pore-clogging soaps or bar cleansers, and you realize how nice your skin feels when it is no longer dry and irritated, you will never go back to the old way again. Just be certain the water-soluble cleanser you select doesn't contain irritating ingredients and won't dry out the skin. Using cleansers that contain exfoliating agents, topical disinfectants, or oil-absorbing ingredients is not the best option because the active ingredients would be washed away before they had a chance to have an effect on skin. Save these ingredients for another step.

Disinfecting. There aren't many options for disinfecting the skin. Alcohol (when used in the right concentrations) and sulfur can be good disinfectants, but they are too drying and irritating, causing more problems than they help, which can generate more breakouts. Plant-derived disinfectants such as tea tree oil (melaleuca) are an option but there are no products currently being sold that contain a high enough concentration to reliably kill bacteria. Benzoyl peroxide is still the best over-the-counter disinfectant to consider and is available in 2.5%, 5%, and 10% concentrations.

If benzoyl peroxide isn't effective, a topical antibiotic or even an oral antibiotic prescribed by a doctor may be the only option left to kill stubborn, blemish-causing bacteria, but an oral antibiotic should be a last resort because of systemic problems and problems with resistant bacteria. Oral antibiotics can indeed kill blemish-causing bacteria, but they also kill good bacteria in the body, causing yeast infections and stomach problems. In addition, *P. acnes* in your body can develop resistant strains in a short period of time, making the antibiotic you're taking ineffective.

Exfoliating. Because blemishes occur inside the pore and involve oil production, an effective 1% to 2% salicylic acid (beta hydroxy acid—BHA) product is a crucial over-the-counter starting point for exfoliating the skin. Salicylic acid is lipid soluble, which means it can exfoliate inside the pore, plus it is extremely gentle. I recommend using BHA in a gel, liquid, or extremely light lotion formula because they are unlikely to contain waxy thickening agents or emollients that can clog pores. Topical scrubs and alpha hydroxy acids (AHAs) can be helpful for surface exfoliation, but they can't affect the pore lining, and it's essential to do that to deal with one of the root causes of a blemish.

Improving cell production. Tretinoins, Differin, and azelaic acid are prescription options for generating healthy cell growth that can change the shape of the pore, allowing for normal oil flow. This improvement can eliminate the environment that allows the blemish to develop.

Absorbing or controlling excess oil. Clay masks are an option for absorbing oil as long as they contain no irritating ingredients. Using milk of magnesia as a facial mask is a simple and effective way to absorb oil. Birth control pills and hormone blockers can equalize hormones, reducing or eliminating the source of excess oil production.

When all else fails. If your breakouts persist after you've tried these over-the-counter and prescription options then you can still try Accutane, which is the only medication that can essentially cure acne. This is the last option in any lineup concerning blemishes only because of its serious side effects if a woman becomes pregnant while using it and because of other health issues (these are discussed in more detail later in this chapter).

SALICYLIC ACID

Referred to as beta hydroxy acid (BHA), salicylic acid can be a judicious starting point in the treatment of breakouts for all skin types. This is a multifunctional ingredient that addresses many of the systemic causes of blemishes (source: *Seminars in Dermatology*, December 1990, pages 305–308). For decades dermatologists have been prescribing salicylic acid as an exceedingly effective keratolytic (exfoliant). Yet, in addition to salicylic acid's incredibly helpful exfoliating properties, it can do even more. Salicylic acid is a derivative of aspirin (both are salicylates—aspirin's technical name is acetyl *salicylic acid*) and so it also functions as an anti-inflammatory (source: *Archives of Dermatology*, November 2000, pages 1390–1395). Combining exfoliation with reduced irritation has many advantages for skin, especially for someone struggling with breakouts. Diminishing or eliminating the redness and swelling blemishes cause can help skin heal, prevent scarring, and decrease the chance of further breakouts.

Preventing pores from becoming clogged is a requisite to preventing blemishes. One way to achieve this is to improve the shape of the pore lining. The lining of a pore is made of skin cells (epithelial tissue) that can become thick and misshapen, preventing the natural flow of oil out of the pore. To act on the pore lining it is necessary to exfoliate inside the pore, dislodging excess skin cells. Exfoliants such as alpha hydroxy acids (AHAs) or mechanical scrubs have limitations for blemish-prone skin due to their inability to penetrate inside the pore. AHAs are water-soluble and can't get through the oil. Mechanical scrubs have particle sizes that are too large for them to have any effect below the surface of skin. Salicylic acid is the perfect answer. It is an effective exfoliant, it is lipid soluble (so it effortlessly penetrates into the pore), and it is an anti-inflammatory so it can actually reduce irritation, swelling, and redness.

Another notable aspect of salicylic acid for breakouts is that it has antimicrobial properties (source: *Preservatives for Cosmetics*, by David Steinberg, Allured Publishing, 1996; Health Canada Monograph Category IV, *Antiseptic Cleansers*). That means it can be effective in killing the bacteria that cause acne. Together, all these properties mean salicylic acid is one of the more multifunctional ingredients in combating the causes of acne.

As wonderful as this sounds, salicylic acid is a tricky product to buy. The concentration must be at least 0.5%, but 1% to 2% is more effective. Additionally, the formula's pH is a critical factor. For salicylic acid to work as an exfoliant on skin, it must be in a formulation with a pH of 3 to 4; if it isn't, it loses its ability to exfoliate skin (source: *Cosmetic Dermatology*, October 2001, pages 65–72). Well-formulated salicylic acid products do exist, and once you've found the right one, it can be a successful part of your battle plan to fight blemishes.

AN OVER-THE-COUNTER ANTIBACTERIAL

Some things go hand in hand: bread and butter, love and marriage, Laurel and Hardy. None of these are the same by themselves. That's also true for exfoliants and topical antibacterial agents when it comes to reducing or eliminating blemishes. Cleaning the skin without exfoliating *and* disinfecting is far less likely to have an impact on skin. You can get pretty good results using one or the other, but together they are a formidable defense against blemishes.

Benzoyl peroxide is considered the most effective over-the-counter choice for a topical antibacterial agent in the treatment of blemishes (source: *Skin Pharmacology and Applied Skin Physiology*, September-October 2000, pages 292–296). The amount of research demonstrating the effectiveness of benzoyl peroxide is exhaustive and conclusive (source: *Journal of the American Academy of Dermatology*, November 1999, pages 710–716). Among benzoyl peroxide's attributes is its ability to penetrate into the hair follicle to reach the bacteria that are causing the problem, and then kill them—with a low risk of irritation. It also doesn't pose the problem of bacterial resistance that some prescription topical antibacterials (antibiotics) do (source: *Dermatology*, 1998, volume 196, issue 1, pages 119–125).

Benzoyl peroxide solutions range from 2.5% to 10%. For the sake of your skin, start with the less potent concentrations. A 2.5% benzoyl peroxide product is much less irritating than a 5% or 10% concentration, and it can be just as effective. It completely depends on how stubborn the strain of bacteria in your pores happens to be.

Despite benzoyl peroxide's superior disinfecting and penetrating properties, some bacteria just won't give up easily, and in those situations a different weapon may be necessary. That's when you should consider prescription topical disinfectants (topical antibiotics).

PRESCRIPTION ANTIBACTERIALS

If your skin doesn't respond to a 2.5% benzoyl peroxide or to the various over-the-counter higher strengths, the next step is a prescription topical antibacterial, meaning antibiotics in a lotion or gel form. Topical antibiotics have limitations. They can have difficulty penetrating the hair follicle and long-term use can lead to antibiotic-resistant strains of bacteria. Erythromycin, tetracycline, and clindamycin are the most popular topical antibiotics.

You can use these antibiotics alone, but a good deal of research points to the greater benefit of combining these with benzoyl peroxide to create a potent and effective treatment. Studies indicate that "topical clindamycin and benzoyl peroxide have each demonstrated clinical efficacy in the treatment of acne vulgaris. When used in tandem, they promise greater efficacy than either individual agent through their antibacterial and anti-inflammatory effects. . . . Benzoyl peroxide [and] clindamycin demonstrated significantly greater reductions in inflammatory lesions . . . and significantly greater overall improvement as assessed by physicians . . . and patients" (source: *Journal of Cutaneous Medical Surgery*, January 2001, pages 37–42). This same assessment was echoed in the *American Journal of Clinical Dermatology* (2001, volume 2, issue 4, pages 263–266).

Another option, considered to be quite effective, is a prescription product called Benzamycin, which contains 3% erythromycin and 5% benzoyl peroxide. This combination boosts penetration, which benzoyl peroxide does best, and combines that with erythromycin's strong antibiotic action (source: *British Journal of Dermatology*, February 1997, pages 235–238).

Basic directions: After you have cleaned your face and used a toner, apply the BHA over the face (or areas of the neck, back, or chest where you tend to break out). Then apply your topical antibacterial. During the day, sunscreen goes on next; in the evening, if you need a moisturizer, apply it minimally only over dry patches or dry areas around the eye.

Warning: Do not apply benzoyl peroxide and a retinoid (such as Retin-A, Renova, Tazorac, Avita, generic tretinoin, or Differin). Benzoyl peroxide inactivates retinoids (source: *British Journal of Dermatology*, September 1998, page 8).

TEA TREE OIL VERSUS BENZOYL PEROXIDE

Please see the section in Chapter 2, Miracles, Frauds, & Facts: An A to Z Guide, on "Tea Tree Oil—Melaleuca."

TRETINOIN FOR BLEMISHES

Retinoid is the general category name for any and all forms of vitamin A. Tretinoin is a form of vitamin A and, therefore, comes under the general heading of retinoids. The best-known products that contain tretinoins are Retin-A, Renova, Retin-A Micro, Tazorac, Avita, and generic tretinoin. These are all basic treatments for blemishes because they change the way skin cells are formed in the layers of skin as well as in the pore. If skin cells have an abnormal shape, they tend to stick together and shed poorly, often getting backed up in the pore. Tretinoin can transform cell production by improving shedding and by unclogging pores, thereby producing a significant reduction in inflammatory lesions. Topical tretinoins and antibacterial agents have complimentary actions, and they work well together when combined. Tretinoins are not able to kill *P. acnes*, the bacteria that cause the breakouts, but an antibacterial agent can. Meanwhile, tretinoins can improve and restore the shape of the pore, opening a clear pathway for the antibacterial agent so it can be more active (source: *Journal of the European Academy of Dermatology and Venereology*, December 2001, page 43).

One of the major drawbacks to the use of tretinoin is the irritation it can cause. For some people this can be so severe as to prevent its use. But there are alternatives. There is a great deal of research showing that adapalene (brand name Differin), another retinoid but different from tretinoin, can be just as effective as tretinoin but without the irritation (see the following section on Differin).

Meanwhile, remember that using any tretinoin product can make the skin more vulnerable to sun damage and sunburn. It is essential to wear an SPF 15 sunscreen that contains one or more of the UVA-protecting ingredients avobenzone, titanium dioxide, or zinc oxide as the active ingredient. Zinc oxide and titanium dioxide are occlusive and can possibly clog pores and avobenzone can be sensitizing for some skin types. It takes experimentation to find the right sunscreen that works best for your skin type.

Basic directions: After you have cleaned your face and applied a topical antibacterial (though not benzoyl peroxide, which with the exception of Differin, inactivates retinoids), you can spread a tiny amount of Retin-A, Renova, Retin-A Micro, Avita, Tazora, or generic tretinoin over the face. If you are going outdoors in the daytime, it is essential to follow this with a sunscreen to protect the face from sun damage. At night you can apply a moisturizer afterward over dry areas or around the eyes.

DIFFERIN

In the world of prescription acne treatments, Retin-A and tretinoins have been in a class by themselves for many years. Now they have some stiff competition in the form of Differin, generically known as adapalene, a prescription-only, topical acne medication from the folks who make Cetaphil.

Remember, if abnormal skin cells in the layers of skin and in the pores are left to do their own thing, they just accumulate there, creating an environment in which blemishes can flourish. Aside from topical and oral antibiotics that primarily address the issue of killing off the bacteria responsible for producing pimples, tretinoin was the only prescription product available that could help exfoliate skin cells (especially inside the pores), literally changing the way the skin cells are produced. It works for more than half of the people who can tolerate the treatment, but therein lies the rub—tolerance—because tretinoin can irritate the skin. Even Dr. James Leyden, an associate of Dr. Albert Kligman, the original patent holder for Retin-A, said, "Retinoid [Retin-A] therapy . . . due to the side effects, has always been a double-edged sword, limiting its use in many patients."

I can relate. When I was young, Retin-A left my face so red and inflamed I thought it was going to blister, especially in the days when I also used strong astringents and bar soaps.

Where does Differin fit into this picture? Differin is a retinoid, a form of vitamin A that has been shown in clinical studies to be significantly less irritating than tretinoin. According to a study published in the March 1996 *Journal of the American Academy of Dermatology*, Differin was also significantly more effective in reducing blemishes and was better tolerated than tretinoin gel. Other more recent studies have come to the same conclusion, which is that, by several measures, adapalene cream and gel were less irritating upon multiple dosing than various tretinoin creams and gels (sources: *International Journal of Dermatology*, October 2000, pages 784–788; *Journal of Cutaneous Medical Surgery*, October 1999, pages 298–301).

It seems that Differin has a radarlike ability to positively affect the skin-cell lining of the pores, substantially improving exfoliation and helping to prevent blockage. Moreover, for those with oily skin, the original Differin comes in a lightweight gel formula that is barely felt on the skin. It contains little more than water and cellulose, a sheer thickening agent. Differin is also available in a cream base for those with dry skin and blemishes.

Should you consider Differin? If you have tried Retin-A or other tretinoins and had difficulty dealing with the irritation, or if you just want to see if Differin can work better for you (which it may), then it is certainly an option.

Basic directions: After you have cleaned your face and applied a topical antibacterial, spread a tiny amount of Differin over the face, or any other part of the body with breakouts. If you are going outdoors in the daytime, it is essential to follow this with a UVA-protecting sunscreen to shield the face from sun damage. At night you can apply a moisturizer afterward, over dry areas or around the eyes.

AZELAIC ACID

The introduction of new and reformulated prescription exfoliants in more-emollient or nonalcohol bases reflects the demand for medications that meet the needs of older women looking for ways to deal with pre- and postmenopausal acne. Differin, the new tretinoins, and azelaic acid all affect the way skin cells are formed and shed in the skin layers and inside the pore lining. The difference with azelaic acid (trade name Azelex) is that in addition to exfoliating the skin, it also performs an antimicrobial action on the skin.

Technically, azelaic acid is a saturated dicarboxylic acid found naturally in wheat, rye, and barley that behaves like a 5% topical benzoyl peroxide gel, a 0.05% tretinoin cream, or a 2% erythromycin cream (a topical prescription antibiotic), meaning it can exfoliate and disinfect the skin at the same time. There is some research that shows azelaic acid to be well-tolerated, and that it may not cause as much overt irritation, redness, or swelling as tretinoin (source: *Acta Dermato-Venereologica*, November 1999, pages 456–459). However, other research indicates that irritation is a possible side effect.

Unlike the tretinoins, azelaic acid is not likely to cause sun sensitivity. It is most definitely an ally in the battle against breakouts, particularly if skin is naturally sensitive to the sun or if irritation is an issue.

Azelaic acid's efficacy can be enhanced and improved when it is used in combination with other topical medications such as benzoyl peroxide 4% gel, clindamycin 1% gel, tretinoin 0.025% cream, and a gel combining 3% erythromycin with 5% benzoyl peroxide. Furthermore, another study has shown that azelaic acid plus benzoyl peroxide achieves greater efficacy and higher patient satisfaction ratings of convenience than [single] therapy with erythromycin–benzoyl peroxide gel (source: *Journal of the American Academy of Dermatology*, August 2000, Supplemental, pages 47–50).

Basic directions: After you have cleaned your face and applied a topical disinfectant, spread on a tiny amount of azelaic acid. If you are going outdoors in the daytime, it is essential to follow this with a UVA-protecting sunscreen to shield the face from sun damage. At night you can apply a moisturizer afterward, over dry areas or around the eyes.

ORAL ANTIBIOTICS

If topical exfoliants, retinoids, and antibacterial agents don't provide satisfactory results, an oral antibiotic prescribed by a doctor may be an option to kill stubborn, blemish-causing bacteria. Several studies have shown that oral antibiotics, used in conjunction with topical tretinoins or topical exfoliants, can control or reduce many acne conditions (source: *International Journal of Dermatology,* January 2000, pages 45–50). As effective as oral antibiotics can be, they should be a last resort, not a first line of attack. Oral antibiotics can produce some unacceptable long-term health problems. Some dermatologists tend to give the negative side effects of oral antibiotics short shrift and prescribe them as if they were nothing more than candy for their acne patients. Oral antibiotics are anything but candy. They kill the good bacteria in the body along with the bad, and that can result in chronic vaginal yeast infections as well as stomach problems.

A more worrisome side effect is that the acne-causing bacteria can become immune to the oral antibiotic. According to an article in the *American Journal of Clinical Dermatology* (2001, volume 2, issue 3, pages 135–141) "The main cause for concern following the use of systemic antibiotics is the emergence of antibiotic-resistant strains of *P. acnes.*" Similarly a paper presented at the General Meeting of the American Society for Microbiology in May 2001 (http://www.asmusa.org/memonly/abstracts/AbstractView.asp?AbstractID=47544) stated that "antibiotic treatment in patients with severe acne causes development of antibiotic resistance. . . . The prevalence of antibiotic resistance to tetracycline, erythromycin, clindamycin and trimethoprim-sulphamethoxazole . . ." was found after two to six months. "When patients with acne are treated with antibiotics, the risk of development of antibiotic resistance should be realized. The use of antibiotics to treat acne should be restricted and other regimens should be tested."

This means that if you have been taking an oral antibiotic to treat your acne for longer than six months it can stop being effective. This loss of effectiveness leaves many women puzzled when initially the antibiotic they were taking gave incredible results but then stopped working.

An even more serious argument against taking oral antibiotics was discussed in the *American Journal of Clinical Dermatology* (July-August 2000, pages 201–209), which stated: "At a time when there is global concern that antibiotic resistance rates in common bacterial pathogens may threaten our future ability to control bacterial infections, practices which promote the spread of antibiotic-resistant bacteria must be fully justified."

The decision to use oral antibiotics should not be taken lightly. The course of action you take should be discussed at length with and monitored by both you and your dermatologist.

BIRTH CONTROL PILLS FOR ACNE?

If you are a woman (sorry, guys) looking for a way to reduce breakouts, you might want to discuss your skin problems with your gynecologist instead of your dermatologist. The FDA has approved low-dosage birth control pills (Ortho Tri-Cyclen and generic norgestimate/ethinyl estradiol) for use in the treatment of acne. In Canada, Diane-35, a combination of cyproterone acetate and ethinyl estradiol is approved for the treatment of acne (source: *Skin Therapy Letter*, 1999, volume 4, number 4). Depending on your lifestyle and medical history, you could solve two problems with one prescription.

How does the birth control pill work on acne? Increased oil production can be caused by the body's androgen (male hormone) production, which can be highest just before menstruation starts. It appears that low-dosage birth control pills can decrease the presence of excess androgens, thereby decreasing breakouts. They work particularly well when used in conjunction with other therapies such as topical antibacterial agents or tretinoins (source: *Skin Therapy Letter*, February 2001, pages 1–3). For a lot of women this is no surprise. Many have noticed an improvement in their skin after they started taking birth control pills.

According to a double-blind, placebo-controlled study published in *Fertility and Sterility* (September 2001, pages 461–468), other "low-dose birth control pills can be an effective and safe treatment for moderate acne." The double-blind, placebo-controlled, randomized clinical trial found that the birth control pill containing levonorgestrel (Alesse) reduced the appearance of acne.

Low-dose oral contraceptives also result in a low occurrence of estrogen-related side effects like nausea, headaches, and breast tenderness, in addition to low, if any, weight gain (source: Medscape press release, September 7, 2001).

Is taking birth control pills to control acne right for you? There are risks associated with taking birth control pills, and these should be taken into account before you make a final decision. These risks include increased chances of heart attack, strokes, blood clots, and breast cancer (and these are compounded if you smoke), not to mention possible side effects such as vaginal bleeding, fluid retention, melasma (dark-brown skin patches), and depression. All that may not be a worthwhile trade-off for clear skin. But if you are already considering or using the pill for birth control, this remedy may be worth looking into.

ACCUTANE

Looking back, my only regret is that I waited so long. I tried. I really tried. I patiently waited for my skin to clear up. Spent untold dollars on dermatologists and followed their instructions. Diligently wiped antibiotic lotions over my face and took oral antibiotics for years. Exfoliated with baking soda, faithfully used Retin-A, and slathered on sulfur masks. I used milk of magnesia masks twice a week, and sometimes wore it under my makeup to soak up oil during the day. For most of that time my skin did improve, but it never really stopped breaking out and I still had to put up with oily, wet-looking skin. Besides, despite the improvement I saw from using antibiotics and the other treatments, I didn't want to stay on them forever. Adapting to the antibiotics was a risk I wasn't willing to continue taking. Who knew how much longer I would continue breaking out? It had been going on since I was 11, and by then I was 38.

I had known about Accutane for a long time. I knew it had some pretty serious, even dangerous, side effects, and that most dermatologists didn't prescribe it very often, and then only in the most serious cases. My acne and oily skin were serious to me, but not as bad as the pictures I had seen of the cystic acne cases that responded brilliantly to treatment with Accutane. Then, in 1990, a woman I worked with and two of her friends started taking Accutane, and they not only lived through it, their skin looked flawless. More than flawless—radiant (at least in comparison to what it looked like before).

"Considered the biggest breakthrough in acne drug treatment over the last 20 years, Accutane is the only drug that has the potential to clear severe acne permanently after one course of treatment" (source: *FDA Consumer* magazine, March-April 2001, http://www.fda.gov).

I was convinced that I needed to research the topic for my newsletter, *Cosmetics Counter Update*. What a remarkable decision that turned out to be. A dermatologist I had heard about at my health cooperative, Group Health in Seattle, Washington, told me it was possible, in fact, highly probable, that I could have clear skin for the rest of my life if I took Accutane. I told him I had heard controversial things about Accutane and was hesitant to try yet another prescription drug for my acne.

And this one sounded even more serious than antibiotics. He responded with a fascinating saga.

Accutane (its generic name is isotretinoin) is a drug derived from vitamin A, and is taken orally. It essentially stops the oil production in your sebaceous glands (the oil-producing structures of the skin) and literally shrinks these glands to the size of a baby's. This prevents sebum (oil) from clogging the hair follicle, mixing with dead skin cells, rupturing the follicle wall, and creating pimples or cysts. Normal oil production resumes when treatment is completed and the sebaceous glands slowly begin to grow larger again, but never (or at least rarely) as large as they were before treatment.

"Because of its relatively rapid onset of action and its high efficacy with reducing more than 90% of the most severe inflammatory lesions, Accutane has a role as an effective treatment in patients with severe acne that is recalcitrant to other therapies" (source: *Journal of the American Academy of Dermatology*, November 2001, Supplemental, pages 188–194).

In a large percentage of patients who complete a four- to six-month treatment with Accutane, acne is no longer considered to be clinically significant. In other words, for all intents and purposes, *their acne is cured*! Does this mean if you take it you'll never break out again? You may once in a while, but an occasional pimple here and there is hardly anyone's definition of acne. Especially anyone who, on a daily basis, had numerous breakouts, lots of blackheads, and oily skin.

The remaining percentage of patients who take Accutane do experience recurrences. For this group, when the breakouts return, typically three to six months after treatment, they are often milder and easier to treat, and can on occasion be cured with a second or third treatment with Accutane. Of course, there is a percentage that receive no benefit from taking Accutane, no matter how many treatments they take.

By the way, dosage and duration depend on the severity of the patient's acne, but treatments generally last sixteen weeks. If a second treatment is necessary, an eight-week rest period is required between treatments. Interestingly, acne continues to improve even after the course of treatment is completed, although doctors do not know exactly why.

[Accutane] is the treatment of choice for severe nodulocystic acne. It represents the sole agent that effectively addresses all of the pathophysiological factors in the production of acne" (source: *Seminars in Cutaneous Medical Surgery*, September 2001, pages 162–165).

So what's the catch with this "miracle" drug and why don't doctors prescribe it to everyone? Accutane is controversial for many reasons, but principally because of its most insidious side effect: It has been proven to cause severe birth defects in nearly 90% of the babies born to women who were pregnant while taking it. Before physicians knew about this alarming hazard, when it was first prescribed in France back in the 1970s before enough research had been conducted to establish its safety, more than 800 babies out of 1,000 births were born seriously deformed. The only way to avoid this risk is to abstain from sex during treatment or, according to the information provided with every prescription, to use a minimum of two forms of birth control. If you are taking a birth control pill, you still need to use a condom or diaphragm. You will need to discuss with your physician how long to continue using the extra birth control precautions after you are done taking Accutane. Generally, Accutane's effects do not last very long once you stop taking it.

If you *aren't* pregnant, are there still risks? Absolutely. Commonly reported, although temporary, side effects of Accutane include dry skin and lips, mild nosebleeds (your nose can get really dry for the first few days), hair loss (I lost a small amount of hair that grew back when I finished the four months of treatment), aches and pains, itching, rash, fragile skin, increased sensitivity to the sun, headaches (mild to severe—mine were fairly mild), and peeling palms and hands.

A study in the *Journal of Cutaneous Medical Surgery* (April 2000, pages 66–70) followed 124 people through their course of treatment with Accutane. "The majority of patients experienced persistent dryness of lips. Dry eyes affected 40% of patients; this continued throughout treatment in 25%. Contact lens wearers were more likely to develop conjunctivitis. Lower back pain was reported early in about 30% of patients and fewer than 10% of patients would develop it later in the course of treatment. Joint pain was noted in 16.5% of patients at the first visit and there was little change with ongoing treatment. Hair loss was experienced in a small percentage but was rarely noted on more than one occasion. Headaches occurred in less than 10% and were occasionally severe, but most often intermittent and recorded at a single visit. Depression occurred in 4% of patients and tended to persist throughout the treatment. All these patients completed the full course of treatment." The study concluded that "patients treated with [Accutane] experienced a predictable series of side effects. Some occurred fleetingly, but several persisted for the duration of treatment."

More serious, although much less common, side effects include severe headaches, nausea, vomiting, blurred vision, changes in mood, depression (discussed more in this chapter), severe stomach pain, diarrhea, decreased night vision, bowel problems, persistent dryness of eyes, calcium deposits in tendons (doctors don't know yet whether this is significant), an increase in cholesterol levels, and yellowing of the skin.

Understandably, many people, doctors included, are scared off by these side effects, above and beyond the risk to pregnant women. That's why dermatologists recommend Accutane only to patients with chronic acne (large, recurring cysts or blemishes that can permanently distort the shape and appearance of the skin), or sometimes to people with less-severe acne that has not responded successfully to other forms of treatment. Many doctors won't prescribe Accutane at all.

Although the high risk of birth defects and the other side effects should be taken seriously, it seems a shame that Accutane has been kept away from many acne patients. It is the most effective, short-term drug for acne available today. All other acne treatments require ongoing, tenacious adherence to the program and they don't offer a cure. The public is largely misinformed about Accutane's potential dangers as well as its potential benefit. Many doctors believe that if it weren't for the proven risk of birth defects, Accutane would be prescribed almost as frequently as antibiotics. Not surprisingly, it is prescribed much more frequently to men.

Given what I have learned, I wish somebody had told me about Accutane 20 years ago! It would have saved me a lot of time, money, and heartache. Although oral and topical antibiotics, exfoliants, gentle cleansing, staying away from products that aggravate breakouts, and using milk of magnesia to absorb excess oil can work successfully for lots of people, for many people the question remains, "When will I outgrow acne and how long will I have to struggle with the pain of breakouts?" Sadly, there is no telling if you're *ever* going to outgrow it. People who don't outgrow it, and lots of women don't, are looking at years of applying topical solutions and taking oral antibiotics that sometimes work well and sometimes don't.

ACCUTANE PREGNANCY WARNINGS IGNORED

Despite warnings and information regarding Accutane's detrimental effect on fetuses, women are still becoming pregnant while taking it. According to an August 17, 2001, FDA press release, the Centers for

Disease Control and Prevention (CDC) reported that "despite prevention efforts some women who take Accutane, a prescription medication given for severe acne and known to cause birth defects, still become pregnant while on this medication." The CDC also reported that a symbol intended to remind women that they must not get pregnant while taking these medications is commonly misinterpreted. The two studies, "Continued Occurrence of Accutane-Exposed Pregnancies" and "Interpretations of a Teratogen Warning Symbol," were published in *Teratology* (2001, volume 64, issue 3, pages 142–147 and 148–153). (Teratogen refers to a substance or process that causes developmental malformations and birth defects.) Both of these studies indicate that there are serious problems related to women either not understanding or not being fully informed about the risks of becoming pregnant while taking Accutane.

The press release went on to say that "since 1988, the CDC and the Food and Drug Administration (FDA) have worked closely to help educate health care providers and women of reproductive age who may be prescribed Accutane. The devastating birth defects caused by Accutane include: brain defects, heart defects, and facial defects such as babies born without ears." Women who want to take Accutane are supposed to have two negative pregnancy tests before beginning the medication, use two forms of effective birth control during treatment, and have repeat pregnancy tests every month during the course of medication. It turns out that many women do not follow these recommendations. Moreover, many doctors do not inform their patients that this is required despite the fact that more women are taking Accutane for their acne than ever before.

In response, the FDA has established new restrictions designed to prevent women from becoming pregnant while they are taking Accutane. According to the FDA, the new requirements for being allowed to take Accutane, or for a doctor's ability to prescribe the drug, will include mandatory monthly pregnancy tests. Pharmacists will be allowed to fill only a one-month supply at a time, requiring proof of a negative pregnancy test from the patient. Physicians will have to place an "Accutane Qualification Sticker" on their prescriptions to establish that the patient has had a negative pregnancy test.

You can find more information about the CDC's work on Accutane and birth defects at http://www.cdc.gov/ncbddd/bd/accutane.htm. For more information about the FDA's review of Accutane and birth defects, please see http://www.fda.gov/cder/drug/infopage/accutane/default.htm.

DEPRESSION FROM ACCUTANE

According to an article in the *Journal of the American Academy of Dermatology* (October 2001, pages 515–519), "The Food and Drug Administration (FDA) has received reports of depression and suicide in patients treated with [Accutane]. . . . From 1982 to May 2000 the FDA received reports of 37 U.S. patients treated with [Accutane] who committed suicide; 110 who were hospitalized for depression, suicidal ideation, or suicide attempt; and 284 with nonhospitalized depression, for a total of 431 patients. Factors suggesting a possible association between [Accutane] and depression include a [limited time] association between use of the drug and depression. . . . Compared with all drugs in the FDA's Adverse Event Reporting System database to June 2000, [Accutane] ranked within the top 10 for number of reports of depression and suicide attempt."

In contrast to this report, a paper presented at the 59th Annual Meeting of the American Academy of Dermatology (March 27, 2001, Washington, DC) stated that "up to the current time, a rate of 12 suicides per 8 million isotretinoin-treated patients has been documented. Half of these patients were on concomitant [other] medications. A small number of patients have reported that depression subsided when isotretinoin was withdrawn and recurred with treatment resumption. In the United States, 64 suicides occurred between 1991 and 1999 in patients who at one time took isotretinoin. Thirty occurred during treatment, 24 after treatment was stopped (6 months–10 years), and 10 occurred in patients whose treatment status was unknown.

"These numbers must be compared with general suicide statistics in the United States. In total, 30,000 suicides occur per year (in the general population, the rate is 11.4 per 100,000). Eighty percent are males. Suicide is the third leading cause of death in the 15- to 24-year age group (6000 per year). So when isotretinoin patients are observed, the 64 total suicides must be compared with an expected suicide rate of more than 10 times that number (670). These data suggest that in these patients the suicides were likely due to factors other than isotretinoin treatment. The isotretinoin suicide rate of 1.8 per 100,000 is well below that of the general population, as noted above. In addition, in the isotretinoin patients, there was no alteration in the typical U.S. pattern of suicide in terms of gender distribution, relationship to depression, underlying psychiatric disorders, or lack of warning signs (typical of youth suicide)."

Despite the controversy, Hoffman-La Roche, the makers of Accutane, is adding a warning about depression to the product information insert. Hoffman-La Roche is also removing copy from their ads that suggests Accutane can relieve the "psychological trauma" and "emotional suffering" associated with acne. The lengthy package insert for Accutane did include warnings about depression but not about possible suicide or psychosis.

As is true with any medication, all the pros and cons must be considered before starting treatment. If you or the teen you are responsible for already have a history of depression, then the potential for exacerbated depression must be taken into account and discussed with your physician.

HANDLING THE SIDE EFFECTS OF ACCUTANE

How do you deal with some of the side effects when taking Accutane? It helps to be prepared. If you take Accutane, stay out of the sun! This drug makes the skin photosensitive even if you are wearing sunscreen (and you must wear sunscreen). Any prolonged sun exposure can cause severe redness and fever. Treat dry areas of the face with a moisturizer. If your nose becomes dry, apply a thin layer of petroleum jelly on the skin inside the nose, and do it frequently. That will make a big difference. Do not use any skin-care products that can cause irritation or dryness. Avoid bar soaps, washcloths, AHA and BHA products, scrubs, hot water, and facial masks. If you are using tretinoin, Differin, azelaic acid, or topical antibiotics, I suggest you stop using them unless your doctor recommends that you continue. Dry eyes can be treated with artificial teardrops; do not use products like Visine that simply constrict blood flow and can dry out the eyes even more. Headaches and body aches are eased quite nicely with ibuprofen. Be sure to drink plenty of water. If you have any concerns, discuss them at once with your physician.

Pay attention to your mood. If you find yourself feeling excessively depressed, hostile, angry, or have even a fleeting thought of suicide speak to your doctor immediately. It is also essential for your doctor to monitor your blood. Cholesterol can shoot up dangerously high and liver function must be monitored. It is extremely important that you stay in close contact with your physician during the entire time you are taking Accutane.

HORMONE BLOCKERS FOR ACNE?

Using a testosterone-blocking drug to reduce the hormone levels responsible for activating oil production is controversial; it's also an approach to treating acne and oily skin that is not very well-researched. The most frequently prescribed hormone blocker is known as spironolactone (brand name Aldactone). It is an option only for women, however, because without testosterone men start to develop female characteristics such as enlarged breasts and softer skin. But because testosterone can be one of the primary causes of acne, curtailing its presence in the body may have positive results—namely, acne clears up and oil production slows.

What kind of results can you expect? A study described in the *Journal of the American Academy of Dermatology* (September 2000, pages 498–502) looked at " . . . 85 women with acne treated consecutively with spironolactone. . . . Results: Clearing of acne occurred in 33% of patients treated with low doses of spironolactone; 33% had marked improvement, 27.4% showed partial improvement, and 7% showed no improvement. The treatment regimen was well-tolerated, with 57.5% reporting no adverse effects." Another study, reported in the *Archives of Dermatology* (September 1998, volume 134, number 9) reviewed " . . . 38 patients: 4 with severe acne (with cystic lesions), 32 with moderate acne, and 2 with mild acne. Improvement in acne, defined as a lessening in severity of acne classification, was observed in 32 (97%) of 33 patients who continued to follow up while receiving therapy. Of the 32 patients with improvement in their acne, all 4 patients with severe acne improved to moderate acne, 26 of 27 patients with moderate acne improved to mild acne and in 2 of those the acne disappeared, and both patients with mild acne experienced complete resolution. One patient had no improvement in her acne."

While those statistics aren't exciting, they may be of interest for women who have not responded well to other treatments. But the side effects of Aldactone are as daunting as those for Accutane. The list of adverse effects include abdominal cramping, nausea, diarrhea, headache, reduced sexual drive (libido), dry mouth, excessive thirst, unusual tiredness, unusual muscle weakness, skin rash, deepening of voice, irregular or no menstrual periods, and slowed heart rate, plus enlarged breasts in men, and breast tenderness in women.

Moreover, hormone blockers require long-term use to effectively treat acne. When you stop taking them, the testosterone returns and so can the acne. Because hormone blockers require repetitive, continuous use, at least for treating acne, I strongly recommend trying Accutane before trying hormone blockers. Although Accutane's side effects can be more serious than those of the hormone-blocking drugs, use of Accutane is very short term, involving only a few months, and it can be a permanent cure.

WHAT ABOUT ORAL SUPPLEMENTS FOR ACNE?

Very little, if any, research points to vitamins, herbs, or minerals of any kind or in any combination as having an effect on breakouts. What little research does exist shows zinc to be a valid option to consider. A handful of studies have compared oral antibiotics to zinc, with zinc showing some benefit. A study reported in *Dermatology* (2001, volume, 203, issue 2, page 40) evaluated "the place of zinc gluconate in relation to antibiotics in the treatment of acne vulgaris. Zinc was compared to minocycline [an antibiotic] in a multicenter randomized double-blind trial. 332 patients received either 30 milligrams elemental zinc or 100 milligrams minocycline over 3 months. The primary endpoint was defined as the percentage of the clinical success rate on day 90." The study concluded that "minocycline and zinc gluconate are both effective in the treatment of inflammatory acne, but minocycline has a superior effect evaluated to be 17% in our study."

In conjunction with other treatments, zinc may prove to have even better results. But zinc is not a benign supplement. High doses of zinc can be toxic. Avoid taking more than 100 mg of zinc per day from a supplement (source: http://www.drweil.com). It is also recommended that you take a daily multivitamin because increased levels of zinc mean that the body requires more copper and manganese.

Of course, zinc is not a cure-all for your acne, and it probably works best in tandem with other, topical agents.

Pantothenic acid (vitamin B_5) is touted as being effective for acne. However, there is only one study supporting this notion and it dates from the early 1980s (source: *International Journal of Dermatology*, 1981, volume 20, pages 278–285). There is no current research showing this to be an effective treatment.

Vitamin A is another oral supplement thought to be helpful for acne. In one study, showing it to have a positive impact, the participants were given 300,000 IU per day. Considering that the usual recommended daily amount is 10,000 IU, the 300,000 IU is a large enough amount of vitamin A to be possibly toxic and is not recommended.

At this time there is no reliable research pointing to any oral supplement other than zinc as being helpful in the treatment of acne.

FACIAL MASKS FOR BLEMISHES

Some facial masks, particularly masks that are part of a skin-care routine for acne, contain sulfur, which can have some benefit as a disinfectant for breakouts. However, it is an unnecessary (compared to other options) and fairly strong substance to use to disinfect the skin, especially when you leave it sitting on your face in a facial mask for a period of time. There are gentler ways to disinfect the skin. Sulfur has pretty much been abandoned as an option for treating breakouts since the 1980s, given the other successful and less irritating topical choices available.

Masks are a poor choice for dealing with blemishes anyway, because when breakouts are the problem, the bacteria that cause the eruptions must be killed daily or even twice daily, depending on the severity of the problem. Sulfur masks are usually applied too sporadically to effectively prevent breakouts.

For someone with oily skin, I recommend a mask of plain milk of magnesia (no mint or cherry flavors, please), the kind you buy at the drugstore for an upset stomach. Milk of magnesia is just liquid magnesium. Magnesium, like clay, is an earth mineral, but, unlike clay, magnesium has some disinfecting and anti-inflammatory properties and can absorb more oil for its molecular weight than clay can. Clay masks are an option as long as they contain no additional ingredients that can cause irritation.

REMOVING BLEMISHES

This isn't a pretty topic, but it is a fact of life and human nature that just leaving a blemish or blackhead alone is almost impossible. Fortunately, gently removing a blackhead or blemish with light-handed squeezing can actually help the skin. Removing the stuff inside a blackhead or especially a pimple relieves the pressure and reduces further damage. Yes, squeezing can be detrimental to the skin, but it's the way you squeeze that determines whether you inflict harm. If you oversqueeze, pinch the skin, scrape the skin with your nails, or press too hard, you are absolutely doing more damage than good. Gentle is the operative word and, when done right, squeezing with minimal pressure is the best (if not the only) way to clean out a blackhead or blemish.

Although I never recommend steaming the face (heat can overstimulate oil production, cause spider veins to surface, and create irritation), a tepid to slightly warm compress over the face can help soften the blackhead or blemish, making it easier to remove. First, wash your face with a water-soluble cleanser, pat the skin dry, then place a slightly warm, wet cloth over your face for approximately ten to fifteen minutes. Once that's done, pat the skin dry again. Using a tissue over each finger to keep you from slipping and tearing the skin, apply even, soft pressure to the sides of the blemish area, gently pressing down and then up around the lesion. Do this once or twice only. If nothing happens, that means the blemish cannot be removed, and continuing will bruise the skin, risk making the infection or lesion worse, and cause scarring. Again, only use gentle pressure, protect your skin by using tissue around your fingers, and do not oversqueeze.

Be sure to use a 2.5% benzoyl peroxide solution after you're done, and if you wish you can follow up with a facial mask of plain milk of magnesia to soothe the skin and reduce inflammation. Do not remove blackheads or blemishes more than once or twice a week or you can cause too much irritation.

WHAT ABOUT PORE STRIPS?

Pore strips in all their varying incarnations are meant to remove blackheads. You place a piece of cloth with a sticky substance on it over your face, as you might do with a Band-Aid, wait a bit for it to dry, and then rip it off. Along with some amount of skin, blackheads are supposed to stick to it and come right out of your nose. There is nothing miraculous about these products, nor do they work all that well. The main ingredient on these strips is a hairspray-type ingredient. If the instructions are followed closely you can see some benefit in removing the very surface of a blackhead. In fact, you may at first be very impressed with what comes off your nose.

Unfortunately, that leaves the majority of the problem deep in the pore. What has me most concerned about pore strips is they are accompanied by a strong warning not to use them over any area other than the intended area (nose, chin, or forehead) and not to use them over inflamed, swollen, sunburned, or excessively dry skin. It also states that if the strip is too painful to remove, you should wet it and then carefully remove it. What a warning!

Also, despite the warning on the package, I suspect most women will try these strips wherever they see breakouts. If I didn't know better, I know I would. The way these strips adhere, they can absolutely injure or tear skin. They are especially unsafe if you've been using Retin-A, Renova, Differin, AHAs, or BHA; having facial peels; taking Accutane; or if you have naturally thin skin or any skin disorder such as rosacea, psoriasis, or seborrhea.

YOU STILL NEED SUNSCREEN

There is no way around it: Even if you are battling blemishes, you still need to minimize sun damage by using an effective sunscreen. In fact, it's especially important because, as part of that battle, you should be exfoliating the skin, which can make it more susceptible to the sun's rays.

Unfortunately, the last thing someone with oily skin needs is another product on her skin. Most sunscreens, even those that claim to be oil-free, contain ingredients that can cause blemish flare-ups. The few sunscreens that are indeed lighter-weight tend to be alcohol-based, posing new problems, because alcohol can be an irritant. Plus the sunscreen ingredients themselves can cause breakouts, particularly so-called non-chemical sunscreens, which contain titanium dioxide or zinc oxide. Even though titanium dioxide and zinc oxide are superior sunscreen agents, doing their work with little to no risk of irritation, they are occlusive and can clog pores. Other types of synthetic sunscreen ingredients can cause irritation and also result in breakouts. So you're between a rock and a hard place. Yet you still need sunscreen. In my opinion, the best option in this situation is to wear a foundation with a reliable SPF (preferably SPF 15) that uses either avobenzone, titanium dioxide, or zinc oxide as one of the active ingredients.

A foundation that contains sunscreen is less of a problem than moisturizers when it comes to causing breakouts, regardless of the ingredients. Foundations are designed to stay on top of the skin, rather than be absorbed. Additionally, it means using one product instead of two, if you were going to wear a foundation anyway. The fewer products you put on your skin, the better, and this is doubly true for someone afflicted with breakouts or oily skin. And please, if you do choose to wear a foundation that contains sunscreen, don't forget that the other parts of your body that are exposed to sun during the day need sunscreen, too.

The bottom line: It takes experimentation and diligence to find a comfortable sunscreen for any skin type, but even more so for someone with oily skin and a tendency toward breakouts.

BATTLE PLANS FOR FIGHTING BLEMISHES

The following battle plans are presented in order, starting with the most commonly available products with the least potential for side effects such as irritation, and working up to stronger products, some available only by prescription. The first battle plan may be all you need to help your skin. As you see how your skin responds, you can experiment with the various options for each category. **The most important element for all these skin-care battle plans is consistency. It takes a minimum of three weeks to six months to see a consistent improvement in your skin.** Remember that spot treatment doesn't work. You have to maintain consistent gentle cleansing, exfoliation, disinfecting, and reduced oil production to change the way your skin behaves.

If irritation or skin sensitivity occurs, you may need to cut back on the exfoliant, disinfectant, and/or facial mask you are using. That doesn't mean the skin-care routine isn't working for you (or that it won't eventually work), but perhaps your skin can't handle the frequency of application, at least not in the beginning. In that case you may need to reduce how often you apply the AHA, Retin-A, or Differin from twice a day to once a day or every other day, and the same is true with the disinfectant and facial mask.

Note: The following plans include the types of products needed to gently cleanse (without further clogging pores or increasing the presence of bacteria), exfoliate, and then disinfect. (The products are not presented in the order in which you'd apply them.)

Plan A. Gentle cleanser; 1% or 2% salicylic acid—exfoliant; 2.5%, 5%, or 10% benzoyl peroxide—disinfectant; and milk of magnesia—facial mask.

Plan B. Gentle cleanser; 8% or 10% AHA—for those who can't use salicylic acid for exfoliation; 2.5% or 5% benzoyl peroxide—disinfectant; and milk of magnesia—facial mask.

Plan C. Gentle cleanser; 1% or 2% salicylic acid—exfoliant; tretinoin (Retin-A, Tazorac, or Avita) or Differin in the evening; 2.5%, 5%, or 10% benzoyl peroxide—disinfectant, in the morning (do not apply at the same time the Retin-A, Tazorac or Avita is applied); and a milk of magnesia facial mask.

Plan D. Gentle cleanser; azelaic acid—antibacterial and exfoliant; and a milk of magnesia facial mask.

Plan E. Gentle cleanser; tretinoin (Retin-A, Tazorac, Avita), Differin, or azelaic acid; a topical prescription antibacterial; and a milk of magnesia facial mask.

Plan F. Gentle cleanser; tretinoin (Retin-A, Tazorac, Avita), Differin, or azelaic acid; a topical prescription antibacterial; oral antibiotic; and a milk of magnesia facial mask. (**Please note:** Oral antibiotics can eventually result in development of resistant acne bacteria and are therefore best considered as short-term treatment.)

Plan G. When all else fails, Accutane.

BATTLING BLACKHEADS AND LARGE PORES

I understand the frustration of battling blackheads. Insidious and glaring, blackheads make skin look mottled and unclean. The truth about blackheads (usually accompanied by oily skin) and whiteheads (usually accompanied by dry skin) is hard to accept. What is the truth? The truth is they are just hard to get rid of. It is hard to win the battle against clogged pores! However, because there are only a handful of options for dealing with this annoying skin malady, it's relatively simple to explain.

Pores that are functioning normally produce a normal amount of sebum (oil) and easily distribute the oil to the surface of skin. Hormones, almost exclusively, regulate the amount of sebum production. When a normal amount of oil is produced it moves effortlessly through the pore and out onto the surface of skin, where it melts into an imperceptible film that forms a protective barrier over the face.

Hormones can cause too much oil to be produced, or skin cells can block the exit path of the oil, or, when you have pores that are malformed, the oil in the pore can get clogged, and then blackheads or whiteheads form. Further exacerbating these conditions is the buildup in the pore of skin-care or makeup products—mixed in with skin cells, they can get trapped in the sticky sebum sitting in the pore. When sebum and skin cells sit in a pore that is not covered over by skin, they are exposed to air, which causes the sebum and skin cells to oxidize and turn black. If the sebum and skin cells are sitting in a pore that is covered by skin, they are not exposed to air and remain clear, forming a slight white bump under the skin.

What's behind all this is primarily a genetic predisposition accompanied by the conditions mentioned above randomly occurring in any one of the thousands of pores we have on our face. Not to mention unknown reactions to the over 50,000 cosmetic ingredients we may come in contact with from products we use.

To clear up the confusion, the following are battle plans against blackheads and whiteheads, because with some effort they can be reduced, and, depending on how your skin reacts, maybe even reduced a lot.

Other than avoiding products that are too emollient (meaning thick or greasy creams) and not using moisturizers when you don't need them, there are really only four essentials for dealing with whiteheads and blackheads.

1. **Gentle, water-soluble cleansers** (and avoiding bar soap). The ingredients that keep bar soap in its bar form can clog pores, and irritation can cause skin cells to flake off before they're ready and accumulate in the pore. It's actually getting harder and harder to find a cleanser that isn't gentle. Be careful of cleansers that are too emollient and leave a greasy film on the skin, which can cause further problems.

2. **Gentle exfoliants** that can both remove the excess skin cells on the surface of the face (so they don't build up in the pore) and exfoliate inside the pore (to improve the shape of the pore, allowing a more even flow of oil through it). Keep in mind that the inside structure of the pore itself is lined with skin cells that can build up, creating a narrowed shape that doesn't allow natural oil flow. But don't get carried away with this step. Removing too many skin cells (overdoing it) can cause problems and hurt skin. Exfoliation is essential for both dry and oily skin when you are trying to eliminate blackheads or whiteheads. The only difference is that someone with dry skin will want an exfoliant that has a more moisturizing base. The best option for exfoliating skin both within the pore and on the surface of the skin is a salicylic acid (beta hydroxy acid—BHA) lotion, gel, or liquid. Salicylic acid can

penetrate the pore to help improve the shape of the pore lining, allowing an unobstructed path of oil flow.

3. **Absorbing excess oil.** This step is more for those with oily skin. It's really not an option for those with whiteheads (milia) and dry skin because with milia the problem is more due to trapped oil than it is to excess oil. For those with oily skin, you all know I prefer milk of magnesia (a few companies, including mine, have cosmetic versions of this). Clay masks are an option as long as they don't contain other ingredients that are irritating. The handful of silicone-based oil-absorbing products meant to be worn under makeup, from companies like Lancôme and Clinique, get mixed reviews from women but are worth a trial run.

4. **Improving cell production** can help the pore function more normally. Effective considerations for all skin types are tretinoins (Retin-A, Tazorac, Avita, Renova), Differin, and azelaic acid. These can be used by themselves or with a BHA product. Research has definitely established that Retin-A, Renova, and Differin have positive effects on how pores function, and these products should be considered for very stubborn cases or when blackheads are accompanied by breakouts.

For those with oily-skin troubles, certain low-dose birth control pills may be an option to reduce the hormone levels that create the excess oil that is at the root of the problem. And, when all else fails, Accutane can be considered. Be aware that many doctors are reluctant to prescribe Accutane for "merely" oily skin and blackheads. The fact is, for those with that kind of persistent skin problem it does not feel like a "mere" problem in the least, and Accutane can be a cure.

Blackheads can be made to seem less noticeable with pore strips, but only when the instructions on the box are followed exactly and they are not overused. Pore strips do not affect pore function.

For all skin types, AHA peels, microdermabrasion, and laser resurfacing can significantly affect the appearance of blackheads and whiteheads; however, they don't necessarily improve pore functioning (it depends on the depth of the treatment); rather, they temporarily get rid of the surface problem, making your skin look better.

Topical disinfectants (such as benzoyl peroxide) or topical antibiotics available by prescription are unwarranted and would be wasted in the treatment of blackheads and milia because bacteria are not involved in these conditions.

WHAT ABOUT EMPTY, ENLARGED PORES?

Once a pore is emptied and the unsightly blackhead is removed it can take a period of time for the pore to heal and close up. Maintaining the regimen of gentle cleansing, exfoliating, and absorbing oil can go a long way toward making this happen. If your skin can tolerate Retin-A, Renova, or Differin, these products can help promote healing by further improving cell production in the pore. However, even after all this, an empty, open, but permanently damaged, pore can be an unattractive, left-over by-product of the original problem. If you have patiently adhered to all the "right" steps, there is very little else that can be done to change the damage. Time will tell if the effects of improving pore function can shrink a pore, but it does take time, and not everyone will have the same results. Microdermabrasion, AHA or BHA peels, and laser resurfacing can improve the appearance of pores, but these are considered tempo-rary fixes and are not noted for actually changing or correcting the problem. Most likely the improvement is caused by the skin's swelling which makes the pores look smaller. Again, it is hard to determine suc-cess rates because there are no published results from long-term studies available.

The struggle to cover up large pores is nothing less than maddening. The very nature of a depression in the skin makes it difficult, if not im-possible, to keep the indentation from showing. Especially if your skin is still oily, and even if you use an extremely matte foundation, such as Revlon's Skin Mattifying Makeup or regular ColorStay, Lancôme's Teint Idole, or Estée Lauder's Double Wear or Double Matte, the oil can still cause some shifting, creating a look of pooled foundation in the pore.

I apologize for sounding dismal about this, but when there are limita-tions in the skin *and* in the world of makeup, searching for better options or alternatives can waste money and only increase your frustration. Here is a game plan to tackle the problem. It isn't foolproof and it won't work for everyone, but these are the best options available.

1. Avoid moisturizer over the open-pore areas of the face before applying makeup—even if you have dry skin. Any extra "slip" on the skin will cause makeup to pool in the pore. If the skin is dry and flaky, be more diligent in the evening about treating your skin. Then in the morning use a toner with water-binding agents that can help soothe skin and reduce any dry feeling, yet not add anything that can make skin feel

slippery. That means it is essential that your foundation contain your sunscreen, because an additional sunscreen under the foundation will almost certainly cause slippage.

2. Do use a matte or ultra-matte foundation. Even if you have dry skin, these stay on far better than other foundations, are somewhat impervious to oil production, and, therefore, prevent the foundation from slipping into the pore.

3. Consider wearing a tiny amount of milk of magnesia under your foundation over the open-pore area. This is a bit like applying spackle that has minimal to no movement. It can absorb oil at the same time and the foundation glides over it, creating an even surface. This works better under matte foundations than under ultra-matte foundations.

4. For more stubborn problems, touch up your makeup several times during the day with oil-blotting papers. Then dust the face with a pressed powder designed to be worn as a foundation. Pressed powder foundations apply a slightly thicker layer of powder than normal pressed powders do, and can better hide the pore. But do this only with a brush; never use a sponge or pad to apply powder because they can place way too much product on the face, making things look cakey and thick.

chapter *10*

BATTLE PLANS FOR WOUNDS AND SCARS

HOW SKIN HEALS

Whether it is a paper cut, scratch, cut, sore, lesion, or a really bad wound that requires stitches, one of the more amazing aspects of skin is its capacity to heal. Damaged skin regenerates and repairs itself. Only in certain circumstances, usually a result of some illness such as diabetes, is that not true. When skin is injured, a multifaceted, complicated number of reactions take place. Many factors affect how long a wound takes to heal, and the way the wound heals affects how the skin will look, meaning what kind of scar will result. And that's not to say a scar is a bad thing—rather it's a sign that the body's repair system has kicked in so the fissure in your skin, no matter how small or big, closes up and mends.

Basically, skin goes through three fundamental and essential stages of repair. In the first stage, the scab is formed, and it's almost always accompanied by swelling, redness, and some tenderness or even pain. During the next stage, new skin tissue is formed under the scab. The final stage involves the rebuilding and reforming of the outer and inner layers of skin. Each of these stages of skin repair needs different kinds of help to aid in the healing process. What you do during the first days of a wound versus what you do after the scab has formed, or when the scab eventually comes off, is vital to the final appearance of the skin.

Stage 1, Inflammation. As soon as a cut or break in the skin has occurred, the body begins its job of preventing further injury. Signals are sent out for the blood to begin clotting and to call skin cells in to start protecting the damaged area. While the skin is working on its initial repair response, the immune system is trying to remove any foreign matter or bacteria that may have invaded the injury.

Stage 2, Regrowth. Now the body is busy producing collagen and reforming the substances that constitute the intercellular matrix. Intense collagen growth and the tightening of the surrounding tissue are the reason why we see an edge around a wound while a scab is being formed.

Stage 3, Renewal. With the inflammatory reaction calmed, and after the new skin tissue in the form of a scab and then a scar has been achieved during regrowth, it is time for the skin to focus on returning to normal. As time passes the scar becomes less noticeable, redness decreases, and the skin texture normalizes.

How your body goes about this process is genetically determined, but outside influences can also affect the way your skin responds to being injured.

WHAT TO DO WHEN YOUR SKIN IS INJURED

Does applying aloe, vitamin E, or a variety of marine plants from algae to seaweed help heal wounds, prevent scars, or reduce the scarring you already have? There's no single substance or product that can address the complex issue of wound healing and scars, but there is a battle plan you can follow to minimize scarring as much as possible. Although aloe and algae can't hurt a scar and may indeed be helpful, what is more important is the overall way you treat the wound from its beginning, when the skin is injured, to the end, when the scar has formed.

Skin's unique, but unfortunate, response to injury is scarring. But skin, almost miraculously, also regenerates quickly, essentially renewing itself in two to four weeks. Depending on your genetic makeup and the depth of the injury, scarring can range from a slightly reddish discoloration to a thick, raised red or darkened scar (described as hypertrophic or keloidal), to serious disfigurement. Even so, the way you initially take care of a wound makes all the difference in the world.

Whether it is from acne, getting cut, or an operation, when skin damage first occurs you should allow it to "breathe" as much as possible. Do not gunk up the area with creams, lotions, or vitamin E capsules.

Rubbing creams and lotions on a wound can damage fragile skin in the first stages of healing. Keep the damaged skin clean but don't overclean it; using a gentle cleanser is the best way to do this. If you suspect there is a risk of infection, consider using an over-the-counter antibacterial such as Bacitracin.

At this stage, a little pure aloe vera gel or a very sheer, lightweight moisturizing gel is just fine, but *little* is the operative word here. In the beginning, keep the injured site out of sunlight altogether, as opposed to loading up on sunscreen. Heavy creams will suffocate the skin and prevent it from healing. Once the wound is healed, keep it out of sunlight as much as possible; and when it's not possible, remember it's imperative to protect the area with sunscreen. Sun damages skin and doesn't promote healing. Smoking is a skin destroyer and will also prevent healthy healing of wounds.

Here's what to do when you have a wound.

1. Wounds or lesions that don't require immediate medical attention (that is, if the wound does not require stitches and is not a chronic nonhealing ulcer) should not be completely or heavily occluded when the damage first occurs (source: *Archives of Dermatological Research*, November 2001, pages 491–499). After cleansing, it is best to cover the wound with a light, thin bandage. In other words, avoid heavy bandages, creams, salves, or oils that can impair the skin's initial healing process. Depending on where the wound or lesion is, it can be OK to wear a very lightweight bandage during the day or very lightweight moisturizers to protect the skin from getting reinjured, but, if you don't have a lightweight bandage, take the coverings off at night or apply a lotion that lets air get to the wound.

2. Let a scab form and don't pick or touch it—ever! Any manipulation or removal is a serious impediment to the healing that is taking place underneath and can cause scarring that would otherwise not have taken place.

3. Do not soak the lesion in water. Too much moisture saturation prevents wound healing.

4. It is important to keep the wound clean to prevent infection. Using a gentle cleanser is essential. Topical Bacitracin is an option if you suspect a risk of infection, but use it minimally because it is very thick and occlusive and can prevent air from getting to the wound.

5. Do not irritate the skin! The skin's primary, natural reaction to a

wound is inflammation, which makes blood surge to the area to aid in healing. However, inflammation must be kept to a minimum and it should not be exacerbated because it can further damage skin. Anything you do to irritate the skin more makes matters worse. That means no soaps (they're too drying), no highly fragrant products (fragrant plant extracts and synthetic fragrances are all irritating), and, as always, no alcohol, peppermint, menthol, citrus, eucalyptus, clove, camphor, or mint.

6. Use sun protection! Leaving a wound unprotected to sun exposure impedes the skin's healing process *and* causes further skin damage.

7. If you do want to apply something soothing to the skin, use a very lightweight moisturizing lotion or pure aloe vera gel. Aloe's benefit for wound healing is mostly anecdotal; however, because aloe allows skin to breathe and can be soothing, it is still a great option to consider in the beginning. A moisturizer with antioxidants is the best way to help the wound continue healing.

AFTER THE WOUND HAS HEALED

After the wound has healed you can use slightly more emollient products with antioxidants to keep free-radical damage to a minimum. Sunscreens in a light moisturizing base are essential, not only to keep the skin moist, but also to allow the skin to continue healing. There is some evidence, although the relevant studies used small samplings, that AHAs and tretinoins (such as Retin-A, Renova, Tazorac, Avita, and generic tretinoin) can significantly reduce the appearance of scarring by exfoliating the surface skin (using AHAs) and by stimulating normal cell production (using tretinoin). Exfoliation can reduce the thick, discolored appearance of scar tissue. Tretinoins, over time, *may* help generate collagen production to possibly shore up some of what was lost from the injury.

Exfoliation, antioxidants, and sunscreens can all help minimize scarring after the skin has healed. None of them will get rid of a scar, but the possibility of reducing the appearance of a scar is not to be ignored. Basically, there are no miracle skin-care ingredients or products when it comes to healing skin or reducing the appearance of scars. Instead, practice good skin care: Don't overmanipulate the site, protect it from the sun, keep the area disinfected, keep heavy emollients off the skin, and, as much as possible, let the skin handle its own healing process.

As to nutritional issues, some of these definitely play a factor in healing wounds and scars. A list and description of oral supplements (i.e., systemic treatments) that have been shown to help heal wounds and scars is presented on the Web site http://www.drweil.com.

The following list describes topical factors for healing wounds and scars. The most important thing, both for healing a wound and trying to improve the scar's appearance, is patience. It can take up to two years—sometimes longer—depending on the depth of the lesion or wound, and it can depend on how diligent you are about caring for your skin with the following steps.

1. Once the skin has healed completely and the scab is gone, you can use nonfragrant plant oils or a lightweight moisturizer to keep the skin moist. The point here is to keep skin pliant and soft to help the skin's healing process (dry skin can fissure and tear, which can cause further skin damage). Topically applied vitamin E has not been shown to be of any special help in healing wounds or scars and may make matters worse.

2. Now that the skin is healed, it is helpful to remove the surface layers of skin where scar tissue may be forming. It is also helpful to improve skin-cell production, which may have been damaged from the wound (which is completely dependent on the depth of the lesion—meaning how many layers of skin were affected and how well you have left the scab alone). For gently removing the surface layers of skin, consider using an effective salicylic acid product (BHA is preferred over AHA because BHA is composed of salicylic acid, which has anti-inflammatory properties, and reducing or preventing inflammation is essential for the healing process) as well as tretinoin (Retin-A, Renova, Tazorac, Avita) for improving cell production.

3. Once the wound or lesion is completely healed (this can take several months or up to two years), there are several options for dealing with the resulting scar. For surface discolorations and minor irregularities, microdermabrasion is an option. Acid peels (including AHA peels or trichloroacetic acid peels) as well as laser resurfacing are also significant options for reducing or eliminating scars.

4. For a thickened, raised scar, silicone sheets are still a primary option. It is believed that both the silicone and the pressure from the sheets encourage hydration, softening, and compression of the scar. Keep in mind that the silicone sheets may need to be worn for prolonged pe-

riods of time to gain the best and most lasting results. For further explanation of this option, refer to "Silicone Sheets for Keloidal Scarring," below.

VITAMIN E FOR SCARS?

The simple answer to that question is, "Probably not." A report of research published in *Dermatologic Surgery* (April 1999, pages 311–315), in an article titled "The effects of topical vitamin E on the cosmetic appearance of scars" concluded that the " . . . study shows that there is no benefit to the cosmetic outcome of scars by applying vitamin E after skin surgery and that the application of topical vitamin E may actually be detrimental to the cosmetic appearance of a scar. In 90% of the cases in this study, topical vitamin E either had no effect on, or actually worsened, the cosmetic appearance of scars. Of the patients studied, 33% developed a contact dermatitis to the vitamin E. Therefore we conclude that use of topical vitamin E on surgical wounds should be discouraged." The study was done double-blind "with patients given two ointments each labeled A or B. A was Aquaphor, a regular emollient, and B was Aquaphor mixed with vitamin E. The scars were randomly divided into parts A and B. Patients were asked to put the A ointment on part A and the B ointment on part B twice daily for four weeks." Antioxidants are definitely an option for skin, but, for preventing scars, vitamin E directly applied on skin does not appear to be one of them.

SILICONE SHEETS FOR KELOIDAL SCARRING

Even though you've done all you can to help heal the skin, thicker raised keloidal scars can set in. One way to treat this kind of scarring is with a pliable sheet of silicone. Some examples of silicone sheets are ReJuveness *($39.50 to $95, depending on the size)*, Syprex Scar Sheet *($20 to $40 depending on the size)*, and Curad Scar Therapy Cosmetic Pads *($16.99)*. It is not clear how these sheets of silicone oil work. They may increase the amount of water in the scar, and continuous rehydration of scars may soften the tissue, making them more elastic and pliable, thus encouraging the flattening process (source: *European Journal of Dermatology*, December 1998, pages 591–595). But they do work, and rather successfully (although I use the word "successfully" with caution).

Silicone sheets appear to be most effective for hypertrophic or keloidal scarring. As wonderful as this sounds, there are disadvantages. Users purchase one relatively inexpensive sheet of silicone that is worn over and over again. The sheet must be kept clean, which requires care and maintenance time. The sheet must be worn over the scar for prolonged periods of time, so you might not want to wear one on your face or other exposed parts of your body, at least not during the day. Also, the silicone sheet can stick to the skin and skin reactions such as rashes or irritation can occur.

As mentioned, you must wear the sheet for long periods—for hours at a time, over a span of at least two to nine months—to see a difference. But patience pays off. The longer you wear it, the more likely it is that the scar will dissipate to some extent. Of course, these sheets work best over new scars, but they can make a difference with old ones, too. Even acne scarring—thick, raised scars, not pits—can be reduced if the scars have been present for less than sixteen years. As wonderful and hopeful as this all sounds, be aware that the word "reduce" is imprecise. Do not try these if you are hoping for extraordinary results, of the kind the advertising implies. Dr. Loren Engrav, associate director and Chief of Plastic Surgery for the University of Washington burn unit at Harborview Medical Center, explains that the "silicone strips are standard treatment for helping dissipate scars, and though the results may be good, they are absolutely not a miracle."

Some women buy silicone sheets to use over stretch marks, but there is no clinical evidence that this product will have any effect on them whatsoever. These sheets create a flattening process, while a raising process is what would be required for stretch marks.

LASERS FOR SCAR REPAIR

"A variety of lasers can be used to treat scars and stretch marks effectively. It is of paramount importance that the type of scar be properly classified on initial examination so that the most appropriate method of treatment can be chosen. Classification also allows the laser surgeon to discuss with the patient the anticipated response to treatment. The 585-nm pulsed dye laser (PDL) is the most appropriate system for treating . . . keloids, [red] scars, and stretch marks. The PDL carries a low risk of side effects and complications when operated at appropriate treatment parameters and time intervals. Atrophic scars are best treated with ablative CO_2 lasers and Er:YAG lasers; however, [growing or worsening] keloids and [deteriorating] scars should not be vaporized because of the high risk of scar recurrence or progression. The appropriate choice and use of lasers can significantly improve most scars. As research into laser-skin interaction continues, further refinements in laser technology, coupled with the addition of alternate treatment procedures, will allow improved clinical efficacy and predictability" (source: *Dermatologic Clinics*, January 2002, pages 55–65).

OPTIONS FOR KELOIDAL SCARRING

Effecting treatment of keloidal scarring is best approached with a multitherapy course of action. Using only one method is not as successful as combining two or more options.

Cryotherapy, or cryosurgery, uses extreme cold, in the form of liquid nitrogen, to get rid of the unwanted tissue. This method doesn't cause bleeding or scarring but it can leave behind a white mark that often doesn't regain normal skin color. It works best on some raised scarring but can be less successful on keloids. Ultrasonic treatment uses high-pulse sound waves to reduce collagen buildup.

Scar massage is not recommended because, while it can break down the material in the skin creating the raised scar, the massage can also stimulate collagen production, which caused the scar in the first place. Corticosteroids can be injected into the raised scar to inhibit production of the cells that are responsible for generating the scar tissue. Interferons are known to reduce the production of major scar-forming growth factors (source: *Rehab Management*, August-September 2001, http://www.rehabpub.com/features/892001/3.asp).

Topical verapamil hydrochloride is a relatively new option for the prevention and treatment of keloidal scarring. One study showed "keloids were cured in 54% of the cases in the first group . . . [and] in the remaining 36% of patients in the first group in whom keloids recurred, there was an improvement in size and above all in consistence" (source: *Dermatology*, 2002, volume 204, issue 1, pages 60–62).

STRETCH MARKS

Whether from pregnancy or weight loss, the striated tracks that can show up on skin are frustrating to women. One treatment that seems to show promise for improving the appearance of stretch marks is the use of topical tretinoin, especially if it is applied as soon as the skin alteration is noticed (sources: *Archives of Dermatology*, May 1996, pages 519–526; *Advances in Therapy*, July-August 2001, pages 181–186). While these studies show promise for improving the appearance of stretch marks, the word "improve" needs to be qualified. These studies were done on a small sampling of women and the improvement was evaluated as good, but the stretch marks did not disappear. What does show the most promise for reducing or even eliminating the appearance of stretch marks is laser resurfacing or chemical peels. These are discussed in Chapter 13, Cosmetic Surgery.

Note: Some types of laser resurfacing are considered problematic for women with darker skin colors.

MEDERMA

An article in the *Archives of Dermatology* (December 1998, pages 1512–1514, "Snake oil for the 21st century") from the Department of Dermatology, Harvard Medical School, stated that "With the current promulgation of skin 'products' and their promotion and even sale by dermatologists, and the use of treatments of no proven efficacy, this association between dermatology and quackery is set to continue well into the 21st century. The list of offending treatments includes silicone gel sheets and onion extract cream (Mederma) for keloids."

Another study (source: *Cosmetic Dermatology*, March 1999, pages 19–26) concluded that there were no discernable differences between skin treated with Mederma and skin that was treated with a placebo. Nevertheless, Mederma advertises itself as promising to get rid of scars.

Mederma, which uses onion extract as the scar-changing ingredient, contains water, thickeners, onion extract, fragrance, and preservative. There is no research showing onion extract to be effective as a skin-care ingredient. A customer service representative for Mederma told me that the onion extract "prevents the release of histamines which causes scarring." Even if onions could prevent the release of histamines, however, histamines have everything to do with allergic reactions but nothing whatsoever to do with scarring. The body produces histamines in response to an allergic reaction; the body sends them in to fight the allergen that causes the redness, swelling, and itching. While histamines can cause the skin to react, that reaction isn't related to the breakdown of collagen and elastin that causes scarring. If anything, because onions release a

complex mixture of sulfur-containing oils together with sulfur-free alde-
hydes and ammonia, all of which are more or less intensely volatile
(that's what makes your eyes burn and tear when you cut into them),
onions can be a potent skin irritant.

WHAT ABOUT SCARS FROM ACNE?

Severe and even mild acne can often lead to some form of scarring. A permanent scar is a defect in the skin caused by an injury to the area, such
as an acne lesion. The key word here is "permanent." Most of the acne
lesions that people call scars are really not scars at all, but instead postinflammatory redness—red spots left behind after the blemish heals.
What is frustrating about this redness is that it takes time for it go
away—anywhere from six to twelve months, depending on the depth of
the original lesion and how you cared for the lesion. However, there are
ways to facilitate healing. Following the guidelines for treating wounds
that were presented in previous sections of this chapter will make a huge
difference in the way the skin heals.

Permanent scars develop as the skin attempts to heal itself by surrounding the acne lesion with new skin. The epidermis (outer layer of
skin) grows in from the sides to the center, and underneath the sebaceous
gland. When the acne finally heals, a depressed pit can remain in the
skin. Scarring is unpredictable—it's impossible to know how much a particular person will scar, if at all. Early treatment of lesions is the best
prevention for acne scarring.

The best way to prevent scars is to not do anything that makes matters worse. Untreated or improperly treated acne is likely to cause the
worst scarring because the problem is never mitigated and the skin has
no chance to heal. Harshly attacking blemishes and creating deep scabs
and sores that take a long time to heal are surefire ways to guarantee a
scar will be permanent. Using heavy or irritating facial products will also
hinder the healing process. In addition, because many women don't
know how to treat acne, they use ineffective topical disinfectants and exfoliants, which can also impede the skin's ability to repair itself. Unprotected sun exposure can exacerbate scarring, too. Yet, if you are good
about not picking and oversqueezing blemishes from the outset, scarring
can be greatly reduced. Even so, the most meticulous state-of-the-art acne
skin-care routine can still result in scars. Most acne scars do fade with
time, but that time can seem like an eternity when the face is yours.

Once acne and breakouts have been reduced or eliminated, the brown, pink, or purple discolorations left by acne lesions can fade a great deal in the next six to twelve months, depending on your skin color. You can speed up that fading by continuing to use a product with AHAs, BHA, or tretinoin (which are all helpful in the treatment of acne and breakouts anyway).

Once acne has healed, small areas with shallow scars or pit-type scars can be injected with dermal fillers (various substances used to lift or fill the depression), but these are not permanent fixes and require repeated treatments.

Chemical peels such as salicylic acid (beta hydroxy acid—BHA), alpha hydroxy acids (AHAs), and trichloroacetic acids (TCAs) can improve the appearance of surface scarring. (But these peels are unwarranted for scarring if the acne is still active.) Just don't expect an AHA or BHA peel to improve the appearance of deep scarring. For larger areas of the face, laser resurfacing is absolutely the treatment of choice (sources: *Facial and Plastic Surgery*, November 2001, pages 253–262; *Aesthetic Plastic Surgery*, January-February 2001, pages 46–51).

Microdermabrasion can improve the texture and color of skin, but it requires deeper microdermabrasion treatments to obtain visible improvement in acne scarring (source: *Dermatologic Surgery*, June 2001, pages 524–530).

Skin-lightening lotions with hydroquinone or other skin-lightening ingredients do not work well, if at all, on acne scarring. These lotions prevent melanin production; they do not have much effect on what gives acne scars their color.

chapter *11*

COMMON SKIN DISORDERS

SPECIAL CONCERNS

As if the issues surrounding skin type (normal, oily, sun-damaged, blemish-prone), skin sensitivities, and allergic reactions weren't enough, a large percentage of the population deals with medical conditions that add to skin-care woes. These problems make selecting the appropriate skin-care routine extremely tricky. It becomes a challenge to find the right combination of products that will benefit the skin and not make matters worse. The most common skin disorders are eczema, psoriasis, seborrhea, and rosacea. Early identification goes a long way toward reducing the symptoms of these skin afflictions because it can help sufferers avoid buying products that are likely to exacerbate the condition. Almost without exception, these skin disorders require a dermatologist's care; they cannot be treated at the cosmetics counter or with over-the-counter products from the drugstore. Finding the right skin-care and makeup routines that work with each of these conditions is important, but it's equally vital that they complement, and not undo, the benefit of the medical treatments for the specific disorder.

ROSACEA

Rosacea is no fun. It is a stubborn skin disorder that is frustrating and extremely difficult to treat. Thought to afflict at least 30% to 50% of the population, it is frequently misdiagnosed by dermatologists and physicians. Rosacea develops over a long period of time, starting with what first seems like a tendency to blush easily, a ruddy complexion, or an extreme sensitivity to cosmetics. The distinctive redness or flushing, which appears in a characteristic butterfly pattern over the nose and cheeks, is the first likely indication that rosacea may be what your skin is struggling with. Though bothersome, the subtle initial redness is often ignored by women as being just a skin-tone or color problem and not a skin disorder.

Another challenge with identifying rosacea is that pustules (pimples) and papules (red raised bumps) that resemble acne are often present. That makes rosacea look like acne and that means it's often misdiagnosed. Unlike most acne conditions, rosacea is rarely, if ever, accompanied by blackheads. The distinctive flushing and extreme skin sensitivity also differentiate rosacea from acne. The final toll on the face is the presence of flaky patches that may or may not be accompanied by either dry or oily skin, or possibly by both at the same time. Rosacea can be extremely confusing for a woman because the dry, flaky skin responds minimally or not at all to moisturizers and the acnelike bumps and whiteheads respond minimally, or not at all, to typical acne treatments.

Even more confounding, when rosacea first develops, it may appear, disappear, and then reappear a short time later. This fluctuation also makes diagnosis difficult. Yet, despite its evasive beginnings, the condition rarely reverses itself (meaning there is no cure) and almost always becomes worse without treatment.

What usually happens is that the skin doesn't return to its normal color and stays persistently red. Other symptoms, such as enlarged blood vessels, flaky patches, oily skin, skin sensitivity, and breakouts, become more and more visible. As rosacea progresses, pimples appear on the face in the form of small, solid red bumps and pus-filled bumps. In more advanced cases of rosacea, a condition called rhinophyma may develop. Rhinophyma is characterized by a bulbous, enlarged red nose and puffy cheeks. It may also involve thick bumps that develop on the lower half of the nose, spreading to the nearby cheek areas. However, rhinophyma rarely occurs in women.

For years rosacea was referred to as "acne rosacea." That only added to the confusion because rosacea is completely unrelated to acne. However, because the papules and pustules that can accompany rosacea look like acne, many doctors misdiagnose it and end up prescribing medications that make matters worse instead of better. Most acne treatments (tretinoin and topical antibacterials) can increase rosacea's red, flaky appearance. That's why the right medication is crucial for relieving the cause of the disorder. You and your doctor need to know exactly what you are dealing with to be sure you are receiving the right treatment. Understanding the difference between acne and acne rosacea can make a huge difference in the health of your skin.

There are only a handful of treatments for rosacea, and they are all available by prescription only, including topical application of MetroGel, MetroCream, MetroLotion, and Noritate. The active ingredient in each of these is metronidazole, which is considered the primary treatment for rosacea (source: *Skin Therapy Letter*, January 2002, pages 1–6). Occasionally, azelaic acid and oral antibiotics are also an option. Because you must experiment until you find what works best for your skin, all of these should be considered when creating your own battle plan for treating rosacea.

What causes rosacea? Surprisingly, no one really knows, but it is suspected that some kind of microbe under the skin is responsible for the symptoms. Killing off this microbe seems to be the most helpful way to improve the appearance of skin and (if caught early enough) keep matters from getting worse. The active ingredient metronidazole may work in this capacity due to its antimicrobial activity on the skin. If the microbe is left to flourish, the resulting chronic inflammation (redness, swelling, breakouts, flaking skin) is believed to account for some of the symptoms of rosacea (source: *Advances in Therapy*, September-October 2001, pages 237–243).

BATTLE PLAN FOR ROSACEA

Red, flushed cheeks; swollen, almost bulging, oil glands; dry flaky skin, often with an oily layer underneath; overly sensitive skin that reacts to everything; and red, pimple-like lumps—this is what rosacea can look like. It can be a combination of symptoms, or a variety, or just one. Regardless, if left untreated, rosacea almost always gets worse and it just doesn't feel pretty when you have it.

Rosacea is much like any other pervasive skin disorder, from breakouts to eczema, because there are no easy answers. Cosmetics companies looking for your money have a penchant for claiming that their line has the answer to your problems, but these products often have no relation to the needs of someone struggling with rosacea (exfoliants, anti-irritants, antifungal ingredients, and so on). But the hope that the next product can make a difference is just too tempting for most women looking for the magic bullet. In reality, even well-formulated products, meaning primarily those that are free of topical skin irritants, can be a problem for rosacea.

So where do you begin when you're dealing with rosacea? Because rosacea is so often misdiagnosed, the place to start is with a dermatologist who has experience with this disorder. Next come skin-care considerations, to be sure the products you are using aren't making matters worse, and then lifestyle considerations, because what you do can cause flare-ups.

Treatments: As stated above, no one really knows what causes rosacea but it is suspected that a microbe under the skin causes the symptoms. Killing off the microbe seems to be the most helpful way to improve the appearance of skin and, if caught early enough, keep matters from getting worse. **The handful of prescription-only topical medications that exist that can combat the microbe responsible for rosacea include MetroLotion, MetroGel, MetroCream, Noritate, and azelaic acid** (source: *Journal of the American Academy of Dermatology*, June 1999, pages 961–965). The success of these topical medications, when combined with an oral antibiotic, can be significant. (When considering an oral antibiotic you must consider the risk of the microbe adapting to it after prolonged use. If that happens, that specific oral antibiotic won't be effective to help deal with other types of infections you may encounter.)

Isotretinoin (Accutane). This medication has been shown in several studies to be effective for those with treatment-resistant rosacea, and it is effective in a low dose of about 0.5 to 1.0 milligram per kilogram of body weight. (Accutane is always prescribed based on the weight of the patient.) No one is quite sure how Accutane works for rosacea but the success rate is good, and after treatment the swelling and distortion of the oil glands are often resolved (source: *Archives of Dermatology*, July 1998, pages 884–885).

Accutane is also considered an option for treating the occurrence of rhinophyma (nose swelling) that often takes place in cases of advanced rosacea. Rhinophyma is the distorted appearance of the nose resulting from overgrowth of its oil glands. Ironically, rhinophyma has been traditionally associated with alcoholism, yet there is no evidence to support this association. Generally, rhinophyma is best treated surgically, though systemic isotretinoin may also be an effective option (source: *Facial and Plastic Surgery*, 1998, volume 14, issue 4, pages 241–253). For an assessment of warnings and risks associated with Accutane, see the "Accutane" section on page 240 in Chapter 9, Battle Plans for Blemishes.

Gentle skin-care products. Because redness, irritation, and skin sensitivities are part and parcel of rosacea itself, anything exacerbating those things will cause more problems. Gentle cleansers, a soothing toner with anti-irritants, lightweight moisturizers with antioxidants and anti-irritants, and nonchemical sunscreens (with zinc oxide and titanium dioxide) are the basics. The National Rosacea Society (http://www.rosacea.org) surveyed 1,000 of its members who identified alcohol, witch hazel, fragrance, menthol, peppermint, and eucalyptus as contributing to flare-ups. It isn't always easy to identify those substances on a label when they are listed under the Latin names that are required by the FDA for ingredient labels. Moreover, there are many fragrant components and lots of other potentially irritating skin-care ingredients in many products. Even if you've been diligent in checking your products you can still run into problems because it is often hard to determine what is causing your own specific flare-ups. Yet as difficult as it is to pinpoint exactly what ingredients may trigger rosacea, the ones listed in Chapter 3, Skin Care Basics for Everyone, in the section "How to Be Gentle," on page 78, as being likely to cause irritation give you a good idea about what to avoid. Keep in mind that not everyone responds the same way to any of these ingredients, but avoiding these as much as possible will at the very least reduce the redness and dry flaky skin.

Salicylic acid treatment. I feel strongly that anecdotal information is correct when it points to the benefits of using a gentle toner or moisturizer that contains 1% to 2% salicylic acid (BHA) in a base with a pH of 3 to 4. Salicylic acid is an exfoliant that helps to remove the built-up layers of dry, flaky skin on the face and, because salicylic acid is related to aspirin (both are salicylates), it can also have anti-inflammatory properties on the skin, reducing redness and swelling.

Lifestyle factors to avoid. Several lifestyle factors can make rosacea worse, although these are not the same for everyone because people have different reactions to the same ingredient or external elements. These catalysts can include hot liquids, spicy foods, exposure to extreme temperatures (including cooking over a hot stove), alcohol consumption, sunlight, stress, saunas, hot tubs, smoking, rubbing or massaging the skin, irritating cosmetics, and anything else that overstimulates the skin and blood vessels.

Other irritants to avoid. Rosacea can also be exacerbated by AHAs (though not for everyone), Retin-A, Renova, Differin, exfoliants of any kind (including scrubs and washcloths), and clay-based facial masks. The less you do, meaning the fewer products you use, and the fewer ingredients in each, the happier rosacea-afflicted skin is going to be.

Ocular rosacea. This condition refers to rosacea of the eye and, according to an item in the March 2001 issue of *Cosmetic Dermatology*, it is significantly underdiagnosed and untreated. In fact, it is believed that 60% of those who have rosacea on their face will have involvement in the eye area too (source: www.emedicine.com). They note that: "Of an estimated 13 million U.S. adults [with rosacea], 89% of 2,010 rosacea sufferers . . . indicated they also experienced discomfort or redness of the eyes in varying degrees." Those with ocular rosacea most commonly experience irritation of the lids and eye, as well as sties and chronically red eyes. In rare cases, ocular rosacea can also affect the cornea. This condition can be treated, usually with soothing eye drops (but not Visine) along with oral or topical antibiotics, but it requires a dermatologic evaluation before any action is taken.

The *Rosacea Review*, an online newsletter of the National Rosacea Society, at http://www.rosacea.org/rr/index.html, is an excellent source for detailed and ongoing information concerning treatment and research for rosacea.

LASER TREATMENT FOR ROSACEA

The following letter I received from a reader sums up the issues around laser treatment for rosacea.

Dear Paula,

I have rosacea and have had four PhotoDerm laser treatments by a top dermatologist in the Houston area. After the fourth treatment, I was quite discouraged, as the veins on my nose still showed, and overall I still had a great deal of pinkness. I went to her about it, and she patch-tested the side of my nose with a stronger laser setting. The veins are still there, and I still look sunburned.

I have now moved to a midwestern city. They still seem to be discovering current beauty treatments here and there isn't a PhotoDerm laser to be found. I am also seriously questioning whether this treatment is viable for rosacea. At $1,600 later, I'm not too keen about trying the supposedly magic fifth treatment anyway!

What do you suggest for me? If you say PhotoDerm is still an option, is there a way I can find out (other than the yellow pages) who is professionally certified in it where I live? I don't have a problem with breakouts, so my MetroGel doesn't do a lot for me.

Frustrated in St. Louis

Dear Frustrated,

As helpful as PhotoDerm can be for treating rosacea, not everyone gets the great results you've heard about. According to an article in the *Journal of Cutaneous Laser Therapy* (April 1999, pages 961–965), "A total of 200 patients were treated with an intense pulsed light source (PhotoDerm VL) using various treatment parameters. The patients were treated for facial veins (primarily telangiectasia), facial hemangiomas, rosacea, and port wine stains. Results: Of the 188 patients who returned for follow-up after 2 months, 174 achieved 75% to 100% clearance in one to four treatment sessions. The post-treatment side effects were minimal and well-tolerated by the patients. There were no instances of scarring or other permanent side effects." While that statistic is impressive, there were still 26 people who weren't happy with their results. Statistically it was wise for you to consider this treatment, but after four sessions it is clearly not one that will work for you (assuming of course that the physician you saw knew what she was doing).

There are other options for your skin, but they involve deeper laser resurfacing. You would need to discuss this with a plastic surgeon or dermatologist with a well-established practice in working with lasers. To find one in your area refer to http://www.plasticsurgery.org (The American Society of Plastic Surgeons) or http://www.aad.org/DermProfile/index.html (American Academy of Dermatology).

One other point: You seem to be under the assumption that MetroGel is meant to treat "breakouts," and that is not the case. MetroGel is meant to deal with the symptoms (and theoretically the source of the problem) for rosacea. Whether it is redness, flaking, enlarged pores, or breakouts, MetroGel (active ingredient: metronidazole) should be considered an option.

PSORIASIS

Psoriasis is a chronic recurring skin disease, identified by the presence of thickened scaly areas and papules (small, solid, often-inflamed bumps that, unlike pimples, do not contain pus or sebum). These bumps are usually slightly elevated above the skin surface, sharply distinguishable from normal skin, and red to reddish brown in color. They are usually covered with small whitish silver scales that stick to the cystlike swelling and, if scraped off, may bleed. The extent of the disease varies from a few tiny lesions to generalized involvement of most of the skin. Often the elbows, knees, scalp, and chest are involved. Psoriasis affects over seven million people in the United States alone, but for most people it tends to be mild and unsightly rather than a serious health concern, which is probably why fewer than two million people seek medical treatment for it (source: *OTC Journal Newsletter*, October 15, 2001, online at http://www.otcjournal.com/profiles/astr/20011015-1.html).

No one knows for certain exactly what causes psoriasis, although recent studies suggest it may be related to an immune system problem, which triggers inflammation. The resulting intense inflammation causes the skin to shed too rapidly. Psoriasis is the recurring growth of too many skin cells that are not able to shed properly, accompanied by inflammation and redness. A normal skin cell matures in 28 to 45 days, while a psoriatic skin cell takes only 3 to 6 days. Both men and women can get psoriasis at any age, so it isn't unusual to start noticing red, swollen, flaky bumps on your skin late in life.

Psoriasis appears in several forms. The scaly, papule kind called plaque psoriasis is the most common. Other forms include guttate psoriasis, typified by small dotlike lesions all over the body; pustular psoriasis, with weeping lesions and intense scaling; and erythrodermic psoriasis, characterized by severe sloughing and inflammation of the skin. Psoriasis can range from mild to moderate to severe and disabling. On occasion, some people who have psoriasis experience spontaneous remissions, but no one knows why or when that may happen.

Sadly, there is no cure for psoriasis, but there are many different treatments, both topical and systemic, that can clear it for periods of time. Experimenting with a variety of options is essential to find the treatment that works for you, but all require a doctor's attention.

BATTLE PLANS FOR PSORIASIS

Of the various therapies available to treat psoriasis, it is generally best to start with those that have the least-serious side effects, such as topical steroids (cortisone creams); coal-tar creams, lotions, cleansers, or shampoos; and careful exposure to sunshine. If those methods are not successful, you can proceed to the more serious treatments involving oral medications. More often than not, successful treatment requires a combination of methods.

Topical Treatments

Natural sunlight can significantly improve, or even clear, psoriasis. Ultraviolet (UV) light from the sun suppresses the skin's immune response and, therefore, reduces inflammation, slowing the overproduction of skin cells that causes scaling. Daily, short, nonburning exposure to sunlight clears or improves psoriasis in many people. Therefore, sunlight may be included among initial treatments for the disease (source: National Institutes of Health, Department of Health and Human Services, *Questions and Answers about Psoriasis*, January 2002, online at http://www.niams.nih.gov/hi/topics/psoriasis/psoriafs.htm).

Regular daily doses of sunlight, taken in short exposures with adequate sun protection, are strongly recommended. Sun protection is vital not only to prevent sunburn, which may make psoriasis worse, but also to reduce skin damage from the sun's UV radiation. This outdoor approach to treating psoriasis is often referred to as **climatotherapy**. Some people travel to Florida, Hawaii, the Caribbean, or the Dead Sea in Israel (where special clinics offer treatment solariums and supervised medical assistance) to use swimming and natural sunlight as their psoriasis treatment (some people believe immersion in salty, mineral-laden water may also have some unknown benefits). In some countries, medical plans actually cover trips to these types of sunny climates and mineral spas for subscribers with psoriasis.

When you can't get to sunshine, medically supervised administration of UVB lamps may be used to minimize widespread or localized areas of stubborn and unmanageable psoriasis lesions. UVB light is also used when topical treatments have failed, or in combination with topical treatments. The short-term risks of using controlled UVB exposure to treat psoriasis are minimal, and long-term studies of large numbers of patients treated with UVB have not demonstrated an increased risk of skin cancer, suggesting that this treatment may be safer than sunlight. (Sunlight has both UVA and UVB radiation; UVA causes skin cancer, while UVB mainly triggers sunburn.) UVB treatments are considered one of the most effective therapies for moderate to severe psoriasis, with the least amount of risk. There are even sources of UVB light therapy, called narrow-band

UVB, that give off only the part of the UV spectrum band that is most helpful for psoriasis and reduce the risk associated with wideband UVB light.

Treating psoriasis with **coal tar** is a very old and effective remedy. It is a topical medication available both over the counter and by prescription; the difference is in the potency and amount of coal tar the medication contains. Coal tar inhibits certain skin substances that incite cell proliferation, thus reducing the appearance of psoriasis. Coal tar can be combined with other psoriasis medications (like topical steroids) or with sunshine (UV). However, coal tar can make the skin more sensitive to UV light, and extreme caution is advised when you combine coal tar use with UV therapy (or exposure to the sun) to avoid getting a severe burn or causing skin damage. Other downsides to coal tar are the irritation it can cause, the smell, and its tendency to stain clothes.

Anthralin, much like coal tar, is a topical prescription medication that has been used to treat psoriasis for decades. Though anthralin's action on skin is not clear, it appears to inhibit cell proliferation. It has few serious side effects but can irritate or burn the normal-appearing skin surrounding psoriatic lesions. Anthralin also stains anything it comes into contact with. It is prescribed in a range of concentrations, but the most effective form is a hard paste that is very difficult to apply, requiring a great deal of patience; also, it can't be used over inflamed lesions, and must not get on the face. There are a variety of regimens for its use, but the negative side effects and cumbersome and time-consuming application process often make it a less-than-desirable option.

A study in the *American Journal of Clinical Dermatology* (2001, volume 2, issue 2, pages 95–120) reviewed the efficacy and studies involving the topical application of **calcipotriene** (trade name Dovonex), a derivative of vitamin D3 used to treat mild to moderate psoriasis. (It is not the same compound as the vitamin D found in commercial vitamin supplements.) Calcipotriene acts not only to inhibit cell proliferation and enhance cell differentiation in the skin of patients with psoriasis, but also appears to have effects on immunologic markers that are thought to play a role in the cause of the disease. In several well-designed, short-term studies in adults, the efficacy of calcipotriene ointment (50 micrograms twice daily) was similar or superior to the efficacy of several other antipsoriatic agents in adult patients with mild to moderate psoriasis. Calcipotriene is generally well-tolerated in short- and long-term studies in adult patients, with the major side effect being irritation. In addition, calcipotriene ointment proved beneficial in combination with other topical, phototherapy, or systemic antipsoriatic treatments, reducing the dosage and/or duration of some of these treatments and potentially improving their benefit/risk ratio. Calcipotriene ointment is valuable as a first- or second-line therapy option for the management of mild to moderate psoriasis and also in combination with other antipsoriatic agents for more severe psoriasis. Other forms of vitamin D3 creams include **calcitriol** and **tacalitol**.

Topical corticosteroids (cortisones) have been used for years as the first-step approach in the treatment of psoriasis. Cortisones reduce inflammation and itching and potentially reduce cell buildup. Brands differ in potency, and the more powerful a drug the higher the risk of more severe side effects, which include burning, irritation, dryness, acne, thinning of the skin, dilated blood vessels, and loss of skin color. Less potent drugs should be used for mild to moderate psoriasis, saving the high-potency drugs for more severe conditions. An effective regimen uses high-potency cortisones, such as halobetasol (Ultravate), daily until the psoriasis plaque flattens out, after which they are applied only on the weekends. Another high-potency corticosteroid, mometasone (Elocon), needs to be administered only once a day and is as effective, or more effective than other corticosteroids while having a lower risk of severe side effects. These very potent drugs carry a small risk of causing hormonal problems for a period of time after the drug has been withdrawn. The larger the area treated with corticosteroids, the higher the risk, especially if the area is covered by heavy material or is bandaged. Also, in most cases, resistance to these drugs eventually develops; and the disease can recur after treatment is stopped (source: http://my.webmd.com/content/article/74/89271.htm).

Topical retinoids such as **Tazorac** (active ingredient tazarotene) have been shown to have a positive effect on psoriasis (source: *Cutis*, January 1999, pages 41–48), particularly in combination with other treatments (source: *International Journal of Dermatology*, January 2001, pages 64–66).

Salicylic acid (beta hydroxy acid) in strengths of 1.8% to 3% is approved by the FDA as an over-the-counter treatment for psoriasis, because it is a keratolytic, meaning it softens and removes scaly skin layers of psoriatic lesions. Removing these skin layers is important because it allows other topical medications to better penetrate skin. Also, because of salicylic acid's chemical relationship to aspirin, it has anti-inflammatory properties and can reduce the redness associated with psoriasis. Salicylic acid is available in many forms, and it is often combined with other topical medications to enhance their effectiveness (source: http://www.psoriasis.org). The primary concern in choosing a well-formulated salicylic acid product is to be sure the concentration is stated clearly on the product, and that the pH of the product is no higher than 3.5.

Systemic Treatments

Methotrexate is an anti-cancer drug that can reduce the overproduction of cells. It is an established and highly effective systemic treatment for severe psoriasis and has been widely used during the last three decades. For this reason, the long-term adverse effects of methotrexate are well-known. The most frequent adverse effects that occur during methotrexate therapy are abnormal liver function test results, nausea, and gastric complaints. The most feared adverse effects are liver damage and the suppression of bone marrow activity. However, liver problems associated with methotrexate are related to a high cumulative dose. This means that rotating types of therapy or using methotrexate intermittently instead of continuously can reduce the risk. Most people tolerate low-dose methotrexate therapy relatively well, provided they work closely with their physician and watch carefully for adverse effects and drug interactions during treatment. The long-term clinical efficacy and relative safety of methotrexate remain impressive (sources: *American Journal of Clinical Dermatology*, January-February 2000, pages 27–39; *Clinical Rheumatology*, 2001, volume 20, issue 6, pages 406–410).

Cyclosporin (trade name Neoral) is a strong immune-suppressant drug and a primary medication used to prevent the rejection of transplanted organs such as liver, kidneys, and heart. In skin diseases, cyclosporin acts by reducing inflammation in the skin and reducing cell proliferation by blocking immune factors that may be generating the problem. Studies have shown cyclosporin to be highly effective and well-tolerated in short-term treatment of severe psoriasis (source: *American Journal of Clinical Dermatology*, 2001, volume 2, issue 1, pages 41–47). However, this is a serious medication. Temporary side effects of cyclosporin can include headaches, gingivitis, joint pain, gout, body-hair growth, tremors, high blood pressure, kidney problems, and fatigue. Of serious concern is the

National Toxicology Program's *Eighth Report on Carcinogens*, 1998, which warns that cyclosporin is "known to be a human carcinogen based on studies in humans." All of these factors must be weighed and carefully assessed before deciding on this course of treatment.

Etretinate (trade name Tegison), **acitretin** (Soriatane), and **isotretinoin** (Accutane) are retinoids. Etretinate and acitretin are similar to isotretinoin, except that etretinate and acitretin are approved by the FDA for use in the treatment of psoriasis, while isotretinoin is approved by the FDA for use in treating acne. How retinoids work in the treatment of psoriasis is not completely understood, although they are thought to block the overproduction of skin cells. The substantial amount of data on the clinical effectiveness of etretinate was obtained empirically from numerous multicenter trials and individual reports (sources: *Journal of the American Academy of Dermatology*, December 1992, pages S8–S14; *European Journal of Dermatology*, November-October 2000, pages 517–521).

While none of these retinoids are to be used when a woman is pregnant, the risks associated with etretinate are considered even more problematic. All systemic retinoids have the strong potential to cause major fetal abnormalities, including neurological and skeletal deformities. It is essential that effective contraception be used for at least one month before and throughout treatment. However, because etretinate can remain in the blood for up to *three years* after treatment, birth control must be continued for an indefinite period of time following therapy. It has not yet been determined how long it is necessary to wait before becoming pregnant after you stop taking etretinate to ensure that none of the drug remains in your system (source: FDA Web site, http://www.fda.gov/cber/bldmem/072893.txt). As a result of the risks associated with etretinate, particularly the length of time it can stay in the system, acitretin and isotretinoin are considered safer and just as effective choices for severe psoriasis (source: *Journal of the American Academy of Dermatology*, November 2001, pages S150–S157).

Severe fetal abnormalities do occur if a woman is or becomes pregnant while taking either acitretin or isotretinoin (Accutane), but because these drugs don't remain in the system for long after you are finished with treatment, no long waiting period is required before becoming pregnant. Specifics regarding how long to wait after treatment before considering having a baby should be discussed with your physician.

Etanercept (trade name Enbrel) is an antitumor medication that is used in the treatment of rheumatoid arthritis. It has also been found useful in the treatment of psoriasis. Etanercept appears to be a promising agent that can be used in combination therapy for the treatment of psoriasis (source: *British Journal of Dermatology*, January 2002, pages 118–121).

5-fluorouracil (brand name Efudex) is a chemotherapy drug that may be effective in the treatment of psoriasis affecting the nails. Psoriatic-affected nails are quite common for those with psoriasis—up to 50% of those with psoriasis have it in their nails, too. There is no consistently effective treatment for psoriasis of the nail, though there are a handful of studies showing a topically applied 5% 5-fluorouracil cream can be beneficial (source: *Cutis*, July 1998, pages 27–28). For risks associated with 5-fluorouracil please see the section on "Actinic Keratosis" on page 153 in Chapter 4, Sun Sense.

Combination Therapy

The most typical combination therapy for psoriasis is something called PUVA. PUVA involves the use of a prescription medication called Psoralen and exposure to ultraviolet light A (UVA)—hence the initials PUVA. It is also called "photochemotherapy." The drug Psoralen, which can be taken orally as a pill or applied topically to the skin, makes the skin more sensitive and receptive to the wavelength of UVA light (320 to 400 nanometers). This combination suppresses the growth of abnormal skin cells. The good news is that PUVA can eliminate or dramatically reduce psoriatic lesions for the majority of people who use it, and there is evidence it can provide extended remissions. The bad news is that Psoralen and UVA light are phototoxic and carcinogenic. Getting rid of psoriasis can mean a lot, but putting your skin at risk for premature aging and cancer may be trading one problem for another. In light of the risks involved, PUVA should be considered only for extreme or disabling psoriasis, after other treatments have failed (sources: http://www.psoriasis.org; *Cutis*, November 2001, pages 345–347; *Biochemical Pharmacology*, January 2002, pages 31–39).

All of the above treatments, both topical and oral, are often used in varying combinations for the best results. Frequently, several combination treatments are used in rotation to reduce the potentially harmful side effects of each one. Discovering whether any of these will work for you, alone or in combination, takes patience and a systematic, ongoing review and evaluation of how your skin and health are doing. Successful treatment, as is true with all chronic skin disorders, requires diligent adherence to the regimen and a realistic understanding of what you can and can't expect. It is also important to be aware of the consequences of the varying treatment levels. For example, continued long-term use of topical cortisone creams can cause skin thinning, stretch marks, and built-up resistance to the cortisone medication itself, so that it actually becomes an ineffective treatment. Exposure to sunlight without adequate protection (particularly from UVA radiation) can cause skin cancer. Oral steroids can have serious withdrawal effects, including increased bouts of psoriasis. Accutane causes birth defects if a woman becomes pregnant while taking it. Several systemic psoriatic treatments can cause liver problems, nausea, and severe irritation. Each option has its own set of pros and cons that need to be researched and discussed at length with your physician.

For more information on the current status of available treatment visit the Web site for the National Psoriasis Foundation (NPF) at http://www.psoriasis.org/.

SEBORRHEA

Seborrhea is a skin disease of the sebaceous (oil) glands marked by an increased secretion of sebum (oil) or a thickened sebum discharge. It can resemble acne and blackheads. One of the differences between acne and seborrhea is that in seborrhea the increased oil production is often accompanied by a scaly, thickened skin, especially on the scalp, and the oil itself can have a strange, viscous texture. However, in seborrhea—and sometimes in acne—the sebum (a firm waxlike substance in the pore that liquefies into oil on the surface of the skin) in the sebaceous gland accumulates, causing the gland to become swollen and filled to the brim. When this overproduced sebum is covered over by skin, it forms a small, firm mound called a whitehead. When the sebum is exposed to air (not covered by skin) and the duct fills with dead skin cells, the sebum turns dark and the blemish becomes a blackhead. The size of the eruption, the texture of the oil, and the flaky skin are what differentiate seborrhea from acne.

Seborrhea can show up wherever there are lots of oil glands. The scalp, sides of the nose, eyebrows, eyelids, behind the ears, and middle of the chest are the areas most commonly affected. Other areas, such as the navel and the skin folds under the arms, breasts, groin, and buttocks, may also be involved. The swelling, breakouts, and accompanying yellowish, greasy-appearing scales make this skin disorder hard to miss.

Seborrhea is identified by excessive yellowish, thickened scaling, accompanied by excessive oiliness, and is possibly triggered by a yeast organism (yeast is a type of fungus) present in the hair follicle (source: *British Journal of Dermatology*, March 2001, pages 549–556). Seborrhea can occur at any age, but typically it is seen in infants, when it is called "cradle cap." Because yeast, or some other form of fungus, likely triggers seborrhea, antimicrobial agents capable of targeting this type of organism have been shown to have a high success rate.

Prescription medications for the treatment of seborrhea include ciclopiroxolamine 1% in a cream base. This is an antifungal that has been shown to be effective in a well-controlled study (source: *British Journal of Dermatology*, May 2001, pages 1033–1037). Topical metronidazole (Noritate, MetroLotion, MetroGel, and MetroCream) also can have significant positive results, and is very effective in the treatment of seborrhea (source: *Journal of Family Practice*, June 2001, volume 50, issue 6). An oral medication, terbinafine, has been identified as beneficial in the treatment of seborrhea as well (source: *British Journal of Dermatology*, April 2001, pages 854–857).

Several over-the-counter topical treatments for seborrhea include zinc pyrithione 1% (Dandrex, Zincon, Head and Shoulders, Denorex); coaltar preparations (DHS, Neutrogena T-Gel, Ionil T, Tegrin, Esorex), ketaconazole (Nizoral), selenium sulfide 1% (Selsun Blue), and selenium sulfide 2.5% (Selsun). As in the treatment of psoriasis, UV light therapy can be of benefit for those who suffer from seborrhea, but it carries the same risks mentioned above for psoriasis. Topical steroids are often of limited use because they can cause thinning of the skin.

Treating seborrhea takes patience and experimenting to find what works for you. All of these medications, either alone or in combination, are options for achieving the best results.

ECZEMA

On a personal note, I suffered from eczema for many years. At one point in my life almost 80% of my body was affected, and the resulting itching and scratching, sores, irritation, and discomfort were more awful than I can put into words. For years I struggled with medications and a varying assortment of cortisone creams and bar soaps, from Basis to Aveeno, until the day my dermatologist found the right cortisone strength and I started to stay away from topical irritants; then my skin finally settled down—but the problem didn't go away until much later in life.

Eczema, also known as contact dermatitis, atopic dermatitis, irritant dermatitis, allergic dermatitis, and a host of other designations, is without question a difficult, uncomfortable, often painful skin disorder. When you have it, you generally know it by the cracked, abraded, blistered, crusted, weepy, reddened, patchy, dry skin surface, accompanied by persistent, almost unbearable itching and the tendency for everything you touch to make matters worse. A simple act like washing your hands, applying eye makeup, or wearing scratchy material can instigate a flare-up that feels interminable.

Almost anything can trigger eczema, and sometimes nothing at all can precede a bout of oppressive itching, scratching, and rashes. Wool (from clothing to carpets), shampoos, hair dyes, nail polish, jewelry, plants, undergarments (elastic waistbands and spandex bras are special villains), deodorant, tight socks, nylons, pet allergies, excessive heat or air conditioning (which increases dry and itchy skin), bathing too often (which leaches moisture out of the skin), using harsh or mild soaps, hot water, vigorous rubbing or massaging, chlorinated water, salt water, and even sweat (this triggered my eczema almost instantaneously) are all possible offenders. In the world of cosmetics, preservatives, irritants (such as peppermint, menthol, alcohol, camphor, eucalyptus, fragrance, and essential oils), bath salts, bubble bath, scrubs, AHAs, BHA, and loofahs are all potent eczema triggers.

Despite this daunting list, everyone is different, and what irritates your skin might not irritate someone else's. There is no exact science to discovering what causes your skin to react; rather, it is a process of paying attention to what you come into contact with, seeing what makes things worse for your skin, and then eliminating or avoiding those things at all costs.

Generally, dry skin (an impaired surface skin barrier) is more prone to the sensation of itching and chapping, so finding a reliable way to deal with dry skin is almost always the starting point for the treatment of eczema. To this end it is important to keep bathing time short, avoid bath salts or bubble baths, use lukewarm to warm water (avoid hot water most of all), and avoid bar soaps of any kind (they all contain potential irritants). Using fragrance-free, gentle liquid cleansers that also contain moisturizing agents, and applying and reapplying moisturizers quickly afterward can help a lot.

Unquestionably, moisturizers minimize dryness and are a mainstay in treating mild to chronic dermatitis. It is believed that regular and frequent use of emollient moisturizers can reduce the amount of topical steroids needed in the maintenance treatment of eczema. The more emollient the cream the better, and when fatty acids are included in the formula it's particularly helpful. Fatty acids are ingredients such as triglycerides, oleic acid, linoleic acid, evening primrose oil, borage oil, fish oil, flaxseed oil, coconut oil, and palm oil (source: *Skin Pharmacology and Applied Skin Physiology*, March 2002, pages 100–104). While using a moisturizer twice daily is considered adequate, it is essential to keep a moisturizer with you at all times so that you can reapply it every time you wash your hands. During the day it is essential that you apply an emollient moisturizer with an SPF 15 or greater that contains UVA-protecting ingredients on exposed areas of your body. In the case of eczema, because of the risk of irritation and skin sensitivity, the UVA-protecting ingredients should be only titanium dioxide and zinc oxide with no avobenzone or other synthetic sunscreen agents of any kind. Synthetic sunscreen agents have a potential to cause skin irritation.

For years topical corticosteroids (cortisone) have been the drug of choice for treating eczema. These products are available in a vast range of strengths and molecular structures that allow for varying skin penetration and potency. The risks associated with prolonged use of a potent corticosteroid are that it may result in skin deterioration and adaptation (that means it stops having an effect on the skin). Because of these risks, newer nonsteroidal treatments for eczema have been formulated and have been approved by the FDA. However, if these newer treatments are not effective for you, concerns about skin breakdown (which happens with any long-term cortisone use) and adaptation should not limit your use of a good potent steroid. It is still a valid way to get control of the dermatitis. As much as possible, try to minimize the frequency of cortisone application, using it only as necessary to keep the irritation abated. But don't cut back too far because there is a point of no return where if you don't use enough your skin becomes an itchy, rashy mess.

BATTLE PLAN FOR ECZEMA

An announcement in the December 2000 *FDA Talk Papers* reported the approval of a new drug for the treatment of a form of eczema called atopic dermatitis. For anyone struggling with this itchy, red, oozing, sensitive-skin condition, this is definitely worth looking into. The drug is called Protopic and contains the active ingredient tacrolimus in a 0.1% and 0.03% concentration ointment for adults and a 0.03% concentration ointment for children two years of age and older. It is a nonsteroidal (meaning not cortisone) ointment indicated for patients with moderate to severe eczema and for whom standard eczema therapies such as cortisone creams have not worked or are not considered healthy. (With repeated use, cortisone can cause thinning of the skin and prematurely aged skin.) According to the *FDA Talk Paper*, "The FDA based its approval on the results of three 12-week studies which indicated that 28–37% of patients using Protopic experienced greater than or equal to 90% improvement of their skin condition, as measured by physicians, and two one year studies that indicated that the drug is safe for intermittent long term use." In addition, the drug has been tested in 28 worldwide trials on more than 4,000 adults and children. What makes tacrolimus unique is that it has been used primarily orally to prevent transplant rejections due to its action as an immunomodulator. In other words, by suppressing the immune system it prevents the body from rejecting a transplanted organ. It is thought to work in some cases of moderate to severe dermatitis because of its effect in preventing the skin's own immune reaction from causing red, itchy, inflamed rashes. (In other words, in this form of eczema, it's as if the person's own immune system is attacking the skin, causing the itching, blistering, and irritation.) By stopping this immune reaction, it eliminates the problem.

The study goes on to note that "common side effects associated with this drug include temporary stinging or burning sensations where the drug is applied, which may lessen if the diseased skin heals. There was evidence from an animal study that Protopic may accentuate the adverse effects of ultraviolet light on the skin. Therefore sun protection at all times is vital" (but you already know that sun protection is vital all the time regardless of what else you put on your skin).

Another interesting study on eczema, presented in the *Archives of Dermatology* (January 2001, pages 42–43), reported research in Japan that demonstrated that two-thirds of the patients with eczema improved after a month of drinking a liter of oolong tea daily. According to the study "118 patients . . . were asked to maintain their dermatological treatment. However, they were also instructed to drink oolong tea made from a 10-gram teabag placed in 1000 milliliters of boiling water and steeped for 5 minutes. After 1 month of treatment 74 (63%) of the 118 patients showed marked to moderate improvement of their condition. A good response to treatment was still observed in 64 patients (54%) at 6 months." The study concluded that "The therapeutic efficacy of oolong tea may well be the result of the antiallergic properties of tea polyphenols." While the study didn't look at the effect of tea drinking if the topical treatments were stopped, the patients did receive some benefit. So by combining topical treatments (moisturizers and possibly Protopic) with some oolong tea, perhaps the positive effects of both will add up, and those with eczema can breathe a sigh of relief.

part III

MORE BEAUTY SOLUTIONS

chapter 12

HAIR REMOVAL

HAIR-BRAINED IDEAS?

From the onset of adolescence, the desire to get rid of unwanted body hair becomes an almost daily obsession. Whether it is shaving legs or under-arms, struggling with dark hair above the lip or on the chin, or dense hair growth on the arms, finding a way to effectively and efficiently deal with this problem is a recurring issue. Most of us realize that if a beauty need exists, lots of cosmetics companies are more than willing to manufacture products with claims to solve it. However, most of these end up sounding far more effective than their actual performance. Infomercials and ads in fashion magazines seem to have the answer for the hair you're longing to get rid of, but alas, these products either can't live up to their claims or they are just standard depilatories or waxing options that offer little to no improvement over what has been around for years. Believe me when I say I would love to find an easy way to achieve a smooth bikini line or a hair-less upper lip without trouble or bother, but hair removal just isn't that simple. Here are all the available options, each with its own pros and cons. Depending on your budget, available time, and the area you want to make hair-free, you can check these over and choose what works best for you.

DEPILATORIES

Depilatories literally melt and dissolve hair with strong ingredients like calcium hydroxide and sodium or calcium thioglycolate. There are many reasons why this group of products is not great for everyone; the most compelling is they risk causing serious irritation or (in the extreme case) possible burns to the skin and eyes. It is essential to test the depilatory on your arm first as a precaution against allergic reactions or skin sensitivities. Hair and skin are similar in composition, so chemicals that destroy the hair can also destroy the skin.

Depilatories, much like shaving, remove only the hair on the surface, which means the hair comes back in just a few days. To get the best results from your depilatory, first apply warm to hot (but not too hot) compresses, which help soften the hair and open the pores (where the hair is growing), allowing the depilatory to be absorbed better. Then apply an extremely thick, generous layer of the depilatory completely over the entire length and base of the hair shaft and let it stay on for the full recommended time, but no longer than between four and fifteen minutes, depending on how fine or coarse the hair is. Because depilatories dissolve the hair, applying pressure can help remove more of the shaft. Instead of simply washing the depilatory away, use a washcloth and wipe the cream off, using a firm back-and-forth motion.

Depilatories should never be used for the eyebrows or other areas around the eyes, or on inflamed or broken skin.

The FDA issued a recall on September 13, 1997, for The Art of Beauty Epil-Stop Hair Removal Cream *($49.95 for 4 ounces)*, manufactured by International Chemical Corporation, Amherst, New York. Previously, on September 4, 1997, the California Poison Control Office had issued a press release warning that Epil-Stop "is adulterated in that it has high pH levels which may cause skin irritation and burning." Check out the FDA home page at http://www.fda.gov for more information.

Epil-Stop (not to be confused with EpilLight, a pulse-light laser device) was advertised on television, magazines, and over the Internet, with claims about removing hair and stopping hair growth naturally and painlessly. It turns out that Epil-Stop worked like any other drugstore depilatory—by dissolving hair with a high-pH ingredient base. Unlike other drugstore products, however, Epil-Stop took their pH to a still higher level, so that it ate away not only the hair but also the skin.

HAIR-GROWTH–INHIBITING PRODUCTS

Ultimate Hairaway *($39.95 for 2 ounces)* is a prime example of how the cosmetics industry doesn't have to relay honest information. This is supposed to be a hair-growth-inhibiting product and it claims to be all-natural, yet the ingredient list is as far from natural as you can get. It contains water, extractable fruit derivatives (whatever that's supposed to mean), polypropylene glycol, glycerol, disaccharides, urea, dithiothreitol, EDTA, methylparaben, and propylparaben. What could be inhibiting hair growth in this product? It isn't the natural-sounding fruit derivatives. It's probably the dithiothreitol. Dithiothreitol is related to thioglycolic compounds, standard and highly alkaline ingredients that can dissolve hair and potentially irritate skin, similar to any depilatory.

Depending on your sense of humor, you may find it terribly funny that Ultimate Hairaway suggests that you "first remove hair from the roots, as with waxing, sugaring, tweezing, or electrolysis" before you apply their product. They claim Ultimate Hairaway isn't a depilatory, which is why the hair has to come off first. Rather, it is supposed to inhibit hair growth, eventually letting you phase out the need for hair-removal procedures. Given the variable cycle of hair growth and the fact that you are supposed to use another method to remove the hair, it would be a long time before you had any idea this product wasn't working. Tweezing and waxing already make hair growth seem slower because when hair has been removed from the root, it has to grow longer to get back to the surface. Moreover, electrolysis has long been a hair-removal method known to stop hair growth because of the impact of the treatment on the hair follicle, but Ultimate Hairaway fails to mention that.

Another claim Ultimate Hairaway makes is that it works like "male pattern baldness, inhibit[ing] hair growth." While that comment simplifies the issue, the description in the brochure is much more complicated and hard to follow. According to the booklet, "the top of a healthy papilla ['papilla' is a term that refers to the bump or bulge where a hair grows] is naturally cornified . . . ['cornified' refers to the conversion of skin cells into a keratinized material, such as hair or nails]. When the hair is removed, the sides of the papilla are exposed and susceptible to the treatment. [That may be true, though I doubt it; but regardless, the papilla isn't where the hair grows from.] . . . Male pattern baldness is caused by renegade type apocrine glands, which develop and connect to the duct of the sebaceous gland and introduce naturally occurring secretions into the hair follicle. The opening of hair follicles at the skin's surface is often blocked by shampoo, conditioner, gels, hair spray, sweat, oils, sebum, etc. This blockage disallows these natural secretions to escape. These acidic secretions, having no place to go, seep their way to the base of the hair follicle and slowly cornify the sides of the papilla, preventing penetration of hair cells. Ultimate Hairaway can duplicate the cause of baldness on the desired area." Wow!

Let me try to interpret this mumbo jumbo. First, male pattern baldness is caused by the hormone dihydroxytestosterone (DHT), which binds to the base of hair follicles and causes them to shrink and deteriorate. "Apocrine glands" refers to any glandular secretion, anywhere in the body. I have no idea what that has to do with the hair shaft because it isn't how the hair follicle functions (unless they are referring to DHT, but they don't say that). Then they start talking about how some hair-care products can clog a hair follicle and, I suppose, cut off its blood supply and reduce growth. Now, that is true, but hardly something you would want to encourage, because you would also be clogging the pores at the same time. The rest of the stuff I can't decipher. I've never heard of this acidic secretion issue that cornifies the hair follicle itself. It sounds like their product is supposed to block the pilosebaceous unit (the hair follicle and oil gland combined are the pilosebaceous unit) to stop unwanted hair growth. Are they suggesting that you can artificially create acidic secretions in the hair follicle (secretions I haven't seen any evidence of) to stop hair growth? Does that mean AHAs (which are highly acidic) can stop hair growth?

None of this is substantiated by one ounce of published research, and none of the dermatologists I spoke to confirmed or even understood what the company's statement means.

Perhaps the final joke is the last statement in the Ultimate Hairaway brochure: "If you prefer to shave to control unwanted body hair, simply apply [Ultimate Hairaway] twice a day for one week and then once a day thereafter until the desired results are acquired. Shave as necessary." See, they were talking about mechanically removing hair by shaving (or any other method) all along; it just took them a very long time to say that.

There are many more products boasting hair-inhibiting ability, such as Derma Nude Advanced Moisturizing Spray *($39.95 for 4 ounces)* and Hair No More Advanced Hair Growth Inhibitor Soothing Gel *($29.95 for 2 ounces)*. These two are representative of many I've seen. While they don't seem to contain anything irritating or painful, the claims that they are all pure and natural are purely nonsense. Both include water, propylene glycol, glycerin, aloe vera, green tea extract, enzymatic plant extracts, EDTA, and DMDM hydantoin. DMDM hydantoin is a form of formaldehyde (source: *Contact Dermatitis*, April 1988, pages 197–201) and propylene glycol is also a synthetic ingredient. Further, enzymatic plant extracts are not a legal or approved ingredient description name. The FDA requires all cosmetic ingredient lists to comply with Cosmetic & Toiletry Fragrance Association (CTFA) rules or the International Nomenclature Cosmetic Ingredient (INCI) names. With vague wording like this, there is no way consumers can actually know what they are putting on their skin. Enzymes sound natural, so the consumer assumes it must be gentle, but that is a leap of faith you might want to think twice about before you jump into this quagmire of misleading and invalid information.

WAXING

Waxing is an excellent and inexpensive way to deal with most hair removal on the body or face. Waxing leaves the area smoother than shaving does because it pulls the hair out below the top layer of skin, which makes it grow back slower and less uniformly. You can do waxing at home by yourself, and beauty supply stores sell all the equipment you need, from the wax to spatulas, strips of cotton, and anti-inflammatory lotions. There are even hair-remover kits with strips of wax or waxlike ingredients that you just peel off, place on the skin, and then rip off. No heating or mixing. This is by far the most convenient and easiest way to peel off hair from large areas such as the legs, bikini line, and arms. For smaller areas such as the upper lip, a wax that is melted in the microwave (instead of on the stove) and applied with a small spatula offers the most control.

In hot waxing, a thin layer of heated wax is applied to the skin in the direction of the hair growth. The hair becomes embedded in the wax as it cools and hardens. The wax is then pulled off quickly in the opposite direction of the hair growth, taking the uprooted hair with it. Cold waxes work similarly. Strips precoated with wax or a cool, sugar-based substance are pressed onto the skin in the direction of the hair growth and pulled off in the opposite direction.

Before you consider doing this yourself, visit an aesthetician with experience in this method of hair removal. It's tricky to get the technique right, and getting it wrong can mean a sticky mess on your body, in your kitchen, and around your bathroom. It also smarts a bit when the hair is ripped off. You can't wax again until the hair grows out to a noticeable length.

SUGAR FORMS OF WAXING

The best known "sugaring" method of hair removal is Nad's Gel Hair Removal *($29.95 for one kit)*. Thanks to its many reruns in late-night and early-morning infomercials, this is a product many women are now familiar with. What makes this kind of hair removal different is that it literally uses sugar instead of wax. With its thick, caramel-like consistency, it works identically to regular waxing, only instead of spreading a wax substance over the skin, you're spreading caramel.

I have to say this is one of the first products I've ever run into where the claim of being 100% natural and organic is 100% true. Nad's ingredients are honey, molasses, fructose, vinegar, lemon juice, water, alcohol, and food dye. Now that's what I call natural. But does that make it better than waxing, as the company claims? First, waxing isn't unnatural—after all, wax is a natural substance. And as far as hair removal is concerned the effect is identical. You spread the Nad's caramel gel over the hair you want removed (there needs to be some hair length or there won't be anything for it to grab). Then you rip it off and out comes the hair, same as waxing.

However, there are two main positives to sugaring over waxing. First, sugaring's mess washes away while wax has to be peeled or scratched off (and that isn't easy). Plus sugaring doesn't require heating while waxing often does, and adding heat is far more damaging to skin! Easy cleanup and a relatively easier application (no risk of burn) are the incredible benefits of sugaring.

But before you jump on the Nad's or other sugaring hair-removal system bandwagon, you should know a few more details about the claims that accompany the sugaring method, as some aren't true. Nad's states, "when you use Nad's, the hair is extracted, including the roots so regrowth is softer, finer and slower." That isn't true. Hormones and genetics determine hair growth and hair thickness, not the hair-removal method. What does happen when you "tweeze" out hair is that because it has been removed closer to the root the new hair takes longer to grow back to the top of the skin, unlike with shaving, where the hair is removed only from the surface, so the hair pops back out faster. Also, because each hair follicle has a different rate of growth, there will be less of it as it grows back than what was present when you first waxed or sugared, making the hair seem softer.

There are also claims that sugaring prevents ingrown hairs. Ingrown hairs are unrelated to the way hair is removed. Ingrown hairs occur when a hair that has been removed below the skin's surface has trouble finding its way back to the surface. That applies to hair removal in general, regardless of whether you shave, tweeze, sugar, or wax.

Another claim: "Because of the natural substances in Nad's, there is little chance of irritations. Redness for a short time is normal, depending on how sensitive your skin is." Natural or not, ripping out hair hurts, and for some skin types that can be a problem. What is better about sugaring, however, is that the stuff doesn't have to be heated and so, as a result, it's less irritating—but that isn't because it's natural.

TWEEZING

Tweezing is not only a painful option, but also an extremely time-consuming one. It is OK for occasional stray hairs or very small areas, but it is not the best for large areas or areas with dense hair growth. Tweezing works virtually the same way as waxing—pulling the hair out from the root—which means the effects last far longer than shaving. Some women worry that tweezing will increase the growth or make the texture of the hair heavier, but it won't. If plucking (or waxing and shaving) altered hair growth, we would all have bushy eyebrows! Actually, pulling out hair can eventually shut down the hair follicle by causing repeated shock and injury, though this takes a very, very long time. For the most part, any texture change is a result of the initial grow-back phase, when the hair reemerges from the pore.

BLEACHING

Bleaching is a great, inexpensive option if the issue is not the density of the hair but its darkness. This method is particularly effective for the upper lip or other parts of the face, neck, and arms. There are many options for facial bleach products at the drugstore or on the Internet. One of the best Internet sources for a range of inexpensive options is http://www.folica.com. Please be aware that this site also sells an **array** of products that exaggerate their claims or simply mislead as to what they can really do for skin.

ELECTROLYSIS

Electrolysis is the only permanent form of hair removal, at least so far, but it requires repeated treatments that can take up to a year and it can be pricy, especially when you take into consideration the time commitment. The biggest hurdle is finding an extremely skilled technician to achieve satisfactory results. Before you see someone, check out the clients who have had permanent success with this tricky, but effective, method of hair removal.

There are two types of devices that use electric current to remove hair: the needle epilator and the tweezer epilator. (Tweezer epilators are discussed on the next page). Needle epilators introduce a very fine wire under the skin, and into the hair follicle. An electric current travels down the wire and destroys the hair root at the bottom of the follicle. The loosened hair is then removed with regular tweezers. Every hair is treated individually. Needle epilators are used in electrolysis because this technique destroys the hair follicle. Thus, this is considered a permanent hair-removal method. The hair root may persist, however, if the needle misses the mark or if insufficient electricity is delivered to destroy it. However, the stimulus for hair growth can never be permanently removed. For instance, you can't control hormonal changes that may cause new growth (source: FDA *Consumer* magazine, September 1996).

The major risks of using electrolysis include electrical shock, which can occur if the needle is not properly insulated; infection from a nonsterile needle; and scarring resulting from improper technique. In addition, there are no uniform licensing standards regulating the practice of electrolysis. Only 31 states require electrologists to be licensed, and among those the license requirements vary from as few as 120 hours to 1,100 hours, which means that to set up shop many electrologists only need a machine and very little else.

The American Electrology Association and the Society of Clinical and Medical Electrologists have certification programs based on a written exam. A list of licensed and certified electrologists is available from the International Guild of Professional Electrologists, 202 Boulevard Street, Suite B, High Point, NC 27262; (800) 830-3247 or on the Web at http://www.igpe.org/.

HOME ELECTROLYSIS

Technically, these devices work the same way as those that the professionals use (they also carry the same health risks). However, the risks for the home-use machines are not very great because the voltage and current output are not very high, and that means they aren't as effective. I know we've all seen those little machines you can buy via mail order (for about $100) that claim to remove hair painlessly and permanently. They've been advertised for years and years. I remember them from when I was a kid. The chances of operating these successfully yourself are at best slim. You probably would end up just tweezing instead of zapping the hair because getting the device to work right is extremely tricky and incredibly time-consuming. Given the time it takes for a hair to grow back, it could take months before you knew if it was really working (source: FDA *Consumer* magazine, September 1996).

Perhaps the most advertised at-home product is IGIA's Hair Removal System *($119)*. It is supposed to be a "painless home electrolysis system that helps keep hair from growing back! Unlike common [tweezing] and depilatory devices that can cause skin irritation, this system uses mild radio frequency pulses that is absolutely safe and is delivered through the tweezers to remove hair without touching the skin." Well, that much is true. This overpriced machine delivers low-voltage radio waves through the hair shaft. Does that kill off a hair follicle? There is no research indicating that these machines do anything but tweeze the hair. The low voltage makes these machines extremely low risk, but they are also ineffective. What a waste. Still, in comparison to the other IGIA products, this one is the safest of the bunch. Keep in mind that even though these kinds of self-electrolysis machines have been advertised for years and years, there are other truly effective options to try.

SHAVING

Shaving is fine, but we all know the problems associated with it. Shaving is the method most of us go back to for our legs and bikini line, but the hair grows back way too fast and the stubble or redness it can cause on the thigh and crotch is obnoxious. There are ways around the redness, such as shaving with a good topical lotion like a hair conditioner or body wash and applying a nonfragranced moisturizer afterward. Also, one of the best options for preventing red bumps is applying aspirin topically to the skin. Aspirin has potent anti-inflammatory properties even when applied to the surface of skin. Simply dissolve one or two aspirins in about ¼ cup water and then apply the solution with a cotton ball to the area you just shaved. This works on any part of the body you shave. You will be impressed by the results.

On the legs, using a mild scrub of baking soda mixed with Cetaphil Gentle Skin Cleanser can help keep flaky skin at a minimum, which means you can get a closer shave. Skin should never be shaved while dry; wet hair is soft, pliable, and easier to cut. Contrary to what many believe, shaving does not change the texture, color, or rate of hair growth. Hair density is genetically and hormonally determined; it has nothing to do with what you do topically to the skin (unless you traumatically damage the hair follicle via injury or burns).

LASER HAIR REMOVAL

Since the advent of the first FDA-approved laser hair-removal system in 1995, its popularity has made laser hair removal a financial cornerstone for many dermatologists and plastic surgeons. The original laser hair-removal machine was **The Soft Light Hair Removal System** developed by Thermolase Corporation. Since then the growing popularity of and demand for this treatment from eager consumers reading ads and articles in fashion magazines has prompted many laser manufacturers to seek FDA clearance for their laser hair-removal machines. The market is growing so quickly that the FDA cannot maintain an up-to-date list of all laser manufacturers whose devices have been cleared for hair removal, as this list continues to change. However, to learn if a specific manufacturer has received FDA clearance, you can check the FDA Web site at http://www.fda.gov/cdrh/databases.html. You will need to know the manufacturer or device name of the laser. You can also call the FDA's Center for Devices and Radiological Health, Consumer Staff, at 1-888-INFO-FDA or (301) 827-3990, or fax your request to (301) 443-9535 (source: FDA Center for Devices and Radiological Health, *Laser Facts*, May 2001, online at http://www.fda.gov/cdrh/consumer/laserfacts.html).

One of the significant FDA regulations regarding all companies that promote approved laser hair-removal systems is that "manufacturers may not claim that laser hair removal is either painless or permanent. . . .

The specific claim granted is 'intended to effect stable, long-term, or permanent reduction'. . . . Permanent hair reduction is defined as the long-term, stable reduction in the number of hairs regrowing after a treatment regime, which may include several sessions. The number of hairs regrowing must be stable over time—greater than the duration of the complete growth cycle of hair follicles, which varies from four to twelve months according to body location. Permanent hair reduction does not necessarily imply the elimination of all hairs in the treatment area." That is a very convoluted way of saying that laser hair removal is not permanent and that there are no studies showing it to be so even after several treatments. However, the consumer is usually not told what the FDA's regulation is.

When laser hair removal arrived on the scene, many exaggerated, largely unsubstantiated claims about its efficacy, risks, side effects, and long-term effects were asserted (source: *Journal of Cutaneous Laser Therapy*, March 2000, pages 49–50). Far more research has taken place since then and there's much more data (both clearer and more precise) regarding statistical analysis of performance and adverse outcomes. For example, a study reported in *Dermatologic Surgery* (November 2001, pages 920–924) used a " . . . 755 [nanometer] alexandrite laser equipped with a cryogen cooling. . . . Eighty-nine untanned patients . . . in the study underwent a minimum of three treatment sessions spaced 4–6 weeks apart [each patient had an average of 5 treatments]. . . . Treatment sites included the [armpit], bikini, extremities, face, and trunk. RESULTS: The patients had a mean 74% hair reduction. . . . The best results are achieved in untanned patients . . ." Several studies have looked at various other laser systems, including some showing more promise for darker skin tones (source: *Annals of Plastic Surgery*, October 2001, pages 404–411).

The risks in laser hair removal can include skin discoloration (either darkening or lightening of skin), swelling, inflammation, and infected hair follicles. Laser hair removal is particularly problematic for those with tans or darker skin colors (source: *Cosmetic Dermatology*, November 2001, pages 45–50). Because of the potential for complications and the plethora of hair-removal machines available, it is essential to have this procedure performed by a physician who is familiar with the research and who can make the correct choice about which procedure is best for you.

VANIQA

Manufactured by Bristol-Meyers Squibb, Vaniqa *($37.50 for 1.05 ounces)* is FDA-approved as a prescription-only topical cream for reducing and inhibiting the growth of unwanted facial hair (it has not been studied for its effect on hair on other parts of the body). On the surface, Vaniqa might sound like a depilatory (those nonprescription, drugstore products that topically "eat" away hair), but Vaniqa's effect on hair and skin is unrelated to the way a depilatory works.

The active drug in Vaniqa is eflornithine hydrochloride, which has been used as an oral medication for certain cancers and to treat African Sleeping Sickness. Many disconcerting side effects are associated with this drug, ranging from anemia to diarrhea, vomiting, and hair loss. The notion that topical application of eflornithine hydrochloride could also effect hair loss probably stems from its hair-loss side effect when taken orally. However, the product information insert for the medication states that, when applied topically, eflornithine hydrochloride, "is not known to be metabolized and is primarily excreted unchanged in the urine with no adverse systemic side effects."

The information insert for Vaniqa explains that eflornithine hydrochloride affects the skin because it "interferes with an enzyme found in the hair follicle of the skin needed for hair growth. This results in slower hair growth. . . . [However] Vaniqa does not permanently remove hair or 'cure' unwanted facial hair. . . . Your treatment program should include continuation of any hair removal technique you are currently using. . . . [Further] improvement in the condition occurs gradually. Don't be discouraged if you see no immediate improvement. Improvement may be seen as early as 4 to 8 weeks of treatment . . . [and] may take longer in some individuals. If no improvement is seen after 6 months of use, discontinue use. Clinical studies show that in about 8 weeks after stopping treatment with Vaniqa, the hair will return to the same condition as before beginning treatment."

There are warnings that accompany this cream and there is still research to be done. Note that the insert warns, "You should not use Vaniqa if you are less than 12 years of age." Plus, there are animal studies that showed definite fetal problems. That means pregnant women should not use this drug, and lactating women probably should not either, though there is no research about that risk. Also, "Vaniqa may cause temporary redness, stinging, burning, tingling or rash on areas of the skin where it is applied. Folliculitis (hair bumps) may also occur," as well as acne.

So, should you consider Vaniqa? Well, that depends on how you look at the statistics, because clearly for some women it may work well to reduce the amount of facial hair. In addition, you must consider how often you have to use other methods such as tweezing, shaving, or waxing. And it sure beats the expense of laser hair-removal treatments.

What about those statistics? Vaniqa does not work for everyone. "In two randomized double-blind studies involving 594 female patients, approximately 32% of patients showed marked improvement or greater after 24 weeks of treatment compared to 8% [with a placebo]." It is important to note that 42% to 66% of those women in the study showed no improvement or actually believed their condition got worse. If you think it's worth it to find out if you fall into the group of those who might have success with Vaniqa, it may be worth the risk. Just keep in mind that this isn't a slam dunk. More than half of those who use it won't be happy with the results.

HAIR-GROWTH SCAMS

An article in the October 25, 1999, issue of *The Rose Sheet* reported that the National Advertising Division (NAD) of the Better Business Bureau was taking action on unsubstantiated claims for hair-regrowth products being sold by Dr. Adam Lewenberg. Full-page ads in the *New York Times* stated astounding results and a "90% success rate" from using Lewenberg's products, which each sell for around $70 for 2 ounces. "NAD found the study used by Lewenberg not to be adequate for the claims. It was not a controlled clinical study, but rather the advertiser's anecdotal reports of personal observations." What is particularly dismaying is that Lewenberg's formula is merely minoxidil with tretinoin! Both of these are readily available, either over the counter (in the case of minoxidil) or from a dermatologist (in the case of tretinoin, which is the active ingredient in Retin-A and Renova). Tretinoin and minoxidil are indeed options for hair growth, but the statistics are incredibly overblown. Regardless, if you want to give these a trial run, it doesn't require Lewenberg's products, and you'll spend far less money to boot.

HAIR-REMOVAL WARNING!

All treatments for hair removal are contraindicated after any facial peel or laser procedure. It can take six to eight weeks for the skin to completely heal after a peel. Any trauma to the skin during the recovery period can cause discoloration or even scarring.

Hair removal is also extremely problematic if you are using AHAs, BHA, topical retinoids, azelaic acid, or taking Accutane. These treatments can make skin more susceptible to tears, wounds, and irritation. This can all prove damaging and uncomfortable.

chapter *13*
COSMETIC SURGERY

CUTTING AND PASTING

Sometimes money is the root of expensive mistakes. Just because celebrities are doing something doesn't mean you should jump in and do it, too. Yes, lots of celebrities have had their looks altered by cosmetic surgery, but often you can tell at a glance who got a bad face-lift, because their faces have been cut and pulled so tight they look constantly surprised or incessantly half-smiling. Michael Jackson is a classic example of facial cosmetic surgery run amok, but we've all seen others who seem shockingly unattractive, or strangely altered as a result of having had skin pulled too tight, or overfilled with dermal implants, or Botoxed into an expressionless-looking zombie. A number of famous women have had their chests augmented and enlarged to the point that their breasts seem to enter the room a full minute before they do, or stand out like rocks from the chest, but that doesn't mean you should, too.

In short, what you don't know about plastic surgery (namely, the pros and cons and all your options) can hurt you—not just your appearance, but also your health and your pocketbook. To help you think about this, I'd like to give an overview of what is available, along with what you need to know about the risks and/or benefits of different procedures.

Before I get to the details involving the various corrective medical procedures available, I want to address the most important consumer challenge of all: Who should do your surgery, regardless of what you decide to have done. Given the growing number of doctors with cosmetic or plastic surgery practices (and if you live in Southern California or Florida, their advertisements are about as prevalent and insufferable as those for car dealerships), it is very difficult to know where to go and how to get started.

Most women use one of four methods to select a cosmetic surgeon: articles in fashion magazines, finding out where celebrities went (everybody loves knowing where the "stars" are going for anything and everything, regardless of how they look), getting a referral from a friend or a friend of a friend, and, last but not least, checking out the doctors who advertise their services.

Though I wouldn't call these the worst plans of action, they should just be the beginning of the process. You need to know more before you can make an informed final decision. Take the time to gather detailed consumer information. Draw up a comprehensive list of questions to ask so you'll know what all your options are, which procedures will meet your needs, what are the risks or disadvantages, and which doctors are performing the safest and most reliable current procedures. The latest method doesn't necessarily mean the best when it comes to surgery—you don't want to be someone's test case.

Shockingly, many physicians downplay any risks. A quick review of several cosmetic surgery Internet sites reveals a scarcity of information regarding what can go wrong during or after a procedure. Yet each and every medical or cosmetic corrective procedure has risks. Yes, the risks are few and far between, but an average of about 1% to 4% (depending on whose statistic you use) of all patients have some sort of problem or negative outcome. When you consider that over 7.4 million procedures were performed in 2000, that would mean there were at least 74,000 problems. It is wise for you to decide if you want to chance being one of those who may fall within that statistic.

Being proactive about any surgery is incredibly important, but let me reiterate that it is even more vital with cosmetic surgery. After all, this surgery is usually elective and completely up to you; there is (or ought to be) nothing life-or-death about these procedures. Furthermore, cosmetic surgery is a very lucrative business—most surgeons get paid up front before you go under the knife or laser. So, before you hand over your hard-earned money, your very appearance, and your well-being, you have to be knowledgeable about every detail.

COSMETIC SURGERY VERSUS PLASTIC SURGERY

What is the difference between a cosmetic or plastic surgeon and a board-certified plastic surgeon? A lot! Training and credentials in surgery are the issues in contention. Although a doctor may offer cosmetic, plastic, or aesthetic surgery, he or she may not be board-certified to perform that surgery. The person could literally be a gynecologist, pediatrician, or dermatologist with no training in cosmetic surgery whatsoever. Board-certified means the doctor has gone through very specific and extensive training in a specialized field and passed a difficult examination by a board of experts in that field. A non–board-certified cosmetic or plastic surgeon may be self-taught and may lack formal training in that field. Board-certified plastic surgeons consider this an issue of public safety, and I think that's an understatement. They suggest that going to anyone but a board-certified plastic surgeon is a huge mistake, asking, "Would you want your plastic surgery performed by someone who has never had any formal plastic surgery training?" Good question.

According to the American Society of Plastic and Reconstructive Surgeons (a professional association), many physicians who today practice plastic or cosmetic surgery received their formal training in another specialty—often a nonsurgical specialty—or had surgical training for another area of the body. One clear distinction with board-certified plastic surgeons is that they will have privileges to perform plastic surgery at an accredited hospital. Though most cosmetic surgery procedures are done in a doctor's office, you want to be assured that your surgeon has the level of skill accepted by an accredited hospital. It is completely fair to ask any doctor you see for cosmetic surgery whether he or she is board-certified and which hospitals he or she is affiliated with. Then check to be sure the hospital is accredited and the doctor's certification is current and recognized by the American Board of Plastic Surgery (ABPS), the only board recognized by the American Board of Medical Specialties (ABMS) to certify physicians for the full range of plastic and reconstructive procedures. To verify a surgeon's certification status, contact the American Board of Plastic Surgery at (215) 587-9322 or visit the board's Web site at http://www.abplsurg.org or the American Board of Medical Specialties at http://www.abms.org or by phoning (800) 776-2378 (source: American Society of Plastic Surgeons, online at http://www.plasticsurgery.org).

Of course, there are great dermatologists and lousy board-certified plastic surgeons practicing plastic surgery. But the odds of getting someone who is inexperienced are greatly reduced when you take the time to find out if that person is board-certified. To be certified by the ABPS, a physician must have at least five to six years of approved surgical training, including a two- to three-year residency in plastic surgery. He or she must also have been in practice for at least two years and pass comprehensive written and oral exams in plastic surgery.

For more information about a physician in your area who provides these kinds of services, call the Society for Dermatologic Surgery at (800) 441-2737 or the American Society of Plastic Surgeons at (888) 475-2784.

WHAT TO ASK

Once you've dealt with the issue of board certification, ask lots of questions and look for answers that make you feel comfortable and make the most sense to you in light of the research you have done. Not all cosmetic surgeons will come up with the same game plan for your face. Each surgeon has techniques he or she prefers, sometimes regardless of whether they represent the best or most current technology. That's not necessarily bad. Some surgeons use the latest technology not because it is better or has proven more effective but due to pressure from their "elite" clients, who expect what's new regardless of the risks.

One of the most important questions you can ask the surgeons you interview is how often per month they perform the specific procedure or procedures you are considering. It is best (but not essential) to get a doctor who specializes, as opposed to a doctor who tries to do it all.

Likewise, it is also imperative to ask how many surgeries the doctor performs in a day. If the doctor schedules more than three procedures a day, most likely another doctor or nurse will do the prep work and/or the finishing work. That may not mean poor results, but it does mean the doctor is not giving you his or her full attention. Make sure the doctor you are consulting will be the only doctor working on your face or body, and that he or she will never leave the operating room during your procedure.

It is also valid to ask if the doctor charges for redos and touchups. Though it isn't something doctors like to admit, going back in for finetuning or to correct mistakes is common, and you don't want to be charged to have the doctor repair what you don't like.

Be insistent about understanding every nuance of the postoperative procedure. Many complications can occur when the patient doesn't realize her part in the healing process. For example, scar tissue can cause problems for a breast implant. One of the ways to minimize that risk is to keep your breasts tightly bound and your arms firmly at your sides, with little to no movement and no lifting for four to seven days.

WHAT CAN GO WRONG

Negative outcomes are another complex issue. Both patients and physicians have a tendency to ignore the downside of cosmetic surgery. Paying attention to the risks of cosmetic surgery takes the glamour out of the process, so dangers are downplayed almost to the point of being entirely ignored. Even when a doctor does broach the perils of cosmetic surgery, they are often mentioned in an offhand style or glossed over completely in a vague and patronizing manner. Do not turn your face over to a surgeon who doesn't discuss, at length, all the risks involved with the cosmetic procedure you are interested in!

For example, if you are interested in a CO_2 ablative laser peel, you should be told about the risk of scarring or skin discoloration. About 2% of the patients who have a laser peel may develop some amount of scarring (source: *FDA Consumer* magazine, May-June 2000, http://www.fda.gov). You may also not be told that, in one study, 22% of the patients who underwent laser resurfacing considered their results to be disappointing and 77% of the patients (even those who had good results) stated that they would be unwilling to undergo another resurfacing procedure (source: *Facial Plastic Surgery*, August 2001, pages 187–192).

Another fascinating article in *Facial Plastic Surgery* (2000, volume 16, issue 3, pages 215–229, "Prevention and Correction of the 'Face-Lifted' Appearance") discussed some of the known problems of various facial cosmetic surgery procedures. "The unopposed tension of lateral vector face-lifts [traditional face-lifts] allows the cheek tissues to descend eventually over the tightened jawline, creating a "lateral sweep" or pulled appearance of the face. . . . Following conventional blepharoplasty [plastic surgery of the upper and lower eyelids], the lower eyelid contour becomes deeper, and often a hollow appearance develops. . . . Unwanted and unattractive results are not the fault of the surgeon or the patient but are caused by the surgical technique. As a primary rejuvenative procedure, a composite [face-lift] will deliver an impressive result that will disallow the ultimate lateral sweep and hollow eyes. In patients that have the unhappy signs of surgery this procedure can effectively correct the face-lifted appearance."

Cosmetic corrective or plastic surgery procedures can produce amazing results and literally erase years off your face or create the appearance you've always wanted, but do not assume there aren't risks, because there are. What you don't know means you can end up unhappy and, in plastic surgery, you won't get your money back.

WHEN TO DO IT

The options for changing your body and face are almost limitless, and the results can be stunning. Traditional surgical procedures that cut off leathery, thick, lined, and sagging skin long abused by the sun can subtract years from a person's appearance. Laser resurfacing can create smooth skin and remove skin discolorations. Dermal fillers can plump up wrinkles and acne scarring. Endoscopic face-lifts can rejuvenate the face using tiny incisions without any cutting and pasting of the skin.

In the past, most people waited until they were well into their late 50s and 60s, with noticeably aged skin, before they jumped into the fray of cosmetic surgery. All that has changed with the advent of relatively non-invasive, low-cost procedures such as laser resurfacing, Botox, and dermal fillers. Indeed, having some procedures done at a younger age, before you "need it" means having healthier-looking skin for years as opposed to an abrupt change when you finally decide you can't take it any more and search out a plastic surgeon.

Women in their early 40s and 50s may want to undergo cosmetic surgery to deal with sagging corners of the mouth, slight pouching or sagging of the chin and jawline, and folds along the forehead. Though hardly aging by some standards, these irksome signs of middle age are easy to modify. Cosmetic surgery at this relatively young age slows the way skin will continue to age.

There are also endless options for cosmetic procedures that are just about maintenance or reshaping the face. Whether it is acne scarring, excess fat or skin, surfaced face veins, skin discolorations, hair removal, or changing the appearance of your nose or lips, facial enhancement has a plethora of options to offer.

Some cosmetic surgeons suggest that when you are younger, laser resurfacing, endoscopic face-lifts, and mini-tucks (doing a section of the face as opposed to an overall face-lift) are the best ways to put off the need for a full face-lift or eye tuck until you're much farther down the road. They claim that if you do things as they crop up there's less trauma, better healing, and, because younger people generally have more elasticity and fat in their skin, the results should last longer. Whether or not less-invasive procedures or minor procedures decrease the need for eventual major surgery is not yet known, but there is something to be said for having the face you want now as opposed to later.

We are in a new era of accessibility to cosmetic surgery. Some people are pleased to know their face doesn't have to look as old as they really are, and that they can have a choice about what to do about it. As long as the results are impressive (and they are), people will want to stay young-looking via any procedure that is relatively nonrisky and permanent (although all cosmetic surgery has duration limitations). That's not bad or good, it is just a legitimate option for creating the look you want. Plus, it beats wasting money on creams and lotions that do nothing for the wrinkles. As one plastic surgeon I spoke with noted, "Women have been buying wrinkle creams by the truckload, and yet they still get wrinkles and I'm still in business because none of those cosmetic products work to stop or change wrinkling."

PRETREATMENT

Some women have been told that before they have a chemical peel, laser resurfacing, or any cosmetic surgical procedure they need to purchase special products weeks ahead of their treatment. The claim is that these will prepare the skin, improving the outcome and healing process. Most typically you will have been sold an AHA solution of some type, a skin-lightening product (hydroquinone-based), and a vitamin C concoction, along with the recommendation to pick up a prescription for Retin-A or Renova. However, an article published in *Cosmetic Dermatology* (March 2000, "Pre-Treatment of Skin for Laser Resurfacing: Is It Necessary?") states: "Retinoic acid derivatives [tretinoin such as Retin-A or Renova] have been studied most thoroughly and have been shown to accelerate wound healing. On the other hand, the preoperative use of AHAs, hydroquinone, and ascorbic acid [vitamin C] has proven to be of no apparent clinical benefit. Since these compounds appear to affect only superficial epidermal melanocytes [skin cells] (which are vaporized upon . . . laser irradiation) . . . they have no effect on the lower layers of skin." That means you can save your money on expensive pretreatment products being sold by the physician.

However, you will want to consider using a topical tretinoin cream. A study published in the *Archives of Dermatological Research* (November 2001, pages 515–521) concluded that wound healing is greatly improved with the pretreatment of topical tretinoin, but that is different from the cosmetic products many doctors are selling these days.

Although cosmetic skin-care products are not helpful for use as a pretreatment, at least in terms of helping your skin handle the procedures better, the ongoing use of well-formulated AHAs, BHA, skin-lightening products, and sunscreen can go a long way toward helping you keep the results you achieved and also ensuring that your skin is as healthy as it can be all the time.

POSSIBILITIES FROM A TO Z

The pages that follow include procedures from the neck up listed alphabetically. The risks and gains are best contemplated cautiously and from a consumer's point of view (weighing the pros and cons), not by how your friend looks after she had it done. These procedures are not a guarantee of happiness, just a way to buy the kind of face you want. (If that designer suit didn't make you happy, don't expect a face-lift to provide peace of mind!) Every plastic surgeon I spoke with suggested that the patients most pleased with the results of their surgery were the ones who had the most realistic expectations. What are unrealistic expectations? Expecting to end up looking like a supermodel or believing you will now find the perfect relationship. Plastic surgery should be about your self-esteem associated with societal standards of beauty—nothing more and nothing less.

Important details: Keep in mind that everyone scars differently, and it often has little to do with the skill of the surgeon. You could be left with lines wherever an incision was made. In general, the paler your skin, the more prone you may be to red, welt-like scarring, and the darker your skin, the more prone you may be to thick, dark, keloidal scarring.

There are serious risks with all surgical procedures, and recovering from the more serious operations, such as face-lifts, can be a daunting, frightening experience. Studies indicate that 97% of people who experience some kind of cosmetic surgery are quite pleased with the results. However, the 3% who are unhappy can be devastated. For example, eye tucks can damage the tear ducts or permanently destroy eyelashes, face-lifts can leave painful scars and pockets of dimpled flesh, and laser or chemical peels can render skin tone uneven.

Many doctors love to use computer imaging to "close the sale" on the cosmetic procedure they are recommending. A picture of your face or body is taken and scanned into a computer program, allowing the surgeon to then demonstrate how you would look pulled a little here, tucked a little there, and lifted a little all over. As impressive as this is, it is only a computer image and not real life. It is a great tool for getting an idea of what you can expect, but it isn't an exact blueprint. Don't let it be the deciding factor in your final decision.

All cosmetic surgery procedures have limitations as to how long the change will last, depending on skin type, age, the surgeon's technique, and postoperative care (including using sunscreen). Do not expect any cosmetic surgery to be permanent, especially laser peels, dermal filler injections, chemical peels, and Botox (discussed below).

Note: As indicated below, prices for these procedures vary widely. The region of the country you live in, the popularity of the surgeon, the specific techniques used (the more invasive or complex, the more expensive), the combination of techniques, and discounts given for doing more than one procedure can all greatly affect price.

Botox (Botulinum Toxin A) ($300 to $1,000)

The following section on Botox is the only place where I share my personal experience with a cosmetic corrective procedure. I believe my experience was extremely representative, and after all the research I've seen, I thought it would be helpful and maybe a bit fun. What happened, to mention just one thing, was that for a period of time I couldn't look too surprised. At least not for three to four months after I had it done. Botox is the brand name of the nontoxic form of botulinum toxin type A. In 2001 botulinum toxin type B (see next section) was launched, with the trade name Myobloc. When injected into specific muscles, both these treatments prevent movement by partially and almost completely paralyzing them. The resulting inability to use particular face muscles causes certain wrinkles to disappear completely. This helps eliminate almost all of the wrinkles of the forehead, in the crow's feet area (by the eyes), and the lines that run from the nose to the mouth (the nasolabial folds). As outlandish and frightening as this sounds, in reality it is no more bizarre than any other cosmetic corrective procedure. It is also important to mention that the results from Botox are truly astounding, and I mean really astounding, which explains the growing popularity of this medical procedure for the treatment of wrinkles. Over 800,000 Botox treatments were administered in 2001.

Botox is not anything new. Since 1973 it has been used by ophthalmologists to treat patients with disabling eye ticks, as well as to treat crossed eyes. It is also used by other medical specialists to treat spasmodic neck muscles, spasmodic laryngeal muscles, multiple sclerosis, cerebral palsy, some post-stroke states, spinal cord injuries, nerve palsies, Parkinson's disease, facial spasms, and, most recently, migraine headaches. This extensive use (and the corresponding research) has shown that Botox has a great success rate, with minimal risk of detrimental side effects. In rare cases, depending on what parts of your face were injected, you may experience temporary facial or eye drooping, bruising, or jaw and neck weakness, but it lasts only for the duration of the Botox, so it goes away in three to six months.

From my own experience, the Botox injections, about ten of them in various points of my forehead, did hurt. One injection site bruised and two others were sore for three days. The bruising was completely gone after five days and so was the soreness. I did have a consistent, though mild, tension headache for several days. I think this was from repeatedly testing the results by trying to raise my eyebrows or frown. I couldn't look in mirrors often enough, straining to raise my eyebrows to see how it was going, plus my friends and those in my office wanted to see the results. Though everyone could tell my forehead wrinkles and the wrinkles between my eyes were gone they couldn't tell the difference when it came to the way I use my forehead and eyebrows. It was amazing to me that no one could tell I wasn't able to squint or look surprised. Once I stopped my facial demonstrations the headaches seemed to disappear.

After the first day I couldn't raise my eyebrows. It took several days before I could no longer furrow my brows. After the first injections, I had a consistent feeling of heaviness in my eyes and I thought they looked somewhat puffy under the eyebrow area (that did not happen on subsequent injections). This feeling lasted about a week. One interesting and unexpected side effect is that putting on eye makeup is now a little tricky because I can't raise my eyebrows to adjust my eyelid and crease area to get a flat area to apply eyeshadow.

The bottom line, or should I say the bottom un-line, is that my forehead is unusually smooth and the wrinkles are practically gone! It is the most amazing thing I've ever experienced. Studies have shown that repeated injections can create a buildup effect, making the results last longer. This one is too tempting to ignore—which explains its rise in popularity.

Note: The physician who performed the procedure on me warned that there are physicians advertising or offering inexpensive Botox treatments for under $400. He feels strongly that, given the raw material cost of Botox (over $300 to treat the forehead area alone), if a physician isn't charging enough they could very possibly be using a watered-down Botox solution, resulting in poor or extremely short-term results. It takes just a little mathematics to realize that a doctor would be operating at a loss if he didn't charge appropriately for the Botox treatment. If the solution costs $300, you have to add in the doctor's expenses like rent, assistants, liability insurance, equipment, and on and on. There are no doctors providing cosmetic Botox treatments as a charity. As is true in any cosmetic or medical procedure, this is not an arena where you should expect to get both good results and a bargain.

Myobloc (Botulinum Toxin B) ($300 to $1,000)

Myobloc (botulinum toxin type B) was approved by the FDA in December 2000 "for the symptomatic treatment of patients with cervical dystonia (CD) to reduce the severity of abnormal head position and neck pain associated with CD." Cervical dystonia is a neurological movement disorder in which a person's neck and shoulder muscles are subject to contractions that force the head and neck into abnormal and sometimes painful positions, making it difficult for some people to function normally in their daily activities.

For those receiving Myobloc treatments for CD, the side effects may include dry mouth, dysphagia, dyspepsia, and injection site pain. These adverse effects are generally mild to moderate, transient, self-resolving, and more common only with higher doses. The side effects are also related to the location of the injection site and the muscles involved and not the drug itself. Myobloc was formerly known as BotB and is marketed outside the United States as Neurobloc.

For facial wrinkles, people who are resistant to Botox might find Myobloc more suitable and effective. However, the question of whether to choose Botox over Myobloc is not a simple one. According to Mike A.

Royal, MD, in an online research paper entitled "The Use of Botulinum Toxins (BT) in the Management of Myofascial Pain and Other Conditions Associated with Painful Muscle Spasm," (http://www.pain.com), "The recent addition of the Elan Pharmaceuticals product, Myobloc™ (BTB—Botulinum Toxin Type B) also raises the important issue of choice. Although the net effect of each BT is to block acetylcholine release, one cannot take data derived from clinical studies of BTA (Botulinum Type A) and apply it to BTB by making some adjustment for potency differences. Each BT has a different structure, different mechanism of action (although the net effect may be the same), different formulation, different storage and handling guidelines, different FDA-approved uses, different dosing concerns, and possibly different antibody development concerns. BTA has been around much longer and all of the published pain and headache clinical research used BTA."

The same holds true for wrinkles. Clearly, Myobloc can be effective for wrinkles but the information for this is limited. As this book goes to press, we know far more about the success of Botox (BTA) for wrinkles than we do about Myobloc. I would wait to jump on the Myobloc bandwagon. You don't need to be the guinea pig for this one.

Cheekbone (Malar) Augmentation ($2,000 to $3,500)

Improving the shape of the face is an option separate from the issue of facial rejuvenation. For many women a more sculpted face is an aesthetic goal, and, therefore, cheekbone augmentation is a more common procedure in facial plastic surgery practices. Cheekbones are reshaped and built up by placing a plastic implant over them. This procedure is considered a safe, relatively simple technique with generally good results (source: *Facial and Plastic Surgery*, February 2000, pages 35–44). The implant is usually inserted via an incision within the mouth, but it may be done through a lower eyelid or brow incision. Perhaps the biggest mistake made during this procedure is overcompensation which causes a fake-looking visage because of cheekbones so enlarged that they look like they belong on someone else (think Disney's Cruella de Vil.)

Alternatively, the buccal fat pads, which are located above the jawline near the corners of the mouth, just below the cheekbone, can be removed in individuals with an excessively round face. This procedure imparts a more contoured look, sometimes referred to as the "waif look," à la Kate Moss. However, plastic surgeons warn that, in many individuals, removal of the buccal fat pads can lead to a more drawn, hollow-cheeked look as aging progresses, something that naturally occurs to the face as it grows older.

Chemical Peel ($500 to $2,700 depending on the type of peel)

Peel solutions may contain alpha hydroxy acids, beta hydroxy acid, tricholoracetic acid (TCA), or phenol as the peeling agent. Each of these are categorized by the concentration and the resulting depth of the peel on the skin. Fine lines and wrinkles, skin discolorations, reduction in the appearance of skin discolorations and scars, along with overall improvement in skin texture and subtle rebuilding of the skin's collagen are all possible outcomes of chemical peels. There are definite drawbacks to consider, but this is largely dependent on the depth of peel. The risk of complication is directly related to the amount of benefit desired. Superficial peels have little to no associated risks, although prolonged redness, swelling, and increased skin sensitivity do occur. When more significant results are desired, the complications increase proportionately. Skin discoloration in medium and deeper peels (called hypopigmentation) is typical for most Caucasian patients. Many more complications and scars are recorded from TCA peeling than from phenol, perhaps because of the care with which phenol peels must be performed and the implied safety of TCA (source: *eMedicine Journal*, February 14, 2002, volume 3, number 2).

Chemical peels are performed by the application of the specific solution that peels away the skin's top layers, either on the entire face or on specific areas. Often, several shallow to medium-depth peels can achieve results similar to one deep-peel treatment, with less post-procedure risk and a shorter recovery time.

Alpha hydroxy acids (AHA) use glycolic acid as the chemical ingredient. Various concentrations can be applied, but most commonly 30% to 70% concentrations are used. The lower the concentration, the less impressive the results. AHA peels are effective in improving skin texture, causing some collagen and elastin rebuilding, somewhat reducing the appearance of acne scarring, and reducing the appearance of skin discolorations (source: *American Journal of Clinical Dermatology*, March-April 2000, pages 81–88).

AHA peels are not medical procedures and as a result are not regulated by the FDA. A physician usually performs higher-concentration peels, but this is not always the case. In lower-concentration peels, often performed by aestheticians, repeated treatments are necessary to achieve and maintain the results seen immediately after the peel is performed.

Beta hydroxy acid (BHA) or salicylic acid peels are not as popular as AHA peels, yet they are equally as effective and have specific advantages for some skin types. A solution of salicylic acid can work in a way that is similar to a glycolic acid peel, but irritation is much reduced. Salicylic acid is a compound closely related to aspirin (acetylsalicylic acid), and it retains its aspirin-like anti-inflammatory properties. A deep BHA peel can be superior for many skin types because the irritation and inflammation are kept to a minimum due to the analgesic action of the BHA compound. Salicylic acid is also lipid soluble; therefore, it is a good peeling agent for blemish-prone skin with blackheads. The most common concentrations used today are 20% to 30% (source: *Dermatologic Surgery*, March 1998, pages 325–328).

Trichloroacetic acid (TCA) peels in concentrations of 10% to 35% have been used for many years and are considered effective and safe (source: *Dermatologic Clinics*, July 2001, pages 413–425). It can be used for peeling the face, neck, hands, and other exposed areas of the body. It has less bleaching effect than phenol (see the next paragraph) and is excellent for "spot" peeling of specific areas. It can be used for medium or light peeling, depending on the concentration and method of application. TCA peels are best for fine lines but are minimally effective on deeper wrinkling (source: *eMedicine Journal*, December 5, 2001, volume 2, number 12). However, at higher concentrations, such as 50% and above, TCA has a tendency to scar and is less manageable than other agents used for superficial peels.

Phenol is sometimes, though rarely, used for full-face peeling when sun damage or wrinkling is severe. It can also be used to treat limited areas of the face, such as deep wrinkles around the mouth, but it may permanently bleach the skin, leaving a line of demarcation between the treated and untreated areas that must be covered with makeup. "Although phenol produces the most remarkable resolution of actinic damage and wrinkling among the various [chemical peels] . . . it also possesses some of the more significant [serious side effects]. Many have abandoned phenol in favor of other agents or laser resurfacing. . . . Hypopigmentation may occur in all skin types, noticeably lightening patients with darker skin and making lighter-skinned patients appear waxy or pale. A clear line of demarcation may be present between treated and untreated skin" (source: *eMedicine Journal*, July 20, 2001, volume 2, number 7). Given the positive results that can be achieved with other resurfacing procedures and the extreme risks associated with phenol, this method is actively discouraged and rarely used.

Buffered phenol offers yet another option for severely sun-damaged skin. One such formula uses olive oil, among other ingredients, to diminish the strength of the phenol solution. Another, slightly milder formula uses glycerin. A buffered phenol peel may be more comfortable for patients, and the skin heals faster than with a standard phenol peel, but it is still a risky procedure that can depigment the skin.

Chin Augmentation (Mentoplasty), Chin Reduction ($1,700 to $5,000)

Chin augmentation can strengthen the appearance of a receding chin by increasing its projection. (Look at pictures of Michael Jackson when he was young, then look at a recent picture; it's hard to ignore his mega-chin implant.) The procedure does not affect the patient's bite or jaw, and can be done using one of two techniques. One approach is to make an incision inside the mouth, move the chin bone, and then wire it into position; the other requires the insertion of an implant through an incision inside the mouth, between the lower lip and the gum, or through an external incision underneath the chin. Hydroxyapatite granules, a bone substitute made from coral, can also be used to enhance facial contours, such as forming a more prominent chin or cheekbones. The substance also has reconstructive uses in craniofacial surgery.

From another perspective, even if the shape of the chin may not be an issue, excess skin can start pouching along the jawline, creating the appearance of a double chin or a turkey neck. A chin tuck can help shore up this sagging by cutting away surplus skin and using liposuction to remove the excess fat. The scar is hidden just under the jaw.

Collagen Injections ($325 to $1,400)

See "Dermal Fillers," on page 320.

Cosmetic Tattooing ($750 to $1,500)

Cosmetic tattooing, or micropigmentation, can be used to create permanent eyeliner, eyebrow color, or lip color. It can also be used for permanent blush or eyeshadow, though this is uncommon. Other uses include re-creating the coloration of the areola around the nipple following breast reconstruction; restoring the color of dark or light skin where natural pigmentation has been lost through such factors as vitiligo (a whitening of the skin from an autoimmune response), cancer, burns, or other scarring; and eliminating some types of birthmarks or previous tattoos.

As a general rule, I do *not* recommend tattooing as a cosmetic way to create permanent eyeliner, eyebrows, colored lips, and especially not for blush. As seductive as permanent makeup sounds—who wouldn't love to avoid drawing on eyebrows and eyeliner, or constantly reapplying lipstick—remember that fashions change and the face ages. Permanent eyebrows that look nice and even when you're in your 40s can sag as your skin ages, and the same is true for the eyeliner and blush. Additionally, your personal style preferences can change. A pink or red lip color imprinted on your mouth may look good today, but in five or ten years it can look strange and out of date. Many cosmetic surgeons I've interviewed have commented that removing tattooed-on lip liner, eyebrows, and blush has become a lucrative business due to the large number of botched applications.

Dermabrasion ($1,000 to $2,500)

Dermabrasion is a procedure in which a high-speed wheel, similar to a rotary sander using fine-grained sandpaper, is used to abrade the skin. As a method of resurfacing, dermabrasion can provide effective treatment for treating deep acne scars and deep facial wrinkling. Its benefit is the absence of heat damage that lasers and chemical peels can cause. However, some expected side effects, both transient and long-term, are considered normal and do occur. Transient effects can include spot bleeding for several days after surgery, swelling, breakouts, and hyperpigmentation. Hypopigmentation, the more permanent loss of skin color, occurs in 20% to 30% of patients. Possible scarring can also occur but that is true for any of the deeper chemical peels and ablative laser resurfacing (source: *eMedicine Journal*, October 17, 2001, volume 2, number 10).

Despite these daunting considerations dermabrasion may still be recommended for deep acne scarring, providing there is a real understanding about the risk of depigmentation.

Dermal Fillers

Whether it's called tissue augmentation, injectable fillers, soft-tissue fillers, implants, or filler injections, one of the more popular ways to improve the appearance of wrinkles or acne scars is to fill them in with a variety of substances. These fillers work by literally being injected or implanted into a wrinkle or a scar where the material (either synthetic or natural) then fills in the depression (temporarily or semipermanently), creating a smoother impression. Almost all fillers can also work to plump up lips or alter the shape of the face, but their primary use is to fill in wrinkles and acne scars.

Filling in wrinkles or scars using any form of tissue augmentation is often done in combination with other cosmetic procedures. These can range from Botox injections to laser or chemical peel resurfacing (as well as face-lifts) to achieve optimal results in obtaining the smoothest looking skin you can get. If you're considering injectable fillers of any kind the following information will help give you a realistic guideline for comparisons, risks, and expectations. It is vital to understand that with any cosmetic corrective procedure there isn't one best option. Quite the contrary—there are many excellent alternatives available, with the final decision determined by your doctor's skill, your budget, how much risk you're willing to take, and what kind of realistic results you're looking for.

When it comes to filling in wrinkles with injectables or any filler substance, each type has its own limitations and benefits. Once again, there isn't a single best or foolproof method. Injectable fillers and tissue augmentation are not reliable options for extreme wrinkling, particularly the crisscrossed or interwoven wrinkles that appear on the cheeks or the lines around the mouth. The effects are also rarely permanent, requiring subsequent procedures at different intervals (typically three months to a year). Some of the fillers can feel hard or look noticeable under the skin, while others can distribute unevenly and look lumpy. In addition, many of the fillers being used today are new and there isn't a great deal of information about long-term results.

I know it's a lot of work trying to understand such a confluence of complicated information regarding all your options. But weighing the pros and cons of each alternative and then discussing them with your doctor *is* truly the best way to get the results you want and not be disappointed.

Note: One of the risks that all injectable or tissue fillers present is a possible reaction to the needle or device used to place the material in the skin. Side effects can include pain, bruising, inflammation, discoloration, and swelling. These often resolve within a few days to a few weeks. On rare occasions discoloration can last for up to a year if a blood vessel was affected.

Animal-Derived Collagen Injections
   Brand names: Zyderm, Zyplast, Fibrel
   Major risks: Allergic reactions can occur. It can have a hard feel under skin, and may look lumpy or uneven under the skin.
   Stability: Benefits can last three to six months.
   Results: Appearance improves immediately.
   Cost: $300 to $800 (subsequent injections may cost less).

Collagen is found in all living tissue, and its basic function is to provide support and structure for the skin. The FDA approved injectable collagen in 1981. For most of the 1980s and 1990s, collagen injections were one of the primary methods used to fill in wrinkles. Zyderm and Zyplast are derived from cow collagen; Fibrel is derived from pig collagen. Injectable animal collagens are used less frequently in Europe than in the United States due to the risk of their association with bovine spongiform encephalopathy (Mad Cow Disease). Collagen injections derived from animal sources are now used less frequently than other dermal fillers in the United States, but that is largely due to a substantial risk of allergic reaction (according to the FDA, "about 3 percent of the population is allergic to collagen") and the short duration of the results.

Because of the potential for allergic reaction (particularly for cow collagen), it is essential to have a pretest at least four to six weeks prior to treatment. A small amount of the collagen is injected into the arm or thigh and the area is monitored closely for any signs of inflammation, swelling, irritation, rashes, or itching. Once it has been determined that you are not allergic to the material it can be injected into the wrinkle underneath the skin. Repeated injections may be necessary until optimal results are achieved.

Human-Derived Collagen Injections
   Brand names: Dermalogen, Autologen, Isolagen
   Major risks: Minimal to no risk of allergic reaction, but the area injected can have a hard feel under skin and may look lumpy or uneven.
   Stability: Benefits can last three to nine months and possibly longer, though there is no research establishing exact length of time.
   Results: Appearance improves immediately.
   Cost: $500 to $1,000 (subsequent injections may cost less).

Dermalogen is derived from human cadaver collagen, Autologen is derived from your own skin's collagen, and Isolagen is made of cells that are actually cloned from your own skin. The primary benefit of human-derived collagen injections is that there is almost no chance of having or developing an allergic reaction.

Autologen can be harvested during cosmetic surgery procedures such as tummy tucks, face-lifts, and breast augmentation or reduction. The skin removed from those procedures is sent to a laboratory where it is processed to become injectable collagen filler. Depending on the results you are trying to achieve you may receive a series of injections over a period of a year. Some doctors claim that Autologen achieves permanent results, but that has not been proven, and for many women is definitely not the case.

Isolagen, as futuristic as it sounds, is made of cells cloned from your own skin. It's done by simply removing a small piece of skin (about the size of a dime) from your neck or behind your ear. The skin is sent to a lab that, in about four to six weeks, can grow your own injectable collagen from it. Generally, three to four injections are delivered over a two-month period. Each subsequent injection produces increased improvement. After the last injection, continued improvement may still be seen because, unlike all other injectable procedures, Isolagen uses live cells and that stimulates further smoothing out of wrinkles for a period of time.

Note: Isolagen was available in the United States from 1996 to 1999. During that time the FDA categorized Isolagen as a graft, and it was, therefore, not subject to any regulatory scrutiny. In 1999, the FDA reclassified Isolagen as a drug, which meant it could no longer be used in regulated surgical medical procedures. The company that makes Isolagen has filed a New Drug Application with the FDA, and clinical trials are pending. That process can take up to four years before it meets the FDA standards for drug acceptance. However, there are patients currently involved in clinical trials who are receiving Isolagen injections (source: *Skin & Allergy News*, May 1999).

The process of creating Dermalogen is similar to that for creating both Isolagen and Autologen. Dermalogen, however, is derived from skin tissue removed at the time of death, much as other organs are removed from human donors. All three—Autologen, Isolagen, and Dermalogen— are thought to last longer than animal-derived collagen, but that is yet to be proven. A primary benefit of Dermalogen over Isolagen and Auto-logen is that it doesn't require any skin removal (at least not from you); and there's no waiting time for preparation.

Fat Transfer Injections

Technical names: Autologous Fat Transplantation, fat injections, Microlipoinjection, Fat Grafting

Major risks: There are risks associated with liposuction procedures. From the injection itself there can be some local swelling, redness, and bruising. Scar-tissue buildup is possible, and it is possible to tem-porarily lose sensation in the treatment area due to nerve damage or swelling. Long-term or permanent loss of sensitivity is possible. There is also the risk of an asymmetrical appearance.

Stability: Your body will absorb about 65% of the fat within the first six months. The remaining 35% can remain in place for longer, but exactly how much longer varies greatly from person to person. For some reason some people's bodies just can't hold on to the injected fat, even when it's their own.

Results: Appearance improves immediately, though doctors often overfill the area to improve the chances of long-term results.

Cost: $450 to $3,000.

Getting rid of your own fat and then injecting it into your wrinkles to eliminate them does sound like the best of all worlds, but fat injections are a more complicated process than other injectables. So even though the concept of redistributing fat from an area where you don't want it (like the thighs and buttocks) to areas where it may be of better use (like wrinkles) is very appealing, the benefit of fat transplantation is limited by the dramatic reabsorption of fat grafts.

The first step is to remove fat from your own body, and it's usually taken from the abdomen or buttocks. It is important that the fat being used has a soft texture so it can more easily adapt and be contoured to the shape of the face. Once the fat is extracted it is processed to make it usable, so it can be injected precisely underneath the wrinkle to fill in and reshape the area. This injection process is repeated until the desired en-hancement is attained.

Another added benefit of fat injections is that when physicians extract fat from a liposuction procedure, breast augmentation, a tummy tuck, or some other reduction surgery, they can store the fat in a freezer to be used in future fat-injection procedures.

Because of the amount of absorption that takes place within the first few months of treatment; many physicians overfill the treated area to help improve the long-term results. This overfilling can create a strange appearance by making the face look swollen and puffy. The puffiness does diminish over a period of weeks, but be aware that this is a potential problem for the short term.

Hyaluronic Acid–Derived Fillers

Brand names: Restylane, Hylaform, Perlane, Rofilan Hylan Gel

Major risk: Hypersensitivity can occur in 1 out of every 2,000 treated patients. There have also been cases of persistent inflammation and noninfected abscesses, which may persist for up to a year, or until the injected material is fully reabsorbed.

Stability: Benefits can last three to six months and occasionally for one year.

Results: Appearance improves immediately.

Cost: Still in trial stages so pricing is not available.

Restylane, Hylaform, Perlane, and Rofilan are not yet approved by the FDA for use in the United States. However, a handful of doctors have been selected to test them on patients willing to sign a waiver while the products go through the FDA's process of being accepted as approved medical treatments for wrinkles. All of these fillers are derived from nonanimal sources of hyaluronic acid. Although hyaluronic acid is a part of human skin, these injectable substances are synthetically modified. Even though a pretest is thought not to be necessary, it is generally best to go through the process anyway to be certain you do not have a special or unique reaction to this substance. None of these new fillers are permanent and they are eventually reabsorbed into the body.

Hylaform, Perlane, Rofilan, and Restylane have many similarities. The primary difference is in their consistency: Hylaform, Perlane, and Rofilan are viscoelastic gels, which means that they are more viscous and pliable than Restylane. This makes them better for treatment of deeper lines than for superficial wrinkles, where they can feel thick and be visible under the skin. Restylane, on the other hand, is better for treatment of superficial wrinkles.

Human Donor Tissue Implants

Technical name: Acellular Cadaveric Dermis

Brand names: AlloDerm, Micronized AlloDerm, Cymetra

Major risk: There can be some local swelling, redness, and bruising (mainly from the injection itself), but this is usually short-lived. The implant area can feel hard for a period of months and even longer for some patients.

Stability: Benefits can last one to two years, though maybe less for areas of the face that have the most movement.

Results: Appearance improves immediately, but continued improvement takes place as production of your own body's collagen is stimulated.

Cost: $1,000 to $1,500.

Acellular Cadaveric Dermis is essentially the use of donor tissue obtained from dead bodies. Much as donor organs are removed from cadavers at the time of death, skin tissue can also be surgically removed and then processed to be used as filler material for wrinkles or to improve facial contours. The donated human tissue goes through a treatment process until it is finally freeze-dried in a way that preserves the integrity of the dermal matrix. When it is ready to be used it is rehydrated and surgically inserted under the skin where recountouring is desired. Once implanted, AlloDerm merges with your own skin and stimulates your body to produce its own collagen until it essentially becomes a part of your skin. Although Alloderm is not widely used as a filler for wrinkles, it has been successfully used in thousands of skin-graft operations and is considered exceptionally safe, stable, and reliable for creating natural-looking results.

Fascia Injections

Technical name: Irradiated Human Cadaveric Preserved Fascia Lata

Brand name: Fascian

Major risks: Depending on the amount of material and the size of the needle used, the injected site can become swollen or bruised. The area may also feel thick or lumpy, though typically this softens in time. Allergic reactions are rare.

Stability: Benefits can last three to six months.

Results: Appearance improves immediately.

Cost: $800 to $1,000.

Fascian, much like Alloderm (reviewed on page 326), is obtained from donor tissue from dead bodies. In this case the donated material is fascia, the substance covering your muscles (and some organs) in large, thick, white sheets, keeping them compact and supported yet limber. Fascia's unique property is that it is a firm yet pliable type of human tissue, with qualities that make it adaptable for use in improving the appearance of skin. The main drawback of this procedure is its expense when compared with the length of time results remain, which is not much longer than other injectables.

Synthetic Implants
   Brand names: Gore S.A.M., Softform
   Major risks: Unpleasant firmness and risk of the implant breaking through the skin. Thinner strands of Gore S.A.M. (Subcutaneous Augmentation Material) and Softform may reduce the risk of overfirmness. Synthetic implants are not recommended for lip enhancement due to the potential for an uneven or hard, unnatural appearance of lips. Your body can reject the implant. Scarring can occur.
   Stability: Benefits can be permanent.
   Results: Appearance improves immediately, but as your own skin tissue meshes with the implant further improvement is often seen.
   Cost: $1,000 to $4,000.

For those of us who live in the Northwest, Gore-Tex is a well-known, durable, synthetic fabric that works well in all weather conditions. It is essentially a form of Teflon. Gore-Tex has remarkable flexibility, and in the form of Gore S.A.M. created by the same company that developed Gore-Tex (W. L. Gore and Associates), it can be used for cosmetic corrective procedures. The actual implant material is called expanded polytetrafluoroethylene (ePTFE). Implanting threadlike strips of Gore S.A.M. under the skin around the lips or along the nasolabial folds (the lines that run from the nose to the mouth) can improve the appearance of the face.

Gore S.A.M. is porous, and therefore allows the body's own tissue to attach itself to the implant, creating a very durable, stable implant. However, Gore S.A.M has limited uses. For example, those with thin skin would find that the implant can easily be felt or even seen under the surface. It also should not be used on the lips because of the risk of stiffness, making the mouth look unnatural.

The Softform implant is made from the same material as Gore S.A.M.

The major difference between Softform and Gore S.A.M. is that Softform threads are hollow, as opposed to Gore S.A.M., which is porous. Softform's hollow form allows your own tissue to grow through the cylinder to help make it more stable and durable.

Artecoll

Brand name: Artecoll

Major risk: Artecoll has the same potential for allergic reactions as collagen injections.

Stability: Benefits can be permanent, but this is still under investigation.

Results: Appearance improves immediately, but continued improvement takes place as your own body's production of collagen and connective tissue is stimulated.

Cost: Still in trial stages so pricing is not available.

Artecoll is a combination injectable made up of a synthetic substance called polymethylmethacrylate (PMMA) and collagen (similar to Zyderm and Zyplast, reviewed on page 322). Artecoll is not approved as an implant material in the United States. The FDA has only recently accepted it for research as an Investigational Medical Device (IDE) for wrinkles, which means that only a handful of doctors are approved to use it. While Artecoll is relatively new in the treatment of wrinkles, it has been around for the past 50 years as a bone substitute and it is approved in Canada and Europe as an injectable filler for wrinkles. It is thought to have fewer reactions than other injectables, but this is yet to be established definitively.

Artecoll is injected in the same manner as collagen, and has the same initial results. With Artecoll, however, after the collagen is absorbed or broken down by the body, the synthetic material PMMA remains, stimulating the formation of new collagen and connective tissue in the area surrounding the PMMA. One or two applications are enough to obtain good results. The results are thought to be permanent, but this is yet to be proven.

Silicone Injections

Brand name: Dermagen

It is amazing to me that silicone injections are still being used to fill in wrinkles. According to the FDA, silicone injections are approved only for limited ophthalmic use and are prohibited for any other purpose. We tend to think of silicone in relation to breast implants or breast augmentation. Dow Corning has settled some very sizable lawsuits due to complications resulting from their medical-grade silicone breast implants. However, there are some doctors who still use injectable silicone as a wrinkle filler for the face. While the exact potential for damage to the body is an extremely controversial question, there is no doubt that silicone in the body can become encapsulated as the body tries to reject it, creating a serious and persistent inflammation that has strong potential for becoming infected and destroying surrounding skin tissue. I would not encourage anyone concerned with filling in wrinkles to pursue this procedure.

Ear Surgery (Otoplasty) ($2,000 to $3,000)

If you've worn heavy earrings for most of your life, your earlobes may be swinging down closer to your shoulders than you ever thought possible. A simple, 30-minute earlobe reduction can be performed in a plastic surgeon's office or at the same time as a face-lift. Aesthetically speaking, or at least to be sure your earlobes don't wobble, the earlobe should not be more than 25% of the total length of the ear. If it exceeds this, an L-shaped wedge can be cut away, and the earlobe edges can be brought together and sutured.

The earlobes can also protrude from the head. This protrusion can be part of the entire ear sticking out or be caused by an oversized ear shape that looks out of proportion to the shape of the head. Earlobe surgery can achieve an appearance that makes the ear more in balance with the face. One way to accomplish this is to position the ears closer to the head by reshaping the cartilage (supporting tissue). Otoplasty can be performed on children as early as age five or six.

Eyelid Surgery (Blepharoplasty) ($2,500 to $5,000)

Eyelid surgery is one of the more popular cosmetic surgeries because it is relatively simple, it requires minimal postoperative recovery, and the results can be stunning. This operation involves cutting away the fat that causes bags beneath the eyes and removing wrinkled, drooping layers of skin on the eyelids. Blepharoplasty is often performed along with a face-lift or with other facial rejuvenation procedures, especially forehead lifts. Incisions follow the natural contour lines in both upper and lower lids, and the thin surgical scars are usually barely visible and blend into the eyelids' natural lines and folds, although it depends on how your skin scars. A talented surgeon can avoid some of the typical mistakes, such as creating a scar that sits above the fold of the upper eyelid, overpulling the skin, or removing too much of the fat pad areas, which would create a sunken, drawn appearance (source: *Facial Plastic Surgery*, 1999, volume 15, issue 3, pages 173–229).

Transconjunctival blepharoplasty, a variation of eyelid surgery, is performed by making an incision inside the lower eyelid. It avoids any scarring on the lower lid and may reduce the possibility of the eyelid pulling down, a postoperative complication in some patients. It is a useful technique when fat only, and not skin or muscle, needs to be removed from the eyelid area.

It is important to note that eyelid surgery may not be indicated if a forehead lift (of the endoscopic type) can produce a more positive effect without risking the eye area or obvious scarring. This option should absolutely be discussed with your surgeon.

Endoscopic Face-Lift ($2,500 to $5,000)

An endoscope is a small surgical instrument that can be inserted under the skin through small incisions, allowing a surgeon to perform a cosmetic corrective procedure via microsurgery. The endoscope itself is a miniature camera with a light fitted on one end of a long tube. When inserted under the skin the camera transmits magnified images to a television monitor. During the procedure the surgeon watches the screen as the endoscope functions as the doctor's under-skin eye. Simultaneously, the surgeon inserts and uses other surgical instruments, including scalpels, scissors, or forceps to actually perform the operation. Endoscopic face-lifts are an optimal way to minimally impact the skin and yet achieve impressive results similar to the results of traditional face-lifts. But without cutting and pasting sections of skin how does an endoscopic face-lift work?

It turns out that a good deal of the skin's tendency to sag over time is a result of the face's muscles and fat pads shifting down and in toward the center of the face. This is what happens with the deepest furrowed lines on the face, particularly the forehead and the nasolabial folds from the nose to the mouth.

Let's say your jawline is beginning to sag. Using the somewhat simple surgical procedure called endoplasty, the surgeon makes a mere quarter-inch cut underneath the chin and at each edge of the jaw, and then, via microsurgery (the surgeon watches what is being done via a television screen), sutures the platysma muscle, which extends from jawline to jawline under the chin, back where it belongs.

Similar to the reason skin sags, the deep frown lines and vertical creases in the midforehead result from a literal slippage of the forehead muscles downward and inward, as well as just simple frowning and movement of the forehead. The same endoscopic technique used to anchor the platysma muscle can be used on the forehead muscles, and an additional separating of the muscles between the eyebrows can reduce the fold lines there. This operation can be done via three tiny incisions inside the hairline, allowing the surgeon to anchor the slipped muscles back in place and to cut away a small section of the muscles between the eyebrows.

There is a great deal of research showing that endoscopic face-lifts not only achieve impressive results—as good as, if not better than traditional cut-and-paste face-lifts—but also have minimal to none of the risks associated with traditional surgical procedures (sources: *Facial Plastic Surgery*, 2000, volume 16, issue 3, pages 283–298; *Plastic and Reconstructive Surgery*, January 2002, pages 329–340; *Facial Plastic Surgery Clinics North America*, August 2001, pages 439–451; *Aesthetic Plastic Surgery*, January 2001, pages 35–39).

Note: While reanchoring the muscles of the jaw and forehead can eliminate or decrease sagging, forehead lines, and the nasolabial folds (the fold of skin from the nose to the mouth), laser surgery is the treatment of choice for smoothing out fine lines all over the face, principally around the eyes and the mouth. Laser surgery can also slightly decrease sagging, but its main function is to smooth out lines. Although laser surgery can take three weeks to heal, endoscopic surgery takes only about 48 hours, although it is often accompanied by a postoperative headache that can last for a few days.

Face-Lift (Rhytidectomy) ($5,000 to $10,000)

Here's what one respected source has to say about this procedure: "Although there are a multitude of techniques currently used for performing face lifts, there is no general agreement as to which, if any, of these techniques is most effective. There may never be a definitive answer to this issue because of the highly subjective nature of aesthetics, variability among surgeons, differences in patient anatomy, and specific patient desires" (source: *Plastic and Reconstructive Surgery*, 1998, volume 102, pages 878–881).

An article in the *Journal of Plastic and Reconstructive Surgery* (October 2000, "National Plastic Surgery Survey: Face Lift Techniques and Complications") stated that "15 percent of [cosmetic] surgeons perform . . . [superficial] skin-only procedure[s], and 74 percent said they address the SMAS [superficial musculoaponeurotic system]. Nine percent of surgeons prefer a composite or deep-plane lift. Only 2 percent generally perform a subperiosteal-lift; about half of those use the endoscope." (See page 320 for endoscopic face-lifts.)

The art of the face-lift is extremely complicated and the choices read like a menu with too many entrees. A traditional face-lift can dramatically reduce sagging skin on the face, neck, and jaw. As impressive as this cosmetic procedure can be in creating a youthful, taut visage, it can also create an overly pulled, masklike appearance, with the face drawn up in a stretched, permanent smile (à la The Joker of *Batman* fame). This is one cosmetic procedure where you want to see the doctor's work on someone else up-close and personal.

During this complicated, elaborate procedure, incisions are made in the hairline both in front of and behind the ears (the exact design of the incisions may differ from patient to patient, and surgeons' personal techniques can vary widely). For younger patients, more limited incisions may be appropriate. When necessary, fatty deposits beneath the skin are removed or repositioned, and sagging muscles are tightened. The slack in the skin itself is then taken up and the excess cut away. Scars can usually be concealed, but when things go wrong, thick, obvious scars may be seen or the hairline behind the ear or along the forehead may be altered in such a way that it creates an unnatural, strained appearance.

Most face-lifts also involve repositioning the muscles and fat pads of the cheek that have slipped forward, causing deep lines near the mouth (laugh lines), as well as sagging the muscle along the chin. Face-lifts that tighten only the skin without repositioning the muscles and fat pads can cause the face to look gaunt and unnatural. Face-lifts also have limitations as to the areas of the face they can affect. Other areas require a forehead lift, chin tuck, or endoscopic repositioning of those muscles and fat pads. Likewise, wrinkles by the eyes and mouth are not affected by a face-lift alone and require additional procedures (such as laser resurfacing) that are often done at the same time the face-lift is performed. Here is a menu of options for face-lifts a doctor can select from.

Classic or Traditional Face-Lift

This is what most of us think of when we think of a face-lift. Sagging, wrinkled skin is cut away and repositioned to create a smoother and tighter visage. Cutting skin is only one part of this procedure; to create the most natural finished appearance, the muscles and fat pads under the skin need to be repositioned so the realigned skin is formed over a youthful base.

SMAS-Lift (Superficial Musculoaponeurotic System)

The SMAS face-lift is a term that has become familiar to those looking into plastic surgery. SMAS refers to the superficial musculoaponeurotic system. The skin on the face is composed of the superficial layers of skin, both the top and lower layer as well as the underlying layer of fat. Beneath the skin, fat, and muscle is a gliding membrane composed partly of connective tissue and partly of muscle. This gliding tissue is the SMAS, which is responsible for our ability to have facial expressions. Realigning this structure is considered a valid option for re-creating a youthful appearance for the face. However, when you cut under the muscle layer you can negatively affect nerve endings, and that is the major risk of this procedure. However, if you pulled only the top layers of skin and fat, the muscle layer (which also sags and causes an aged appearance to the face) would not be corrected. Many surgeons feel that addressing the SMAS layer of skin is necessary to avoid giving a flat or unnatural appearance to the face (source: *Plastic and Reconstructive Surgery*, 2000, volume 105, pages 290–301).

Subperiosteal Lift

Periosteal refers to the thick membrane that covers the surface of bones. The subperiosteal lift is a technique used for the mid- and upper-face area, an area that is not helped by the typical face-lift (cutting and pasting skin around the ear area) or by endoscopic face-lifts (that reposition fat tissue and muscles without cutting and pasting). This is an aggressive technique that removes all the tissue and muscles attached to the bone and reshapes it into a more youthful position over the face. The benefit of the subperiosteal approach to the midface is the ability to lift the center of the face, improving the appearance of the nasolabial folds, smoothing the cheek area, and tightening the eye area (source: *Plastic and Reconstructive Surgery*, September 1999, pages 842–851). However, any time work is done deeper under the skin the risk of impairment to nerve endings increases.

Neck Lift

A woman's neck area is often the place that can look the most aged. Traditional face-lifts do not address this area. Sagging of the neck results when the platysma muscle loosens and becomes elongated. Typically, when an SMAS-lift is performed the platysma muscle is reshaped and repositioned at the same time. Excess skin and fat can also be cut away at this time (source: *Plastic and Reconstructive Surgery*, 1999, volume 104, pages 1093–1100).

S-Lift or Mini-Lift

This technique may be helpful for minor jowling or sagging skin. One source describes its objective this way: "To develop a safe and effective method to lift the jowl either as a single procedure or combined with other rejuvenation methods, S-shaped incisions are marked and then cut from the area just in front of the tragus [the front part of the ear]" (source: *Dermatologic Surgery*, January 2001, pages 18–22). Once the small S-shaped flap of skin is cut and lifted away from the face it is tightened and repositioned along with the underlying muscles and fat tissues. If necessary, excess fat can be removed from this area at the same time.

Temporal Lift

The temporal face-lift refers to the area along the sides and top of the forehead. This technique is also referred to as a brow-lift. It is meant to smooth out the lines of the forehead and some of the eye area by repositioning the forehead skin along the hairline. At the time of the cutting and pasting for this area, the muscles of the forehead would also be repositioned (source: *Facial Plastic Surgery*, February 2001, pages 57–66).

Deep-Plane Lift

A deep-plane face-lift simply refers to how deep under the skin the surgeon works to perform any given face-lift procedure. Although it is similar to the SMAS-lift, the deep-plane face-lift goes even deeper. It involves lifting and repositioning the various layers of the face—skin, fat tissue, muscles, and other structures—as a single unit rather than separating and lifting them individually. Because of its complexity, this procedure is not widely performed. However, while it is technically demanding, the results are considered more satisfactory than those of a traditional or more superficial face-lift (source: *Ophthalmology*, March 2000, pages 490–495).

Fat Implants
See "Dermal Fillers," page 320.

Forehead Lift (Brow Lift—Transblepharoplasty brow lift) ($3,000 to $5,000)

The forehead lift is designed to correct or improve wrinkling, as well as sagging of the eyebrow area that often occur as part of the aging process. The procedure may also help to smooth horizontal expression lines in the forehead, smooth vertical frown lines between the eyebrows, and reduce the sagging appearance of the eyelids. Behind the hairline, incisions are placed above the ear and over the top of the head, although in some cases incisions may be made in front of the hairline. Forehead lifts are often (and usually should be) accompanied by repositioning the muscles of the forehead, which are partly responsible for the furrowed lines of the brow. The major downside of this procedure is that the hairline may be pulled farther back than desired.

Laser Resurfacing Procedures ($1,200 to $7,500)

Issues involving cosmetic corrective surgical procedures are complicated as it is, but when the topic turns to laser resurfacing what you find is a large tangled mess—one that's almost impossible for the consumer to wade through. An article in the *Archives of Facial Plastic Surgery* (January-March 2002, pages 6–7, "Laser Madness in Facial Plastic Surgery") summed up the problem beautifully: "In facial plastic surgery, many articles written by physicians promoting . . . facial resurfacing lasers appear in both peer-reviewed and non–peer-reviewed journals. These articles may read more like advertisements than science, overestimating the advantages of laser surgery, while underestimating the disadvantages and complications. Furthermore, the public's fascination with high-tech procedures related to cosmetic surgery has further exacerbated the unchecked outbreak of laser madness. . . . Promoters [of facial resurfacing with the CO_2 laser] have greatly exaggerated the advantages of laser facial resurfacing over other methods of resurfacing. A better result is not guaranteed simply by using a laser, despite suggestions to the contrary by advertisers. Laser facial resurfacing may be appropriate in patients with severely photodamaged skin and deep wrinkles who are willing to have a prolonged painful healing period and accept the risks of permanent pigmentation changes. . . . Currently, it is unclear who is benefiting from laser madness in medicine. Is it the patient, the physician, or the laser company?"

Why the controversy? It will become clear in just a moment!

Lasers and light-emitting machines are all about electrical wavelength, energy output, and pulse-width variations. The length of each of the waves used relates to the structures it will affect, such as blood (veins), melanin (skin pigment), and water (found in skin cells). The energy output tells you how powerfully that wavelength will impact the targeted structure. Pulse width indicates how long the wavelength will be in contact with the structure. Each machine has variations on each of these parameters, and can, therefore, target different aspects of skin.

There are basically two types of laser resurfacing options, ablative and nonablative. Nonablative laser treatments use lasers that are noninjurious and do not cause damage to skin tissue. Nonablative lasers include the N-lite laser, Nd:YAG laser, Flashlamp laser, Pulsed-Light laser, and CoolTouch laser. Ablative laser resurfacing uses extreme heat generated by laser pulses that can injure and damage skin even as they may benefit it. In fact, part of the effect that ablative lasers have is a direct result of the damage they cause. Ablative lasers include the CO_2 Pulse laser, the Er:YAG laser, and the Q-Switched Ruby laser.

Ablative laser resurfacing can absolutely make a remarkable difference in the appearance of skin, particularly in terms of long-lasting improvement in the appearance of deep wrinkles, surface wrinkles, and skin discolorations. But as wonderful as that sounds there are risks and complications that can occur with ablative laser resurfacing. These include swelling, scabbing, oozing, bleeding, flaking, redness, and irritation that can last for an extended period of time, and there is also a definite risk in terms of even longer-term skin discoloration and scarring.

Nonablative laser resurfacing is performed by plastic surgeons and dermatologists alike, and has none of the side effects associated with ablative laser resurfacing. That means no downtime and none of the risks associated with ablative laser resurfacing. However, nonablative resurfacing doesn't produce the same dramatic results ablative resurfacing can. According to an article in the July 2000 issue of *The Journal*, online at http://www.lasernews.net, "Nonablative [laser resurfacing] leads to improvement in photodamaged skin and rhytids (wrinkles) without any obvious wound. . . . However, at the present time, the clinical improvement seen with such techniques is less than that following the inelegant ablative laser resurfacing techniques." Not only are the results of nonablative laser resurfacing subtle, but it requires multiple treatments to achieve any kind of noticeable outcome.

For ablative resurfacing involving a laser peel, the quality of the postoperative techniques is almost as important to the success of the procedure as the skill of the physician performing the peel. In fact, one complication of laser surgery is improper or inadequate home care. The side effects of a laser peel can be daunting. The skin oozes, crusts, and needs to be cleaned and dressed for about two weeks before you look even vaguely normal. Because the top layer of skin has been stripped away, the raw, exposed skin must be cleaned and treated very carefully. The patient can easily do this wrong, causing infection, delayed healing, and irritation.

Although it may sound weird, some physicians require patients who have undergone a laser peel to wear a clear silicone bandage (much like Saran Wrap) over the entire treated area for five to seven days. The silicone bandage prevents any interference from the patient except for gentle cleaning around the mouth, eyes, and nose, which are understandably left unbandaged. But there are problems with this type of wrapping. It can be uncomfortable for the patient, oozing can occur at the edges of the bandage, and it just plain looks strange. (On the other hand, peeled skin looks strange no matter what you do to it.) Antibiotics, special cleansing procedures, and general skin-care instructions are of vital importance in reducing the risk of complications.

To help you make more informed decisions when interviewing a dermatologist or plastic surgeon about laser resurfacing (also called photorejuvenation), you need to have a better understanding of the various laser and light-emitting machines available and their preferred functions on the skin. If a doctor has only limited access to a variety of machines or has only one or two at his disposal, he might not be inclined to let you know each machine's limitations.

The following is a list of the more popular lasers and light-emitting machines in use and their known or ideal benefit for skin, along with their associated risks.

Ablative Laser Resurfacing

CO_2 **Pulse Laser (trade names Feather Touch and Ultra Pulse):** This is one of the oldest ablative laser-resurfacing machines around. While it can deeply resurface skin, creating more lasting and noticeable results than any other laser, it is also associated with the most severe damage and risk to skin. After treatment, skin can take one to two weeks to heal and can be red for one to two months. Risks of scarring, skin discoloration, and uneven texture can occur, though many doctors would insist that this happens less than 2% of the time and rarely when a doctor is experienced in the use of this kind of procedure.

Erbium:YAG Laser (or Er:YAG Laser): This ablative laser has a far less invasive effect than the CO_2 Pulse laser. The skin may take only four to five days to heal and the redness usually dissipates after one to two weeks. There is minimal risk of scarring and minimal risk of skin discoloration. While all lasers can be used around the eye area, the Erbium:YAG laser can be used to spot treat the eye area for dark circles because it doesn't affect skin colors (it won't cause hypopigmentation or hyperpigmentation).

Q-Switched Ruby Laser: This laser is minimally ablative, especially in comparison to the CO_2 Pulse and Erbium:YAG lasers. Its primary use is to selectively remove skin pigment, such as freckling, sun-damage spots, and actinic keratosis (precancerous brown skin lesions) without damaging the surrounding skin tissue. It is also especially useful for removing tattoos and some birthmarks. The Q-Switched Ruby laser was the original machine used for temporary hair removal. It can take several treatments to see the desired results.

It is interesting to point out that one of the popular uses for the Q-Switched Ruby laser is to remove cosmetic tattoos. Many physicians believe that the incidence of poor work from inexperienced or poorly trained aestheticians who tattoo lip liner, eyeliner, and eyebrows is so rampant that eliminating their mistakes constitutes a large portion of the laser work many doctors do.

Nonablative or Coblative Laser Resurfacing

Pulsed Dye Laser, Short- and Long-Pulsed: This nonablative laser gives impressive results in eliminating surfaced capillaries on the face, port wine marks, hypertrophic scarring (thick or raised scars), and hemangiomas (red dots on the surface of skin). Because the Pulsed Dye laser is nonablative it doesn't cause skin damage, but it almost always causes temporary bruising. It can take several treatments to see the desired results.

Long-Pulsed YAG Laser (trade name Lyra): This nonablative laser's unique feature is that it has a built-in cooling device that protects the top layer of skin. It is especially suited to those with darker skin tones because it will not affect pigment. It can take several treatments to achieve the desired results. The laser is currently the laser of choice for hair removal.

CoolTouch Long-Pulsed YAG Laser: This nonablative laser is noted for its ability to build collagen. It is typically used for wrinkles and acne scars, and it can take several treatments to achieve the desired results. The results for this are very subtle and result in only a slight improvement.

Long-Pulsed Alexandrite Laser (trade names GentleLASE and Cool Pulse): This nonablative laser is another option for hair removal, but it is best suited for those with light skin and dark hair. This machine also more easily and quickly covers large areas of skin. It can take several treatments to achieve a subtle improvement.

Intense Pulsed-Light Device or Flash Lamp (trade names PhotoDerm and Quantum): This is not a laser, but belongs in this category because of its place in "photorejuvenation" procedures. The Flash Lamp creates a pulse of intense light that is used most frequently as a method to remove hair, reduce or eliminate surfaced capillaries or veins, hemangiomas (red dots on the surface of skin), and superficial brown spots, as well as to tighten the skin. The number and degree of side effects are considerably less than with laser treatment. It can take several treatments to see desired results.

1064 Nanometer Long-Pulsed Nd:YAG Lasers (trade names Vasculite, CoolTouch, Varia, and CoolGlide): These lasers are noted for their treatment of surfaced leg veins. Although bruising can occur, there is no associated skin damage or risk with these devices. However, it is extremely painful and the outcome can vary from person to person. It takes multiple treatments to achieve the desired results. Although new surfaced veins can emerge, the ones that were zapped are gone forever.

The following is a summary covering a range of laser machines and the skin conditions they address.

Skin Condition	Laser or Light-Emitting System
Wrinkles and lines	CO_2 (carbon dioxide) Erbium:YAG CoolTouch Long-Pulsed YAG
Brown spots	CO_2 (carbon dioxide) Nd:YAG Q-Switched Ruby

Deep pigmented lesions	Q-Switched Ruby Nd:YAG Pulsed Dye
Scars and stretch marks	CO_2 (carbon dioxide) Pulsed Dye CoolTouch Long-Pulsed YAG
Tattoos	CO_2 (carbon dioxide) Nd:YAG Q-Switched Ruby
Hair removal	Nd:YAG Long-Pulsed Alexandrite Intense Pulsed Light (PhotoDerm) Long-Pulsed YAG

Lip Augmentation or Reduction ($2,500 to $4,000)

While thin lips may not seem like a cosmetic issue, for some women looking for perfection, fuller lips are considered more attractive. Aside from dermal fillers (reviewed above), one of the more interesting methods for augmenting the lips is to surgically advance the lip forward via incisions placed inside the mouth. Fat implants or collagen injections (see "Dermal Fillers," page 320) may then be positioned under the lining of the lip to add additional plumpness. Neither collagen nor fat is permanent, however, and the procedure must be repeated periodically to maintain results.

A lip lift is a technique that surgically lifts the corners of an aging mouth to eliminate the pronounced droop and unhappy facial expressions that often develop with advanced age. Cutting away small diamonds of skin just above the corners of the mouth raises the border of the lips into a slight smile.

If thin lips have a fashionable downside, it isn't hard to imagine that overly full lips can also be viewed as unattractive. In lip reduction, a small section along the top lining of the lip is surgically removed to narrow the lips to the desired proportion. The small scars on the outside of the lips are often barely noticeable, though it all depends on how you scar.

Microdermabrasion ($300 to $1,000)

Microdermabrasion machines require the lowest level of approval from the FDA for a medical device because they are considered Class 1 medical devices, which means they are subject to the least amount of regulatory control. Type 1 devices can be sold and used without any supportive clinical efficacy data (source: FDA Classification of Medical Devices, http://www.fda.gov/cdrh/dsma/dsmaclas.html#class_1). Often, consumers are given a range of erroneous information regarding microdermabrasion's credentials.

For all intents and purposes microdermabrasion, including both "superficial" and "deep" treatments, is similar to an intense topical scrub. The machine delivers a flow of aluminum oxide crystals onto the skin that are then suctioned off the skin through the same tube that was used for delivery. The process produces varying levels of mechanical exfoliation. Superficial microdermabrasion is completely noninvasive (no downtime), readily available, and reasonably quick and safe, which probably explains its increasing use. Deep microdermabrasion disturbs the surface of the skin and can cause oozing, redness, swelling, and discomfort. Because of the risks, only a physician should perform deep microdermabrasion treatments, though that is not always the case.

What makes superficial microdermabrasion a "lunchtime" process is that in most cases the redness and irritation caused by the treatment fade in a matter of minutes to just a few hours. Though the irritation can be minimal, there is some tightness, skin peeling, and, rarely, the skin can appear swollen and red, which can last from a few hours to a few days for more sensitive skins. All this can make skin look somewhat less wrinkled or scarred, at least for a short period of time. Superficial microdermabrasion requires repeated treatment to see results and the results are not long-lasting. It can take from four weeks to three months before the improvement diminishes.

How effective is any of this? There is no easy answer for this one because the studies don't agree. For example, a study published in *Dermatologic Surgery* (November 2001, pages 943–949), "quantified the effects of microdermabrasion on photodamaged skin in 10 individuals. Their subjects underwent once-weekly microdermabrasion for a series of 5–6 treatments (using the *Parisian Peel* device). During the 5- to 6-week treatment period, patients were assessed at each visit." The study concluded, "In general, quantifiable results were modest and transient. . . . Seven of

10 patients showed at least mild (1%-25%) improvement of their pho-todamaged skin after completing 5–6 treatments. . . . Seven of 10 patients reported subjective improvement; intriguingly, all 3 patients who re-ported no improvement had the most severe baseline wrinkling."

However another article, in *Skin & Allergy News* (November 1999), stated that "microdermabrasion's versatility and potentially destructive power was demonstrated in a histologic study presented at the annual fall meeting of the American Academy of Facial, Plastic, and Recon-structive Surgery. . . . Used conservatively, the system works well in treating basically, anything that's minor. . . . Under the microscope, a low number of passes equated with negligible histologic evidence of mean-ingful skin changes. But increasing passes resulted in extreme damage down to the dermis [deep microdermabrasion]. Of note, deep ablation with the microdermabrasion machine produced serum exudate [oozing] and bleeding, and left histologic evidence of aluminum oxide crystals embedded in the dermis."

That's not to say there can't be some noticeable results from micro-dermabrasion. But to suggest it doesn't have risks or that you will end up with wrinkle-free smooth skin is either deception or ignorance on the part of the person performing the service. And it goes without saying that the results are under no circumstance permanent.

It is useful to distinguish a bit more clearly what the differences be-tween superficial and deep microdermabrasion procedures are. Superfi-cial microdermabrasion is the procedure that we commonly call microdermabrasion. It is the procedure performed at spas, as well as physician's offices, by aesthetic, paramedical, and medical personnel alike. It involves superficial abrasion of the skin's surface (the nonliving skin cells that occupy the top three to five layers of skin only). This cell layer has no capillaries and is nonpigmented, hence its disruption causes no bleeding, crusting, or skin discoloration. It is known that normal skin can take on a dull or thick appearance and fine lines seem more apparent because the surface skin cells slough unevenly. Regular superficial mi-crodermabrasion treatments with an appropriate system can even out and slough skin. This can modestly improve skin texture and some su-perficial scarring and discoloration.

Deep microdermabrasion should be performed only by physicians and involves disruption of part of or the entire epidermis. Because the skin cells of the epidermis have capillaries and varying degrees of melanin, their disruption can cause bleeding, crusting, and skin discolorations, particularly in darker-skinned individuals. It was believed, when micro-dermabrasion technology was newer, that this deeper disruption of the skin, akin to traditional dermabrasion, causes dermal remodeling of collagen and should, therefore, reduce the appearance of acne scars, pits, and deeper wrinkles. But as I mentioned, confirmation of this has yet to be established and clinical correlation remains controversial.

Nose Reshaping (Rhinoplasty) ($4,000 to $6,000)

Rhinoplasty is usually performed to alter the size and shape of the bridge and tip of the nose. Reshaping is generally done through incisions inside the nose, but sometimes an incision across the central portion of the nose between the nostrils is also made. Narrowing the base of the nose or reducing the size of the nostrils involves removing small wedges of skin at the base of the nostrils. The nose is reduced, or sometimes built up, by adjusting its supporting structures, a process that involves either removing or adding bone and cartilage. The skin and soft tissues are then redraped over this newly created structure.

An open rhinoplasty technique can sometimes benefit patients who need more complex correction or who are undergoing a secondary rhinoplasty procedure. A small incision is made outside the nose across the columella (the tissue that divides the two nostrils). This enables the plastic surgeon to turn the outer tissue of the nose back, providing a view of the structures inside. Additional incisions, like those used in the traditional closed approach, are made inside the nose as well. The scar from the incision on the outside of the nose eventually becomes barely visible.

chapter *14*
HAND AND NAIL CARE

SERIOUSLY DRY HANDS

Struggling with dry hands can be painful. Even if you are diligent about keeping them protected when doing housework or gardening, and unfailingly apply moisturizer whenever the opportunity arises, you can still suffer from bone-dry, cracked, parched hands. Clearly, it is essential to protect your hands from dish detergent, laundry detergent, excessive washing (medical professionals have a rough time with this one), and irritating ingredients, and also when doing potentially irritating manual work. Wearing gloves to prevent contact with irritating products and ingredients is of the utmost importance. However, a significant number of women may find they are allergic to latex gloves. About 10% of the population have negative reactions, ranging from mild to severe, if they come in contact with latex. If this turns out to be a problem, ask your physician or pharmacist where you can find nonlatex gloves.

The faster you get an emollient moisturizer on your hands after washing, and the longer you can keep it on, the better. It helps to keep small tubes or bottles of emollient moisturizer all over the house, including near the kitchen sink, in the bathroom, at the bedside, and in the garage. Keep more in your car, purse, briefcase, and desk drawer. That way it is never out of reach for a quick application. The best moisturizers for daytime are moisturizing sunscreens whose active ingredient is either avobenzone, titanium dioxide, or zinc oxide. Titanium dioxide and zinc oxide provide an occlusive barrier that can act as a protective layer to retain moisture in the skin while keeping the sun's rays off the skin. (Bear in mind that brown "sun spots" on the back of hands and arms are a direct result of relentless, daily, unprotected sun exposure.)

Moisturizers such as Palmer's Cocoa Butter Formula, Eucerin Dry Skin Therapy Plus Intensive Repair Cream or Lotion, Curel Extreme Care Body Lotion, Jergens Advanced Therapy Lotion, and countless others are all excellent for use at night. The best approach is to apply moisturizer every chance you get. It is also incredibly helpful to purchase an over-the-counter cortisone cream such as Lanacort or Cortaid to help treat cracks and fissures that may occur, but cortisone creams are only to be used intermittently, not on a regular basis.

HARD AS NAILS

While some women have naturally great nails, others search endlessly for anything that will help make their nails strong, thick (but not too thick), and long (sometimes too long). Sadly, you can't fool Mother Nature. What is genetically predetermined cannot be permanently transformed. If you are lucky enough to have strong, fast-growing, perfectly shaped nails with smooth, even cuticles, only trauma and damage to the nail bed will change the health and appearance of your nails. If you have naturally brittle, soft nails and thick cuticles, there is also no way to alter what you've inherited. There is a lot you can do to make your nails look and feel better (there's plenty you can do to make matters worse, too), but changing the way your nails naturally grow is as impossible as changing the way your hair grows.

I know there are dozens of nail products made by everyone from Revlon and Sally Hansen to Barielle, Orly, and Cutex, plus new ones being introduced monthly, all claiming they can repair the irreparable. Don't any of them work? If they did, we'd all have long, beautiful nails. Yet millions of women have struggled with weak, brittle, soft nails, trying an endless assortment of strengthening, lengthening, and fortifying nail products, only to give up in frustration. It is almost impossible for a woman who wants to improve the appearance of her short, fragile nails not to wonder about all of the products that claim to feed the nails, engorge them with vitamins, or build them up from the outside in. **I would love to say those claims are legitimate and tell you which ones perform the best, but all the claims are bogus; changing the way a nail grows can't** be done by putting something on it topically. Also, there's no research showing that vitamin supplements such as biotin can change the way the nails grow, either.

Physiologically speaking, the nail is simply a protective covering composed of dead cells filled with a thick protein called keratin, quite similar in essence to the hair. Although the part of the nail you can see is dead, the matrix (the part of the nail under the skin) is very much alive. The white crescent area of the nail is called the lunula and is part of the matrix. The nail grows out from the matrix and as the growth of new cells builds up and dies it is pushed forward and out toward the surface. The cuticle is the protective layer of skin between the outside environment and the matrix. Keeping the cuticle intact is perhaps the single most important element in preserving the health of the nail.

Despite the nail's basic attributes, several long-standing myths about getting the talons of your dreams make the coffee-klatch rounds every now and then. Perhaps you've heard some of these nail delusions before, such as that tapping your nails on a hard surface will help nails grow and make them stronger. That isn't true in the least. You can't strengthen the nail by exercising it, assuming the nail needs the same training as a muscle. If anything, tapping will do just the opposite of what you want. Repetitive pressure or strain on the nail will lead to breakage and splitting. Another inane nail fiction is the notion that eating gelatin makes nails healthier. Gelatin probably got its reputation as a nail builder because of its relationship to protein. Like your nails and your hair, gelatin contains protein, but no form of food goes directly to the nail or hair to help it grow. There are no studies or data demonstrating that eating gelatin will improve the condition of anything. Eating a balanced, low-fat, nutritious diet (meaning lots of fresh fruits, vegetables, and whole grains) is certainly an important factor in overall good health, but feeding the nail directly isn't feasible.

Fluoride

Several nail-care products want you to believe that "What's good for your teeth is great for your nails," so you can "harness the power of fluoride with strengtheners, base and top coats, and cuticle care." If only that were possible! It would be a dream come true to have a product that could make nails as strong as teeth, or even relatively as strong. Alas, unless you were born with naturally strong nails, fluoride isn't going to help your nails the way it helps teeth.

First, teeth are unrelated to nails. Teeth are made of a bony substance composed of various mineral compounds, mostly calcium phosphate. Nails have no mineral content but rather are composed of hardened keratin, basically the same substance that comprises skin and hair. Further, fluoride doesn't "strengthen" teeth, but rather, according to the American Dental Association, has varying influences that work with saliva and the growth of developing teeth to prevent decay. One function of fluoride is to reduce the constant reaction taking place between the tooth's surface, saliva, and bacteria in the mouth. When we eat sugar or starchy foods the number of bacteria in the mouth increases, which raises the acidity of our saliva, which in turn slowly, over time, demineralizes the surface of the tooth. As the acidity subsides, the tooth's surface becomes remineralized. Fluoride reduces the presence of bacteria in the mouth, which reduces the acidity of the saliva and in turn reduces or eliminates tooth decay. None of that, to put it mildly, has anything to do with nail growth or nail problems.

One more point: Given that almost all of us drink and wash with fluoridated water, our nails are constantly exposed to fluoride. If fluoride were important for healthy nails—which it isn't—the amount we get in our drinking water would be more than enough.

The nail-care industry has tried to build up many ingredients in the effort to convince us that we can grow stronger nails. For years protein was a big one that showed up in nail-care products, though protein can't feed the skin or nail from the outside in. Diligently applying most nail-care products does help, but it is the protective coating they provide that does the trick, not these impressive sounding, do-nothing special ingredients.

Calcium

Perhaps the last piece of nail improbability is the belief that applying calcium to your nails will make them strong. Calcium, along with lots of other minerals and vitamins, shows up in many nail-care products owing to the assumption that you can feed the nail from the outside in. You can't feed the nail directly, though even if you could, calcium and other minerals are unlikely ingredients for this purpose. Calcium and minerals may help build strong bones (bones are primarily calcium), but that is unrelated to the content of nails. The notion of having nails as strong as bone does make calcium sound appealing. However, even by itself calcium can't build bone; the body needs other minerals to use the calcium.

Moreover, there is virtually no calcium in nails; they're made of keratin and that's about it.

CUTICLE CARE

Although trying to affect the matrix and change the inherent growth of the nail with nail-care products is a waste of time and money, there are many things you can do to improve your nails. Without question, the most important element to pay attention to is the skin around the nail, namely the cuticle. **The best way to keep your nails healthy, whole, and as free from problems as possible is to push your cuticles back as little as you can. The less you manipulate and cut your cuticle the better off your nails will be.** Aside from inherited problems and physical trauma (getting smashed by a hammer or door can permanently alter the physical attributes of the nail), damage from overpushing or overtrimming the cuticle is the number one cause of nail problems. I know this may seem shocking and contrary to much of what you've heard, but excessively pushing back the cuticle and cutting it off is a huge no-no. Removing too much cuticle can damage the nail.

Overtrimming the cuticle can destroy the integrity of the matrix, which is the source of healthy nail growth. There is no way around this one. The cuticle is the body's form of protection for the area between the exposed dead part of the nail and the living matrix where the nail grows from. Anything that damages this seal puts the nail at risk.

If you cut too much cuticle away it can result in weak, brittle, ridged, dented, peeling, or unevenly growing nails (where one part of the same nail grows at a different rate), and once these problems occur, they won't go away until the nail grows out and that can take anywhere from three months to a year. Orange sticks and metal cuticle tools, even when padded with cotton on the tip as most manicurists do, can cause damage to the nail if they are not used carefully.

Almost every dermatologist I interviewed agreed that cuticle damage negatively affects nail growth. You can test this for yourself. Stop manipulating, pushing, or overtrimming your cuticles. For the next six months, simply take care of your nail shape (I'll explain more about that later in this chapter) and only minimally trim hangnails or excess skin around the nail. Do not overmanipulate the cuticle in any manner whatsoever. Within a relatively short period of time you are likely to see a radical change in the growth of the nail. I know this is a hard one to get used to but it will pay off in the long run.

Another thing you can do for the cuticle is to moisturize it as often as possible, and during the day be sure you use a moisturizing sunscreen with avobenzone, titanium dioxide, and/or zinc oxide. It doesn't have to be a special nail or hand moisturizer with sunscreen—as long as the SPF is 15 or greater and the active ingredients are the ones I've been mentioning it will do just fine. If the cuticle becomes dry and flaky (or sun damaged), the protective barrier for the matrix will break down, which can absolutely and quickly hurt nail growth. In some ways it is almost impossible to keep the cuticle moist and healthy. Think about how often you wash your hands and use them every day for everything from office work to housework to sports. Also, the hands are incessantly exposed to the sun and it is difficult to keep them constantly protected with sunscreen. Yet doing so is essential. **In short, don't overdo trimming cuticles, keep nails protected from the sun, and use a moisturizer to prevent dryness.**

MANICURES AND PEDICURES

While leaving the cuticle alone is the best thing you can do for the growth of the nail, leaving the length of the nail alone is also a wise part of nail care. The part of the nail that extends past the quick is long dead and vulnerable to damage. Overfiling can tear at the nail's structure, and that can never be replaced. Once filing tears or starts lifting the fibrous nail material, it can begin a cycle that is hard to stop. Nails are softened by water, and soft nails are more susceptible to damage and tears. Shape the nails only when they are completely dry. It is also essential to avoid metal or extremely coarse nail files. Use the gentlest file with extremely gentle pressure to achieve the shape you want. You'll use up more nail files faster than you did before, but stronger nails will be the result of the extra expense and trouble. You've probably heard the one about filing in one direction only. That is completely unnecessary. Regardless of the direction you file, if you don't do it gently you will damage the nail.

When you do take the time to indulge in a full manicure or pedicure, it is essential to **keep it simple.**

The following is a great system for creating the perfect manicure or pedicure.

- First, remove any previously applied nail polish. **It doesn't matter whether you use a nail-polish remover that contains acetone or not. It also doesn't matter whether the nail-polish remover contains moisturizing ingredients. If a nail-polish remover can remove nail polish it is going to be harsh stuff, but that is the price of nicely painted nails.** Use as little nail-polish remover as necessary to remove the polish. Never soak the nail in nail-polish remover! Nail-polish remover is extremely drying and damaging to the entire nail, especially the cuticle. Keeping contact with nail-polish remover to a minimum is crucial for the well-being of the nail and cuticle.
- Gently file the nails into the shape you want, using the least-abrasive emery board you can find. **Avoid shaping your nails into long talons or severe shapes (too square or pointy).**
- Softening the cuticle around the nail is necessary only if you plan to remove just a tiny bit of excess cuticle. Soak the nails in plain warm water for no more than three minutes. **Oversoaking hurts the nail and the cuticle. Avoid soapy or detergent-filled water, which only dries the skin and damages the cuticle.** If the hands or feet are dirty, wash them first and that's it. Minimal contact with cleansers is best for any part of your body, including the nails!
- **Trim the cuticle and avoid pushing it back as much as possible, being exceedingly careful not to pull, lift, tear, rip, force, or cut into the cuticle in any way.**
- **Trim the nails carefully, using sharp manicure scissors or nail clippers.** Nails are definitely easier to trim after bathing or soaking. Fingernails should be given a slightly rounded edge to protect the nail growth; toenails should be trimmed straight across, slightly above the quick. Avoid cutting nails too short because doing so increases the chance of developing ingrown toenails.
- **Moisturize the cuticle with an emollient moisturizer.** Almost any moisturizer for dry skin will do. It is not necessary to purchase special cuticle creams: They contain absolutely nothing special for the nail or cuticle.
- Before you polish your nails it is essential to remove the moisturizer from them. **Moisturizing ingredients prevent nail polish from adhering to the nail.** Use nail-polish remover just over the nail's surface to take off any moisturizer. Avoid getting nail-polish remover on the cuticle; that's the area you want to keep the moisturizer on.
- Polish your nails in layers, allowing them to dry between coats. A min-

imum of three coats is standard. **If you have weak or brittle nails, place one or two coats of ridge-filling nail polish on the nail as the base coat.** This is the best way to shore up the nail. Two coats of a colored nail polish are next, followed by a top coat to add shine and luster.

- **Allow plenty of time for the polish to dry.** Quick-dry polishes and some quick-dry top coats of polish often contain alcohol, which can cause the polish to peel and chip more easily, so you want to avoid those. Using a quick-dry oil or spray after you're done polishing is a great way to ward off smudges, but these won't prevent nicks or dents in the polish, so be careful.
- **Do not dry your nails with a blow dryer or any other heat source.** Heat causes the polish to expand and lift away from the nail.
- **Touching up polish every other day with a layer of top coat can help make a manicure last longer.** Carry a bottle of top coat in your purse, and when you have a moment or break in your day, quickly do a once-over. A single layer dries quickly and makes all the difference in keeping up appearances.

NAIL POLISH THAT LASTS

After spending way too much money on nail-care products and nail polishes, many women complain that for this kind of money their nails should be ten times stronger and the polish should last ten times longer. A nice thought, but that isn't the case. Price has no relation to how long a nail polish will last. Nail polishes are produced by only a handful of manufacturers, so there are no secrets, and the formulations vary only slightly because only a handful of ingredients will stay on the nail.

Lots of women complain that if they want their nails to look good it takes practically a full-time effort, and they can't live life like a normal person. I myself have gone around walking like a surgeon to be sure my nails don't come in contact with any surface anywhere. Though it doesn't take money to improve the appearance of your nails, it does take diligence and care. Those two things can't be avoided. Unfortunately, some polishes do tend to chip more than others (but this is determined by formulation, not cost). I wish I could offer some insight into which formulations work best, but no matter how many surveys I do or how many cosmetics chemists I interview, I have found no consensus as to which products last better. More often than not, polish longevity has to do with the process of applying the layers in the right order, including base coat (preferably a ridge-filler-type product), color, and top coat; applying layers that are thick enough but not too thick; allowing plenty of time for drying; and then treating your nails carefully (wearing gloves, avoiding water, having minimal contact with soaps or cleansers, and not using the nails as tools).

Polishes are often given names like SuperWeave Base Coat, Color Lock No-Chip Sealer, Strong Wear Nail Strengthener Polish, Extra Life Top Coat, Nail Building Base Coat, Color Shield, Fortifier Hydrating Base, or Nail Protector. They are all great names that promise wonderful things they can't even begin to deliver. Take Markron's Five Minute Nail Miracle, for example. This product isn't even a minor miracle. It contains standard nail-polish ingredients and tiny amounts of protein and amino acids, as well as formaldehyde. Nails are dead, and all the protein and amino acids in the world won't help them live. Formaldehyde can toughen nails, but it can also seriously dry them out and damage the cuticle. What kind of miracle is that?

I wish I could find a line of nail polishes that last, but it doesn't exist. So many factors affect how well your nail polish holds up. For example, Do you wear gloves when you clean? What kind of daily work do you do with your hands? Are your nails oil- and cream-free before you start polishing? I also get frustrated trying to separate one nail product from another because they have so much in common. The resins, lacquers, and basic products are all essentially the same. Most women experience about the same amount of wear from product to product, and it's about one to three days. All nail polishes begin to chip on the third to fourth day after application, regardless of the claim on the label (but you already knew that, didn't you?). Reapplying your top coat daily and avoiding fast-drying nail polishes will increase the chances of having your polish last. Finding the discipline to do that isn't easy, but it is the cheapest and most reliable way to make a manicure stick around until the end of the week.

By the way, it is completely unnecessary and actually a bad idea to store nail polish in the refrigerator. Condensation and cold negatively affect nail polish, making it too thick to use reliably.

DIBUTYL PHTHALATE

Dibutyl phthalate (DBP) is a very common ingredient in almost every nail polish being sold. It is used as a plasticizer and is a key component in giving nail polish its unique properties. But a lot of women are giving their nail polishes a second look since the Centers for Disease Control and Prevention (CDC, http://www.cdc.gov) published the *National Report on Human Exposure to Environmental Chemicals—Results for Mono-butyl phthalate* [which is] *(metabolized from Dibutyl phthalate)*. Basically the CDC found measurable levels of phthalate in the urine of the participants in a study looking at the issue of phthalates. However, the CDC stated that "Finding a measurable amount of one or more phthalate metabolites in urine does not mean that the level of one or more phthalates causes an adverse health effect. Whether phthalates at the levels of metabolites reported here are a cause for health concern is not yet known; more research is needed" (sources: CDC, http://www.cdc.gov/ nceh/dls/report/results/Mono-butylPhthalate.htm; *Environmental Health Perspectives*, December 2000, volume 108, issue 12).

In animal tests, dibutyl phthalate has been shown to produce detrimental effects. The Environmental Working Group (EWG, http://www.ewg.org), a nonprofit environmental research organization, found that "DBP is a developmental and reproductive toxin that in lab animals causes a broad range of birth defects and lifelong reproductive impairment in males [when] exposed in utero and shortly after birth. DBP damages the testes, prostate gland, epididymus, penis, and seminal vesicles. These effects persist throughout the animal's life."

There are no similar studies or research showing any of that to be true in humans. In 1985, the Cosmetic Ingredient Review (CIR) board (http://www.cir-safety.org/) deemed dibutyl phthalate safe for use in cosmetic products. More recently, a press release issued on November 30, 2001, titled "Statement by the Phthalate Esters Panel of the American Chemistry Council on the Cosmetic Ingredient Review Expert Panel Assessment of Phthalate Esters," noted that "The Cosmetic Ingredient Review (CIR) Expert Panel is reviewing the use of three phthalate esters (also known as phthalates) in cosmetics. It is anticipated that the Expert Panel will complete its review in the first half of next year."

As this book goes to press, phthalates in general are still under investigation, and the jury is still out on whether or not phthalates are really harmful when used in cosmetics. In checking every line of polish I have ever seen, from Dior and Hard Candy to Lancôme and Chanel, I have yet to find one that didn't contain it, so unless you give up polish there is no way to avoid this ingredient. I wish I could be more definitive about what to recommend, but for now I will continue to monitor the study results as they become available and report on what is published in my print and online bimonthly newsletter *Cosmetics Counter Update*, and my online biweekly *Beauty Bulletin*.

FAKE NAILS—REAL PROBLEMS

The long and short of artificial nails is that there are risks associated with having them applied. I won't get into the aesthetic issue here, though it is a mystery to me why women can consider this a valid expenditure of their hard-earned money or believe that anyone thinks these are real—that's another story altogether. What is of more concern is the number of women every year who see a physician because of nail-related disorders that are directly related to the application of artificial nails. The most typical problems are horizontal nail grooves that develop close to the cuticle. This abnormality, according to an article by Dr. Zoe Draelos in the January 1998 issue of *Cosmetic Dermatology*, is seen in chemotherapy patients and women who wear artificial nails. When it's unrelated to chemotherapy, this nail damage is probably a result of the drill used by the manicurist to buff out the acrylic nail, or to rough up the real nail to allow better adhesion of the fake nail. It is far less damaging to use an emery board to file the nail, but salons are using the drill procedure to speed up an otherwise time-consuming process.

The thinning of the nail plate is another problem that occurs, especially when the acrylic nails are finally removed. To address this, it is quite typical for the manicurist to recommend oils, vitamins, or other treatments ranging from calcium to oxygen infusions, none of which will improve the appearance of the nail. The weakened, fragile part of the nail is long dead, and there is nothing that can be done to change the damage that took place when the artificial nail was applied and the repeated damage with each reapplication. The only option is time, enough of it to grow out the damage, assuming that you are not doing anything else to your nails to cause more damage to the nail or cuticle.

Inflammation of the nail area is almost always a direct result of the chemicals used to apply artificial nails, but it can also be an allergic reaction to the acrylic material. However, if the inflammation persists or swells, it is essential to use a topical disinfectant such as Bacitracin. If the swelling continues or becomes more painful, it is imperative to see a physician who can treat the possible infection.

Another typical and more painful problem is something called onycholysis, which is the separation or loosening of a fingernail or toenail from its nail bed. What makes acrylic nails often more amazing than your own nails is, according to Dr. Draelos, "that the adhesion between the artificial nail and the natural plate is stronger than the adhesion between the natural nail plate and the nail bed." If you twist your nail, it is far easier to have your own nail become detached from your skin than it is for the artificial nail to pop off your natural nail. This means you need to avoid misuse (and not think the artificial nail can withstand any amount of pressure). It is imperative to pay attention to any loosening of your own nail and to be careful how you use the artificial nail. Because the artificial nail may be stronger than your own, it can put your real nail at risk.

One other possible problem for fake-nail wearers is infection. If you see a yellow or green discoloration, you can attempt to treat it yourself with Bacitracin. But if this doesn't produce any improvement then it is essential you contact your physician.

NAIL STRENGTHENERS

If only nail-strengthening products really existed! What I wouldn't give for that, and I've tried them all. As it turns out, many of the products that claim to strengthen nails contain extremely drying ingredients such as formaldehyde or toluene, which do toughen the nail temporarily, but also make it more brittle. Formaldehyde goes by other names on ingredient lists, so watch out for names like toluene, toluene sulfonamide, and toluene sulfonic acid. Toluene and toluene-like ingredients are illegal in the state of California because of the serious health risks they pose, including cancer and respiratory problems.

Some formaldehyde-free nail strengtheners just coat the nail, like the ridge-filling products. So-called strengthening creams contain thick, waxy ingredients, like lanolin, that smooth over the nail and are hard to wash off. If you are good about reapplying these several times a day (sans polish, of course, because they can't penetrate polish), you might just see a change in your nails because they help protect the cuticle and prevent the nail from drying out, but it takes discipline. Keep in mind that you can't wear polish over any kind of moisturizing product because polish won't adhere to a moist, lubricated surface. You can apply these products over polish; but then they won't help the nail, although they can moisturize the cuticle.

NAIL DO'S AND DON'TS

Surprisingly, there are more don'ts than do's when it comes to taking care of your nails. Most dermatologists will tell you that what you don't do to your nails is far more important than what you do to them when healthy, strong nails are what you want. This list summarizes some of the things I've mentioned earlier, but the information bears repeating, given the amount of deceptive nail information and the number of nail products being sold and advertised all over the cosmetics world.

- **Do coat the outside of the nails with nail polish or ridge fillers,** which can help protect the nail and prevent breaking and splitting, at least while the manicure lasts.
- **Do moisturize the cuticle area** to prevent cracking and peeling, which can hurt the matrix.
- **Do wear gloves** to protect nails and cuticles from housework, gardening, and doing dishes.
- **Do be cautious when doing office work.** Nails and cuticles can take a beating from filing, opening letters (use a letter opener), typing (use the flat of your finger pads on the keyboard instead of the tips of your nails), and handling papers.
- **Do apply a hand cream frequently,** especially after you're done washing your hands, and pay attention to the cuticle area.
- **Do wear a sunscreen** during the day on the hands and cuticles to prevent sun damage, which can hurt the nail, and reapply every time you wash your hands.
- **Do meticulously clean all nail implements** and change nail files often. Bacteria and other microbes can get transferred by the nail tools you use, causing infection or harm to the matrix.
- **Do disinfect any tears or cuts to the cuticle, and treat ingrown nails as soon as possible.** Nail infections are not only unsightly, but also can cause long-lasting damage to the nail. Any drugstore antibacterial ointment, such as Polysporin, Neosporin, or Bacitracin, will do.
- **Don't use nail products that contain formaldehyde or toluene.** They pose health risks for the nail and for your entire body as well.
- **Don't use fingernails as tools** to pry things open.
- **Don't use your fingers as letter openers.** That destroys the cuticles, which destroys the nail matrix and affects nail growth and strength.

- **Don't soak nails for long periods, and never use any kind of soap or detergent when soaking.** Nails and cuticles that become engorged with water weaken, and the longer soap or detergent is in contact with skin and nails (despite the advertisements for Palmolive dish detergent) the greater the potential for damaging the nail and cuticle structure.
- **Don't overuse any kind of nail-polish remover.** Use a minimal amount on the nail and avoid getting too much on the cuticle and skin.
- **Don't push the cuticle back too far.** Leave the cuticle alone as much as possible. Trim only the part of the cuticle that has started to lift away from the nail.
- **Don't allow any manicurist to touch your hands with utensils that have not been properly sterilized.** The importance of this step cannot be stressed enough. Risking your health and well-being for a manicure is just not worth it, and that is a definite possibility with bacteria-laden nail instruments!
- **Don't pull or tear at hangnails.** Always gently cut them away, leaving the cuticle intact and as untampered with as possible.
- **Don't ignore nail or cuticle inflammation.** Disinfect the skin as soon as you can with an antibacterial or antifungal agent. Any change to the nail's appearance (see the next section) needs to be checked out by a dermatologist.

WHEN THE NAIL GETS SICK

There are times when nail care requires a dermatologist. Fingernails and toenails are extremely vulnerable to infection and damage. If you have been diligent about leaving your cuticles alone and avoiding all the don'ts and performing most of the do's in the list above and you are still having nail problems, make an appointment with your dermatologist. Nails that are brittle, discolored, dull, abnormally thick, distorted, crumbling, loose, or subject to unusual debris under the nail are a medical problem, not a cosmetic one.

It is quite normal for the skin to host a variety of microorganisms, including bacteria and fungi. Some are useful to the body. Others can multiply rapidly and lead to infections. Specifically, fungal infections are caused by microscopic plants (fungi) that thrive on the dead tissue of the nails and outer skin layers, particularly the cuticle.

Fungal nail infections are most often seen in adults, can be difficult to treat, and often recur. Toenails are affected more often than fingernails. People who frequent public swimming pools, gyms, or shower rooms; people who perspire a great deal; and people who wear tight, occlusive shoes are most likely to develop toenail infections because the fungi flourish in warm, moist areas. Prolonged exposure to moistness on the skin, minor nail injuries, and damage to the cuticle area can also increase susceptibility to fungal infection. Please be aware that fungal and bacterial infections are extremely contagious and can be spread through direct contact with another person who has the problem, and even through contact with contaminated towels, shower and pool surfaces, and nail implements such as cuticle clippers, nail clippers, orange sticks, and cuticle pushers.

Nail infections can be cleared with the persistent use of a prescription antifungal or antibacterial cream or lotion. Because nails grow slowly, treatment must be continued for three to six months for fingernails and six to twelve months for toenails (the time it takes to grow a new nail). There are oral medications for these problems, but they are best discussed with your doctor.

In terms of preventing problems for the feet, it is essential to keep them clean and dry. Change shoes and socks frequently. Dry the feet and hands thoroughly after bathing. Powders such as baby powder or talcum may help keep the feet dry. Of course, avoiding any damage to toenails and fingernails is of utmost importance.

To minimize the risk of damage to the nails, keep them smooth and properly trimmed. Trim the fingernails weekly. The toenails grow more slowly and may be trimmed as needed, about once a month. Nail-polish remover of any kind can weaken and dry the nails. Nail polish may coat and protect the nails slightly, but if you choose to use it remember that all polishes are basically identical, despite advertising claims to the contrary. Nail strengtheners can discolor or break the nails and damage the nail, too. Artificial nails may produce allergic reactions under the nail and can create a perfect environment for bacterial or fungal growth.

INGROWN NAILS

Ingrown nails are another inelegant but typical nail problem. Often they are the result of cutting the nail too deeply or filing the nail too much, setting the scene for abnormal growth. Pain, swelling, infection, and discharge can result when the nail edge then grows into the surrounding skin. Many women love to wear shoes that crunch their toes into unnatural positions, and this, too, can interfere with nail growth and impair a normal healing process.

How can you prevent ingrown nails? Give your toenails plenty of room. That means wearing shoe styles that do not force the foot into an unnatural shape. Also, when you trim your fingernails and toenails, it is essential to avoid radically changing the natural shape of the nail by overfiling or by cutting the nail below the tip of the finger or toe. Also, do not cut or push the cuticles; damage there can significantly affect the nail's growth.

If an ingrown nail does become infected, thoroughly clean the area and try to minimally trim away the portion of the nail that is digging into the skin. Overcutting can simply re-create the problem, so be cautious. Disinfect the area with an over-the-counter antibacterial ointment like Polysporin, Neosporin, or Bacitracin. If the problem does not improve, it may require medical care.

part IV

MAKEUP:
WHAT THE PROS KNOW

chapter *15*

MAKEUP APPLICATION STEP BY STEP

MAKEUP: A PHILOSOPHICAL APPROACH

A documentary produced by the British Broadcasting Corporation went into entertaining detail and analysis of this salient point. *The Human Face* was written and directed by comedy legend John Cleese and features some rather candid comments from dermatologist Dr. Vail Reese on how we perceive skin flaws while watching films, and the way we make character assumptions based on things like facial asymmetry or scarring. According to Reese, "you'll have the clear complected individual as the hero, while any skin defect can be used by film makers to identify to audiences: Watch out for this one. So skin becomes a reflection not just of health, but of moral content. It is true that people with bad skin are not evil. We know that rationally. But studies have shown that subjects who interacted with those with clear skin and then those with facial scarring showed that there was more hesitation, more avoidance, more fear associated with the people who did not have good skin." In terms of cosmetic adornment, Vail commented that "makeup is used to minimize any discoloration of the skin, any irregular contours, and then better allow attention to be drawn to certain features such as the eyes or the mouth, which we as humans want to accentuate" (source: http://www.skinema.com *Skinterview*, March 2001).

I have always believed that beauty is more than skin deep and that physical beauty has little meaning compared with the importance of an individual's positive contribution to the world we live in. A capacity for compassion, kindness, creativity, and an enduring respect toward each other, the environment, and all living creatures is infinitely more meaningful than how we look. Yet, it would be foolish to ignore that personal appearance has an enormous consequence in life. Whether you can or should judge a book by its cover, for the most part, most everyone does. I don't know if Brad Pitt, Jennifer Aniston, Tom Cruise, or Julia Roberts are good people, but they are simply stunning to look at. Looking beautiful has power in our society and often determines the way people relate to each other. Ignoring the significance of that impact may be virtuous, but it is utterly unrealistic.

Applying makeup can be about looking well-groomed and feeling more beautiful and it can be exciting and fun. When done right, it can also express a great deal of personal power and élan. In the following pages I explain how to apply makeup with panache and sophistication so you can, if you choose, add to or improve this concept of beauty in your life. I personally feel less is best when it comes to makeup, but I know women's choices and tastes range from no makeup at all to the whole nine yards. Whatever your choice, if you do want to wear makeup, applying it deftly can make the difference between looking attractive and looking out of date, out of place, or just plain unattractive.

Throughout this chapter, I try to guide you through the maze of options and help you create a beautiful makeup look for yourself that feels comfortable and fits like a glove. **Although fashion statements can be taken to extremes—from following the whims of everything the fashion magazines portray or your favorite celebrity decides to get into, to holding on to looks that are long gone—ignoring fashion is a mistake. Finding your own balance between fashion, comfort, and personal style is the most logical and beautiful choice.**

DRESSING YOUR FACE—WHAT'S IN FASHION?

In many ways, makeup application is infinitely less complicated than skin care. Caring for your skin involves sorting through complex technical, medical, and physiological issues, while makeup is a more subjective and introspective art form. Makeup has little to do with hard facts and everything to do with skill and fashion. Discovering your personal preferences and honing your application technique are the essence of makeup application. **For the most part, makeup application is about experimentation and self-determination, because there are essentially no dos or don'ts, no have-tos or must-nots, no absolute rights or wrongs.** By way of illustration, you may decide that blue eyeshadow, dark brown lipstick, white foundation, and false eyelashes create the fashion statement you want to make, while I unequivocally recommend you avoid doing any of that. Yet wearing that makeup combination won't hurt you in the least. It may prevent you from being taken seriously or from getting the job you want, but that depends on what you want in life or what your career choices are.

When fashion is the topic, there are enough opinions and viewpoints to fill thousands and thousands of pages in hundreds of women's magazines every single month, year after year. With such a storm of possible options screaming at us from the pages of *Vogue, Glamour, In Style,* and all the rest, choosing a direction may seem impossible. One model may wear a minimal sweep of tan blush on her cheeks, a hint of lipstick, taupe eyeshadow used both on the lid and crease, and a thin coating of mascara. Another model may have on an elaborate blend of contour shading; blush on top of that; an array of eyeshadow colors; dramatic, thick liner across the upper lashes and another thick sweep of liner along the lower lashes; and lots of mascara. The variations are endless. To make things even more confusing, each month there are new announcements about what is fashionable and what isn't. One month red lipstick is hot, the next month it's mauve, and the next pink, and then you read that blue eyeshadow is coming back and you have to avoid wearing anything more than a hint of blush. Following these dictates can be maddening, not to mention expensive and perhaps inappropriate for you.

So where do you fit in? There are no hard and fast rules, though I know that's what we all want to hear—a clear path of exactly what to use to make us look picture perfect. In the long run, the final decision is yours amongst an array of choices. **I will show you how to build a basic and classic makeup application, one that most, if not all, makeup artists use repeatedly in one form or another.** Once you get these basics down— how to choose and apply concealer, foundation, powder, contour (if you want), blush, eyeshadow (one is plenty, but you can choose more), eyeliner (optional), eyebrow color (if needed or desired), mascara, lip liner (optional), and lipstick—wearing as little or as much color or using as many of these steps as you feel comfortable with is completely up to you. That's not to say I won't be throwing in my opinions of what I think works and looks best. If you use lip liner that smears, eyeshadows that streak and flake, mascara that clumps, blush that goes on choppy, eyeliner that smudges, or concealer that creases into the lines around your eyes and mouth, you and your makeup will not look beautiful in the least—and the goal is to look and feel more beautiful.

As you look at fashion magazines and study the various makeup applications, styles, and images portrayed, decide which ones will help you with your career or any other aspect of your life that is important to you. The world is complicated enough—who needs to waste time wondering what to wear every season? It is far more powerful and beautiful to stick with classic looks that facilitate and enhance your ability to handle job interviews, get ahead in your career, raise a family, and concentrate on financial matters than it is to chase every new trend that comes along. The fashion headlines and headshots may look beautiful, but if they don't fit with your lifestyle and goals, let them be beautiful for someone else who has time and money to burn.

The pictures in this chapter demonstrate a full makeup application, and depict a progression of colors—neutral tones across the cheeks and eyes going from light to dark—that can fit almost any face. Makeup professionals the world over use this pattern time after time, and you can see it on the covers of most fashion magazines and on news anchors, TV personalities, and celebrities. It can be adjusted to include a wide variety of colors and intensities to achieve the look you want. This type of makeup application has been around for more than 25 years (it was established by makeup artist extraordinaire Way Bandy back in the early 1970s, who was my guru when I started) and it's used today by most professional makeup artists, including the late Kevyn Aucoin, who not only cited Bandy as his main influence but often used Bandy's style as a blueprint for his own makeup applications.

DOES MAKEUP CHANGE WITH AGE?

Whether or not you choose a new approach to your makeup based on your age is entirely dependent on what you're doing at the moment and how that makes you feel. Just because more and more candles are finding a way onto your birthday cake, you don't have to hightail it to the nearest cosmetics counter for a makeover. If you have reached a point where you truly feel comfortable and confident in your own skin, what you adorn it with should reflect this. For most women, this may mean a sheer foundation that matches their skin exactly, a neutral-toned, crease-less concealer that does not play up wrinkles, a light dusting of sheer, nonshiny powder, soft matte eyeshadows in a variety of neutral hues, lightly defined and shaped brows, a great mascara that makes the most of your eyelashes, a softly blended blush color that adds vibrancy and color to your cheeks, and a lipstick color that seems "just right" no matter what other makeup you use. Sticking with well-chosen, adeptly applied and blended makeup in flattering shades gives a timeless look that can make ordinary features stunning.

However, if you breezed through your teens and twenties choosing makeup on a whim or enjoyed using bold, shiny eyeshadows, obvious blush, overly greasy or glossy lipsticks, heavy or mismatched foundation and too-thick concealer, and a kaleidoscopic array of eyeshadows and liners that were "out" as soon as you discovered they were "in," then you really should consider making adjustments to your routine. The same holds true if you feel as if you've been a slave to the latest makeup fads or styles, be they a retro Marilyn Monroe look with liquid-lined bedroom eyes and pouty red lips or the Crayola crayon–colored eye-shadows and spiky mascara seen in countless ads for sephora.com. You may discover that changing to a classic, well-blended finish where no one aspect of your makeup is more important than another is a refreshing, freeing style you can make your own. I'm all for self-expression—and when you're younger the limits of this are justifiably something to test—but as an adult, if your goal is to be taken seriously and be respected, why not think twice before heading to the office or grocery store wearing taxicab-yellow eyeshadow, clumpy mascara, and blue lipstick?

Being a certain age—be it 30, 40, 50, or beyond—doesn't mean you have to overdo or undo your makeup. Regardless of how the years add up, you need to find a style that makes you look and feel beautiful, and that means finding colors that enhance your appearance and practicing blending techniques that make it all look natural and smooth instead of contrived and painted on.

WHERE TO BEGIN

Three of the most difficult aspects of makeup are choosing the right colors, discerning the differences between products, and learning the correct application techniques. Though these major issues need to be ad-dressed, they are still only part of the picture. Wondering where to put your blush or how to blend your foundation before you know what type of foundation or what color of blush you should wear is putting the cart before the horse. Before you even choose specific makeup colors, discriminate between products, or deal with application, it is important to have a clear idea of the makeup look and style you want to create. Just as you would choose clothes to wear that are appropriate for where you are going—you wouldn't put on a jogging suit to go to a formal dinner or wear a long gown for a grocery run—the same guidelines are true for makeup.

Color, style, and fashion are all essential elements in clothing, and they are also essential to putting together a great makeup look. Too often women shop for or apply makeup with only one of those things in mind. Shopping for a lipstick or eyeshadow color without taking into account the other items in your makeup wardrobe is a mistake. Instead, decide what kind of makeup wardrobe you want to create and then go about choosing compatible colors, products, and application techniques to fit that concept. Think of the makeup staples you will need, such as black mascara, a healthy blush color, taupe or tan eyeshadow, and a suitable red lipstick. These items are akin to wardrobe staples such as a crisp white shirt, blue jeans, or the standard black dress—always fashionable and classic.

The way you see yourself, the way you want to be seen, what you do for a living, what you do in your leisure time, what colors are in your wardrobe, what style of clothing you are comfortable in, and how much time you are willing to spend creating a particular look all affect the way you choose and wear makeup. Those elements should set the course for choosing the right colors and products. So let's think a bit about the image you want to create.

CHOOSING MAKEUP ACCORDING TO YOUR IMAGE

The first part of this makeup self-analysis is to take a close look at you. How do you want to be seen? What do you do for a living? What occupies most of your time during the day? The external image you want to project in your business life and personal life is what wearing makeup is all about. Too often we dress our face without thinking about how it affects our image. My favorite example of this is in the movie *Working Girl*, which stars Melanie Griffith, Sigourney Weaver, and Harrison Ford (it's a great rental if you haven't seen it). Griffith's appearance changes dramatically as her character decides to become more "professional" in order to fulfill her career aspirations. In addition to changing her wardrobe, she changes the way she wears her makeup and hair. To look more polished and put-together, she *softens* her makeup look. Griffith goes from wearing strong pastel-colored, heavily applied eyeshadows to softly applied, neutral taupes and browns. She stops wearing heavy black eyeliner on the lid and lower lashes in favor of a more subtle shade of dark brown. Her lipstick changes from cranberry red to a neutral coral-tan, and her boldly applied blush is replaced by a soft neutral tone. The striking difference in her looks is a beautiful example of how makeup can affect the image you project—and how others perceive you.

Rather than just randomly selecting a lipstick, stop and consider not only whether it's the right color for your skin tone, but also whether it is too soft, too sheer, too noticeable, too sexy, not sexy enough, or has enough flair or subtlety to support the image you want to project. **Problems with how you apply makeup can be solved with technique, but understanding how you want others to see you comes from a sense of purpose and an understanding of what you want out of life.**

BEFORE YOU START

Because makeup goes on poorly over skin that isn't perfectly clean and smooth, the first step in applying beautiful makeup is to start with a clean face. Following the skin-care recommendations described earlier in this book will help you get your skin closer to where it needs to be. Women with dry skin should also wear moisturizer under their foundation (preferably a moisturizer with a good SPF if the foundation doesn't contain one). Women with normal to oily skin should avoid wearing moisturizer under their foundation. Moisturizer of any kind only adds to an active oil flow, and will make skin look greasy that much sooner. (It is, however, completely acceptable to wear a minimal amount of moisturizer over dry areas such as the under-eye area or cheeks.)

The only reason to use a moisturizer is to smooth and lubricate dry skin or dry areas. In spite of what you hear from cosmetics salespeople, moisturizer does not and cannot protect the face from a foundation, nor is that necessary. It's a good sales gimmick, but it's not the truth. There is nothing "bad" inside a foundation that your face needs to be protected from. Moisturizers are absorbed into the skin, and once they are, for all intents and purposes, they're gone, and they can't prevent anything else you put on your face from going where it wants. Besides, whatever protection you think you're applying when you put on a moisturizer is likely wiped away as you apply your foundation (including sunscreen, which should be the last thing applied to the face).

I know this idea of wearing a moisturizer only when you have dry skin borders on heresy, but in the long run it makes the most sense for your skin, especially if you wear a water-based or emollient foundation. What you might not know is that most water-based foundations (and definitely emollient foundations) contain many of the exact same ingredients as your moisturizer, so it isn't necessary to double up products. If you're wearing a moisturizer (with or without SPF 15) and a water-based foundation at the same time, your face can become too slippery and the rest of your makeup will tend to slide right off by lunchtime.

If you believe a moisturizer does help your foundation go on more smoothly, the problem might actually be a different one—such as the way you apply your foundation, the type of foundation you're using, or your skin-care routine, which may be drying out your skin and leaving a rough feeling rather than a smooth one. Before you reach for the moisturizer, make sure another product you're using isn't negatively contributing to the way your foundation applies. And remember, it may not be a single product but a combination of products that's contributing to a less-than-smooth skin surface.

A good way to judge whether your skin needs moisturizer during the day is to notice how long your skin feels dry after you wash your face. A slight amount of dryness immediately after you wash your face is typical. However, if this feeling lasts longer than 15 or 20 minutes, you should wear a lightweight moisturizer under your foundation. If your skin tends to feel extremely dry after you wash your face with a gentle, water-soluble cleanser, wear a more emollient moisturizer under your foundation. If your skin tends to become drier as the day goes by, that, too, is a good reason to wear a moisturizer.

Note: Either your daytime moisturizer or your foundation must be rated SPF 15 and contain UVA-protecting ingredients of avobenzone, titanium dioxide, or zinc oxide. There is no reason to wear two products, a sunscreen and a moisturizer, when so many products combine both beautifully. An exception to this point is that if you opt to use a foundation with effective sunscreen and intend to spot-apply or use it minimally, it is essential to pair this with a sunscreen for proper UV protection.

Now you can start applying your makeup.

LESS IS BEST!

Never use more than you have to—either in the intensity of the colors you choose or the number of products you wear. Many steps in applying makeup can be consolidated or eliminated without affecting your overall makeup look in any way.

Frequently a salesperson at the cosmetics counter insists that you need an absurd number of products to be properly and attractively made up. Yet more complicated doesn't mean you will look any better. If anything, a more complicated makeup routine can mean more chances for mistakes, which can cause you to look overdone as well as waste your valuable time and money.

Speaking of doing too much, so-called foundation primers, eyeshadow bases, blemish cover-ups, and color correctors—to name just a few—are, with rare exceptions, completely unnecessary. They complicate the process of applying makeup by requiring additional blending and allowing too many colors and products to interact on the skin at the same time, leaving a thick, gunky mess and sometimes contrasting colors on the face. Your SPF 15 foundation (or foundation with an SPF 15 sunscreen/moisturizer underneath) and/or concealer can quite nicely accomplish all the functions those extra products are supposedly designed to perform, without any of the extra fuss and expense.

Foundation primers are seen in many of the newer makeup artistry lines, such as Laura Mercier, Vincent Longo, and NARS. Basically, these "primers" are nothing more than lightweight, silicone-based moisturizers. The silicone allows the product to spread easily over the skin, and to some extent can help smooth the skin's texture and remedy mild dry patches that could spell trouble when you apply most types of foundation. These primers also tend to have a soft matte finish on the skin once they dry down, and that can make your foundation a bit easier to control and blend because the skin will be much less slippery than if you had applied an emollient moisturizer. Still, primers are truly optional and their benefits do not outweigh the extra step and expense. The only reason to consider one is if you have normal to oily skin and need the extra smoothness these can provide in order to make your foundation look its best. It is best to test these out via sampling before investing in a full-size tube so you can be sure you're making the purchase because you like what it does for your skin—not because you get suckered into the marketing pitch that makes it sound so important for skin.

Eyeshadow bases are sold to the consumer to help eyeshadows stay in place longer. The eye area is indeed a tricky place to get color to last, but there are ways to make it stay without specialty products. Besides, most eyeshadow bases are very similar to cream-to-powder concealers or foundations. Placing a matte or semi-matte face foundation on your eyelid and applying loose powder over it works just as well. Also, if your eyeshadows tend to smear or slip into the eyelid crease, you can greatly reduce the problem by not placing a moisturizer or greasy foundation on your eyelid.

Blemish cover-ups are sold to consumers solely on the basis of something I call "acne anxiety." The promise conveyed by the word "cover-up" is that this product really can hide a blemish, but nothing could be further from reality. Most cover-ups are heavier than your foundation, and they look thick and obvious over a blemish. And if the blemish cover-up doesn't match your foundation exactly (and most don't), it will look like a different layer of color (usually a shade of peach or ash) placed over the blemish, bringing still more attention to the very problem you are trying to hide. Even if the cover-up is the same color as your foundation, you will probably place too much extra makeup over the lesion. Your foundation by itself is more than sufficient to cover the redness without bringing more attention to the area. I totally understand the desire to want these facial sore spots to disappear. Unfortunately, there is only so much you can do to cover up a blemish before you start making matters more obvious by layering on too much makeup.

It is especially problematic to apply concealer only over blemishes and nowhere else, without any foundation. The natural color and texture of your skin just doesn't resemble most foundations or concealers. Spot application looks, well, spotty! That doesn't hide anything, and it can look particularly strange in daylight.

Some concealers and cover-ups are dubbed "medicated" and are meant to cover and heal blemishes, but they are not effective for this purpose. I have yet to find one that contains ingredients that can disinfect, exfoliate, or absorb oil, all critical components for controlling breakouts.

Plus, these types of products don't cover any better than normal concealers.

Color correctors are those bottles of pink, mauve, peach, green, or yellow liquid meant to be worn under your foundation to alter skin color. Thankfully, these impractical, useless products are becoming harder to find, though some cosmetics lines are steadfast in making you believe you need them. The notion is that if your skin is pink or ruddy, you need to tone it down or counteract it with a yellow-tinted color corrector. If your skin is olive or sallow, you would change it with a pink or mauve color corrector. It's an interesting concept, but a waste of time.

The ingredient lists for most color correctors are very similar to those for moisturizers, which means they are easily absorbed into the skin. Once they are absorbed, you are left with a slight tint of pink, green, mauve, or yellow on the face. Supposedly this means you have now changed your skin tone for the better. In fact, once the liquid has been absorbed, the result is often so minor as to have little to no real effect on skin tone at all. For the sake of argument, though, let's say there is a noticeable change. The tint of the color corrector on your skin would mix with your foundation and you could end up with a very strange shade of foundation. A good foundation in a neutral, soft yellow-tone base should be able to correct and even out all skin tones without adding another layer of makeup on your face.

THE CLASSIC FACE

Classic makeup encompasses all of the following elements: concealer, foundation, powder, contour (optional), blush, eyeshadow, eyeliner, eyebrow color (if needed), lip liner (optional), and lipstick. For each of these steps, you want to find a corresponding product that is best for your skin type and the coverage or look you want. Each step also requires an application and blending tool so you can achieve a smooth, flawless appearance. **Along the way, you can eliminate steps that seem excessive or too complicated, and decide how much makeup you want to wear and what colors are suitable to your needs.**

The first two steps in applying a complete makeup are to reduce the darkness under the eyes and to apply a foundation to even out the skin (it's sort of like putting on panties and a bra). Once that's done, the eyeshadows and blushes can blend on smoothly over an even palette instead of over varying skin textures and colors. Whether you start your application with the concealer or the foundation depends more on personal preference than anything else, although the color of the concealer is another factor. For the sake of organization, I'll start with the concealer.

CONCEALER

Generally, a concealer is thought of as a product that covers blemishes or facial imperfections, as well as dark circles under the eyes. Concealer can also be used to highlight certain areas of the face, especially if it is a lighter texture and color. Concealers with thicker consistencies are best for covering problem areas such as dark circles under the eyes or extreme redness on cheeks or noses. Concealers with a lighter or thinner consistency are better for minimal coverage and for highlighting areas of the face you want accented. Throughout the rest of this book I refer to all products that provide extra coverage (over and above what foundations can do) or make certain areas of the face lighter as concealers.

The primary purpose of concealers is to offset the natural shadows that occur under the eyes, and, in more elaborate makeup applications, to highlight certain areas of the face such as the center of the nose, forehead, top of the cheekbones, or center of the chin. Principally, the under-eye area needs concealer most because the eye is set back in its socket, which lies in a shadow created by the surrounding bone structure. In addition, the skin around the eye tends to be thinner than the skin on the rest of the face, so pigment discolorations and surface veins show through easily, making the under-eye area look dark and dull. The first thing you need, then, is a lightweight, flesh-tone concealer that is a shade or two lighter than your foundation (see the photograph on page 441).

However, if you don't have dark circles under the eye area, you don't need a concealer. If your foundation is opaque enough to even out the skin tone under the eyes, you don't need an extra product for that area.

The logic behind using a lighter flesh-tone color is the same basic rule you learned in Art 101: When you need to make paint a lighter color, you add a lighter color than you started with. Any other color, or the same color, or a darker color would defeat the purpose. Blue, yellow, or shades that are the same as your foundation color will not make the under-eye area lighter. Standard shades can cover discolorations, which is fine, but applying a lighter shade is the only way to correct the darkness caused by shadows. Also, a slightly lighter under-eye area can make the face look brighter and more awake. **Foundation may be all you need to even out minimal discolorations under the eye, cheeks, or nose, or for minor facial discolorations.**

When you shop for an effective concealer, it is critical that the concealer be the same basic, natural skin tone as your foundation, only one or two shades lighter. That way you can be assured that the foundation and concealer will blend together under the eye. If you choose a concealer that is a very different color than your foundation, you will simply end up with a third color where they overlap and intersect.

The only time you wouldn't use a lighter concealer is when the area under the eye is naturally lighter or the same color as the rest of the face. In that case, it's fine to apply your foundation with no concealer. In fact, it may sometimes be necessary to apply a concealer that is slightly darker than your foundation to reduce having a whitish goggle effect around the eye.

I prefer to apply concealer first and then the foundation. If you are using an ultra-matte foundation, the concealer blending on first prevents streaking and staining. (It's hard to blend anything over ultra-matte foundations.) You can apply your concealer in a small arc around the inside corner of the eye or, for a more involved makeup application, you can apply it in a sweep under the entire eye and out on the upper cheekbone. Blend this out evenly, taking care not to spread it onto areas where you don't want it. Be sure you are using a pat-and-blend method of application, as this will ensure that the concealer covers where it is supposed to and is not inadvertently wiped away. The foundation is then applied lightly over this area and blended out over the face. You may also want to try applying your foundation first and then sparingly applying concealer to the under-eye area if it is still dark. The trick is to make sure the foundation and concealer edges merge imperceptibly on the skin.

The most typical problem with a concealer is applying it smoothly over the under-eye area without making it look too white. It is important to always blend the edge of the concealer away from the eye until it disappears. Also, try to concentrate the concealer along the inside corner of the eye and down, as opposed to out. The less concealer you put at the back corner of the eye (unless that area is dark), the lower your chances of looking like you're wearing a white mask over the eyes.

At times when you wish to wear as little makeup as possible, try using only a minimal amount of concealer that is closer to your true skin tone than the concealer you normally use. Or try a lighter shade of foundation than you normally wear and apply it only in the under-eye area. This can make a world of difference in making you look rested and polished, but not made up. Again, the trick is to blend extremely well so that there is no discernible edge between the concealer area and the part of the face where there is no makeup.

In the past it was almost impossible to find concealers in a good selection of colors that also didn't crease into the lines around the eyes. Now the tide has turned, and many cosmetics lines have excellent shades and textures to choose from. When shopping for a concealer, the primary things to look for are (1) a neutral skin tone that is one or two shades lighter than your foundation, but not so light that it looks obvious when blended on in the under-eye area, (2) a smooth texture to ensure easy blending, (3) coverage that suits your needs, and (4) staying power, so it doesn't crease into the lines around the eyes.

Types of Concealers

Concealers come in six different forms: stick concealers, creamy liquid concealers, cream concealers, matte-finish liquid, matte-finish cream-to-powder, and finally the ultra-matte liquid concealers, which blend on smoothly and creamily and dry quickly into an unmovable layer.

Stick concealers: Stick concealers come in swivel-up tubes like lipsticks.

Examples: Cover Girl CG Smoothers Concealer *($5.69)*, NARS Concealer *($16)*.

Application: Stick concealers are applied to the under-eye area much the way a lipstick is applied to the mouth. They can be applied over or under your foundation, depending on how much coverage you want—under the foundation provides less coverage and over the foundation provides more. Dab the stick over the area in dots and then blend with clean fingers or a concealer brush. Avoid wiping it on from the stick in an opaque streak of color. That tends to build up too much makeup and it also pulls the eye area, causing sagging. If the skin under the eye area is dry or wrinkled, it does help to first apply a lightweight moisturizer and then apply the concealer. Be careful the moisturizer isn't too greasy and that you don't put it on too heavily, to ensure that the concealer doesn't slip into facial lines. If you have applied too much moisturizer, use a tissue to dab off any excess before you apply the concealer.

Pros: Depending on their consistency, stick concealers can provide more complete coverage and control for very dark circles under the eye. They tend to go on thickly and don't spread easily, which means you can better control the application.

Cons: The texture of many stick concealers is rather dry and thick, which makes them difficult to blend without overpulling the skin under the eye. They also go on too heavily, which can create an obviously made-up look. Other stick concealers are quite greasy; they can look less obvious because they blend so easily, but the texture often causes slippage into the lines around the eyes. For these reasons, this is the least common type of concealer you will encounter.

<u>**Creamy liquid concealers:**</u> Creamy liquid concealers generally come in small squeeze-tube containers or long, thin tubes with wand applicators.

Examples: Prescriptives Camouflage Cream *($16.50)*, Lancôme Effacernes *($21)*.

Application: Use your finger or the wand applicator to transfer the liquid concealer in small dots or to place a light coat of color under the eye area. Blend gently along the under-eye with either your finger or the sponge applicator, concentrating the largest amount of concealer over the darkest areas. If the skin under the eye area is dry or wrinkled, it helps to first apply a lightweight moisturizer and then apply the concealer. Be careful the moisturizer isn't too greasy and that you don't put it on too heavily or it will surely make the concealer slip into facial lines.

Pros: Depending on their consistency, creamy liquid concealers provide very light, even coverage and have the least tendency to crease into the eye area. They can also be easily layered if more coverage is needed, and they tend to not cake up on the skin.

Cons: Depending on their consistency, creamy liquid concealers can have too much movement and be hard to control. It is important when applying an under-eye concealer to keep the color and coverage just where you want it. If the concealer is too greasy or loose, it can spread too easily, highlighting parts of the face you don't want highlighted. Some liquid concealers go on too thinly, offering very little coverage, but if you don't want a lot or don't mind building coverage, these are the way to go.

<u>**Cream concealers:**</u> Cream concealers usually come in small pots and typically have a smooth and creamy texture. Occasionally these may have a dry, thick texture.

Examples: M.A.C. Studio Finish Concealer SPF 15 *($12.50)*, Stila Eye Concealer *($16)*.

Application: Depending on their consistency, cream concealers can go on easily with your fingertips, a concealer brush, or a sponge, placing the color in dots under the eye area. Blend the concealer out under the eye area, concentrating the application over the darkest areas. If the cream concealer has a dry, thick texture, it can be very difficult to blend and can look heavy and obvious on the skin. If the skin under the eye area is dry or wrinkled, it does help to first apply a lightweight moisturizer and then the concealer. If the cream concealer is very emollient, use minimal moisturizer under the eye area and dab off the excess. Most moisturizers can make cream-type concealers slip even more easily into facial lines. The emollient cream concealers should be set with loose powder immediately after blending to help promote crease-free wear.

Pros: Cream concealers can have a very pleasing creamy and moist consistency, but they can also be rather thick and heavy. Depending on the consistency, they can go on well and provide even, often opaque, coverage. They are especially good for someone with very dry skin who wants more coverage. Cream concealers can also be used as foundations in a pinch.

Cons: If the cream concealer is too thick or greasy, it will crease into the lines on your face. If it is dry and thick, it can be difficult to blend and can also easily crease into facial lines. This is never the type of concealer to use over breakouts.

Matte-finish liquid concealers: Matte-finish liquid concealers typically come in a squeeze tube or a tube with a wand applicator.

Examples: Paula's Select No Slip Concealer *($7.95)*, Elizabeth Arden Flawless Finish Concealer *($14)*.

Application: Use your finger or the wand applicator to transfer the liquid concealer in small dots to the under-eye area, then quickly blend using a soft patting motion. If the skin under the eye area is dry or wrinkled, it helps to first apply a minimal amount of lightweight moisturizer and then apply the concealer. Although these are not as tricky to apply as ultra-matte concealers, they still demand adept blending for the best results.

Pros: Depending on their consistency, matte concealers can provide light to full coverage. They typically do not crease or migrate, and they tend to outlast cream and cream-to-powder concealers. They also work well as a base for eyeshadow if you have trouble with your eyeshadows fading or creasing. Matte-finish concealers work well over blemishes.

Cons: If you have prominent lines around and under the eyes, matte-finish concealers can make them look more pronounced. Some matte concealers go on quite thick and dry, and are difficult to blend easily or dry too quickly.

Matte-finish cream-to-powder: Matte-finish cream-to-powder concealers usually come in compact form and often look like small versions of cream-to-powder foundation.

Examples: Clinique City Base Compact Concealer SPF 15 *($13.50)*, Lancôme Photogenic Concealer SPF 15 *($20)*.

Application: Use your finger, a concealer brush, or a sponge to dab the concealer onto the undereye area or over other discolorations.

Pros: This type of concealer is very easy to apply. It provides the glide and blendability of a cream concealer with the long wear of a matte concealer. Concealers like this work well anywhere on the face, especially if more extensive coverage is needed. Some versions contain effective sunscreens.

Cons: Despite the initial matte finish, the ingredients that create the creamy texture tend to cause it to eventually crease—and to keep on creasing. The powder finish can make wrinkles look more pronounced, and this type of concealer is not the best to use over blemishes or dry, flaky skin.

Ultra-matte liquid concealers: Ultra-matte liquid concealers generally come in thin tubes with wand applicators. Although these were once easy to find, many of them have fallen out of favor and have been discontinued because they are so difficult to work with and can make lines under the eye more pronounced; however, they rarely, if ever, crease.

Examples: Revlon ColorStay Concealer *($9.49)*, Maybelline Great Wear Concealer *($4.69)*.

Application: Use your finger or the wand applicator to transfer the liquid concealer in small dots to apply a light coat of color in the undereye area. You must blend these on very quickly and accurately because they dry in seconds. Once these ultra-matte concealers dry in place, they don't budge, and there is no way to adjust the blending, so you could end up with streaks or patches of color. Once ultra-matte concealers dry, they do what they say they'll do! If the skin under the eye area is dry or wrinkled, it helps to first apply a lightweight moisturizer and then apply the concealer. Concealers like this should always be applied before foundation. Applying them over foundation is just asking for trouble. However, in most cases you don't have to use an ultra-matte concealer if you're using an ultra-matte foundation because the foundation usually provides enough opaque coverage to cover just about anything.

Pros: Depending on their consistency, ultra-matte concealers provide light-to-medium, even coverage and, if blended on correctly, they absolutely will not crease into the lines around the eyes. They are great if you tend to lose makeup during the day or have problems with makeup slipping. They also make excellent, long-lasting eyeshadow bases for those who have a problem with their eyeshadows fading or creasing throughout the day.

Cons: Because ultra-matte concealers stay so well and are so matte, they can make lines under the eyes look more noticeable. It doesn't always help to apply moisturizer underneath because that can sometimes make the concealer streak and look stained. It is important when applying under-eye concealers to keep the color just where you want it and to blend quickly.

Techniques for Blending Concealer

Regardless of the type of concealer you use, the application remains basically the same. Dab the color on with your fingertips, the wand applicator, or the tube concealer itself in a half-inch crescent from the inside corner of the eye out to approximately one-third of the way under the eye. Apply the concealer only where the eye area is dark. If it's dark all the way out under the eye, then that's where the concealer should go. You can apply concealer to the eyelid too if that area is also dark and could use some lightening. Unless you are using a matte or ultra-matte finish concealer, set the concealer with a light dusting of loose or pressed powder. This will ensure a smooth finish and longer wear (but be careful not to overdo powdering under the eye area because this, too, can make lines look more pronounced).

If you want a more elaborate makeup application, you can apply the concealer along the flat bridge of the nose, along the laugh lines, out along the entire under-eye area, on the top of the cheekbone, and in the center of the forehead and chin for accent and enhancement. These options tend to be complicated and time-consuming, even for women adept at applying their makeup, and you can get almost the same results by applying the rest of your makeup correctly. I used none of those techniques with my makeup as it appears on the cover of this book, and all those areas appear nicely highlighted because of the way I applied the rest of my makeup. If you do choose to highlight these areas, place your highlighter in dots over or under your foundation in these areas and blend well, controlling the color so it does not spread all over your face. Keeping the color contained is the goal if you wish to try this extra step (see photograph on page 441).

Whether you apply the concealer first and then the foundation or the foundation first and then the concealer, carefully blend the concealer out and under the eye in a dabbing motion, with either your finger, a concealer brush, or sponge (I prefer to always use a sponge), making sure you cannot see the edge where the concealer stops and the foundation starts. The trick is to keep the concealer blended only over the area where it is needed. If you have to ask whether or not a concealer brush is really necessary, then chances are you do not need one!

Concealer Mistakes to Avoid

1. If you have noticeable lines around the eyes, do not wear a concealer that goes on too thickly or is too dry; it can cake under the eye and exaggerate wrinkles.
2. Consider my recommendations above for specific concealers that don't crease into the lines around eyes, or be sure to test the concealer first by wearing it under your eyes for a while to see that it doesn't crease and to find how it works with your foundation and skin tone.
3. If the concealer is obvious, you've chosen the wrong shade, applied it too heavily, or haven't overlapped the blending with your foundation.
4. Do not wear a peach, orange, green, rose, or ash shade of concealer.
5. If the skin is dry, apply a lightweight moisturizer under the eye to prevent the concealer from caking or making the wrinkles look more noticeable. A moisturizer that is too heavy or emollient can make almost any concealer slip into the lines around the eyes. Be careful using moisturizer with an ultra-matte concealer, because streaking or splotches of color can result if the moisturizer is too heavy or is applied too thickly.
6. Do not forget to blend the foundation and concealer together so there are no edges where one stops and the other starts. This is best done with a makeup sponge.

FOUNDATION

Personally, I've never been fond of the whole process of smearing foundation all over my face or even part of my face. I totally understand when women complain about feeling "made up" when they wear a foundation. So why do I recommend using foundation at all? Because of the flawless, even base a foundation can provide. If the skin has a uniform color, texture, and appearance, the blush and eyeshadow colors you apply will look smooth instead of choppy. However, and here's the tricky part, **to the extent possible, the face should never look like it has a layer of foundation on it.**

If you are already blessed with a totally even, perfect complexion, you will nevertheless want to consider wearing a foundation because of how it helps eyeshadows and blushes go on more evenly. If you try to blend blushes and eyeshadows without foundation, they will most likely go on choppily or wear unevenly during the day. Foundation keeps those powdered colors in place. Skin itself has no real adhesive properties (think about what would adhere to it if it did!). Foundation, therefore, gives the rest of the makeup something to hold on to evenly. By themselves, blushes and eyeshadows have some ability to cling, but not all that much. Besides, today's foundations offer some incredible options for creating the illusion of even, flawless skin without looking like makeup, and many of the best ones contain effective sunscreen.

Finding the Perfect Foundation Color

I cannot stress this point enough: Your skin and foundation should match exactly. If you are pale, that's OK—accept the fact that you are pale, and buy a light foundation that matches exactly. **Whether you have red hair and fair skin or black hair and dark ebony skin, the foundation must match your underlying skin color exactly. Do not buy a foundation that will make your face look even a shade or two darker or lighter or change its underlying color in any manner.** Even with a difference that slight, you run the risk of a more obvious makeup application than you really want, particularly for daytime wear. Find a foundation that matches your skin perfectly and goes on softly and smoothly.

When I tell you to match the foundation with your underlying skin color, you may be asking yourself, "Exactly what is meant by skin color?"

Traditionally, skin color has been defined by the basic underlying tone, described as olive, when the skin appears ashen or green in color; sallow, when the skin has a yellow or golden shade; and ruddy, when the skin has overtones of pink or red. These categories hold true for all women, including women of color; your underlying skin color will always relate to one of those skin tones. You may have been told that you are a particular "season" and your wardrobe and foundation color should be a specific undertone, either cool (blue tones) or warm (yellow tones). Unfortunately, all that information surrounding skin tone can be misleading when it comes to choosing a foundation color.

If you are told your face has cool undertones, meaning blue undertones, should you wear a blue-toned foundation? Of course not. If your skin color is ashen, choosing an ashen foundation will just make you look greener. If your face is strongly pink or red, applying a pink foundation all over will make you look like you're wearing a pink mask. If you have a sallow skin tone, applying a strong yellow-looking foundation will make you look more sallow. None of those would look natural and flawless the way foundation should look, and none of them would come close to matching your skin's underlying, basic color.

So what to do? When you're purchasing a foundation, it is important to identify your overall, exact skin color and find a foundation that matches it, regardless of the underlying tone. **For the most part, regardless of your race, nationality, or age, your foundation should be some shade of neutral ivory, neutral beige, tan, dark brown, bronze brown, or ebony, with a slight, and I mean very slight, undertone of yellow but without any orange, pink, green, or blue. There are no orange, pink, green, or blue people, and buying foundations in those colors is absurd.**

Why a slightly yellow undertone? Because skin color, more often than not, has a yellow undertone: That's just what the natural color of melanin (the pigment in the skin) tends to be. There are a few exceptions to this rule. Native North American or South American women, a tiny percentage of African-American women, and some Polynesian women do indeed have a red cast to their skin, and in those instances this information about neutral foundations should be ignored. Because their skin has a slightly reddish cast, they need to look for foundations that have a slightly reddish cast to them—but that's only a hint of brownish red, and not copper, orange, or peach.

A few makeup lines are aimed at Asian women. These boast a "unique collection of yellow-toned foundations" appropriate for all skin types, but most specifically, Asian women. I concur that most skin types, including those of Asian women, are better served by yellow/neutral-based foundations and powders. However, plenty of lines have awesome yellow/neutral-based foundation colors. The same principle holds true for African-American women. There are many lines claiming to meet the needs of darker skin colors, but often these lines actually have poor color selections or poor foundation types (the exception to this is Iman foundation colors, http://www.i-iman.com). It is best to find a foundation color and type that works for your skin type rather than limiting yourself to a special line claiming to serve a specific skin color.

Question: If all the fashion magazines and makeup experts talk about foundations being sheer and matching the skin exactly, why do so many women of all ages wear heavy-looking, obvious foundations? It may be confusion about skin tone and foundation color; it may be failure to check the foundation in daylight; or, in some cases, it may have something to do with the fact that many women hate their skin and think a layer of foundation looks better than what exists naturally. Rather than going into the emotional ramifications of disliking your skin, let me just say that covering your face with an obvious layer of foundation only makes matters worse. **What's essential to an attractive makeup application of any kind is to begin with a good, light-textured foundation that blends impeccably; otherwise you will look as if the makeup is wearing you.** Even if you feel that you are in need of a foundation that provides good coverage, *obvious* coverage is a monumental mistake and can negatively affect the entire makeup application. Of course, all foundation is about coverage, but it is also your personal key to enhancing—not masking—your complexion.

An Exception to the Rule of Matching Skin Color

Although you are attempting to exactly match the skin color of your face when you choose a foundation, in some cases it is more important to match the foundation to the color of your neck. If your face is darker than your neck and your foundation matches the face, it will look like a mask because of the difference in color. The opposite is also true. If your face is lighter than your neck and you put on a foundation that matches the face, it will still look like a mask because of the difference in color. In situations like this, match the foundation more to the neck color or to a color in between the color of the neck and the face.

For some women who have serious facial discolorations or scars it can be hard to ignore the need for a heavy foundation application that provides opaque, full, concealing coverage. Unfortunately, a heavy or thick foundation is the only way to achieve this effect. Foundations that make claims about superior coverage that also looks natural are not telling the truth. You can't cover your face with foundation and camouflage the imperfections without seeing what is providing the coverage. But that doesn't mean you shouldn't consider a heavier foundation—just be aware that you are essentially exchanging one problem for another. The advantage is that you do get to choose between two options, and even if that's a dilemma, you are still the best judge of what works and feels best for you.

The Final Decision

Once you have selected a foundation color, there is only one way to be absolutely sure it is right for you: Apply the color all over your face and check it outside in the daylight. Check it from all angles and decide if it matches your skin exactly. If you applied it carefully but there are lines of demarcation at the jaw area; or if it looks too thick or too greasy, or gives the face an orange, pink, rose, or ashen tint; or if it looks heavy and opaque instead of sheer and light, go back to the testers. In fact, you may need to test several types before you find the right foundation.

One practical guideline to narrow down your choices is to test many different colors at once. Begin with several that look like good possibilities and place stripes of each one in a row over the cheek area. The best choice is the one that blends almost perfectly with your skin color. The wrong choices will stand out, with obvious edges that don't disappear into your skin. This technique is a reliable way to eliminate some choices, but I've also seen it go wrong more times than I can count because it doesn't go far enough. Use it only as an elimination process; it does not replace the need to check out the color on your face in the daylight, nor the need to blend the foundation shade over a larger area of your face.

Keep trying on foundations until you find the best one. **Once you've made a selection you feel good about, apply it all over your face, wait at least two hours, and check it again in the daylight. How a foundation wears during the day—Does it change color or become too greasy or dry as the day passes?—can be evaluated only after you've worn it for a**

while. Once you've assessed all these details, in the daylight, you can safely make a final determination as to whether this is the right color or type of foundation for you. Please take the time to follow this procedure. This advice will guide you in the right direction, and, ultimately, it is the only way to guarantee that you'll find the right foundation. If you rely only on the salesperson and the lighting at the cosmetics counters, it will be pure luck if you end up with the right color. And if you get the foundation wrong, regardless of how perfectly you choose and apply everything else in your makeup wardrobe, those will all look wrong, too.

Where to Shop

Although there are many wonderful foundation options available at the drugstore, the almost universal lack of testers is incredibly frustrating. For budget-conscious consumers looking for a reasonably priced foundation, this can be quite a challenge, as you're often left standing in the aisle (under horrendous lighting and with no mirrors in sight) to guess which shade is best for you. For this reason, I encourage you to begin your foundation search at a department store or cosmetics boutique (like Sephora) where testers are the rule, not the exception. You will end up spending more for foundation, but the convenience of testers, mirrors, take-away samples, and (at times) professional guidance is worth it. Once you become more skilled at knowing which shades work for you and which do not, you can venture back to the drugstore to try again. It can be helpful to bring along the foundation you are currently using—assuming the color is a great match—to compare with the drugstore options. Last, since you will still not be able to see the color on your skin until you purchase it and test it at home, be sure you buy only from drugstores or mass merchandise stores that allow you to return opened cosmetics. Safe bets in this regard are Rite Aid and Walgreens.

Types of Foundation

Now that you know how to go about finding the right foundation color, the next hurdle is figuring out the type of foundation best suited to your skin type. Cosmetics counters carry a mind-boggling assortment of foundations these days, including oil-free and matte foundations, water-based foundations, oil-based foundations (these are few and far between), pressed powder–based foundations, cream-to-powder foundations, liquid-to-powder foundations, stick foundations, so-called self-adjusting foundations, and foundations that have shine. Given this range of options, narrowing down your choices can be tricky.

Note: Many of the following foundation types have effective sunscreen protection with an SPF 15 or greater and UVA-protecting ingredients of avobenzone, titanium dioxide, or zinc oxide. That means you can rely on these for sun protection if they are applied liberally and evenly all over the face. If you prefer to wear a sheer, thin layer of foundation or don't want to wear foundation all over your face, then a moisturizer with sunscreen must be worn underneath. To ensure your foundation with sunscreen is protecting you all day, consider setting your makeup or touching up your makeup during the day with a pressed powder that contains sunscreen.

<u>Oil-free and matte liquid foundations:</u> Most of these contain oils (even though the names don't sound as though they do) or ingredients that act or feel like oils, such as silicones. These oils and oil-like ingredients are not necessarily bad for any skin type, but their presence demonstrates that the term "oil-free" is another cosmetics industry contrivance that won't necessarily help you find the best product for your skin type. Keep in mind that what most of these foundations have in common when they are well-formulated is that they dry to a matte finish, with no shine or dewy appearance whatsoever. On the skin, "oil-free," matte foundations look like a traditional liquid foundation, although they are often thicker in appearance and have no shine.

Examples: Clinique Stay-True Makeup Oil-Free Formula *($16.50),* Almay Wake Up Call! Energizing Makeup SPF 15 *($9.99).*

Application: See the "Blending Foundation" section on page 394.

Pros: These foundations are the best choice for women who want balanced coverage with no shine at all, and who like a smooth, matte look. They last much longer on oily skin or oily areas than most other foundations (except for the ultra-matte foundations), which for some women is a very desirable, if not essential, effect.

Cons: There aren't many disadvantages to using this kind of foundation. Some of them can make the skin look or feel dry and flaky, but this is usually true only for those that contain talc or other absorbent ingredients.

<u>Ultra-matte foundations:</u> These are an amazing group of products that truly stay put. Most have a very liquid consistency and are blended on like any other foundation, though precision blending is key. You have to

be very careful about using a moisturizer under ultra-matte foundations. If you use too much, if it's too greasy, or if you don't allow it to be adequately absorbed, it can make the foundation gunk up or streak.

The major drawback with foundations like these used to be the lightning-quick dry time, as that meant blending had to be absolutely perfect from the start or you would end up with a streaky, uneven application. Today's ultra-matte foundations are less tenacious than earlier ones, but they are also noticeably easier to blend and more forgiving of mistakes. The trade-off for this added convenience is that these do not wear as long as they used to, but most women will appreciate the extra "play" today's ultra-matte formulas have.

Examples: Maybelline EverFresh Makeup *($8.75)*, Estée Lauder Double Wear Stay in Place Makeup SPF 10 *($28.50)*, Revlon ColorStay Stay Natural Makeup SPF 15 *($10.95)*.

Application: See the "Blending Foundation" section on page 394.

Pros: These foundations are a superior option if you have seriously oily skin, have trouble with makeup slipping or disappearing as the day goes by, live in a humid climate, exercise but still like your makeup to stay put, or like a completely matte finish. Ultra-matte foundations will outlast any other foundation, with no slippage or movement. If you have very oily skin, these are an absolute must to try.

Cons: Regrettably there are many disadvantages to using oil-free, matte foundations. Primarily the problem is that most of them go on rather heavy and look masklike, leaving the skin feeling very dry and taut. To get this makeup on evenly, you must blend quickly or it will dry in place before you know it, and then it can be difficult to blend further. This foundation type can also be hard to work over when applying cream eyeshadows and blush. Ultra-matte foundations have less movement than more emollient foundations, which means eyeshadow and blush have a tendency to stick to them; that can make blending and correcting mistakes a bit irksome, but not impossible.

Women of color should be careful when choosing ultra-matte foundation. Even if it is the right color, these foundations can tend to look gray and ashen after being applied to darker skin tones. Skin that shows no shine or reflection in general tends to look dull gray with this kind of foundation, and that effect is even more pronounced for women of color.

Ultra-matte foundations like this are also the most difficult to remove. The number of options for ultra-matte foundations is dwindling, as women have undoubtedly had problems with them. This is unfortunate because these ingenious formulations can work so well for truly oily skins.

Water-based and standard liquid foundations: Water-based does not mean oil-free, even if the label says so; what it does generally mean is that the first ingredient is water and the second or third ingredient is some kind of oil or emollient slip agent. These foundations look like a somewhat thick liquid and pour slowly but easily out of the bottle. They are perfect for women with normal to dry skin, and the number of foundations fitting this description and performance abound.

Examples: Laura Mercier Moisturizing Foundation *($38)*, L'Oréal Visible Lift Line-Minimizing Makeup SPF 12 *($9.99)*.

Application: See the "Blending Foundation" section on page 394.

Pros: Most water-based foundations are best for those with normal to dry skin. They are perfect for these skin types to wear without a moisturizer, or they can be worn with a moisturizer or a moisturizer that contains an SPF. The oil or emollient part of these foundations gives them good movement, which makes blending a pleasure and allows blushes and eyeshadows to blend on effortlessly and evenly over the face. Mistakes are easily buffed away with the sponge.

Cons: If you have oily or combination skin, this is not the foundation type for you. Even the little bit of oil or emollients in a water-based foundation show shine almost immediately if you have oily skin. Those who do not have oily skin but have a paranoia about any shine on the face will not like the effects of a water-based foundation, either; and for those with breakout-prone skin, the small amount of oil or emollients in this cosmetic may make you nervous. For the most part, I personally don't believe there are any disadvantages to using water-based foundations and I recommend them wholeheartedly. Water-based foundation is also a great option for women of color. The slight amount of emollient these contain helps create a nice glow on the skin, preventing darker skin tones from appearing dull or ashen. That same glow is also most attractive for women with dry skin.

If you are concerned about the small amount of shine that water-based foundations leave behind on the skin, try adding a light dusting of loose powder. After you've blended the foundation in place, you can apply the powder all over the face to reduce the shine.

Oil-based foundations: Oil-based foundations list oil as their first ingredient and water usually as their second or third ingredient. Oil-based foundations feel greasy and thick, look greasy and thick, **and go on**

greasy, yet can blend out quite sheerly and softly. You can blend an oil-based foundation to a very thin, subtle layer of makeup.

Examples: Alexandra de Markoff Countess Isserlyn Cream Makeup *($47.50)*, NARS Balanced Foundation *($38)*.

Application: See the "Blending Foundation" section on page 394.

Pros: Oil-based foundations can be very good for women with extremely dry or wrinkled skin. The emollient ingredients help the skin look very dewy and moist, which can minimize the appearance of wrinkles.

Cons: Oil-based foundations tend to be very greasy and thick and can look that way on the skin unless you are very adept at blending. They also have a tendency to turn orange on the skin because the extra oil in them affects the pigments in the foundation. This can be true for women of color, too, and it explains why oil-based foundations can look orange after they are worn for a while. The typical recommendation for applying an oil-based foundation is to add water to your sponge so that it goes on thinner, and more like a water-based foundation. But that can be tricky to gauge and can cause the makeup to streak. Why not just use a water-based foundation in the first place and skip the negatives of the oil-based foundation? That would be my recommendation. Additionally, if you wear face powder over this type of foundation, the oil grabs the talc and the face can appear coated and heavily made up even if you blend it on thinly. The same is true for blushes and eyeshadows—they will go on more heavily because of the increased oil on the skin, and they will also become darker once applied. Traditional cream blushes tend to work best over this type of foundation.

Pressed powder–based foundations: These foundations come in a compact and appear and perform much like any pressed powder, which is what they really are, only with a bit more coverage and ability to stay put. Almost all of them have a superior creamy, silky feel, but when applied to the skin they blend on as easily and lightly as any pressed powder.

Examples: Laura Mercier Foundation Powder *($38)*, Chanel Double Perfection Makeup SPF 8 *($45)*, M.A.C. Studiofix Powder Plus Foundation *($22)*.

Application: You can apply these foundations with either a sponge or a brush all over the face, including the eyelids. This is the easiest way to get a smooth, light, and fast application. You might have to worry about a smooth application if you have dry skin, but these powder-based foundations go on evenly for other skin types, providing extremely sheer to medium coverage. For more specifics about blending techniques, see the section "Blending Foundation" section on page 394.

Pros: Powder-based foundations are great for women with normal to oily or combination skin. They blend on easily and quickly, last all day, generally don't change color, and feel exceptionally light on the skin. They are best for those who want a minimal feel and appearance from their foundation. They also work very well over sunscreens, and can help reduce the shine some sunscreen ingredients (even those in a matte base) leave on the skin.

Cons: Women who have dry skin should not wear powder-based foundation. This is also not a good option if you have flaky skin, regardless of your skin type. The powder content makes this type of foundation too drying for someone with dry skin, and the way it goes on can make the skin look more dry and flaky. Also, women with very oily skin might want to be cautious, because powder-based foundations can get a thickened, pooled appearance as oil resurfaces on the face during the day.

Cream-to-powder foundations: These foundations are an interesting cross between a pressed powder and a creamy liquid foundation. They come in a compact and have a very creamy, almost greasy appearance. When you blend them on, the creamy part disappears and you are left with a slightly matte, powdery finish. Cream-to-powder foundations provide much better coverage than pressed powder–based foundations.

Example: Clinique City Base Compact Foundation SPF 15 *($21)*.

Application: Cream-to-powder foundations are best applied with a sponge. Some women have success using a brush, but I think this is a difficult, messy technique. See the "Blending Foundation" section on page 394.

Pros: Cream-to-powder foundations blend on quickly and easily and provide a semi-matte, soft, medium coverage. They work great for someone with normal to slightly dry or slightly combination skin. The consistency doesn't require powdering after you apply it. If you wish to use powder, make sure you apply it as lightly as possible to avoid a caked, heavy look.

Cons: Cream-to-powder foundations can blend on slightly thickly, providing a made-up look rather than a sheer, natural appearance. They don't work well for someone with oily skin because the cream components can be too creamy, making skin look more oily, and they don't work well for dry skin because the powder part can be too powdery looking and cause more dryness. Essentially, they are best for normal skin types.

Liquid-to-powder foundations: These liquidy powders with a gel-like wet feel apply easily and dry to a satiny-smooth, sheer, slightly matte finish. They typically contain water as the first ingredient, along with a slip agent such as glycerin. In contrast to cream-to-powder foundations, liquid-to-powder foundations feel significantly lighter on the skin. They also tend to last longer over combination or oily skins because the creamy, waxy ingredients are either decreased or altogether absent.

Examples: Vincent Longo Water Canvas *($45)*, Aveda Cooling Calming Cover Sheer Face Tint *($18)*, Cover Girl Aqua Smooth Makeup SPF 15 *($8.50)*.

Application: Liquid-to-powder foundations are best applied with a sponge. Some women have success using a brush, but I think this is a difficult, messy technique. See the "Blending Foundation" section on page 394.

Pros: Liquid-to-powder foundations blend on quickly and relatively easily and provide a semi-matte to matte finish with sheer to medium coverage. They work great for someone with normal to oily or slightly combination skin. The consistency means that it doesn't require powdering after you apply it. If you wish to use powder, make sure you apply it as lightly as possible to avoid a caked, heavy look.

Cons: Liquid-to-powder foundations dry quickly and can, therefore, blend on choppy, making application tricky. This type of foundation does not work very well over dry skin because the water portion tends to cling to dry areas, leaving a powder finish that is not easily moved. If you have dry skin and want to try this type of foundation, use an emollient moisturizer or sunscreen beforehand. The product itself must be kept tightly closed between uses because the water component will evaporate if left exposed to air for long periods. Some of the compact liquid-to-powder makeups can chip or break apart if you are not careful while swiping your sponge over the makeup.

Stick foundations: These foundations are essentially cream-to-powder foundations in stick form, and the application, pros, and cons mentioned in that section are the same. The main difference between stick and cream-to-powder foundations is the variety of coverage available from sticks. Whereas cream-to-powder makeups typically provide medium coverage, stick foundations come in formulas that range from full to sheer coverage with either matte or creamy texture. Many stick foundations also feature effective sunscreens, making them a great all-in-one option. In addition, they can do double duty as a concealer, and most product lines offer a wide selection of shades.

Examples: Elizabeth Arden Flawless Finish Stick Makeup SPF 15 *($18)*, and Trish McEvoy Foundation Stick *($38)*.

Application: These can be swiped onto the skin right from the stick and then blended with a sponge, fingers, or—if you're up for the challenge—a foundation brush.

Pros and Cons: Refer to the section for cream-to-powder foundations on page 391.

<u>Foundations with shine:</u> A definite trend in the world of makeup is having your entire face shine, either with a makeup primer that shines, a foundation that has shine, or a powder that shines. Shimmering shine (as opposed to naturally produced shine) seems to be "in" and I have to admit that it does look great in pictures. In real life (and especially in daylight) it tends to look sparkly or extremely artificial, and if you have normal to oily skin, it looks like the very oil you were trying to do away with. Try this one and check it out in daylight before you splurge. It works better as an evening look than for a classic daytime look.

Examples: Revlon Skinlights Diffusing Tint SPF 15 *($11.99)*, M.A.C. Hyper Real Foundation *($24)*.

Application: The method of application varies, depending on if it comes in a stick or has a cream-to-powder, liquid, cream, or powder base (refer to those sections starting on page 387 for more information on performance and texture). Generally, a sponge can be used for all of these. A brush can be used if the intent is to highlight specific areas.

Pros: For dull, lifeless skin, the best of the foundations with shine can indeed add a subtle glow to the face, but the more product applied, the more the glow turns into obvious, sparkly shine or looks somewhat greasy.

Cons: In a word, shine. There's a lot of variation when it comes to how much visible shine you'll get from these products, so pick and choose based on whether you want a subtle glow or high-wattage shimmer.

Self-adjusting foundations: These foundations supposedly can absorb oil, stop oil production, and also prevent moisture loss. I've yet to see one perform as promised, though it would be great if someone came up with one that could!

Custom-blended foundations: If a foundation is blended for you and you only, will that get you the best shade? This style of selling makeup is very enticing. The customer-service interaction is impressive. Your foundation is supposedly mixed and matched for your exact skin color and needs. The premise is that there are only so many ready-made shades and you might be better off having one custom-blended. Unfortunately, the idea sounds better than the reality. The major problem with custom-blended cosmetics is that the success of the match depends on the expertise of the salesperson—and there are huge variations in skill.

As nice as custom-blended foundations sound, the formulations are not necessarily superior to (or sometimes even as good as) standard products. The foundation may be too greasy or too dry and it might turn to rose or peach as you wear it. With so many off-the-shelf foundation products available, in many excellent colors, custom blending turns out to be more an expensive gimmick than anything else.

When should you try a custom-blended product, particularly foundation? When you have tested many standard foundations and are still frustrated with the color of your foundation.

Blending Foundation

When it comes to blending foundation over your face, keep one mantra in your head: Blend, blend, and blend again, and then, just to be sure, blend one more time. All the other details are, well, just details, and not anywhere near as important as buffing off the excess foundation and smoothing out the edges to be sure you have the thinnest possible layer of foundation over the skin (see photograph on page 441).

Exception to the rule: If you are using a foundation that contains an effective sunscreen, a thin or sheer application will not provide adequate protection from the sun. To ensure you will be getting the stated SPF, it is essential to apply the foundation liberally and in an even layer all over the face. If you prefer a sheer or spot application, then you will need to wear a separate sunscreen underneath your foundation or consider a tinted moisturizer with sunscreen or a pressed powder that contains sunscreen.

Keep in mind that the goal of wearing foundation is to create the illusion of smoother-looking skin, not a noticeable mask of color. Of course, the best place to check your blending technique is in broad daylight. Unfortunately, most of us apply foundation in bathroom light, with only minimal exposure to sunlight. Once you get into daylight, even on a cloudy day, the areas you missed, particularly next to the ears, mouth, jawline, sides of the nose, and temples, often look streaked, show a line of demarcation (even when the color matches perfectly), or appear blotchy or smudged. This is not the effect you are trying to achieve! Smoother-looking skin takes diligence and daylight, or the very best lighting you can create in your home, where you apply your makeup. But whenever possible always check your foundation in daylight before showing your made-up face to the world!

I never recommend blending foundation with fingers. Instead, use a sponge. **Painting a wall with your fingers would leave streaks and lines, and the same is true for applying foundation to your skin. Using the flat, smooth surface of a sponge is the best way to get a smooth application.** The best tool is a flat, square or round, one-quarter-inch-thick sponge that doesn't have holes and is not made of synthetic foam rubber. Together, the shape and density of this kind of sponge provide the smoothest application possible. I know that many makeup artists, from Kevyn Aucoin to Bobbi Brown, advocate finger application of foundation. The rationale is that the warmth of your fingers will help the foundation mesh with the skin and provide a more natural look. If you feel more comfortable finger-painting than using a sponge, go for it. But humor me and make sure you always smooth out the edges of your finger-applied foundation with a sponge. I think you will find the results will be well worth the effort.

Be good about cleaning or changing your sponges frequently, particularly if you tend to break out or have rosacea, psoriasis, seborrhea, or eczema. While sponges are great blending tools, they love holding on to bacteria, fungi, and yeast that can aggravate those conditions.

The sponges frequently found for sale or in use at most cosmetics counters are the thick, wedge-shaped, foam-rubber ones. These sponges are compact, but they drag over the skin, and that makes blending difficult. Also, because they're so thick, most of the foundation is absorbed into the sponge, where you can't get to it, which can waste a lot of product. Wedge sponges are used for traditional theatrical makeup. They are great for applying grease stick or pancake foundations, which require more "pull" across the face to apply them evenly, but that is the last thing you need when you're wearing a lightweight foundation. Shiseido,

Sephora Collection, and Paula's Select make some excellent makeup sponges—and these can be washed repeatedly without falling apart.

To achieve an even application with your nice, thin, flat, square or round sponge, shake some of the foundation from the bottle onto the sponge, then transfer the foundation to the face and over the eyes by dabbing the sponge over the skin. You can also use your fingers to transfer the foundation in dots from the bottle to the face and then use the sponge to blend the dots. Start by placing the foundation generously over the central area of the face, including the eyes but avoiding the sides of the face near the hairline, jaw, and chin. The foundation can go on in large patches or small dots all over the nose, eyelids, cheeks, and forehead, but only in this central area. Avoid placing the foundation all over the face unless you want a full makeup application or are using a foundation that contains sunscreen as your only source of sun protection. By concentrating the foundation over the central part of the face, as you blend down and out from the center there will be less foundation at the jaw and hairline. When applying a foundation with sunscreen, apply an even layer all over the face, and use the clean side of your sponge to softly feather the edges of the makeup at the jaw and hairline. The objective is to soften, but not wipe off, the foundation.

Once the foundation is on your face, begin using your sponge to blend the foundation evenly. **Holding the sponge between your fingers and thumb, spread the foundation down and out over the entire face with a stroking, buffing motion, going in the direction of the hair growth.** (Going against the direction of the hair growth on your face coats the hair with too much foundation.) The idea is to blend the foundation color out from the center of the face, where you initially placed it, to the perimeter of the face, leaving no line of demarcation at the jaw or hairline. Use the edge of the sponge *without* foundation (or turn the sponge over to the clean side) to dab or buff away any of the excess that tends to collect under the eye or around the nose. You can also use the sponge to wipe away any of the excess that gathers at the jaw or hairline. When blending the foundation, do not try to force it into the skin. There is a fine line between blending something on and wiping something off. Instead, blend a thin layer over the face, smoothing it with your sponge as you go. Using this technique, you can build coverage as desired. At this point your sponge should not be full of foundation; if it is, you've used too much.

If you did not apply a concealer before the foundation, you can apply it now and blend that into place. Apply the concealer, which is a shade or two lighter than the foundation, over the under-eye area and other areas you want to highlight, then dab it into place with your finger or sponge.

Watch out for the jaw and neck. This is very important. **Never, ever put makeup of any kind on the neck; you do not want your makeup to end up on your collar.** Always double-check your blending. Places on the face that you are likely to miss with foundation include the corners of the nose, the tip of the nose, the corners of the eyes (especially over the concealer), and the edge along the lower eyelashes. Also, some places are likely to end up wearing foundation that shouldn't, including the ears, the jawline, and the hairline—especially blonde hairlines. Be careful to remove this foundation if you've gone past your mark. Both situations can make your makeup appear sloppy.

Your sponge is an exceptional blending tool that you should keep near you at all times. When the edges of your blush or eyeshadow need softening, you can blend out the hard edges with the side of the sponge that was used to spread the foundation over the face. Using the side of the sponge that has foundation on it as opposed to the dry edge allows the sponge to glide over the blush or eyeshadow without streaking or rubbing it off.

Applying a Mini-Application of Foundation

If you dislike the feel of foundation or if you want to wear the least amount of foundation possible, yet you still want the benefits that wearing a foundation provides (mainly helping blush and eyeshadows go on more evenly) there is an alternative. The thing most women don't like about foundation is how it feels when it's applied all over the face. One way to solve that problem is to not apply foundation all over, basically because it isn't necessary. (Of course, if your foundation contains your sunscreen, that does require applying it evenly all over the face.) The key points to remember, aside from the question of sunscreen protection, are that foundation is needed primarily to give the blush and eyeshadows something to adhere to, and to even out skin tone. This means that if your foundation color matches the face exactly—and after you finish this section, it will—you can apply a mini-application of foundation just over the areas where you will place the blush and eyeshadows. This way you won't feel heavily made up and the blush and eyeshadows will still go on evenly.

For a mini-application, place the foundation only over a mask-shaped area between the eyes and mouth, including the nose and cheeks. Coverage is not needed on the chin, forehead, or jaw area. Be sure to blend the edges carefully with your sponge. Apply the concealer the same way you would for a full makeup application. You may also want to consider a tinted moisturizer if you want a touch of color and minimal coverage. Lancôme, Aveda, Neutrogena, and Bobbi Brown all have excellent options for tinted moisturizers.

Blending Over Those Fine Little Wrinkles

If you've started to notice that foundation or concealer is sinking into some of those little wrinkles on your face, especially the laugh lines, lines under the eyes, or near the crow's feet (I have no regard for the person who came up with the term "crow's feet" to describe the lines extending from the back corner of the eyes!), you have to be even more meticulous about how you blend your foundation into place. In this regard, less is best. Blend, blend, and blend again, being sure to remove the excess in those areas with the clean side of the sponge. Continue blending intermittently while you apply your lipstick, blush, and/or eyeshadow to ensure that you have removed the excess.

Minimize your use of moisturizers over the areas where you have lines, and use a foundation or concealer that's neither greasy nor too emollient. Anything with movement and slip gives the foundation a free ride into the lines.

As for those concealers and foundations that claim to deflect, reflect, or somehow improve the appearance of wrinkles: They don't. And the foundation primers sold by some cosmetics lines, which are usually just moisturizers with extra film-forming agents (hairstyling-type ingredients), don't work all that well, either, plus they just add another layer of product to the face, which increases the likelihood of clogging pores, exacerbating breakouts, or creating dull-looking skin. **The truth is, a face without foundation always looks less wrinkled. I'm not sure why this has to be so, but it is. You can test this for yourself.** Go to the cosmetics counter, find the most expensive foundation with the most elaborate claims about making the skin look less wrinkled, apply a sample to one side of your face, and leave the other side naked with just a dab of moisturizer over dry areas. Then check out your face in the daylight. You will be amazed how much more noticeable the lines on the foundation side of the face are. Of course, the foundation side will look smoother and will have a more even tone, the redness and blotchiness will be gone, and the pores will have virtually disappeared. But the wrinkles will be more noticeable than on the side without foundation. That's the agony and ecstasy of foundation!

Foundation Mistakes to Avoid

1. Do not buy a foundation before trying it on and checking it in the daylight.
2. Do not wear foundation unless it matches your skin color.
3. Do not wear a foundation that is lighter than your skin, or you will end up looking chalky or pale.
4. Do not wear pink, peach, rose, orange, or ash-colored foundation.
5. Do not wear oil-based foundations unless you have very, very dry skin. Oil-based foundations can look greasy and appear more orange and pink than other types of foundation.
6. Do not wear oil-free or ultra-matte foundations unless you have very oily skin. Oil-free and ultra-matte foundations can look quite thick and matte and make lines on the face more evident.
7. Cream-to-powder foundations work best for normal skin. The cream part can be too greasy for oily skin and the powder can be too dry for dry skin.
8. Use foundations that have shine for a special evening look.
9. Do not apply a thick layer of foundation; thin and sheer are the operative words when it comes to applying foundation unless you are wearing a foundation with sunscreen, in which case liberal, even application is essential.
10. Do not use your fingers to blend your foundation over the face unless you're willing to go over your handiwork with a sponge.

BRUSHES

Before we go on to powders, eyeshadows, and blushes, it is crucial to discuss the most important blending tools you can use (besides the sponge for blending on foundation)—brushes. Brushes are simply the best way to apply almost all types of makeup, and you'd be hard put to find a makeup artist anywhere who disagrees. Moreover, after years of struggling with those tiny, prepackaged sponge eyeshadow applicators and doll-sized blush brushes, we now have a profusion of brushes to choose from. Whether they're from M.A.C., Prescriptives, Bobbi Brown, Trish McEvoy, Stila, Maybelline, Aveda, Lorac, BeneFit, Paula's Select, or other lines, good brushes are available in an impressive array of sizes, shapes, and sensual textures that facilitate makeup application in ways that feel artistic and effortless. As with anything related to cosmetics, though, a high price does not always mean superior performance. And having more brushes does not mean you will be able to apply your makeup better.

The personal set of brushes you choose is determined strictly by how you prefer to apply your makeup. If your makeup application is elaborate and nuanced, involving several eyeshadows, contour, and highlighting, you need a variety of brushes. If your makeup application is uncomplicated and basic, you need fewer brushes. It's that simple. (The reason makeup artists carry an arsenal of brushes is because they see a vast assortment of eye and face sizes.) All you need is a group of brushes that match the areas of your face and the kinds and colors of makeup you apply. A good, basic collection of the brushes I recommend is shown in the photographs on pages 404–405.

As a general guideline, it is best not to purchase a prepackaged set of brushes unless you know you will use all of them and the particular shapes and sizes will meet your needs.

The general rule to follow when considering what size brush to purchase is: **Does the size of the brush match the size of the area you are working on?** Too small and it will take longer to apply your makeup and it can end up looking striped. Too large and you can end up with a messy application. If you are lining the eye, a tiny thin brush with few hairs and that doesn't scratch or feel stiff is best. If you are filling in the brow, a small angle brush with a slight amount of stiffness to control the color is best. (It should be small and stiff enough to fit through the spaces in the hair and follow the edge of the brow with pencil-like control.) For the eyelid, choose a brush size that fits the curve of your lid, and the same reasoning applies for the crease area. Both should be determined by the size of your eye, and there are countless eyeshadow brush sizes to choose from. To highlight along the brow, a soft, small wedge brush (less stiff than the brow brush), fitting just that area, is best. Try not to use the same brush for both lighter and darker shades of eyeshadow.

How many and which brushes do you need? A full makeup application can require three basic eyeshadow brushes, an eyeliner brush (for liner and brows), a blush brush, contour brush, large powder brush, a lash brush (an old clean mascara wand will do), a brow brush (here a toothbrush will do nicely), and a lip brush.

Here is a good basic group to consider. I recommend **two or three eyeshadow brushes**, including one for the lighter eyeshadow colors and one for the crease. If you want to save time and money, you can use the edge (side) of the eyeshadow brush you use for the lid to place a light color under the brow. If you want the perfect tool, a small, soft **wedge brush** for that area is best. If you are shading the back (outside) corner of the eye with a dark eyeshadow, you may want to select a **smaller eyeshadow brush** than the one you use for the lid or crease. Again, the shape of your eye determines the size of the brush you choose.

If you don't use a pencil, a **tiny, thin eyeliner brush** is best for building either a thick or thin line along the upper and lower lashes. While some makeup artists use thicker brushes that are more square or wedge-shaped for this purpose, I think they are harder to control (they can make a thick line, but it's hard to get them to create a thin line, while a tiny thin brush can do either). If you're unsure, experiment with both styles and see which you prefer. A **wedge-shaped brow brush** can be used just for the brow to apply eyeshadow powder or to smooth out the line of an eyebrow pencil. Personally, I use a tiny eyeliner brush to fill in the brows to keep the shading soft by creating hair-thin strokes. An old **toothbrush** is still the best tool for combing through the brows. For combing through the lashes, I strongly recommend a good, densely packed **used mascara wand** that you wash clean, like the ones in L'Oréal Voluminous, Maybelline Illegal Lengths, and Lancôme Definicils mascaras. Most lash brushes that are sold separately have bristles that are too far apart to be helpful for easy unclumping and separating. Avoid metal eyelash combs—these can be incredibly painful and damaging if you accidentally poke yourself in the eye.

Both the **blush brush** and **powder brush** should have a soft, firm texture and not splay out when placed on the skin or into the color (no brush should be so loose as to splay when used either on the face or in the product). They should also feel soft and silky, yet hold their shape. If a brush is too wobbly, it will be hard to control the color. I often recommend getting two good blush brushes in the same size and using one for powder and one for blush (you don't want to dust color over the face). Many powder brushes, though they may feel incredibly soft and luxurious, are too large, cumbersome, and hard to control. It's nearly impossible to maneuver some of these behemoth brushes under the eye, along the corner of the nose, or along the cheek without hitting other areas of the face that may not need powder, and using too much powder is extremely likely.

If you are looking for a **contour brush** to shade along the temple, jaw, or cheekbone, a smaller blush brush is a great choice. Brushes specially designed for this area come in a variety of sizes, but the flat edge of these specially designed brushes, though impressive in appearance, can create just that, a hard edge, which takes more blending to soften than necessary. Simply use a small, half-inch-wide version of your blush brush; the idea is that this contour/blush brush should fit the hollow of the cheekbone.

I'm not among those who diligently apply lipstick with a **lipstick brush**. I just don't have the time. Generally, I save this precision for special occasions or when I want to use up every last drop in the tube. But if you like this option, look for a brush with bristles that are strong and slightly stiff. Tug hard on the brush and make sure it doesn't move in the least. Look for a brush the size of your lips. Too small and it can take forever; too big and you'll be applying lipstick to your face. You know those retractable metal brushes you see almost everywhere and in every price range? They are all the same, and they are excellent! Retracting the bristles neatly back into place beats trying to keep the little plastic protective sheath on a wood-handled brush. (They never stay on and lipstick ends up getting all over your purse and makeup bag!)

You may notice that some brush collections sport a white, thin, slightly stiff brush sold as a **concealer or highlighter brush**. If you use a lighter shade of concealer for smile lines, under the eyes, on the corners of the nose, in the center of the chin, a dab in the middle of your lips over lipstick, or to spot-cover a blemish, this brush is a consideration. Many makeup artists use this type of brush to do things that most people (including me) do with their finger or their foundation sponge. Supposedly it allows better blending with less drag. It definitely helps you use less product, and also lets you more easily reach tight spaces, such as along the lower lash line, the corner of the nose, and the edge of your lips. One thing it does not help in the least is keeping the concealer or highlighter from creasing into lines, despite what the salesperson will probably tell you.

I am not an advocate of foundation brushes, despite the fact that many lines now offer these as part of their brush collections. Quite simply, using foundation brushes takes longer than using a sponge (or fingers if you're so inclined) and they require more maintenance between uses. Depending on the type of foundation being used, these brushes can create a striped or streaked appearance. If you are tempted to try them, experiment with them before making a purchase so you can be sure you like the final result with whatever foundation you use.

Brush Quality and Care

As you check out the different lines of brushes, the first thing you will hear about is the so-called quality of the bristles, and the salespeople will use this to justify the cost. Depending on the line, you will hear pretentious claims about squirrel, sable, pony, goat, and several other animals that did not give up their coats voluntarily. Synthetic brush hair is an option for those who are 100% vegetarian. However, synthetic brush hair is not preferred for most makeup application other than foundations and concealers. The most reliable synthetic brushes are from Origins, Paula Dorf, and Shu Uemura.

Although natural bristles are definitely softer (and often more expensive) than synthetic, it does not take sable to make the perfect brush, and mixed-hair bristles can make for a stronger, more pliable brush that doesn't lose its shape. Natural hairs tend to get softer over time, which means a firm, well-controlled brush can eventually become floppy and too soft. Salespeople who encourage you to buy the expensive brushes will claim that synthetic hairs get coarser and stiffer, or fall out after a year or two of usage, but that is not true. Synthetic hair brushes hold up as well if not better than natural hair brushes.

Ignore the claims about hair quality and trust your own touch and feel tests. Brush the bristles along the nape of your neck and ask yourself, "Is it smooth? Do the bristles hold their shape? Does it feel too loose, too stiff, or too soft? Does the brush feel densely packed, meaning lots of hairs, or flimsy?" Once you decide which feel you prefer, you can determine which brushes you want to work with.

Now that you have a sense of the feel part of the test, use the touch test to ascertain how the brush will hold up. Simply tug at the bristles, pulling away from the handle end, to see if there is any give. Do any hairs fall out? If you feel any release whatsoever, this is not a well-constructed brush. Some brushes are not well-anchored and bound into the base of the brush. For example, Maybelline's incredibly inexpensive brushes beautifully pass the feel test (they are wonderfully soft and firm), but fail

(continued on page 406)

NOW THIS IS A GREAT BRUSH COLLECTION

1 POWDER BRUSH: Don't get one that's too big or you will end up spreading too much powder over your face or powdering areas you don't want powdered.

2 BLUSH BRUSHES: One for blush and one for contouring.

2 EYESHADOW BRUSHES: One small rounded brush for the crease and back corner of the eye and one large rounded brush for the lid and under-brow area.

1 ANGLE BRUSH: For shaping eyebrows.

1 EYELINER BRUSH: For lining eyes or for shaping eyebrows.

1 TOOTHBRUSH: For combing through eyebrows and eyelashes.

1 CLEAN MASCARA WAND: For combing through eyebrows and eyelashes.

1 RETRACTABLE LIP BRUSH, OR LIP BRUSH WITH CAP

AVOID SHARPLY ANGLED CONTOUR BRUSHES—They can leave streaks.

the touch test (the bristles tend to pull out). In the short term they are a superior bargain, but they won't hold up over the long haul.

Some cosmetics lines still sell the bamboo-handled brushes with white bristles. These are often the sparsest of brushes and are not constructed very well. They are a great example of the type of quality to avoid. Yes, they are attractive, but they are a waste of money. Along a related line, the more elaborately adorned a brush is, the more likely it is to fall apart. Look for simple, solid, streamlined construction.

When it comes to the **shape of the brush**, generally it is best to avoid blunt brushes and brushes with the bristles lined up flat with a severe edge. For most brushes—eyeliner, lip, eyeshadow, blush, and powder—look for ends that are more dome-shaped. Not only do these have a softer feel, but they also allow for a softer, less hard-edged application, which is almost always the goal. The only exception is the wedge brush for the brows or under the eyebrow.

When I'm doing my own makeup for media appearances or doing someone else's makeup, I personally favor brushes with long, elegantly tapered wood handles. But when I try to squeeze these long-stemmed beauties into the small makeup bag I travel with or keep in my briefcase, I realize how cumbersome they can be. For women who want to invest in only one set of brushes, short handles are not only more convenient, they are essential.

When it comes to **caring for your brushes**, some people claim you must wash them frequently. If you are a makeup artist working on lots of people, you should be washing your brushes every day. But for those of us who are working on ourselves only and not changing colors on a daily basis, once a month is just fine (and I won't tell anyone if you don't do it that often). Especially for natural-hair brushes, frequent washing breaks down the hair shaft and that breaks down the brush hairs. Also, washing too often can loosen the glue in the handle that holds the bristles together and keeps them in place. When you clean the brushes, concentrate your effort on the bristles, not the handle.

It is best to use a regular shampoo instead of a special brush-cleaning solution (which is just shampoo anyway). The shampoo shouldn't contain any conditioning agents, which can build up on the brush just like they do on the hair. L'Oréal Colorvive Gentle Shampoo and Paula's Choice All Over Hair and Body Shampoo are great inexpensive options. A conditioner is not necessary when caring for your brushes. Brush hair is extremely healthy. It isn't damaged from dyeing, perming, styling, brushing, and the other things people do to their own hair, which requires the use of conditioners. When washing your brushes, carefully follow these steps.

- Gently but thoroughly wash the brush in tepid water.
- Meticulously rinse the brush.
- Carefully press out the excess water and dab the brush dry.
- Arrange the bristles back into their original shape.
- Let the brush air dry flat on a towel without the help of a blow dryer, which can damage bristles.

Brush Techniques

Brushes can become foolproof tools for applying makeup, yet it is definitely possible to use brushes incorrectly. I've seen enough women use their brushes in a rubbing or wiping motion on the face to know how often it can happen. Many women beat at their faces with a wild brushing motion as they attempt to apply their blush and eyeshadows. There truly is an easier and more effective method. When you wipe, beat, or heavily rub the brush against the face, it may be removing what you just put on, not to mention wiping off the foundation underneath, which can result in a streaky uneven appearance. The best technique is to brush in short, light, purposeful motions that glide over the skin.

If there is a distinct line where the brushstroke was placed or if you feel an urge to use your finger to blend what you've just applied, most likely you are not using the brush properly or your brush is too stiff for a soft application. (You may also have applied your foundation too thickly or used a foundation that is too greasy, or the blush color you've chosen is too strongly pigmented for your skin color.) You should avoid blending anything with your fingers—use your brush or the flat, square, thin sponge you use to apply your foundation. Remember, use your sponge for applying foundation and softening edges of your blush, contour, and eyeshadows.

Something else that is critical to using brushes effectively—even though it may seem insignificant at first—is the way you pick up the powder on your brush before you apply it. **Never smash or rub your brush into the powder. Rather, gently place your brush into the powder without moving the bristles.** You don't want to see the brush hair bend or splay. Always stroke through the powder evenly and always knock the excess powder off the brush before you apply it to the face. This prevents applying too much color to the first place your brush touches. When it comes to makeup, it is always easier to add than subtract!

Brush Mistakes to Avoid

1. Do not use hard or stiff brushes.
2. Do not use a brush that is too big or too small for the area of the face you are working on.
3. Do not use brushes that are too soft or ones with bristles that are too sparse; they won't hold up over time.
4. Do not forget to knock the excess powder off the brush before you apply the color to your face.
5. Do not wipe or rub the brush across the face; instead, gently brush on the color with short, even strokes.
6. Do not forget to use your sponge to blend out hard edges and soften your color application.
7. Do not forget to gently wash your brushes every month or so, unless you are using them on a variety of people, in which case you should be washing or disinfecting them every day.

POWDER

Classic makeup application requires powdering after you've applied your foundation, but powdering doesn't work for all types of foundation. Powdering works best after applying a water-based, oil-based, or matte foundation that isn't all that matte. It is either unnecessary or problematic to apply powder over most oil-free or matte foundations, all of the ultra-matte foundations, or any of the pressed powder, cream-to-powder, or liquid-to-powder foundations. Some stick foundations that dry to a powder finish do not need extra powder, but those that remain creamy do.

If you are using a water-based or oil-based foundation, you may indeed want to apply powder to absorb any excess moisturizer or emollients that may make the face look too moist or too dewy. However, the less powder you build up on your face, the less made-up you will appear. Overpowdering also makes the face look dull and dry, especially if you have dry skin or darker skin tones. Some amount of natural, dewy shine to the face is very attractive. **I think it is a 1950s' notion that the face should not shine at all and that a woman must constantly wipe powder over her face to reduce the shine (and then apply shiny eyeshadows, blush, lipstick, or powder so the skin shines, but artificially).** After a foundation is applied, the slight shine that is left behind (except with oil-free, matte, ultra-matte, and pressed-powder foundations) gives the face a radiant glow. Powder is great for touch-ups as the day goes by to dust down excessive shine (see the photograph on page 441), just avoid over-powdering.

Types of Powder

Loose powder and pressed powder: Loose powder is exactly what the name suggests. It tends to provide a more sheer, light application and can be best for someone with normal to oily skin. Pressed powder is merely loose powder with added waxes or emollients to keep the powder in a solid form. While pressed powder is heavier than loose powder, it is more convenient and a lot less messy. Both loose and pressed powders are perfectly fine options and it is a matter of personal preference which you use. What is essential, though, is to choose a powder that is the same color as your foundation. If your powder is lighter than your foundation, you can end up looking pasty and pale; if your powder is darker, you will look like you're wearing a mask.

Pressed powder with sunscreen: A few cosmetics lines, including Paula's Select, Jane Iredale, and Neutrogena, offer pressed powders that contain effective sunscreens. These powders are nearly identical to regular pressed powders except that they have a slightly thicker texture and provide more substantial coverage, along with an SPF 15 or greater including UVA-protecting ingredients avobenzone, titanium dioxide, or zinc oxide. Because sunscreens must be applied liberally to ensure sun protection, I generally do not recommend relying on pressed powders with sunscreen as your sole source of UV protection. Most women simply would not use enough of the powder to get the designated SPF number, and overpowdering is not an attractive option. Therefore, pressed powders with effective sunscreens are an excellent way to add to the UV protection you get from your sunscreen or foundation with sunscreen, particularly for those with oily skin. For longer days in the sun or times when it is not feasible to redo your makeup to maintain sun protection, pressed powders with sunscreen can be very convenient and extremely practical.

Talc is the basic element in almost all loose and pressed powders, but some companies opt to use mica (which lends a shiny finish), cornstarch, or rice starch (both starches have a light but very dry feel). Keep in mind that using powders made from corn or rice is not the best option if you're prone to breakouts. The bacteria that cause acne thrive on food ingredients like this, so why would you give something you don't want (blemish-causing bacteria) what it needs to grow?

Application: Apply the powder with a large (but not too large), full, round brush. Avoid using a sponge or powder puff, which can put too much powder onto the face. Pick up some of the powder on the full end of the brush, knock off the excess, and brush it on using the same motion and direction as you did for the foundation. Apply everything in the same direction to help retain a smooth appearance.

If you are touching up your makeup later in the day, before powdering, use your sponge, a facial tissue, or special oil-absorbing paper to dab away excess oil from the face. Then apply the powder.

Some makeup artists use a powder puff to press the powder into the skin for a very flat, matte finish. As professional a touch as this may be, it is best only for photographs. A powder puff places too much powder on the skin and can look thick and heavy in real life. Powdering with a makeup sponge has the same effect as using a powder puff, although the pores of the sponge do allow for a slightly less matte look. However, this can still lay too much powder on the skin.

Pros: If you want to reduce shine or moisture on the face, powdering is the fastest, easiest way to get the job done. Sans foundation, powder can lend a polished, sophisticated look to the skin.

Cons: There are really no drawbacks to wearing powder, except overdoing it, using the wrong color, or building up too much powder on the skin. There are also some powders that have sparkles or shine added to them. I have even seen some matte or oil-free powders that contain shine. If powdering is meant to reduce the shine produced from your oil glands or from your foundation or moisturizer, it is a huge mistake to do that with a shiny powder. Clearly, that would defeat the entire purpose. If you do want to use powder to add shine, see the next entry on powder that shines. Other than that, powdering is a basic step for almost all skin types to help keep makeup looking fresh during the day.

Powder that shines: If you want to use something to make the skin look luminescent and shiny, one of the best ways to do that is with powder that has shine. Apply this after your foundation and regular powder, and only dust it over the areas you want to glow, such as the cheeks, chin, center of the forehead, shoulders, neck, and décolletage. Most makeup lines offer at least one shiny powder, and some lines offer several. If you want to try a shiny powder, be sure to check the finish in daylight so you can really see how shiny it is and decide if this is the look you had in mind.

Talc in Face Powders: Friend or Foe?

Talc is often maligned as an awful cosmetic ingredient that should be avoided, but I do not agree in the least with that assessment when it comes to makeup products. The concern about talc is not about how it is used in makeup, but, rather, when it is used in pure, large concentrations in the form of talcum powder. Part of the story here dates back to several studies published in the 1990s that found a significant increase in the risk of ovarian cancer from vaginal (perineal) application of talcum powder (sources: *American Journal of Epidemiology*, March 1997, pages 459–465; *International Journal of Cancer*, May 1999, pages 351–356; *Seminars in Oncology*, June 1998, pages 255–264; *Cancer*, June 1997, pages 2396–2401.)

However, subsequent and concurring studies have cast doubt on the way these studies were conducted or the conclusions they reached (sources: *Journal of the National Cancer Institute*, February 2000, pages 249–252; *American Journal of Obstetrics and Gynecology*, March 2000, pages 720–724; *Obstetrics and Gynecology*, March 1999, pages 372–376).

While more research in this area is being carried out to clear up the confusion, none of the research about the use of talc is related to the way women use makeup. There is no indication anywhere that there is any risk for the face when using products that contain talc. That means you need not avoid using eyeshadows, blushes, or face powders that contain talc. But it absolutely means you should consider never using talcum powder on your children or on yourself vaginally. If you still wish to avoid talc in makeup, it is easy enough to do so simply by checking the ingredient list.

Powdering Mistakes to Avoid

1. **Never buy powder without testing it over your foundation first. Even if the powder is translucent, it always has some amount of color to it, and that color and its extra texture over the skin can greatly affect the appearance of your foundation. Powder should match the color of your skin (and foundation) and not change the color of either. Never powder with a color that is lighter or darker than your foundation.**
2. **Never powder with a white, orange, pink, or coral shade of powder;**

it will make you look either pale or overly made-up.

3. To help prevent a caked appearance don't forget to dab off excess oil from the face before you apply your powder during the day to touch up your makeup.

4. Do not apply more than the sheerest layer necessary to take away excess shine; the face can handle only so much powder before it starts looking thick and heavy.

5. Do not powder more than necessary during the day. Powder only once or twice a day to prevent buildup, even if you are using a pressed powder with sunscreen.

EYESHADOW

I've been watching and evaluating other makeup artists and their eyeshadow techniques for years. Though there are myriad alternatives, eyeshadow design is usually built on an application sequence that allows you to create a flow of colors in either one, two, three, or four steps. The four steps involve applying a succession of colors that can be anything you want them to be, but if the goal is a classic makeup application, the colors proceed gradually from light to darker. The basic technique is to apply the lightest shade either just on the eyelid or all over the entire eye area (including the crease and up under the eyebrow) and then to place each progressively darker shade in a more specific section of the eye area, such as the crease and/or the back corner of the eye (see the photographs on page 442).

Types of Eyeshadow

Aside from powder eyeshadows, other types available include liquids, pencils, cream-to-powder, and creams. Though these can be fun and easy to use, they are hard to blend and control. Makeup artists rarely, if ever, use the liquids or pencils, but some opt for creams as a change of pace from powder eyeshadows. Overall, I don't recommend them. I admit they're fun, but I just wish they worked better to create a more sophisticated blend of colors. Almost without exception, cream eyeshadows crease and fade, and they're not the type to choose if you have trouble making mascara or eyeliner last because their emollient consistency can cause smearing and smudging of these other products.

Using Brushes to Apply Eyeshadow

Eyeshadow should be applied exclusively with brushes, and it's best to use brushes that are designed specifically for eyeshadow. Never use sponge-tip applicators—they drag across the eye and tend to blend colors in streaks. Once you get used to good brushes, you will never go back to the sponge-tip applicators again.

When applying eyeshadow, use the flat side of the brush against the eye. Gently wipe the brush across the eyeshadow, knock the excess off the brush, and apply it with long, stroking motions across the eyelid, crease, or under the eyebrow area. This motion of laying strips of color that overlap and blend together over the eye as opposed to beating the brush back and forth across the eye is the way to achieve an even, well-blended design.

Remember that the size of the brush should match the size of the eye area you are working on. If you have a large eyelid area, use a brush that is wide and full. If your eyelid is small, use a smaller brush that's the same width as the lid. The same rule is true for the crease area (if a specific color is being placed just there) and the under-eyebrow area. Using brushes that match the job is essential to putting makeup on effectively and efficiently. Do not purchase or use brushes that have hard, coarse bristles or you will end up with hard edges where the eyeshadow couldn't be blended, not to mention irritated skin.

DESIGNING THE EYE MAKEUP

Makeup books and cosmetics salespeople describe and demonstrate all kinds of eye-makeup designs—say, a dab of pastel yellow in the center of the lid, teal across the crease, taupe above the teal, pink above the taupe, and gray in the back corner of the lid. Not only do I think those designs are too complicated, I've never, at least not that I can recall, seen a model on the cover of any fashion magazine wearing a multicolor pastel eye design.

The most beautiful makeup applications, the ones you see and admire the most on models and actresses, are neutral, not colorful. Look at any fashion magazine. You're not going to see pastel or vivid eyeshadows on many faces, unless it's a purposely eccentric or bizarre montage. Too many competing pastel or vividly colored shadows make the eye design distracting. Pastel and primary colors (green, blue, red) are hard to blend together, so they stand out. Besides, the general purpose of eyeshadows is to shape and shade the eye, not color it. **The only way to shape the eye is by shading it with neutral shades such as taupe, brown, gray, ash, beige, tan, mahogany, redwood, caramel, sable, charcoal, and black.** Eyeshadows are called *shadows* for a reason—they build shape, movement, and interest via shading, not with color.

The list of appropriately neutral colors and tones available is actually quite extensive. Yet color on the eyelid is best kept as subtle as possible, or you will end up creating an eye makeup design that is more noticeable than your eye. **As a general rule, for a classically applied makeup, the lips and cheeks provide color on the face. More color standing out around the eyes can be overkill.**

Be cautious about thinking you need to choose a design based on the need to correct a perceived facial problem, such as your eyes being too close together, too far apart, too round, or not round enough. There are no standard facial dimensions that define how attractive you or your eyes are. You can end up with a contrived look that allows the makeup to be more noticeable than your eyes.

The best way to choose which design to wear is to decide what image you want to project. The more shading you use, the more dramatic and formal the eye makeup design; the less shading, the more subtle and casual the design. Other considerations when choosing one eye-makeup design over another involve your skill at applying makeup, your personal preference, and the amount of time you want (or have) to spend. For example, if you are new or unaccustomed to wearing makeup, keep your entire makeup look simple until you become adept at the different application techniques. The same thing goes if you have only a few minutes in the morning to put your makeup on—it is best to keep your routine simple. Trying to apply full makeup very quickly can result in mistakes or a sloppy application.

Applying an Eye-Makeup Design

Options for building an eye design are almost too numerous to list. The basic concept is to shade the eye to accent its shape, or to change its shape by using a progression of light to dark colors across the eye, blending one over the other so that you can't see where one stops and another starts. Here I will explain, step by step, how you can use one eyeshadow or several different eyeshadows to create a well-blended, classic eye-makeup design. Even for the most formal eye-makeup design, four different colors should be plenty. Whether you use one, two, three, or four different eyeshadows, they become a full design when worn with eyeliner, temple contour (see the "Contouring" section on page 435), and mascara.

One-color eye-makeup design: This design blends one soft, subtle color all over the eye area, from the lashes to just under the eyebrow, with no patches of skin showing through. You should not wear only a splash of color over the eyelid and ignore the rest of the eye area.

Application: When applying a single color, first place it from the lashes to the crease, making sure that you do not extend the color into the inside corner of the eye (off the lid area) or out beyond the lid onto the temple. Also be certain there are no patches of skin showing through on the lid next to the eyelashes. The entire lid at this point is one solid color.

Next, place the color from the crease up to the brow, following the entire length of the eyebrow from the nose out to the temple area. Avoid leaving a hard edge at the back (outside) corner of the eye where the eyeshadow stops. If desired, fade the eyeshadow as you blend up and out from the crease. This will create subtlety and a soft highlight under the eyebrow. Because the eyeshadow for the one-color eye-makeup design is so soft and subtle, blending and application is quite easy. The best colors for this design include light tan, neutral taupe, beige, pale mauve brown, pale gray, light golden brown, camel, and light auburn. Whatever the color, it should definitely not be obvious.

Two-color eye-makeup design: This is one of the most common, practical eye designs for many women. You can approach this design by applying the lighter color to the eyelid and the deeper color from the crease up to the brow, or you can apply the deeper color to the lid and the lighter color from the crease to the brow. Generally speaking, the under-eyebrow color should be a shade or two darker than the lid color. You do not want it to be a distinctly different color, just a different shade. The lid can be taupe, beige, tan, camel, gray, light auburn, golden brown, or any light neutral shade, and the under-eyebrow color would be a deeper shade of the same color. Women with darker skin tones can wear muted rose, mauve, or peach as long as it doesn't make their eyes look irritated or isn't too obvious. Bright, shiny, or whitish shadows can look dated and make the brow bone look more prominent and heavy.

Which color and what shades go where? **The general rule is that the larger or more prominent the eyelid area is compared with the under-brow area, the darker or deeper the eyelid color can be; the smaller the** eyelid area is compared with the under-brow area, the brighter or lighter the eyelid color can be. The notion is that if the eyelid area is already prominent or large, it isn't necessary to make it appear any bigger by applying a light color to it. If the eyelid area is small, it is appropriate to make it more prominent by wearing a lighter color.

Application: Whichever way you choose to apply this design, the lid and under-brow shades should meet—but not overlap—at the crease. As an option for the two-color eye-makeup design, you can apply the light shade to the lid and the darker shade from the crease up to the brow. Then, using a small wedge brush, you can use the light color again as a highlight just along the lower edge of the eyebrow. This can bring dramatic, but subtle, attention to the shape of the brow and the eye without the need for another eyeshadow color. You can also apply the lighter color from the lid to the under-brow area and use the darker color in and slightly above the crease. Then take the brush and use the darker color to softly shade the back corner of the eye, being sure this shading is an extension of the crease color. For more dramatic variations on this theme, see the design descriptions below.

<u>Three-color eye-makeup design:</u> Start by applying either of the basic one- or two-color eye-makeup designs on page 415. Once you have done that, the third shade, an even deeper color than the two previous colors, is added to the back (outside) corner of the lid or in the crease, or over both the crease and the back corner of the lid.

In this design, the lid and under-brow colors are softer and less intense than the color at the back corner of the lid or in the crease. Regardless of where you place this third, darker color, it can be a beautiful deep shade of brown, charcoal, cedar, mahogany, sable, red-brown, slate, chocolate brown, camel, deep taupe, or even black.

Application: If you apply the third eyeshadow in the crease, the trick is to not get the crease color on the lid, but rather to blend it slightly up into the under-eyebrow area and out onto the temple. Be sure, when sweeping the crease color across the eye, not to follow the down-curving movement of the shape of the eye. The best look is achieved if you blend the crease color out and up into the full back (outer) corner of the eye, and up onto the back of the brow bone.

When you apply the crease color, be sure to watch the angle of your brush as you blend the color from the crease out and up toward the under-brow area. If you place your color with the brush straight up at a 90-degree angle, you will look like you drew on wings. The softer the angle and the fuller the sweep, the softer the appearance, so be certain you blend *out* and slightly *up* from the lid area toward the under-brow area.

If you apply the third color at the back corner of the eye, the color hugs a small section of the lid, blending out and up into the crease and temple area. I explain this step in more detail for the four-color eye-makeup design.

Four-color eye-makeup design: In this design, you again start with the one- or two-color eye-makeup design, then add a darker color to the crease and an even darker color such as black or deepest gray to the back corner of the eye. Shading the back corner of the eyelid involves the arts of placement and blending. Because this area almost always requires a dark color, blending is essential to make it look soft, with no hard edges.

Why bother with a crease color and more shading at the back corner of the eye? The best part of this full eye-makeup design is that it shades, defines, and creates movement by adding a shadow in a curved flowing motion that follows the natural shape of the eye. The difficult part of this design is blending the crease color across the entire length of the eye without making it look obvious, choppy, or smeared. The goal is to tuck the color just in the crease at the fold nearest the nose and have it hug the crease until you get to the back corner of the eye, where you start the movement of the eyeshadow up and out onto the brow bone. Again, this sweep of color should not look like a stripe across the eye.

Application: Be sure to knock the excess eyeshadow off your brush, and apply the color with very small strokes over the back corner of the lid only. The problem here is keeping the color on the back of the lid only. If you don't know how to handle the brush, the back wedge can take up more than half of the eyelid (looking more like a mistake rather than carefully blended shading) or look like a stripe across the temple.

As shown on page 416, when you apply the crease color, be sure to watch the angle of your brush as you blend the color from the crease out and up toward the under-brow area. If you place your color with the brush straight up at a 90-degree angle, you will look like you drew on wings. The softer the angle and the fuller the sweep, the softer the appearance, so be certain you blend out and slightly up from the lid area toward the under-brow area.

Remember, the center or fold of the crease area is always the darkest, so start your brush there and blend out in each direction. Concentrate your efforts on how much of the crease area you want to shade. You can start all the way at the front part of the eye area under the front third of the brow, then follow the crease through the center, blending slightly up toward the brow. As you approach the back corner of the eye, begin your movement up and out toward the temple, aiming toward the eyebrow.

Eyeshadow Tips

1. Matte powder eyeshadows in an array of neutral tones from light to dark are your best bets for a classic, sophisticated eye design that accents the shape and color of your eyes.
2. Unless you're using just one eyeshadow color, use at least two eyeshadow brushes for application.
3. Prime the eyelid and under-brow area with a matte-finish concealer, foundation, and/or powder before you apply eyeshadow. This helps to ensure a smooth, even application and (if you have fair to medium skin) will also neutralize the red and blue coloration of the eyelid.
4. Tap off any excess eyeshadow from your brush before applying—this will prevent overapplication as well as flaking eyeshadow.
5. If you really want to make the color of your eyes pop, choose a contrasting color in a soft tone and apply this to the lids. Blue eyes come alive with pale peach or cantaloupe hues, green eyes seem richer with light bronze or caramel tones, hazel eyes become more alluring with chestnut and golden brown shades, and brown eyes are nicely accented by almost all neutral tones.

Eye Design Mistakes to Avoid

1. **Do not overcolor the eyes; too many bright colors can be distracting, not attractive.**
2. **Do not create hard edges; you should not be able to see where one color stops and another starts. Practice your application and blend well!**
3. **Do not wear bright pink or iridescent pink eyeshadows; they make eyes look irritated and tired. Muted or pale pink is an option, but be very, very careful. If it makes the eye look irritated or "red," it isn't the color for you.**
4. **Do not wear shiny eyeshadows of any kind if you are concerned about making the skin look more wrinkled because they exaggerate the appearance of lines. If you have smooth, unlined eyelids and prefer a touch of shine, apply it sparingly and look for a low-wattage glow instead of distracting glitter.**

5. Do not apply lipstick or blush over the eye area; it might sound like a timesaver, but if you have a lighter skin tone, it can make you look like you've been up all night crying. However, most bronzing powders can work as eyeshadows.

6. Do not match your eyeshadow to your clothing or your eye color. If you have blue eyes, blue eyeshadow would make the blue of your eyes look duller. And complementing your clothing is at best dated; besides, what do you do if you're wearing red or black?

7. Unless your goal is short-lived, messy eye makeup, avoid eye glosses and other greasy colors at all costs. These may look intriguing in photographs, but are more annoying than alluring in real life because they smear and smudge all over the place in a very short period of time.

EYELINER

Do you need to wear eyeliner? As with any makeup step, eyeliner is completely optional. From an artistic perspective, if you are wearing eyeshadow, I almost always recommend wearing eyeliner, unless your eyelids and eyelashes are obscured by the eyebrow area. Eyeliner is a basic part of an eye-makeup design because it shapes and defines the eyes and makes the eyelashes look thicker. If you are wearing only mascara and not eyeshadow, or if you want an extremely soft look, eyeliner is not necessary. If you do decide to wear eyeliner when you are wearing mascara and no eyeshadow, be sure to line the eyes with only a very soft, well-blended eyeshadow color.

As with most aspects of makeup, eyeliner presents a host of options. There are eye pencils (both traditional and chunky), liquid liners, gel eyeliners, cake eyeliners, and powder eyeliners. When it comes to colors, what used to be a simple choice of black or brown has morphed into a range of hues that can be overwhelming. Depending on the look you're after and your personal taste, the color of your eyeliner can be anything from crimson to silver to gold, bronze, or even olive green. Although I strongly suggest staying with tried-and-true colors like black, brown, and gray, the final decision is yours.

Types of Eyeliner

Since you can choose from among several styles of eyeliner, it is more important than ever to be aware of which ones have the best staying power, and which ones it's best to avoid. What kind of eyeliner should you use? Eye pencils are a quick, convenient option, but they do have problems; they tend to smear and unless you are using a twist-up pencil they are tricky to keep sharpened.

My favorite option over the years for applying a line is to use a tiny eyeliner brush with an appropriate color of traditional eyeshadow powder. I recommend using a dark-toned, matte eyeshadow color (almost any medium to deep eyeshadow color can work) and a tiny brush. I often apply the eyeshadow by wetting the brush and using it as "liquid" liner. The application is more controlled, but once it dries you have the soft look and the staying power of a powder without the hard edge that liquid eyeliners can create. A tiny, thin eyeliner brush allows absolute control over the thickness of the line around the eye. Another benefit to using powder and a brush is that you can use the powder as an eyeshadow just by selecting a different brush size.

<u>Pencil eyeliners</u> can often work well if you follow these basic rules.

- Self-sharpening pencils are by far the product of choice. Sharpening regular eye pencils is difficult, and keeping the point sharp without chewing up the pencil can be tricky.
- Remember that not all automatic pencils have a wind-down feature. That means if you wind up the tip of the pencil too high, it cannot be retracted and will likely break off.
- It is easier to apply pencil along the lower lashes than along the upper lid because the eyeshadows on the lid are harder for the pencil to stick to. You may want to consider using a greasy pencil for the lid and a firmer, less greasy pencil for the lower lashes. (If a pencil flattens when you press it, it will blend on more easily—but also will tend to smear more easily.)
- Warm the pencil between your fingers to apply a softer line of color; just remember this is not a surefire way to get a smooth application.
- To get a more precise line, if you have the time, leave the pencil in the freezer for a minute or two.
- Apply matching or similar powder eyeshadow over pencil to get the best of both worlds.

<u>Liquid eyeliner</u>, in general, is the most dramatic option, and when applied correctly (meaning a well-controlled, even line with no patches of

skin showing through) it can definitely have an impact. However, getting the application right is more than half the battle with liquid liners. Even those that have well-tapered and firm but flexible brushes can be difficult to control and apply evenly to both eyes. Yet if you're intent on trying a liquid liner, the easiest (and I use this term loosely) way to apply it is after your eyeshadow design is done and before mascara. Do not blink excessively or touch your eye until you're sure the liner has dried. If you wish to apply liquid liner to the lower lash line (which almost always looks overdone), get the tip of the brush underneath the lashes and draw a thin line using light but steady pressure. For best results, liquid liner should be used only on the upper lash-line. Powder eyeliner is a softer choice for the lower lash-line, and you will lose none of the oomph that comes with well-applied liquid liner. Make sure the liners meet at the outer corner of the eye.

Powder eyeliner can be applied with almost any eyeshadow you have, but by far the best products for this are Bobbi Brown, L'Oréal, M.A.C., Trish McEvoy, and Paula's Select eyeshadows. Choose a dark shade of eyeshadow. Always line the eyes last—after all the other eyeshadows have been applied. Use a tiny, thin, slightly stiff brush. Whether you use your powder wet or dry (both are fine, but dry is softer and wet can be more dramatic), stroke the brush through the color, keeping the bristles together. Do not dab or rub the brush into the color. Move the brush across the eyeshadow in the direction of the bristles, making sure the form of the brush is not destroyed. Knock the excess color from the brush, then apply the color to the eyelid next to the lashes and under the eye near the lower lashes.

Gel eyeliner is similar to liquid liners in almost every respect, except the gels tend to go on sheer and need to be layered to achieve the same depth of color you get instantly from a liquid liner. Some gel eyeliners come in small jars and are painted on with the brush of your choice. These tend to go on like a true liquid liner and often have incredible staying power. Bobbi Brown's Long Wear Gel Eyeliner *($18)* is a good example of this type of eyeliner.

Cake eyeliner has been around for years and most of us have either seen or tried it at some point. Compared to a well-pigmented powder eyeshadow or even a standard liquid liner, cake eyeliner is more of an antiquated choice that has no distinct advantages over other types of eyeliners. If you're a devoted user of cake liner and like the results, stick with it. Otherwise, I encourage you to try other types of liner before considering this one to achieve a softer look with more options for neutral color choices.

Applying Eyeliner

Assuming you have a steady hand (if not, try this sitting down so you can steady your arm by placing your elbow on a table), position the brush, pencil, or applicator so it is as close to the lash-line along the eyelid as possible. Then draw a line from the inner to outer corner using one fluid stroke, following the curvature of the eyelid. Do not extend the line past the outer corner of the eye or hug the tear-duct area of the eye. To start, keep the line as thin as possible, and if a thicker line is desired, repeat the process either across the entire lash-line or simply on the outer third of the lid along the lashes. Making the line along the eyelid a solid, even one, starting thin at the front third of the lid and becoming slightly thicker at the back third of the lid can be an attractive classic look.

You can line all the way across the eyelid if you like, from the inside corner to the outer edge, or you can stop the line where the lashes stop and start. Along the lower lashes, line only the outer two-thirds of the eye. **Be sure the lower liner is a less-intense color than the upper liner. Also make sure that the two lines meet at the back corner of the eye.** As a general rule, avoid lining all the way across the lower eyelashes. Leaving some space on the inside corner of the eye where the lashes end near the tear ducts gives a softer, less severe look. Plus, wrapping a complete circle of eyeliner around the eye tends to create an eyeglasses look and can make the eyeliner a stronger statement than the eye itself.

Makeup artists sometimes recommend that women over 40 not line the inner corner of the eye either on top or on the bottom. I think that's a fine suggestion. Instead, highlighting this area with a light shade of matte eyeshadow can be a very attractive alternative.

How thickly can you line the eye? As a general rule, for a classic look, the thickness and intensity of the eyeliner is determined by the size of the lid—the larger the eyelid area, the thicker and softer the eyeliner should be. The smaller the eyelid area, the thinner and more intense the liner should be. If your lid doesn't show at all, forget lining altogether.

You may have seen or heard a dozen other ideas as to how to apply eyeliner. Halfway across the lid, or one-third, or one-fourth, and three-fourths of the way under the lower eyelashes, or one-third, or one-fourth, and on and on. You are more than welcome to experiment with all these placements, but I encourage you to try the classic way first and see how you like it. Because the major reason to wear eyeliner is to shape the eye and make the eyelashes look thicker and deeper, I believe it is important to line where the lashes are and not just arbitrary sections of the lid. You can always line with a very soft color if you are concerned about overdefining the eyes, but I am not convinced that these "adjusted" lengths of placement look very natural.

Should you apply 1960s-style liquid eyeliner? Overexaggerated eyeliner with wings beyond the corner of the eyes is not a good idea. Depending on the effect you are trying to create, you can use a more definite eyeliner look most anytime of day. But for a more classic look, it is best to keep eyeliner soft by using powder or (if you prefer) by using a pencil and then applying powder over it.

What about applying eyeliner in the rim of the eye? There are many reasons why this is not a good idea. The first is that this kind of application smears in a very short period of time and creates goopy dark specks in the eye. Applying any makeup that is destined to smear in less than an hour or two is not a good idea. Pencil applied along the rim of the eye usually causes the area to become irritated; after all you are putting a foreign substance next to the mucous membrane of your eye. I am equally concerned about the health of the eye area when this technique is used. While there are no studies indicating there are any risks associated with pencil being applied to the rim of the eye, it seems problematic to put cosmetic ingredients (that include coloring agents and preservatives) that close to the eye.

Which eyeliner color should you use? For a classic eyeliner application, choose shades of dark brown, gray, or black eyeshadow for the upper lid and a softer shade of those—tan, taupe, chestnut, soft brown, soft gray, or soft black—along the lower lashes. Eyeliner is meant to give depth to the lashes and make them appear thicker. If the liner is a bright color or a true pastel, attention will be focused past the lashes to the colored line, as opposed to the more subtle flow of color from dark lashes to dark liner. Test it on yourself. Line one eye with a vibrant color, the other eye with brown or black, and see which one looks like it has thicker lashes. Then, if all my attempts to convince you have failed, and you still prefer to use bright or pastel liners, go for it.

Checking for Mistakes

After using powder eyeshadow as eyeliner, check for drippies under the eye and on the cheek. Drippies are those little powder flakes that fly off the brush and land on the cheek. Knocking off the excess from the brush every time helps prevent drippies, but there will always be flakes that end up where they don't belong. The best way to go after drippies is to use your sponge and simply wipe them away. If you do this, your next step is to touch up your foundation if that has gotten smeared.

Some makeup artists recommend applying a thicker layer of loose powder under the eyes and onto the upper cheekbone to catch the inevitable drippies, allowing them to be whisked off with a powder brush. If you have relatively smooth, unlined skin in this area you may want to try this. Otherwise, it can make the under-eye area look dry and enhance lines and wrinkles.

Always double-check the intensity of your eyeliner application and blend away any thickness or color that is more dramatic than you intended. It is not possible to blend or correct mistakes with liquid liners, which is one of the reasons I generally don't recommend them.

If you do choose to wear pencil eyeliner, check for smears under the eye as the day goes by. This is annoying, but letting it go without blending away the smears can make any well-applied eye-makeup design look like a mess.

Eyeliner Mistakes to Avoid

1. Do not use greasy or slick pencils to line the lower lashes; they smear and smudge.
2. Do not use brightly colored pencils or eyeshadows to line the eye; they are distracting and automatically look like too much makeup. All you'll see is the color and not your eye.
3. Do not extend the eyeliner beyond the corner of the eye (no wings).
4. Do not make the eyeliner the most obvious part of the eye-makeup design.
5. Do not line the inside rim of the lids, between the lash and the eye itself; it is messy and can be unhealthy for the cornea.
6. If you do use pencil to line the eye, apply a small amount of eyeshadow over your pencil eyeliner to help set it and keep it from smearing.
7. Do not apply thick eyeliner to small or close-set eyes.
8. Do not use eyeshadow as eyeliner unless you use the proper brush.

9. Do not line the eye with a circle of dark or bright color. Both are too obvious and create an eyeglass-style circle around the eye.
10. Do not overblend, spilling your eyeliner onto the skin under the lower lashes; that makes dark circles look worse.

MASCARA

Mascara is an amazing invention and is considered basic to any kind of makeup application. Many makeup artists, including myself, say that if you're not wearing any other makeup but still want to wear something, wear mascara. On the other hand, many of us—and I'm guilty of this, too—get carried away and wear way too much mascara.

Women overdo mascara in part because the cosmetics industry tells us loudly and clearly that long, thick lashes are to be coveted, but even unadvised we covet someone else's long, beautiful lashes. When we apply mascara, visions of longer, thicker lashes sometimes come into view and then we get carried away and decide to apply more and more. Unfortunately, applying too much mascara increases the chances that the mascara will flake, chip, or smear, and that the lashes will appear hard and spiked. Also, the eyelashes can take only so much weight, and excess weight can break them. Lashes gunked up with tons of mascara do not resemble long, thick lashes—they resemble gunked-up lashes!

The desire for longer, more noticeable lashes brings up the image of that ever-popular device that curls the lashes by squeezing them into a bent-upward shape. The problem with curling lashes is that it can bend the lashes into a severe angle that can look unnatural; and, although it can make them more noticeable (sometimes in an odd sort of way), it can also end up breaking them and pulling them out. Doesn't that defeat the purpose of making your lashes look longer? If you're still gung-ho on doing this, curl lashes only before you apply mascara, never after, or you will end up with broken, strangely bent lashes. The best lash-curlers are the ones with a sponge-tip section where the eyelashes are squeezed for protection. Squeeze gently with even pressure. Hold for a few seconds as you "walk" the curler along the length of the eyelashes, and release slowly. Some fashion magazines recommend heating the rubber pad of the eyelash curler by running your blow dryer over it for a few seconds. This may be worth trying, but be extremely cautious that the pad does not get too hot (touch it with your finger to be sure) because you don't want to fry fragile lashes or burn the eyelid skin.

Types of Mascara

Mascara comes in two basic types: waterproof and water-soluble. Mascaras should not smudge, flake, or clump, and it is not your fault if they do. As is true for any aspect of the cosmetics industry, price does not tell you anything about how well a mascara performs. Drugstore mascaras can be as good as more expensive department store brands, and sometimes even better. **Regardless of where you buy your mascara, you might find that upon opening it, it already seems dried up. This is a recurring problem in the cosmetics world. Take it back immediately and get a refund or another tube.**

Can you extend the longevity of your mascara? If you want to, there are a few possibilities. First, do not overpump the wand into the tube in an attempt to build up mascara on the brush. All that really accomplishes is pumping more air into the tube, which makes the mascara dry up faster. Another solution is to avoid mascaras with a wide-bristled brush. To accommodate the wider brush, the tube opening needs to be larger, and this allows more air inside, again causing the mascara to dry out faster. Don't be fooled by the promise that wider bristles will make lashes longer. If anything, big brushes are clumsy to use, and they make it harder to get to the lashes at the corners without making mistakes. One last thing you may want to try is rotating the mascara wand around the inside of the tube. This will ensure you get any mascara that has been clinging to the sides of the tube and can help stretch mascara a bit further.

<u>Water-soluble mascaras:</u> The problem with some water-soluble mascaras is that they don't come off all that easily with water, even though they should. However, a great water-soluble mascara can go on beautifully and wash away easily. Again, there are many superior mascaras at the drugstore—this is not an area where you need to splurge!

<u>Waterproof mascaras:</u> These cause problems because to remove them you usually need to pull and wipe at the eyes, which can pull out lashes. I understand the desire to go swimming while wearing your makeup or to cry at weddings and not have mascara streaming down your cheeks, especially if you're the bride! Waterproof mascara is fine for occasional use, but wearing it every day can cause more headaches in the long run. Another drawback is that although most waterproof mascaras hold up well under water, they can still break down and smear when they meet the oil from your skin or emollients from your moisturizer or foundation. Do not make the mistake of thinking that waterproof means smearproof.

For those times when you do need waterproof mascara, the most effective way to remove it is with a silicone-based makeup remover that won't leave a greasy film on the skin. To be as gentle as possible, soak a cotton pad with the remover and lightly press and hold this against your lashes (make sure the eye is closed) for a few seconds. This helps loosen the mascara from lashes. Using very light pressure, move the pad down over the lashes and then back and forth, paying close attention not to pull or tug the skin. You can perform this step before or after cleansing.

Applying Mascara

The traditional upper-lash application of rotating the mascara wand by round-brushing from the base of the lashes up to cover all the lashes around the entire eye is the most efficient, expedient method. **Keep an old, cleaned-up mascara wand in your makeup bag to use for removing occasional mascara clumps (it can happen with the best mascaras) and separating lashes.**

Apply mascara to the lower lashes by holding the wand perpendicular to the eye and parallel to the lashes (using the tip of the wand). This prevents you from getting mascara on the cheek. It also makes it easier to reach the lashes at both ends of the eye. If you want a softer application on the lower lashes, wipe the wand down with a tissue and then apply lightly.

Have you ever had mascara end up on the eyelid or under the eye while you're applying it? Wait until it dries completely and then chip it away with a cotton swab or your sponge. Most of it will just flake off, with very little repair work needed. Always check for mascara smudges; they can look very sloppy and distracting.

False Eyelashes

Although I am not a fan of false eyelashes (primarily because you can almost always tell that they're fake), I realize that many makeup artists love to use them, and because they do, women wonder if they should try them, either to be doing the "proper thing" or for fun. Basically, false lashes are available in full sets or as individual lashes. Application always involves the use of an adhesive gel (such as Duo) and must be precise if you want the effect to look convincing. Removing false eyelashes can also be tricky, not to mention hazardous to your real lashes. Remember, there are lots of mascaras available that can come pretty close to giving a false-eyelash effect—you may want to experiment with these before ever considering falsies.

Mascara Mistakes to Avoid

1. Do not wear colored mascara such as blue, purple, or green if you're going for a classic daytime look.
2. Do not wear mascara that smears or flakes; don't put up with those that do, because there are lots that don't.
3. Do not use waterproof mascaras on a daily basis; they can be difficult to remove and hard on fragile eyelashes.
4. Do not forget to apply mascara evenly to lower lashes.
5. Do not overapply mascara; your lashes will look clumpy or like thick-barred windows.

EYE MAKEUP—IS IT SAFE?

Mascara, eyeshadow, and eyeliner are intended to make women more attractive. One thing they shouldn't do is harm the eyes! Yet each year, many women suffer eye infections from cosmetics. At the time of purchase, most eye cosmetics are free from bacteria that could cause eye infections. Problems happen when they aren't adequately preserved against microorganisms or if they are misused by the consumer after being opened. Poor preservation or misuse of an eye cosmetic can allow dangerous bacteria to enter and grow in the product. Then, when the cosmetic is applied to the area around the eye, it can cause an infection.

The Food and Drug Administration has taken numerous steps to make sure that eye cosmetics are free from contamination when they reach you and that they contain preservatives to inhibit the growth of bacteria. The cosmetics industry generally makes products that will not harm you. Nevertheless, the FDA urges you to follow these eleven tips on the use of eye cosmetics.

1. Discontinue immediately the use of any eye product that causes irritation. If irritation persists, see a doctor.
2. Recognize that bacteria on your hands could, if placed in the eye, cause infections. Wash your hands before applying cosmetics to your eyes.
3. Make sure that any instrument you place in the eye area is clean.
4. Do not allow cosmetics to become covered with dust or contaminated with dirt or soil. Wipe off the container with a damp cloth if dust or dirt is visible.

5. Do not use old containers of eye cosmetics. If you haven't used the product for several months, it's better to discard it and purchase a new one.
6. Do not spit into eye cosmetics. The bacteria in your mouth may grow in the cosmetic, and subsequent application to the eye could cause infection.
7. Do not share your cosmetics. Another person's bacteria in your cosmetics can be hazardous to you.
8. Do not store cosmetics at temperatures above 85 degrees Fahrenheit. Cosmetics held for long periods in hot cars, for example, are more susceptible to deterioration of the preservative.
9. Avoid using eye cosmetics if you have an eye infection or if the skin around the eye is inflamed. Wait until the area is healed.
10. Take particular care in using eye cosmetics if you have any allergies.
11. When applying or removing eye cosmetics, be careful not to scratch the eyeball or other sensitive areas.

EYEBROW SHAPING AND SHADING

No aspect of makeup seems to go through such dramatic fashion changes as eyebrow styles. Eyebrows are as representative of each fashion decade as clothes are. We've gone from overtweezed, pencil-thin, tortured brows to overdrawn, thickly penciled brows, to a full, bushy natural look, and now we've settled on very soft, natural, but definitely shaped brows. The best idea is for the eyebrows to be natural in appearance but not bushy or thick, with an expertly defined, but not pointed, arch.

Shaping the Eyebrows

Full, softly shaped eyebrows are easier to keep up but there is a balance between overtweezing and no tweezing. We are talking about natural, not Neanderthal. There is a middle ground between Groucho Marx and Greta Garbo when it comes to the appearance of your brows!

Discovering the best shape for your eyebrows without sacrificing a natural appearance is what you want to accomplish. The eye is framed by the arch, length, and thickness of the eyebrow. Just as the shape of a mustache can change the appearance of a man's face, the shape of the eyebrows can affect the appearance of the eyes. For example, if you tweeze too much off the front part of the eyebrows (near the nose), the eyes will appear smaller. If you tweeze too much from under the eyebrows, increasing the distance between the eye and the eyebrow, you can look permanently surprised.

Which hairs you leave and which ones you remove makes all the difference between attractively shaped brows and misshapen ones. And go slowly—because for some reason, over time, eyebrow hair does not always grow back after it is tweezed (there is no known physiological reason for this, but that is what many women experience). You can use an eyebrow pencil and a diagram to help you line up the following parameters for shaping your eyebrow.

The beginning of the brow should align with the center of the nostril, the arch should fall at the back third of the eye, and, although the eyebrow should be as long as possible, it still shouldn't extend into the temple area (see the diagram on the next page). **The basic rule is that the front part of the brow should never drop below the back part of the brow.** Allowing this to happen, either with the way you tweeze your eyebrows or the way you draw them on, makes you look like you're frowning and overemphasizes the downward movement of the back part of the eye.

What are the best tools? The best tweezers are the ones from Revlon or Tweezerman with tips that are slightly rounded to a soft point. Tweezers that are too pointy can stab the skin; if they're too flat across the top they can grab skin along with the hair. There are lots of other tweezers around in all kinds of shapes or with handles that snap together, but these all pose problems when it comes to reliability and ease of use.

Steps to Shaping a Perfect Brow

1. Before you start tweezing, use a lip or brow pencil to heavily draw on the shape you want; you can adjust it as you decide on the look you want.
2. Once the shape is drawn on, tweeze any hairs that fall outside the line of the brow.
3. Next, brush the brows straight up with an old toothbrush. Any hairs that are too long and floppy should be trimmed with small scissors. Tweezing long brow hairs rather than trimming them can result in gaps in the eyebrow or a patchy look.

EYEBROWS 101

Tweezing a soft natural shape is the goal; eyebrows that are too thick or too thin can take attention away from the rest of your face. Follow these steps to create beautiful eyebrows.

1

Draw on the shape you want with an eyebrow or lip pencil, following the natural growth as much as possible. Take your time with this step, repeating it until you get the look you want.

2

Tweeze hairs that fall outside the brow you penciled on. Use rounded or needle-nose tweezers for accurate removal.

3

Brush eyebrow hairs straight up with an old toothbrush.

4

Trim hairs that are too long with a small pair of scissors.

5

To keep brows in place, smooth the hairs with an old mascara wand and then apply brow gel or clear mascara, or spray the mascara wand with hairspray and then comb it through the brows.

Types of Eyebrow Products and Application

<u>**Powder eyebrow colors or eyeshadows used to fill in the brow**</u> should be applied using a soft-textured powder (either an eyeshadow or a powder designed for the brow; both work great) that matches the brow color exactly and a soft wedge brush or a tiny eyeliner brush (I prefer the control of a small eyeliner brush). Follow the basic shape of the brow, using the same guidelines as for tweezing. Fill in only at the front or underneath the brow, or through the brow itself. Avoid drawing on color above the brow. For a softer look, brush through the eyebrows using a clean, old toothbrush.

<u>**Eyebrow pencils:**</u> These are a perennial option but be careful when deciding which one to use. Eyebrow pencils can produce a greasy, hard look and mat the eyebrow hair, and too often you end up looking like you live in another decade. If you are presently penciling your eyebrows, seriously consider changing to powder. If penciling doesn't look absolutely natural, don't do it. Better to go without any eyebrow makeup at all than to be adorned with a line of pencil above your eye.

Many makeup artists use both pencil and powder to create natural-looking brows for women with little or no eyebrow hair, and this can be a great alternative. This way you can get the control and delineation of a pencil, and then soften and shade the effect with a powder. If you decide to try this, look for brow pencils that have a firm but smooth texture and slightly powdery finish. Avoid using any brow pencil that is painful or that applies color too dramatically or thickly.

Application: To apply the powdered brow color or brow pencil, brush the brow up with an old toothbrush and then apply the color with an angled wedge brush, filling in the shape of the brow between the hairs where needed. If your eyebrows are set high, away from the eye area, and you want to reshape them, place the color directly under the eyebrow. The closer the brow is to the eye area (meaning the height from the brow to the lid or eyelashes is small), the more you should fill in the color in the existing brow itself rather than shading just below the brow. As much as possible, work only with the hair that is there. The idea is to shade rather than draw on eyebrows. Do not place your brow color, whether it is pencil or powder, more than one-quarter inch away from where the natural hair growth stops. It simply looks fake and accentuates the fact that there is no brow there in the first place! What you want is the suggestion, the shadow of a brow—not a line and not an obvious application of color (see the photograph on page 443).

Colored eyebrow gels: These are a fairly recent development and a good option for making the most of sparse, light-colored eyebrows or for giving a thicker look to most other eyebrows. These products look like mascara but they have a much lighter consistency. Examples are Paula's Select Brow/Hair Tint *($8.95)*, Origins Just Browsing *($12)*, and Bobbi Brown Natural Brow Shaper *($16.50)*.

Application: Apply the color through the brow in much the same fashion as you apply mascara to the eyelashes. Brush the wand through your brows, being careful not to get the product on the forehead or other areas of the skin and not to leave the brows standing straight up. It will probably take you a few times to get the hang of it. You also might have trouble at first controlling the amount of gel from the tube to the brow. But if you want your brows to look fuller, give this one a try—it really works. The products mentioned above all have dual-bristled brushes, which can be used for a soft, full look or for more definition. Be wary of brow gels and tints with single- or small-bristled brushes because these can make application trickier (they often produce a lined or spotted effect).

What Eyebrow Color Should You Use?

Generally, you should match the exact color of the brows rather than your hair color or a color you think would look better than what already exists. You don't want to see a difference between the eyebrow hairs and the shadow or gel used to fill them in. However, if you have pale eyebrows and want to darken the brow color, use a soft shade of brown that is as close to your brows' natural color as possible. If you have red hair and brown eyebrows, using a red pencil or red-brown powder will look unnatural; just stick with brown. If you have blonde eyebrows, you could use a slightly darker blonde or taupe color on your brows to make them visible. For those with well-shaped, naturally full brows, a clear brow gel (Cover Girl and Max Factor have good ones) is a great option for lightly grooming the brows without adding any color. You can also spritz some hair spray on an old toothbrush and comb through your brows, or add a dab of nonsticky styling gel to keep unruly brow hairs in place.

What if you don't have any hair at all where the eyebrows are supposed to be? This is the only circumstance that requires applying a brow color that matches the hair on your head. It will look the most natural. Use the wedge brush and powder to follow the bone above the eye, applying to whatever hair is there. Usually there's enough shape to create a natural, shaded impression of a brow. Use a light touch, with short, quick

BEAUTIFUL EYEBROW SOLUTIONS

CORRECT
Arch's high point

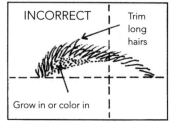

INCORRECT   Trim long hairs

Grow in or color in

L-Shaped Brow

INCORRECT

Grow in or color in

U-Shaped Brow

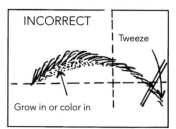

INCORRECT

Tweeze

Grow in or color in

Overextended Brow (back)

INCORRECT

Tweeze

Overextended Brow (front)

Perfectly Shaped Eyebrows: The shape of the eyebrow is correct when the beginning of the brow is aligned with the center of the nostril and the arch falls over the back third of the eye.

L-Shaped Brow
Problem: The arch is over the front third of the eye.
Solution: Grow in or color in the indicated area.

U-Shaped Brow
Problem: The eyebrow has no arch.
Solution: Grow in or color in the indicated area.

Overextended Brow (back)
Problem: The back third of the brow is lower than the front third of the brow.
Solution: Grow in or color in the indicated area and tweeze the end of the brow to align it with the front of the brow.

Overextended Brow (front)
Problem: The front third of the brow is lower than the back third of the brow.
Solution: Tweeze the front of the brow to align it with the back of the brow.

motions, and avoid the temptation to exaggerate the shape by arching it severely or extending it into the temple area. Downplay the fact that there is no hair; it's better not to overexaggerate the area with a strong, eye-catching line. Also, don't place a highlighter or light-colored eyeshadow under the brow to further emphasize the brow. Putting something dark next to something light makes it look even more prominent. Use what you have as the basis for any makeup application, and avoid making any obvious, theatrical changes. Once the brows are softly accented (or left alone), play up your lips or cheeks instead so that these will become the focus rather than your absent or too-sparse eyebrows.

Eyebrow Mistakes to Avoid

1. Do not overtweeze, and never tweeze above the brow, only underneath. Tweezing above the brow can ruin its natural shape.
2. Do not overstate the shape of the brow; minimal brow alteration is best.
3. Do not pluck brows into a thin line thinking it will make your eyes look larger. It will only look strange, contrived, even sinister. It can also give the face a surprised look, and none of this is attractive or natural—or easy to correct once the damage is done.
4. Do not use eyebrow pencil or eyeliner pencil to fill in your eyebrows unless you are adept at making it look very soft and shaded.
5. Do not apply eyebrow powders that are a different color than your own eyebrows; it is best to always match your existing brow color.
6. Do not apply brow color that is obvious or has a drawn-on look.
7. Do not forget that eyebrow color should look shaded and soft, not like a straight, hard line.
8. Be careful of brow colors that look red on the skin, which can make the eyebrow look fake and the skin look irritated. If you're in doubt when choosing between brow shades, go with the more muted option.

CONTOURING

Contouring is the art of creating or increasing shadows in certain areas so the face appears to have more structure and definition. It involves using brown tones of blush or pressed powder to contour along the sides of the nose, at the sides of the forehead, under the cheekbones, and in the center of the chin to add color, definition, and shape to the face. Although contouring is an optional step for most daytime makeup applications, it is still rather intriguing and is worthwhile for some women.

For the most part, the popularity of using contouring to reshape the face has subsided somewhat. The likely reason for its demise is that believable-looking contouring is difficult to master (even more difficult than believable-looking blush). Contouring takes skill and patience, and very few women have the time to deal with it every morning. Women who do decide to take the time often end up with a brown stripe under their blush, and that is not the way contouring is supposed to look! Think twice before incorporating this step into your daily makeup routine until you've practiced and developed the skill to apply this look softly. Without careful application and conscientious blending, what looks sculptural from the front may look odd from other angles.

Contouring is always done as a separate step, using a completely different brush and shade of powder than for the blush application. Shades of pink, red, and orange are used as blushes; only shades of brown are used in contouring. The safest contour shade to use if you have fair to medium-dark skin tones is one that looks like your skin color when it is tanned. A soft or rich golden shade of brown is generally the perfect color to use when trying to produce realistic shadows on the face. Shades of gray-brown can look dirty, and shades of red-brown and mauve-brown can look like bruising on women with fair to medium-dark skin tones. For women of color, particularly African-American women, either an extremely dark shade of golden brown or a deep chocolate brown color can work exceptionally well.

Types of Contour

Contour is essentially blush in a golden brown or reddish-brown color. For the varying types of contour, take a look at the "Types of Blush" section on page 440. The easiest type of contour to work with is applied with powder-based color. Cream and cream-to-powder contour colors can be extremely difficult to control and blend, which can interfere with proper placement—a major no-no when it comes to natural-looking contour color.

Applying Contour

Instead of using a brush designed for contouring, use a brush designed for blush or rouge. (But avoid traditional blush brushes that often come packaged with the blush; they are too small for most cheeks, and so are a poor choice for blush or contour application.) Surprisingly, traditional contouring brushes are also a poor choice for applying contour because they are usually too stiff, have a flat edge, and can leave visible edges when you apply your color. Instead, use the full end of the blush brush when contouring. Knocking off the excess powder before applying, and brushing on the color in short, quick motions going back to the ear will net the best results. Here are some rules of placement to help you most effectively contour your face.

Contouring under or along the jawline: Avoid contouring or shading along any portion of the jawline for daytime. Though this technique can make you look like you've lost a few pounds, you can end up with a line of demarcation around the jaw, negating the trouble you went through to find a foundation that leaves no such line. That means it will not look like natural shading. Nevertheless, shading the jawline or just under the chin can be passable for pictures or possibly for evening, but it must be applied very carefully. Shading under the jawline can also result in shading your collar at the same time. Be careful! Be sure to blend well and soften any noticeable edges or concentrations of color.

Contouring under the cheekbone: Place the center of your brush about one-quarter to one-half inch behind the laugh line, and stroke the color straight back, aiming toward the middle of the ear. The area of application should be approximately a half inch in width, with no definite edges visible. Use your sponge to soften hard edges. The starting point for under-cheekbone contouring is almost always the same regardless of the face shape, because the cheekbone corresponds nicely to the laugh line and middle ear area for most women. You can adjust the angle depending on your preferences. The steeper the angle going toward the top of the ear, the longer the face will appear. If you have a square or round face, you might want to try contouring at a steeper angle. The longer the face (as an oblong or triangular face might be), the more horizontal (straight back toward the middle of the ear) the line can be. This, in effect, de-emphasizes the length of the face. All this takes experimentation, so be patient until you achieve the look you want. Be sure to blend well and soften any noticeable edges or concentrations of color.

Caution: When applying the under-cheekbone contour, be sure never to blend or place the contour color below the mouth area, below the middle of the ear, or onto the cheekbone itself. There is also no need to suck in your mouth to help find your cheekbones—that will only help you find the sides of the mouth, not the cheekbone.

Contouring the sides of the nose: Although most women think that contouring the nose is strictly to make it look smaller or narrower or longer, there is actually a more artistic reason for using this shading technique. If you're applying a full makeup, particularly for evening, and you ignore the nose, you will have color everywhere on your face except for a blank spot in the center of the face. Contouring the nose helps to achieve color balance for the whole face when you choose to wear a formal, full makeup application. It isn't essential, but it's a great trick—and one that can be seen on models gracing the covers of almost every fashion magazine out there.

The goal is to make the contour color look absolutely as soft as possible. The challenge is to restrict the color to the sides of the nose. You never want to accidentally blend the color of the nose contour onto the area under your eyes or onto your cheeks. Take extra care to blend only a small amount of contour color on such an obvious focal point.

The best technique for applying the nose contour is to place the brush itself between your fingers and thumb, so the brush tip becomes somewhat flattened. This way the brush tip can more easily follow along the sides of your nose. (You can use the same brush you use for contouring or a very large, flat eyeshadow brush.) Now, take the index finger of your other hand, place it flat down the center of the nose, and apply the contour color along the side of your finger. Where the brush falls against your finger is the area to be contoured. Once you've done this, remove your finger and softly apply the contour fully around the tip of the nose and on the flare of the nostrils. Continue the contour in a narrow, soft line up under the eyebrow, avoiding the corner of the eye and the area between the eyebrows. Be sure to blend well and soften any noticeable edges or concentrations of color. Blend using very soft, short strokes and pay careful attention so that you do not spread the contour color onto the cheeks (see photograph number four on page 442).

Contouring the temple area: Temple contour is a traditional step that is as basic as applying blush. The difference is that most women don't know about it. Take a look at the cover of any fashion magazine or ad for designer clothes, and you will notice this contouring on most of the models. When temple contour is neatly applied, the eyeshadows at the back of the eye can be blended into it so they don't end abruptly with a harsh edge of color. Without temple contour, the forehead becomes a great bare wall against the colored background of the cheeks and eyes.

The temple contour is placed next to the back third of the eye near the brow bone, directly out and up onto the forehead like a pie wedge, but without the edges. Temple contour can be applied either before or after the eye-makeup design is in place. If you apply the contour after the eye-makeup design, it is important to place the brush directly over the eyeshadows at the back third of the eye and then brush the contour all the way back to the hairline. If you do the contour first, apply it in the exact same place and in the same way, but when you apply the eyeshadows, blend them directly over and onto the temple contour. Either way, the contour softens the back edge of the eyeshadows.

When temple contour looks wrong or unnatural, it's usually for one of three reasons.

1. Forgetting that this step begins at the back third of the under-eyebrow area, right on top of and over the back third of the entire eye area. It does not float on the forehead unconnected to the back corner of the eye.
2. Not brushing the contour directly over the eyebrow itself, which can make the application look choppy instead of smooth and even (you should apply the eyebrow color after the temple contour).
3. Applying the color in a straight one-inch strip next to the eye instead of in a softly blended two-inch pie wedge that is partially blended onto the forehead. Temple contour is a shaded area, like the blush area, and it should never look like a stripe. Be sure to blend well and soften any noticeable edges or concentrations of color.

Contour Mistakes to Avoid

1. Do not use a blush color to contour any part of your face. Contour only with golden brown, chocolate brown, or dark brown shades.
2. Do not use contour under the jaw or at the chin area during the day; it can look too obvious and possibly get on clothing.
3. Do not apply contour as part of your regular makeup routine until you get used to blending it on softly; it should never look like stripes or brown lines on the face.
4. Do not forget to blend hard edges; contour should always look soft and as natural as possible on the face.

BLUSH

Knowing how to choose a great blush color and apply it correctly is essential to successful makeup application. Blush adds life and a hint of healthy color to the face and its importance should not be overlooked when you're deciding how to go about doing your makeup.

Blush is one part of makeup application many women take for granted. The comment I hear most often is, "I've been doing that for years. I know how to put on blush." Yet it is so easy to make mistakes, and I see them all the time. Blush is one of the more prominent parts of any makeup routine, so if you do make a mistake—such as applying it too close to the lines around the eye, applying it like a stripe of color across the cheek, applying the wrong color, or applying it underneath the cheekbones as if it were contour—it is very noticeable. I urge you to take time to learn how to apply blush properly.

I can't say that everyone agrees exactly where you are supposed to place blush! There are many opinions on where it should start, where it should end, and how high or low to place it along the cheekbone. My strong preference—one that is shared by many, as is evident in fashion magazines—is to keep the blush on the cheekbones and away from the eye area, blending the color just on the cheekbones and starting it about one-half inch behind the laugh lines. Some women start the blush no farther into the center of the face than the center of the eye. That can make the blush look very strange. The idea is to blush the entire cheekbone, and that means full across the cheek.

Types of Blush

Powder blushes: Powder blushes are an excellent choice for all skin types. They go on easily, blend beautifully, and come in great colors. A brush is essential for applying these smoothly, softly, and evenly.

Application: To find the area to be blushed, place the full end of your brush about one-quarter to one-half inch behind the laugh line. Starting here, brush downward and back toward the center of your ear, being careful not to place any color below the level of the mouth. Applying your blush by brushing down as opposed to back and forth eliminates a stripe effect. The blush area should be about two inches across, with no hard edges. Always use your sponge to soften edges.

Pros: There are only pros to this type; it works for just about everyone! The only possible negative for powder blushes is due to

(*continued on page 445*)

MAKEUP APPLICATION STEP BY STEP

Jonette
Entrepreneur & Model
"Before"

1 Foundation
Evenly blended application using a thin sponge (see page 394)

2 Concealer
Applied to dark circles and areas to be highlighted (see page 374)

3 Powder
An even, light dusting "sets" makeup and creates a perfect palette (see page 409)

4 Contour
Adds definition and some color (see page 435)

5 Blush
Lightly applied along the entire cheek area, from the "apple" to the back of the ear (see page 440)

6 Eyeshadow
Use an appropriately sized brush for the lid (see page 412)

7 Eyeshadow
. . . and a smaller brush for the crease (see page 413)

8 Liner
Here, a slender brush is used wet with powder (see page 421)

9 Eyebrow
Defined brows help frame the face (see page 429)

10a Lipliner, Lipstick & Mascara Finished Daytime Look
The face is softly accented in neutral earth tones on the eyes and light rosy-brown tones on cheeks and lips. Each feature is played up, but no single feature is more prominent than another. The goal is a flawless gradation of color with no hard, abrupt edges.

10b Modified Eyes & Lips Finished Evening Look
Her daytime makeup was made more dramatic by intensifying the eyeshadow using a darker brown in the crease and back corner of the lid. The eyeliner was deepened with soft black powder eyeshadow. Blush was left alone, and the lips were played up with liner and a classic red lipstick topped with a dab of gloss.

Paula & Jonette

powder's naturally drier texture that can sometimes appear to sit on top of the surface of the skin, although this effect is usually short-lived. It can be eliminated altogether by choosing a silky-smooth, perfectly soft powder blush.

Liquid, gel, cream, and cream-to-powder or stick blushes: These are not my favorites and I recommend considering these carefully. The only real advantage they have over powder blushes is that they tend to mesh better with the skin, which on some women can look more natural—as if it were a "glow from within." Yet in spite of this minor positive point, liquid, gel, and cream-type blushes don't perform reliably for most skin types. They can be very awkward to blend evenly, and they tend to streak whether you use your fingers or a sponge. They can also stain the pores, making the face look dotted with color, and they don't work well over foundation—the foundation gets wiped off as you apply the blush. Still, if you have near flawless, smooth skin (no dryness and not oily), no visible pores, and have a deft touch at blending, you are a candidate for liquid, gel, or cream blush. It does help that many of today's cream blushes are silicone-based, which allows a clean, smooth application and a soft powder finish. Just don't buy anything until you check it out in the daylight and see how it wears during the day.

Application: There isn't one best way to apply these types of blushes. A sponge is my first choice, but some women do fine using their fingers or even a synthetic brush. Use whatever works best for you and always double-check to make sure there are no hard edges to soften. Gel blushes can be the hardest to blend evenly, so you may want to start with cream or cream-to-powder formulas.

Applying Blush and Contouring

If you are applying both blush and under-cheekbone contour, apply the contour color first and then blend the blush on top of and gradually down into the contour color. Then, using your sponge, blend until you meld the colors together into an attractive design. The hallmark of an attractive design is not being able to see where one color stops and the other starts. When done properly, blush and contour add color, depth, and dimension to a face—and that's always attractive.

Choosing a Blush Color

How much color and which color should you use? That is not an easy question to answer. When it comes to a fashion statement the trends seem to change on a monthly basis. One month sheer, almost no blush color is the rage and the next mauve is the style. But by the time the next issue of your favorite fashion magazine is launched, peach, rose, pale red, and apricot blushes may be in style. What to do? Let go of the trends; they are exhausting, and what is trendy may not look good on you. Pale blush can look ghostly on many women, peach can look too sallow for some skin tones, and mauve can look ashen on olive tone skin. In the long run the color that looks best and most natural to your skin tone is the best place to start.

An option to consider when choosing blush color is to go neutral; a soft golden brown, tannish-looking color is a great foolproof choice for many skin tones. I personally use this look for the summer. For darker skin colors, a deeper golden brown works perfectly. Whatever option you choose be sure your lipstick colors match the underlying tone of your blush. In other words, if you are wearing a blush with a blue undertone, the lipstick should be in that same color family; rose blush means rose lipstick; coral blush coordinates with coral or coral/tan lipstick; though a soft tan-looking blush works with almost any color of lipstick. You absolutely do not want to wear pink blush and coral lipstick or mauve blush with orange lipstick. The point is for lipstick and blush colors to work together and not look like opposite, clashing ends of a rainbow.

Your blush color does not need to match your clothing, shoes, or any other accessories, although if you wear vivid clothing colors (fuchsia, turquoise, royal blue) your blush should ideally be in the same tonal family as your clothing to prevent an overly contrasted look.

Blush Mistakes to Avoid

1. Blush and lipstick colors should never clash; they should either complement each other or be in the same color family.
2. Never put blush close to or on the lines around the eye; it makes them look more evident, and if you are using a pink, peach, or coral shade of blush, the eye area can also look red and irritated.
3. Do not apply blush below the mouth or the laugh lines; blush is for the cheekbones only.
4. Do not blush your nose, forehead, hairline, or chin; it can make the face look overly pink or red or made-up. It may look great in professional photographs, but can look blotchy and uneven in daylight.

5. **Do not forget to use your sponge to blend out hard edges or smudges of blush. Blush should always be well-blended, with no visible edges where the blush starts and stops.**

LIPSTICK AND LIP PENCIL

I'd hardly lose the bet if I said most of you already know about lipstick, but I've talked to enough women to know that my next sentence needs to be said. Luckily, it's not complicated: If you're wearing makeup, your lips need lipstick—not lip gloss, but lipstick. Lip gloss doesn't last, but lipstick does. Lip gloss provides a sheer, temporary look that can be great but doesn't go with a full or classic makeup look. Lipstick (cream, matte, or semi-matte lipstick, not overly iridescent) provides a polished and put-together look that can last at least until your second cup of coffee. If your lips are naked while your eyes and cheeks are made up, you will look like you forgot you had a mouth when applying your makeup. For the sake of balance, remember lipstick.

Types of Lipstick

Are there differences among lipsticks? Well, yes! In fact, there are vast differences. As you probably already know from experience, lipstick colors and textures can vary even within the same cosmetics line. Some are creamy; others are dry, greasy, shiny, or flat. Some melt easily; others go on stickily, smearily, evenly, thickly, thinly, and all combinations thereof. I recommend lipsticks that go on creamily, in an even layer that doesn't smear or look thick or greasy. Whether or not to go with a matte or creamy finish is your own personal preference. True matte-finish lipsticks do last noticeably longer than creamy (and especially sheer) lipsticks. The only way to find out which ones you prefer is to be patient and try on various formulas in the colors you like and see how they feel and look. But whatever you do, avoid wearing overly shiny or glittery lipsticks, particularly if you are an adult with a serious career. Glaring iridescence is best reserved for evening, not for daytime.

Note: If your lipstick has a tendency to cake or to dry out as the day goes by, avoid reapplying more lipstick over partly worn-off lipstick. Wipe off all your lipstick first and then reapply. You may also want to apply a bit of lip balm under your lipstick if the problem of caking persists.

What about lipsticks with sunscreen? When it comes to sun protection, ignoring the lips is problematic. Not only is the skin on the lips very thin, it does not contain any melanin—essentially the rest of the skin's built-in defense against UV radiation. Although conventional, opaque lipsticks do provide a barrier (which is one of the reasons skin cancer on the lips is markedly higher in men than in women) for true sun protection, a lip balm with sunscreen applied underneath lipstick, or better yet a lipstick with built-in sunscreen is a must. A few cosmetics companies offer wonderful lipsticks with effective UVA/UVB sunscreens. The ones to look for are: Revlon Absolutely Fabulous Lip Cream SPF 15 *($8.99)*, Almay Protective Lip Tints SPF 25 *($4.99)*, and Cover Girl Triple Lipstick SPF 15 *($5.89)*. When checking an SPF-labeled lipstick, make sure the UVA-protecting elements of avobenzone, titanium dioxide, or zinc oxide are listed as one of the active ingredients. If they don't appear, or if they are listed anyplace other than the active ingredient list, you can't count on getting reliable sun protection.

What about ultra-matte lipsticks? Ultra-matte lipsticks are all essentially identical. They all go on moist and wet, then dry within a few seconds to form a dry, matte layer with no movement or creaminess. The dry texture does prevent transference to coffee cups, glasses, the food you eat, and the significant other you kiss. But it isn't indelible; this stuff does eventually rub off. Actually, it tends to chip or peel off. **Ultra-matte lipsticks are not for everyone, particularly not for those with a tendency toward chapped lips, because they will make the lips even drier.** Ultra-matte lipsticks can feel very uncomfortable during cold, dry winters or in hot, arid climates. Also, while ultra-matte lipsticks tend not to bleed, if you have wrinkles on or near your lips, these lipsticks will accentuate them. Due to trade-offs like this, which are inherent with ultra-matte lipsticks, many cosmetics companies have either reduced the number of or entirely discontinued these products. It seems that most women were not keen on putting up with the drawbacks in exchange for longer wear, and I understand the logic. However, if you have not done so already, you may want to consider the latest ultra-matte hybrids—the ones that use PermaTone technology to create truly long-lasting, comfortable color.

Permanent lipcolor: The world of lipstick changed considerably when Max Factor launched Lipfinity in early 2001. Shortly thereafter, Cover Girl (a sister company to Max Factor, as both are owned by Procter & Gamble) launched the identical (and less-expensive) Outlast lipstick.

What makes both of these products unique is that they use something called PermaTone technology to enhance application, wear, and—most significantly—comfort. PermaTone is a silicone-based ingredient complex that provides semipermanent color by gently attaching color pigments to the lips in a flexible mesh effect. The PermaTone "sets" (after approximately 60 seconds), yet the flexible mesh means the color is able to move and breathe, so that it doesn't dry or cake. Once the color has set, you apply a special top coat, an emollient, clear lip balm that does not disturb the color and provides a soft, glossy finish and comfortable wear. This top coat does not contain ingredients like mineral oil or petrolatum that could break down the color, which is good. But you may definitely need such ingredients to provide some extra help to remove it at the end of the day!

As great as this all sounds, there are some drawbacks to be aware of. First, these formulas offer opaque coverage and are not forgiving of application mistakes. That means you need to get the color on evenly and correctly the first time, or it's back to square one. If your lips are at all chapped, Lipfinity and Outlast will look terribly uneven, so be sure your lips are perfectly smooth and dry—no lip prepping with lip balms or Chap Stick because this will prevent the color from adhering to and setting on the lips. Once you have mastered the color application, you may find you need to reapply the moisturizing top coat frequently, which means you'll be using up more top coat than color (a common complaint from Lipfinity aficionados). Thankfully, you can purchase the special top coat separately. If you're willing to practice with this new breed of semipermanent lipsticks, you will find that unless you're eating very oily foods (such as salad with oil and vinegar dressing), they really do last all day (and often all night or into the next morning!) if properly applied. There is much less chance of cracking or peeling color with these when compared to traditional ultra-matte lipsticks, thanks mostly to the ingenious top coat. Lipfinity and Outlast come in a broad range of shades, and can be removed with plain mineral oil, Vaseline, or most other nonvolatile oils. If long-lasting lip color is important to you, these are a must-try.

Choosing Lip Colors

When choosing lipstick colors, there are three basic rules. (1) Thinner or smaller lips look best with brighter, more vivid colors. Brighter colors may take a bit of getting used to, but they truly make a smaller mouth more noticeable. Occasionally I read about or hear makeup advisors suggesting that women should wear a neutral color on small lips and instead play up the eyes (as if the notion is ever to play down the eyes or ignore the mouth!). Test this technique for yourself before you give in to this nonsense. (2) Avoid darker colors on thin lips; they make the mouth look severe and harsh. (3) Larger lips can wear just about any color, but softer shades look better because darker or vivid colors can make large lips look too prominent.

Applying Lip Color

A lip brush or lip pencil is an optional accessory. You can use a lip pencil to draw a definitive edge around the mouth to follow when applying lipstick, and a lip brush to control your application. A tube of lipstick makes too wide a mark for some lips and too narrow a mark for others. If your lips are small, it is best to use a lip brush; if your lips are large, the only reason to use a lip brush is to improve your accuracy.

If you do choose to work with a lip pencil, always place the color on the actual outline of your mouth. Do not use corrective techniques that make the mouth look larger or longer, especially for daytime makeup. **If you try to change the outline of your mouth with a lip pencil by drawing outside the lips, some time later when your lipstick wears off, the lipliner, which almost always lasts longer than the lipstick, will still be in place and it will look like you missed your lips.** Always line the lips following their actual shape, then fill in the lipstick color, using either the tube or a lip brush.

What about the center outline of the mouth? Do you round the point of the lips or make the point more obvious? As a general rule, a softer appearance is better than a hard one. Leave the points neither rounded nor pyramid-like—someplace in between with a soft arch is best.

To prevent lipstick from gunking up in the corners of the mouth, don't place lipliner or pencil in that area. Stop before you get to the very corners of the mouth. If you feel doing this makes you look as if you have missed a spot, carefully fill in this area with color using a lip brush, but only the smallest amount.

Lip pencils should never create an obvious dark, brown, or clearly visible line around the mouth. Delineations like this keep showing up as if they were the latest thing, and women hold on to the look for some unknown reason, but I've yet to see a professional makeup artist choose this design. **Your lip pencil should not make an obvious line that shows up as a colored border around the lipstick. The goal is to have the lipstick and lip pencil meld so that you can't see where one starts and the other stops.**

If you wear lipliner and you want to help your lipstick last longer, apply the lip pencil all over the lip area, including the outline of the lips, and then apply your lipstick over it. This extra step puts a more permanent color on the lips, so the lipstick won't wear off as quickly as it normally does. **With the exception of Lipfinity and Outlast, there is no such thing as an all-day lipstick.** Even Lipfinity can present some reapplication issues if you eat oily foods, and there is still the issue of touching up with the moisturizing top coat. For years the cosmetics industry has been proclaiming new "all-day" or "long-wearing" lipsticks, yet women continually need to reapply their lipstick. To date it remains impossible for 99.9% of all lipsticks to make it past lunch, or even past midmorning, still looking the same as when you first put them on.

How can you stop lipstick from traveling into the lines around your mouth? The first step is to stop wearing greasy lipsticks and lip glosses. **The greasier the lipstick or lip pencil, the faster the color will slip into the lines around your mouth.** The drier-feeling lipsticks are best for conquering this problem. Powdering the mouth with loose powder before applying the lipstick also helps, but can be a bit messy. Lip pencil will not stop greasy lipsticks from traveling, but can slow them down.

Several years ago, some cosmetics companies came out with new products that were supposed to prevent lipstick from bleeding. I tried a lot of them and many never worked, but I finally found three that changed the way I wear lipstick. Regrettably, all of the options I used to love are no longer made. Refusing to be dismayed by this, I simply found out which company produced the formula (there are only a handful worldwide that make almost all cosmetic pencils) and added the formula I loved to my own line. If you were a fan of products like Coty's Stop It, Revlon ColorLock, or The Body Shop's No Wander, you should consider trying my Long-Lasting Anti-Feather Lipliner in Clear.

Does using a lipstick brush help keep lipstick on longer? Why using a brush would have this effect has never been explained to me in a manner that makes any logical sense, and it simply doesn't work. What does make lipstick stay on longer? When you wear strong, vivid colors that are not greasy, avoid wearing lip glosses, and put on a lot of lipstick!

Lipstick and Lip Pencil Mistakes to Avoid

1. Do not use a lip pencil that contrasts with your lipstick; it has been unfashionable since the 1980s and it almost always looks severe and gives a contrived appearance to the mouth area.
2. Do not wear lipstick that is a different color tone from the rest of your makeup. For example, if you are wearing a rose-toned blush, wear a rose-toned lipstick.
3. Do not use lip gloss in place of lipstick during the day; it can bleed and won't last as long as lipstick.
4. Do not wear noticeably iridescent lipstick; when it wears off, it can look dry, white, and caked; it also looks too distracting for daytime.
5. Do not exaggerate or change the shape of your mouth with your lip pencil or lipstick; it will look like you missed your mouth.
6. If you want your lipstick to last, wear more of it and don't blot; blotting takes off several layers before you've even left the house.

TOUCHING UP

As the day goes by, even the best-applied makeup can slip, fade, and get phone- or fingerprinted. Lipstick can become thick and clumped, too. Long days call for a few quick touch-ups to revive beautifully applied makeup. Following the steps below, in order, will revive the look you started with.

• If you have oily skin, blot away the excess oil by laying either a tissue or one of the face-blotting papers sold by some cosmetics companies over the face and blotting. Perm endpapers also work well. Do this before you do anything else.
• Remove all of your lipstick so you can start over after you have touched up your face makeup. Apply a light layer of lip balm if your lips feel dry.
• Once the excess oil on your skin has been absorbed, take a fresh sponge and smooth out the foundation, blush, and contour (women with dry and normal skin should also follow this step). Use a gentle buffing motion, making sure to smooth things as you go.
• Apply a little extra concealer under the eyes if that area looks a bit dark.
• If you need a little more foundation over blemishes or discolorations, blend it on now, avoiding the blush and contour area.

- Dust a light layer of pressed powder over the face. A pressed powder with an SPF 15 including UVA-protecting ingredients of avobenzone, titanium dioxide, or zinc oxide is an excellent option to ensure all-day sun protection.
- Apply more blush or contour if needed, but *only* if needed, and be careful; color "grabs" more over makeup that has been on the face awhile.
- If you want to touch up your eyeliner, particularly under the eyes where it might have smeared, use a powder shadow instead of a pencil. Use the corner or side of your makeup sponge to remove any smeared eyeliner.
- If your eyeshadows have creased, blot the area gently with a tissue or blotting paper and then use a brush to smooth out the color. Apply a powder over the area to even out the shadows and add whatever color is needed to make the eye makeup look balanced.
- Finally, reapply your lipstick and lipliner.

Note: If you are wearing an ultra-matte foundation, you may find that touch-ups are tricky because ultra-matte makeup doesn't move and re-blending is almost impossible. In that case, you may very well be stuck with starting over. But it's worth a shot to see if you can blend things smoothly and do a simple touch-up. For me, ultra-matte foundations stay so well that my makeup never slips in the least once it's in place.

TURNING DAYTIME MAKEUP INTO NIGHT MAKEUP

All right, you've touched up your makeup, but suppose you now want to change it from your office or daytime look to a knockout evening visage? Here are some ideas to consider.

- Add a dark or black shade of eyeshadow to the back corner of the lid or in the crease.
- Use the same shade of dark or black eyeshadow to create a more dramatic line around the eye.
- Use a wedge or angle brush to add extra definition to the arch of your eyebrows, or add a bit more brow powder to the ends of your brows (but don't overdo it).
- Use a powder that has shine to add some shimmering highlights to the cheekbones, center of the forehead, chin, neck, shoulders, or décolletage.

- A vivid red lipstick always makes a dramatic evening look, especially if you are wearing black.
- Avoid overdoing your blush. Making the cheeks look overly colorful doesn't improve an evening look.
- Avoid applying more mascara, unless you're adept at doing so without creating a clumpy, spiky mess.

BALANCE, PROPORTION, AND DETAIL

Have you ever wondered exactly what it is you admire when you see a well-made-up woman? You may not be able to pinpoint what it is you find appealing, but you probably envy her skill and wish you could figure out how she did it. At the airport a few years ago, I noticed such a woman and watched other women (and a few men) turn their heads and take notice. It wasn't just that she was attractive and her clothes were stylish, but her makeup in particular was impeccable. Her face looked smooth and was accented with rich, though subtle, blush and contour tones. All the colors, from her lipstick to her eyeshadows, softly mingled into a harmonious sweep of light to dark, with just the right amount of shading—not too much and not too little.

That's when it occurred to me that any woman can revitalize her makeup by going over a list of everyday makeup guidelines and just omitting the mistakes that detract from, rather than enhance, her appearance. Recognizing the nuances of a well-done makeup application versus one that is not so good can make all the difference in helping a woman look great all day long. Considering all the time most women spend buying makeup and wearing it, putting it on wrong just doesn't make sense.

Besides the essential rules regarding application and blending techniques, there are only three basic concepts you need to keep in mind to achieve a flattering look: balance, proportion, and detail. **Balance** is about making sure the different elements of your makeup go together and that no one aspect is more prominent than any other. In other words, if you are wearing a dark, rich, brownish red lipstick, you must choose blush in a harmonious color (shiny pink blush is not going to work with a lipstick in that color range). Meanwhile, make sure your eyeshadows accent the eyes so they don't get lost because too much attention is directed toward the lips. When colors and tones are in balance and no one aspect of the makeup shouts over another, you don't notice the makeup as much as you notice the woman. Don't forget little things, like lining the upper lashes if you line the lower lashes (otherwise the line underneath will look too heavy and obvious all by itself). If you choose to wear blush, blend the color well so it doesn't stand out as a visible swipe of color across your cheek.

Proportion is about the total package of selecting what to wear. It's about paying attention to symmetry, to how your makeup colors, wardrobe, and hairstyle work together. If you are wearing a classic, tailored business suit and the eyeshadows you have on range from tan to black, with a wine-colored lipstick and blush, that may indeed be a stunning combination, but a bit too dramatic and overpowering with what you're wearing. The same is true for someone with very light hair and fair skin: The color combination may be dramatic and beautiful, but it will look out of place in sunlight or office light. Proportion is making sure that everything works together, with nothing looking out of synch, so your makeup doesn't upstage you.

Detail is the most essential and perhaps the most difficult area because it takes so much effort and concentration. Pay attention to every nuance of your makeup. If necessary, apply your makeup using a magnifying mirror so you don't leave the house with eyeshadow sprinkles on your cheek or mascara smudges at the back corner of your eyelid. Do not be satisfied with doing a ten-minute makeup application in only five minutes when you're in a hurry. **If you don't have enough time to do your normal makeup routine, be ready to change your look; do only what you have time to apply well.**

I can't tell you how often women have asked me what they can do differently with their makeup, and my responses were that they needed to blend their foundation better because it looked patchy and uneven, or the eyeshadow area looked uncertain or too obvious. Often these women reply, "Things were just frantic this morning, and this was the best I could do." I then say, "I notice you have your blouse buttoned and your skirt zipped up." Typically their answer is, "Of course!" I in turn comment, "Well, even though you didn't have much time, you didn't leave the house undressed. You should apply the same rule to your face." It doesn't mean being late because of your makeup; it means doing less so it goes faster. But whatever you do, take the time to do it right. Because when makeup is sloppy, it just looks wrong.

I use several levels of makeup application, depending on the time I have and what the makeup is for. For me, and I've done this a lot, full makeup for a television appearance takes 20 to 25 minutes. Makeup for a business meeting or a formal event takes fifteen minutes. Makeup for casual daily business or informal get-togethers takes five to ten minutes. Makeup for running to the gym to work out takes a minute and a half (lipstick and mascara only).

Getting Your Makeup to Look the Way You Want It To

- Foundation color should always match the skin exactly—no exceptions. Watch out for lines of demarcation in any light, but most of all in daylight.
- Be sure your foundation is best for your skin type. If you have oily skin, do not use a foundation for dry skin, and if you have dry skin do not use a foundation for oily skin.
- Concealer and foundation should blend together seamlessly. Be sure your concealer is not too light or white and is not a noticeably different texture than your foundation.
- Colors on the face should blend softly and without stop-and-start lines; that is, no stripes of blush or eyeshadow.
- Go light with the powder. After you find a foundation that matches your skin exactly and blend it on smoothly and sheerly, loading your face with powder would negate all your previous efforts. As a rule of thumb, the more wrinkles you have on your face, the less powder you should wear. Shiny powders (even the subtle ones) can magnify large pores as well as wrinkles and lines on the face.
- Powder should either match the color of your foundation or should be transparent and sheer enough to have no color effect on the foundation at all.
- Powder without any added oil is best for oily skin; powder with some amount of oil is best for dry skin.
- Blend, blend, and blend again.
- I know you have been staying away from shiny eyeshadows if you have wrinkles on your eyelids (right?), but many cosmetics lines are busily adding them to their collections and calling them matte, even though they have some shine. I highly recommend staying away from them. No matter how minimally shiny they may appear in the container, once they are on your eyelid, the shine will make the skin look wrinkly, plus

they don't wear as well as matte eyeshadows during the day. Unless that's the look you want (and you can always check this out in daylight) don't wear them.

- Always check for eyeshadow that may have flaked onto your cheek while you were applying it.
- If your eyebrow and eyeliner pencils are smearing during the day, try using powder instead. Why continue using products of any kind that don't hold up during the day?
- Thickly clumped-on mascara does not look like defined, long eyelashes. A neat, clean application will look far more appealing.
- Consider avoiding heavy, greasy lip glosses. Even if you're young, these can look sloppy and messy.
- Greasy lipstick or gloss can look wet and slippery as opposed to creamy and smooth. Be certain your lipstick looks soft, not damp. Also, the greasier the lipstick, the more quickly it will come off.
- Lipliner is a nice touch, and using a lip brush can provide a great professional flair. If you don't have time, you can apply lipstick evenly from the tube and still look terrific.
- Dark lipsticks can be quite attractive, but if they are too dark they can make you look cadaverous unless you are going "Gothic" on purpose. Also, wearing dark lipliner with a lighter shade of lipstick hasn't been in fashion since 1980, and even then it looked peculiar. It is too obvious and makes your mouth look hard and severe.
- When you apply makeup, take into consideration how it will look by midday and at the end of the day. Don't buy products that look great for an hour or two but by lunchtime make you look like you forgot to wash your face the night before. If you have a problem with eyeliner or mascara that smears, reconsider the products you use or the look you are trying to achieve.
- Don't trust the color if it doesn't make sense on your skin. If you buy a gray eyeshadow and it goes on blue, even though it looks gray in the container, it isn't gray, it is blue. Likewise with a foundation that is the right color in the bottle but looks peach, ash, or rose on your skin. Believe what you see on your face, not what you see in the container. If it is not right for you, take it back for a refund or exchange. And always check how the color looks on your skin in daylight—it's the least forgiving, but most realistic, way to gauge if the color you've chosen is a keeper.

CHOOSING COLOR

Finally, we come to the most difficult subject of all to discuss, at least on paper. I would love to have the time to sit down and create a makeup look that works for everyone. That isn't humanly possible, but I do have some rules that can help you create the makeup look you want.

- Foundation matches the skin exactly so there are no lines of demarcation. (I know this is getting repetitive, but I can't emphasize this point enough.)
- Concealer is only a shade or two lighter than the foundation.
- Powder should match the foundation exactly or go on transparent so it does not affect the color of foundation in the least.
- Eyeshadow colors should be neutral shades ranging from pale beige to tan, brown, dark brown, and black (and the thousands of shades in between).
- Eyebrow color should match the exact shade of the existing brow hair, unless your brows are naturally blonde, in which case the brow color should be slightly darker.
- Eyeliner on the upper lid should be a darker color (all the way to black, depending on the look you want) than the line along the lower lashes, which should be a softer shade of brown or gray.
- Blush can be almost any color as long as it coordinates in some logical fashion with the lipstick color, but it must be blended on softly, without any noticeable edges whatsoever.
- Lipstick can be bold to neutral—there is a fantastic range of great colors. When you're choosing, remember that smaller lips should wear brighter shades than larger lips.
- Less is best.
- To create a tanned appearance, use golden brown and chestnut shades for your blush, eyeshadows, contour, and lipstick. Never apply a foundation or bronzer all over the face if that means you'll end up with a line of demarcation at the jaw or hairline.
- It is best not to clash color tones. For example, if the outfit you are wearing is peach or coral, your blush and lipstick should have that same underlying color tone or be neutral enough not to clash.

Color Mistakes to Avoid

1. **Don't wear white or very pale lipstick with a white cast to it. This can look ghostly and ghastly.**

2. Don't wear blue, green, or overly pastel anything, including eyeliner, eyeshadow, and mascara.

3. Avoid navy blue eyeshadow. (Stick with black—it looks smoky, while navy just tends to look ashen.)

4. Don't wear dark brown or black lipstick. (On Dracula it's great; on women it may suggest a cartoonish appearance.)

5. Don't wear shiny eyeshadows (they exaggerate any wrinkles around the eye); they may be fun occasionally, but only if you have smooth, unlined eyelids.

6. Don't wear rainbow-style eyeshadow designs.

7. Don't wear eyeshadow applied as a smudge of black around the eye (unless the members of your rock band insist on it).

8. Don't wear blush and lipstick colors that clash; they should be in the same color family, not glaring opposites.

CORRECTING SOME POPULAR MAKEUP MYTHS

• Some makeup artists declare that you shouldn't be afraid to touch your makeup. The truth is, you should be very careful about touching it. After you've taken time to apply your foundation smoothly with a sponge and your eyeshadows evenly with brushes, there's no reason to use your fingers unless it's absolutely necessary, and only lightly at that. Touching your face during the day will rub off all your nicely applied makeup. In a pinch, clean fingers can be used to soften color or smooth out mistakes, but use a light touch.

• Don't spray water or toner on makeup to set it or freshen things up. It doesn't work. A mist of water can streak foundation, powder, and mascara. How this makeup myth got circulated is anyone's guess!

• Don't change every part of your makeup with every season. If you want to go softer during the spring and summer, that's fine, but it isn't an absolute must. Makeup should reflect how you want to be seen by the world and what makes you feel good—not a seasonal dictate.

• Don't use makeup to correct the shape of anything on your face, especially the lips. Close up and in person you can absolutely tell when lipstick has been applied beyond or inside the natural lip line. If you overcontour, you will look like you have brown stripes all over your face.

• Don't use foundation or color correctors to change the color of your skin. Foundation must match the underlying skin tone exactly. That will soften any skin discoloration or redness. If you have yellow or olive skin there's nothing you can or should do to change it. It's best to accept it and work with it for your own look. Even if you succeeded in changing the color of your face, it would look strange next to your neck and along the hairline.

- To keep pencil eyeliner in place, many makeup artists recommend going over it with a matching powder eyeshadow. That works, but why do two steps when only one is needed? Forget the pencil and just use dark eyeshadow to begin with.

- Glowing skin does look nice, but mostly just in pictures. In real life, the same skin looks like it is covered with glitter. That isn't bad, but it isn't as appealing as the pictures make it seem, and any wrinkles will be illuminated, too. It is an option for an evening out, but that's about it.

- No single set of colors is absolutely right for any skin color. The days of being typed into one color grouping are long gone. Just because you have red hair doesn't mean you *have* to wear corals and avoid blue-red lipstick. It's all up to experimentation and finding what looks best. Quite honestly, most women can wear just about any color they want to, as long as they pay attention to color intensity and application and adjust the details accordingly.

GROWING UP IN THE MILLENNIUM

In our society, for young girls on the perilous journey from preadolescence and adolescence to young adult status, one of the emotional pitfalls is the social pressure and self-awareness that precipitates wearing makeup. Putting on blush, lipstick, mascara, and eyeshadow has become one of the primary rites of passage that marks the moment when changing hormones begin to influence both mind and body. As this new style of expression is developing, teenage anxiety begins to take on a whole new depth (witness a teen's explosive desperation at a single perceived insult or problem). What do you do when the little girl in your life (who is looking less and less like a little girl) wants to start wearing makeup? Particularly when her sensitivities are overflowing but her sophistication is lagging? And it isn't just that she *wants* to wear makeup— she *has* to. To make things even more confusing, teenagers continually demonstrate an inexplicable duality of independence and fierce individualism, while at the same time buying only what everyone else is wearing. How many times have you heard the teen in your life proclaim loudly that she doesn't care what anyone else thinks, while at the same time she refuses to wear anything else but the same style of makeup, shoes, skirts, blouses, sweaters, and dresses her friends or her latest rock-star idol is wearing? Too many to count!

Feeling attractive is an overwhelmingly important aspect of life for many teenage girls. It is often complicated by well-meaning adults who don't quite know what to do or say. "You look beautiful, you don't need to wear makeup" is just as irksome as "A little pink blush, rose lipstick, and brown mascara will make you look beautiful." The first statement, "You look beautiful just the way you are," comes off as a thunderous lie. It discounts what the teenager sees all around her on television and in magazines—that women can look more exciting and glamorous with makeup on (or why else would Mom and the rest of the world be wearing it?). The other comment about adding just a little color here and there suggests that the girl is unattractive and would be better off hiding her face behind a layer of cosmetics (albeit a small one). Then there's the ever-popular, "You can start wearing makeup when you're sixteen and that's that." At best, an arbitrary date like this ignores the specific needs and development of each teen.

What to do? I wouldn't recommend any of the above approaches, that's for sure. Instead, I suggest incorporating all three positions into a compassionate compromise. The goal is to acknowledge the teenager's needs, letting her know they are valid and important. Tell her something along the lines of "I know wearing makeup is important to you and it could look lovely on you. But at the same time I want you to know that I think you are beautiful just the way you are." Then the two of you can decide together what is appropriate, giving in a little as you go. Remember, what you think is important may not be what the teen thinks is important. Gloss yes, lipstick no; blush yes, but only a little; mascara yes, but only brown; concealer yes, but foundation no; and so on. Mostly this process is about being gentle and respectful of the teen's feelings as they arise (and not about trying to control or contradict).

Another option is going together to a professional makeup artist or makeup demonstration. This can be a positive experience as long as you are careful to ward off any attempt on the part of the salesperson to foster insecurity and vulnerability via sales techniques. Let the salesperson know ahead of time, in no uncertain terms, that you don't want her to use any language that suggests something is unattractive or wrong with any aspect of your teen's appearance. If the salesperson wants to introduce something different she can easily say, "I think a softer blush can be an attractive look," instead of "The blush you have on is all wrong for you." Don't let the counterperson get away with "You have small lids and a bright color will make them look larger," when a simple statement such as "A pale brown eyeshadow on the lid is a good color choice for you" can go a long way to build self-esteem instead of makeup addiction and insecurity.

If the age of your teen is of great importance to you in making your decision about when to allow makeup, you can put off the inevitable by intervening with an emphasis on skin care (which is a good starting point in general). Encouraging the everyday use of UVA-protective sunscreen, regular cleansing with a water-soluble cleanser, exfoliating gently with baking soda or an AHA or BHA product, and using 2.5% benzoyl peroxide over blemishes is a great way to start paying attention to beauty issues without getting into makeup, except maybe for mascara or lip gloss. At the same time, it is essential that you take the time to share information about how the cosmetics industry can take advantage of women and stress why it is a waste of money to buy expensive products. That combination is an excellent and beautiful introduction to the world of cosmetics.

You and your teen can even read one of my books or visit my Web site together, marking areas to discuss. If you reach a crossroads and cannot agree, seek out an impartial third party to mediate (preferably not male unless you're looking for a "Who cares?" response!).

Most of us grown-ups started off on the wrong foot with makeup and skin care, somehow learning incorrectly from the outset that it would make us perfect and correct all our flaws (of which there were always too many—eyes too close together or too far apart, nose too broad or too narrow, face too square or too round, skin too yellow or too pink, and on and on). We are now in a good position to hand the next generation a new measure of self-worth and to tell them the truth about cosmetics and what they can and cannot do. That's something the cosmetics industry probably isn't expecting.

chapter 16
PROBLEMS? SOLUTIONS!

WHEN SHOULD I THROW OUT A PRODUCT?

Problem: I've heard a lot of different information regarding when I should throw away a cosmetic. Is there a time limit when products should be thrown away?

Solution: There isn't an easy answer to this question because there are no regulations or agreed-upon guidelines on the expiration times for skin-care or makeup products, and the FDA has no rules on the issue whatsoever. Cosmetics companies generally test their products for stability, but some do one-year assays while others do three-year assays. Clouding the stability testing issue even more is that the cosmetics companies typically look only at temperature variables (freezing or overheating, for instance). The testing doesn't take into account how consumers use the products. Cosmetics that have been improperly stored—for example, exposed to sunlight, left open, or become contaminated (any product packaged in a jar has almost a 100% risk of being contaminated)—may deteriorate substantially before a year is up. On the other hand, products stored under ideal conditions may be acceptable long after the suggested "use by" dates. An additional stability issue, which is not related to stability testing, is that there is no way to tell how long a product has been sitting on a shelf before you buy it.

So what should you do? In general, it's best to toss out cosmetics that you place near the eye (mascara, for example) after four to six months, and to dispose of face products (moisturizers, foundations) after one to two years. The toss time for eye-area cosmetics is more limited than for other products because of repeated microbial exposure during use by the consumer and the risk of eye infections. Some industry experts even recommend replacing mascara after only three months from the date of purchase. Another thing, if mascara becomes dry, discard it. Don't add water or, even worse, saliva to moisten it, because that will introduce bacteria into the product. And if you have an eye infection, consult a physician immediately, stop using all eye-area cosmetics, and discard those you were using when the infection occurred.

Among other cosmetics that are likely to have an unusually short shelf life are certain "all-natural" products that contain plant-derived substances conducive to microbial growth. It's also important, for both consumers and manufacturers, to consider the increased risk of contamination in some "natural" products that contain nontraditional preservatives or no preservatives at all.

Sharing makeup also increases the risk of contamination, and the testers commonly found at department store cosmetics counters are even more likely to become contaminated than the same products in your home. If you must test a cosmetic before purchasing it, apply it with a new, unused applicator, such as a fresh cotton swab. But remember, these are merely suggestions; they are not based on any established research or guidelines (source: FDA *Office of Cosmetics Facts Sheet*, March 9, 2000, "Shelf Life-Expiration Date").

DARK CIRCLES

Problem: I have dark circles that seem to get worse as the day goes by! What can I do to make my concealer last?

Solution: Dark circles can be caused by several factors, and each needs to be dealt with in a different way. Dark circles can be caused by sun damage, veins and capillaries that show through skin, irritation, the natural dark pigment that can occur in this area, and by dry skin that just makes the area look dull and tired. Dark circles can also be the result of natural shadows that fall within the eye area due to the fact that the eye is set back and the brow bone can cast a shadow, making that area appear darker.

Be sure you are using a lightweight moisturizer (gel or silicone-based moisturizers are best) under the eye area; too much moisturizer or too heavy a moisturizer can make your concealer slide off. And always use a sunscreen over this area during the day, or wear sunglasses, to prevent the sun from stimulating melanin (dark pigmentation) production.

Matte-style (rather than creamy or greasy) concealers are best to cover natural shadows or natural dark pigmentation, and concealers such as Revlon ColorStay Concealer *($9.49)*, Maybelline Great Wear Concealer *($4.69)*, and Elizabeth Arden Flawless Finish Concealer *($14)* work particularly well. The color of the concealer must be light enough to cover the dark circles, but not so light that it gives the appearance of a white mask around the eyes. Avoid using greasy pencils along the lower lashes, and stay away from mascara that smears; these can both slide during the day, making the under-eye area even darker. Use only a powder to line the lower lashes, and then the thinnest line possible, or wear no lower liner at all. City pollution can get to your eyes by day's end, too, so you may want to consider using an air filter in your home or office (talk to the building or office managers to see if they are willing to accommodate this request).

If you have allergies that get worse as the day goes on, you may want to consider taking an antihistamine. Although uncommon, food allergies may also be to blame, but this would need to be confirmed by an allergist.

If all else fails, you may want to consider laser treatments for lightening (and in some cases eliminating) dark circles. Traditional skin-lightening products used for sun or hormone-induced skin discoloration do not have any effect on dark circles. For more information on lasers, refer to Chapter 13, Cosmetic Surgery.

LASHES FALLING OUT

Problem: My lashes are falling out! Is there anything I can do to stop this from happening?

Solution: It is natural for lashes to shed and then regrow, but if you are noticing bald spots along your lash line, you may need to change some habits that might be making the condition worse. For example, don't wipe off eye makeup (or any makeup, for that matter) because wiping and pulling at the eyes can pull out lashes. Don't rub your eyes, even if they itch, especially when you are wearing mascara. Also, do not overuse mascara. I know it's tempting to have long, dramatically thick lashes, but the weight of the mascara (and what it takes to remove it later) can be too much for delicate lashes. Waterproof mascaras are the most difficult to remove and often take many lashes with them, so you might want to consider changing mascaras. It is unlikely that you are allergic to your mascara, but on the remote possibility that it may be the cause of the fallout, switch brands and see how that works.

By the way, you aren't using an eyelash curler are you? Over time, that consistent tugging can certainly pull out lashes. Another possibility is that noncosmetic allergies could be playing a part in your eyelash dilemma. Your only recourse, if that turns out to be the cause, is to use antihistamines or eliminate from your environment the allergens causing the problem. For example, if you are allergic to the down in your pillows, use pillows with a synthetic fill. Hay fever can also cause the eye area to swell severely, damaging eyelashes, a problem that could be alleviated by using over-the-counter or prescription antihistamines.

Medically speaking, doctors refer to the loss of eyelashes as *madarosis*. According to ophthalmologist Dr. William Trattler, "While it may seem like mainly a cosmetic problem, the condition can be an indicator of something more serious, such as eye trauma, eyelid infections and even cancer of the eyelid. In addition, metabolic conditions such as hypothyroidism and pituitary insufficiency can cause madarosis" (source: http://ivillagehealth.com).

It is also possible that the eyelash loss can be attributed to the presence of a mite called *Demodex folliculorum*. When it is active in small hair follicles and eyelash hair follicles it can consume epithelial cells, causing the hair follicle to become swollen, inflamed, and plugged. All of this can cause the eyelashes to fall out. Fortunately, this problem is easily treated once correctly diagnosed (source: *eMedicine Journal*, May 11, 2001, volume 2, number 5).

If your loss of eyelash hair is chronic, you should see an eyelid specialist (called an oculoplastic surgeon) and have him carefully examine your eyelid to determine the cause of the madarosis.

SELF-TANNERS

Problem: I tried an expensive new self-tanner from a line called Decleor at Neiman Marcus. It just smelled so much better than the one I was using from Coppertone. Now my palms are striped, one leg is darker than the other, and my knees and elbows look mottled!

Solution: Believe it or not, the Decleor product, though absurdly expensive, is not at fault for your chameleon-like dilemma; rather, it is most likely due to uneven application. First, all self-tanners, regardless of price, use the same ingredient, dihydroxyacetone, to create the color change in your skin. The scent that attracted you to the Decleor product (some women tell me the Clarins, Origins, and Bain de Soleil self-tanners smell great, too) helps mask the naturally sweet smell of this ingredient. However, the fragrance is temporary and fades in a brief period of time. The color, on the other hand, affects the skin cells, and it takes time to get your skin back to its normal color. The cell itself changes color. Sloughing can remove altered skin cells, but at this point you can't quickly slough off all the layers of skin that have been affected. That takes time. Well-formulated AHA or BHA products can make mistakes fade faster and sometimes even remove them entirely. To a lesser extent, you can try baking soda mixed with Cetaphil Cleanser, sea-salt scrubs, and even a washcloth massaged over the problem areas twice a day—but, in most cases, time is the only real cure.

Once your skin is back to normal, you can try again. Remember that when it comes to self-tanners, application is everything! Be patient. Apply the self-tanner only over a clean, dry, exfoliated body, giving special attention to the knees, elbows, and heels. Do not apply self-tanner in a steamy, hot room where perspiration or condensation may make it run. Do one area of your body at a time. Watch what you are doing, and apply the self-tanner thoroughly and evenly. If you miss an area, you are going to look noticeably streaked or blotchy. Wash the palms of your hands as soon as you are done applying the self-tanner, and then stand still until it is completely absorbed, with no after-feel. Some women think that using a fast-darkening self-tanner is best because it changes the skin's color immediately and you can more easily see your mistakes and correct them. Others prefer a self-tanner that changes color slowly, so you can build a tan slowly and evenly. The choice is yours.

SERIOUSLY OILY SKIN

Problem: I have seriously oily skin in the T-zone (forehead, nose, and chin), and it is driving me crazy. I've tried matte foundations, even Lancôme MaquiControle, all kinds of oil-control gels and powders, and my face still feels like an oil slick by midday. Surely there must be something I can do?

Solution: Aside from doing all the right things (see Chapter 3, Skin Care Basics for Everyone), it is essential to be sure you aren't doing anything to your face to make matters worse. For example, if you are using a moisturizer, even an oil-free moisturizer, stop immediately. Your oil glands are already working overtime as a result of hormonal activity, and this oil is also your own built-in moisturizer. There is no reason to add more. If your oily skin is still driving you nuts, my favorite trick is to take milk of magnesia (the one I recommend as a facial mask for oily skin) and apply an extremely thin layer of it over the most oily areas. Let it dry, and then apply your foundation over that. It works great! When it comes to powdering, try loose powder instead of pressed powder in a compact. Even when a pressed powder is oil-free, the waxlike ingredients that keep it in a pressed form can add to a slick feeling on the face. As a last resort, ask your dermatologist about medical options for taming oily skin, which range from birth control pills to hormone blockers and, in extreme cases, even Accutane.

SMALL LIPS

Problem: I have small lips. Any lipstick color I put on seems to make this more noticeable. What should I do?

Solution: The best way to deal with small lips, is to not overline them to make them look larger. That technique of creating a new lipline works great in photographs, but in real life it looks like you missed your mouth. Also, to maintain the look, you have to diligently touch up your lipstick and use your pencil the moment any wears off. What works best is lining just to the outside or edge of your true lipline with a natural-colored lipliner. Do not wear dark lipstick, because dark colors applied to any surface make it look smaller. A true red or any vivid color will make your lips look bigger. Of course you can always consider cosmetic surgical procedures that enlarge lips, but that should be a last resort after experimenting with lipstick options.

FLAKING EYESHADOW

Problem: Whenever I apply eyeshadow, I always find eyeshadow sprinkles on my cheeks and under-eye area. What am I doing wrong?

Solution: Sprinkles are almost inevitable, but knocking the excess powder off the brush before you apply your eye makeup will help a lot. Some eyeshadows are more powdery than others and cause more sprinkles. Eyeshadows made by M.A.C., Physicians Formula, Shu Uemura,

Bobbi Brown, Jane, Iman, and Paula's Select are more reliable in this respect. Another technique that some makeup artists use is to apply foundation and concealer to the eye area first; then the eyeshadow, liner, and mascara; after that, apply foundation to the rest of the face, touching up the concealer if "drippies" have made a mess of things. Although I find that approach time-consuming, it does help eliminate any trace of stray eyeshadow.

BLEEDING LIPSTICK

Problem: I like a sheer lipstick look, but every one I've tried (and I've tried them all) just feathers into the lines around my mouth and looks like a mess! I've tried several of the ultra-matte lipsticks, but they look so hard and dry, and pencils are useless. I'm too young to have this problem. Is there something out there I've missed?

Solution: No, you haven't missed anything; sheer lipsticks (which are just glosses in a stick form), both the expensive and inexpensive ones, are slippery by nature and don't stay put. Pencils are helpful, but they can't block a creamy, glossy lipstick all day. If you have any lines around your mouth—and that's not necessarily related to age—sheer, creamy lipsticks and lip glosses in general will follow those pathways. Your only option is to give up the notion of a completely sheer look. Try a semi-matte lipstick such as Clinique Long Lasting Soft Matte, M.A.C. Matte, or Revlon Absolutely Fabulous LipCream. Once you apply it, blot with a tissue until it looks more or less sheer. I know it won't have the sheen you're looking for, but it also won't travel into the lines around your mouth. Don't try to put a gloss over it; that will only encourage the lipstick to bleed. Matte lipstick isn't a shield that's impervious to the effect of the gloss. Gloss creates movement no matter what it goes over. Perhaps the best option is Cover Girl's Outlast or Max Factor's LipFinity. These are semipermanent lip stains that don't move and really do stay on, and on, and on. These are discussed more fully in Chapter 15, Makeup Application Step by Step in the section "Lipstick and Lip Pencil."

BLOODSHOT EYES

Problem: I have red, bloodshot eyes that just look awful. It seems to have nothing to do with sleep and I don't drink alcohol, so what am I doing wrong, or, better yet, what should I be doing right?

Solution: Many things can cause the blood vessels in the eye to swell and look more obvious. Lack of sleep and alcohol consumption are only two possibilities; there are lots more. For example, contact lenses, exposure to smoke, rubbing the eyes, allergies, dry air (from heat or air-conditioning), makeup particles getting in the eye and causing irritation, bad pollution days, staring at a project or computer monitor all day without giving your eyes a break, and overusing eyedrops can all make the tiny blood vessels in the eye look like roadmaps.

A humidifier in your home or office can help, and so can remembering to blink regularly during the day, especially when working at the computer. Not wearing contact lenses all day, using antihistamines for allergies, keeping your hands away from your eyes, and zealously keeping makeup out of your eyes are all exceptionally helpful. To reduce dryness, the "natural" tear products and eyewashes found at the drugstore are a great option (but use only disposable eyecups; repeatedly using the same eyecup can cause or aggravate problems such as eye infections or irritation). Eyedrops such as Visine used repeatedly can actually aggravate the problem by causing a rebound effect, making the blood vessels swell even more (sources: Visine product warning label; *Ophthalmology,* November 1991, pages 1364–1367). You would want to use Visine-type products only occasionally, not as a regular routine.

PUFFY EYES

Problem: I have puffy eyes every morning that sometimes don't go away until midday. They look awful and I've tried lots of eye products that don't change a thing.

Solution: There are no cosmetics or miracle eye moisturizers that can alter puffy eyes, but lots of things, including water retention, can cause the skin around the eye area to swell. Lack of sleep is probably not as big a factor for puffy eyes as it is for bloodshot eyes. If anything, sitting up instead of lying down would prevent fluids from collecting in the tissues around the eye. Of course, no one should sit up day and night! Sleeping with your head slightly elevated, and making sure you give your neck the support it needs, can help prevent fluid retention. Alcohol consumption and a diet high in salt also can cause water retention and increase the puffiness around the eyes.

Another factor to consider is contact lenses, which can cause irritation and swelling of the eye, so be sure you are wearing the most comfortable type available for your vision correction. As with bloodshot eyes, exposure to smoke, rubbing the eyes, allergies, dry air (from heat or air-conditioning), makeup particles getting in the eyes, allergic reactions to skin-care or makeup products, bad pollution days, leaving makeup on overnight (which can cause inflammation), and using irritating skin-care products around the eyes can all make the eye area swollen.

Be sure to take your makeup off meticulously at night, don't rub your eyes during the day, and take an antihistamine if you have allergies. If you are allergic or sensitive to certain skin-care or makeup products, avoid them.

Preventing dryness around the eyes can also help reduce irritation and swelling that can cause a puffy appearance. If that's your problem, a lightweight, fragrance-free moisturizer will help a lot. Be certain the moisturizer does not contain any irritating ingredients that could make matters worse, such as witch hazel, volatile plant oils, and sensitizing plant extracts like lemon oil or menthol. If you have time in the morning, place cool compresses on the eyes (low temperatures can make the skin contract); if you don't have time for that, leave your moisturizer in the refrigerator so it's cool when you apply it in the morning.

If none of these things help alleviate the problem, it may be that your eyes are just naturally puffy. Most typically this results from overly large fat pads around the eye (everyone has fat pads around the eye) creating a puffy-looking bulge. If that's the case, the only way to get rid of the problem is with cosmetic surgery, which in most cases is incredibly effective at eliminating the problem.

CHAPPED LIPS

Problem: What should I do about my eternally chapped lips? No matter what I use, the chapping never goes away.

Solution: Whether they are responding to cold weather, an arid climate, or are just naturally dry, chapped lips are a pain. Cracking, flaking, and chapping are not only uncomfortable but also unsightly, and lipstick only seems to make the situation worse. You can solve those dry-lips blues with consistency and patience. Chapped lips are not going to disappear in a day, and missing even one day of treatment can drive lips back to dryness.

Lips are more vulnerable to the environment than any other part of the face. This means that keeping your lips moist and sealed against the weather is essential. There are lots of emollient lip products that do just that, and the more emollient they are, the better. Ingredients like lanolin, oils of any kind (including castor oil, lanolin oil, safflower oil, almond oil, and vegetable oil), and shea and cocoa butter are all excellent, especially if they are listed at the beginning of the ingredient list. However, many lip products are little more than waxy coatings that make lips feel thick and protected when they are applied (Chap Stick is a great example), but they don't really moisturize or provide adequate protection from the weather or from the dry heat and air-conditioning you find indoors.

Lots of lip products also claim to be medicated. "Medicated," however, is a dubious term at best, and it has no regulated meaning. These "medicated" products usually contain camphor, menthol, peppermint oil, eucalyptus, but these are not medicines for dry lips! They mostly irritate and can actually make lips burn, which is neither disinfecting nor helpful for lips that are already dry and chapped. Products like Blistex, which includes 0.5% phenol, are the exception, because they truly are medicated; phenol kills anything that gets in its way. However, phenol is strong stuff and actually can trigger serious irritation and dryness all by itself. It is not something I would recommend for anything but extremely limited use.

You may have heard a rumor that lips can adapt to or become addicted to lip balm. It isn't possible. But if the lip balm you are using contains irritating ingredients (and lots of them do), your lips will stay dried up. When a lip product contains irritating, drying ingredients, there is no way the other, more emollient ingredients can help. Likewise, if you are using a lip product that is just waxy, with no emollients or water-binding agents, it can only plaster down the dry skin; it doesn't reduce the dryness.

I am quite fond of BeautiControl's LipApeel. This two-step product exfoliates the chapped skin with a waxy cream you rub over the lips; then, after that's rubbed off, you apply a very emollient balm. It is one of the only really gentle and effective exfoliating products I've ever seen for lips. It's a bit pricey, but it can last for years. BeautiControl's ordering number is (800) BEAUTI-1. I also developed two products for my Paula's Choice skin-care line that work similarly, Protective Lip Balm SPF 15 (with titanium dioxide) and Exfoliating Treatment.

At night you can apply almost any lip balm that contains some of the emollients I mentioned above, but no irritants. **For daytime care, it is best**

to use an SPF 15 lip balm that contains avobenzone, titanium dioxide, or zinc oxide. However, if you wear an opaque lipstick, it may not be essential to have that kind of SPF protection. Research has shown that women who apply lipstick more than once a day are at a much lower risk of getting lip cancer than women who apply lipstick only once a day (source: *Cancer Causes and Control*, July 1996, pages 458–463). Theoretically, opaque lipsticks have enough sun-blocking protection to enable them to screen out the sun's skin cancer–causing rays. Still, you may as well play it safe and use a lip balm or lipstick with sunscreen daily, especially if you are outside for long periods of time in the sun or if you live in a sunny climate.

DRY SKIN AROUND THE LIPS

Problem: For some time now I have had a strange red, dry irritation, just along the skin around my mouth. Moisturizers don't seem to help.

Solutions: One of the first things you can do is determine whether you've developed an allergic reaction to fluoride toothpaste. Fluoride can cause irritation around the mouth. Try a fluoride-free toothpaste for a while and see what happens. If that seems to be the solution, check with your dentist to see how this will affect your dental health.

The dryness and irritation around your mouth could also be caused by a significant other who happens to have a rough beard. There isn't much you can do about that, but occasionally using a little cortisone cream around the area can help minimize the irritation from almost any source. Another possibility is frequent, unconscious licking of the lips. Saliva can be an irritant for the lips, causing flaking and dryness. Lip balm won't be able to keep up with this bad habit.

If the area around the mouth is dry and irritated, that can also affect the lips. What's important here is to treat the root of the problem, which in this situation may require using an emollient moisturizer around the edge of the mouth as well as a lip exfoliant and lip balm for the lip area.

PERIORAL DERMATITIS—
RED BUMPS AROUND THE MOUTH

Problem: I can't seem to get rid of these red, swollen, sometimes crusty bumps around my lips and at the sides of my nose. Nothing seems to help, including over-the-counter acne products and cortisone creams. What can I do?

Solutions: What you describe sounds like an almost classic case of perioral dermatitis. According to the American Academy of Dermatology (http://www.aad.org) "Perioral dermatitis [POD] is a common skin problem that mostly affects young women [20 to 45 years of age]. Occasionally men or children are affected. Perioral refers to the area around the mouth, and dermatitis indicates redness of the skin. In addition to redness, there are usually small red bumps or even pus bumps and mild peeling. Sometimes the bumps are the most obvious feature, and the disease can look a lot like acne. The areas most affected are within the borders of the lines from the nose to the sides of the lips, and the chin. . . . Sometimes there is mild itching and/or burning."

POD is actually quite common and, according to most dermatologists, is increasing in incidence (source: *Australasian Journal of Dermatology*, February 2000, pages 34–38). While little is known about what causes this disorder, there are theories that overuse or chronic use of topical cortisone creams, fluoridated toothpaste, or heavy or occlusive skin-care ointments and creams (especially those with a petrolatum or thick wax base) and foundations may be responsible. Exposure to sunlight, heat, and wind can also make matters worse (source: *eMedicine Journal*, August 1, 2001, volume 2, number 8).

You can experiment by stopping the use of any of the potentially problematic products mentioned above. It would be a great idea to stop using topical cortisone creams, but be advised that this step can initially make matters worse before any improvement takes place. That can feel self-defeating, but be patient, at least for a few weeks, to see if the condition finally improves.

It would also be helpful to find out if fluoridated toothpaste is the source of the problem. You can try brushing with fluoride-free toothpaste such as Tom's of Maine Natural Fluoride-Free Toothpaste *($2.99 for 4 ounces)* and see if that makes a significant difference. If fluoride-free toothpaste turns out to be the solution, check with your dentist to see how this will affect your dental health.

If these experiments lead you to suspect POD is indeed the cause of the bumps around your mouth and nose, it is best to see a dermatologist because there are no cosmetics or over-the-counter medications that can treat the condition. A dermatologist can prescribe topical metronidazole

(MetroGel, MetroLotion, or MetroCream), alone or in combination with either oral tetracycline or erythromycin. Even though topical cortisone creams may be the cause of POD, you may be prescribed a low-potency cortisone cream to reduce the inflammation and to help you wean off the stronger topical cortisone cream you may have been using (source: *Seminars in Cutaneous Medical Surgery*, September 1999, pages 206–209). For more information on POD, visit http://www.aad.org/pamphlets/ Perioral.html (this URL is case-sensitive).

EXPENSIVE VERSUS INEXPENSIVE

Problem: I'm not one to fall for a company's enthusiasm for its products, but surely some companies can have secret or special ingredients and formulas, or use more expensive, superior ingredients. A friend mentioned that her chocolate chip cookies contain flour, sugar, shortening, eggs, vanilla, chocolate chips, and nuts, but they still don't taste like Mrs. Fields'. I have used your inexpensive recommendations and they have worked great, but I am so tempted to buy the more expensive stuff!

Solution: I understand the concept your friend is suggesting when it comes to her cookies. However, some people may prefer Mrs. Fields cookies while others would prefer your friend's. If she does have a secret ingredient, that may taste great to you but not to someone else. When it comes to shopping for makeup and skin-care products, there are unquestionably great formulas out there that work better for different skin types and different needs, in all price ranges, but the notion that expensive is better isn't supported by any of the research I've seen or done. We know this is true, because we've all bought expensive products we didn't like. After interviewing dozens of cosmetics chemists and cosmetic ingredient manufacturers, I have yet to find any that agree with this theory that secret ingredients provide superior benefits for the skin. There are ingredients that can make a difference, but almost without exception they are accessible to every cosmetics manufacturer. Further, even if there were "secret ingredients," keeping them secret wouldn't be legal. According to the FDA, *every* ingredient except fragrance must be included on the ingredient list or the product would be subject to seizure.

I rate lots of expensive and inexpensive products as both excellent to poor, so I've come to know that judging by price alone can hurt your skin and waste your money.

USING DIFFERENT PRODUCTS
FROM DIFFERENT LINES

Problem: I've been following your advice and am using products from several different lines. My skin is doing great, but all the cosmetics salespeople say it is a mistake to mix and match. They say products are designed to work together, and that is what helps the skin best.

Solution: Stop listening to the cosmetics salespeople; they are wrong. If every line had SPF 15 sunscreens with the requisite UVA protection, gentle cleansers with nonirritating ingredients, foundations that aren't peach-colored, and on and on, I would agree that you don't need to mix and match. But I have found good and bad products in every line (and I've reviewed hundreds of cosmetics lines and thousands of products). Many lines don't have adequate sunscreens, have products that contain irritating ingredients, or offer rose, peach, and ashen foundation colors, though they may have superior mascara and blushes. Staying with the same line for all your skin-care or makeup needs almost always ensures that you end up with some bad products! Mixing and matching is the only way to go. You don't wear clothes from one designer, buy furniture from one manufacturer, take medicine from one pharmaceutical company, or eat food from just one company. The only way to develop a successful skin-care or makeup routine is to select what works best for your skin type and needs, not what one line happens to be selling.

FEELING BEAUTIFUL DURING
THE TRAUMA OF CANCER

Problem: I have a dear friend who has just been diagnosed with breast cancer. I want to be a support for her. I know how important feeling beautiful is for her. Any suggestions from you would be truly appreciated.

Solution: I've spoken with many women who have lived through the ordeal of radiation and chemotherapy, and they all agreed that paying attention to how they looked helped their emotional well-being a lot during the trauma of diagnosis and treatment. Having gone through this life-threatening event with my older sister, I had a reason to look further into these issues, and now I have the opportunity to share some solutions and possibilities with you and your friend. Given the number of women who have breast cancer or other cancers, surely most all of us know someone who can benefit from this information. One thing my sister found immensely helpful was talking openly about her cancer experience without embarrassment or reservation. Perhaps your friend or someone else in your life would appreciate that kind of support and openness.

Body care: Because chemotherapy and radiation make the skin ultra-sensitive and even sunburned, as a general rule it is best not to use any types of adhesives, tints, bleaches, waxes, harsh or irritating chemicals, or to take hot baths or showers. Even deodorants and shaving can be problems. Saunas, Jacuzzis, loofahs, strong soaps, and washcloths can also exacerbate irritation. Anything you can do to reduce the hyper-sensitivity will go a long way to making the skin feel soothed and less irritated.

Instead of bar soap, which can be extremely drying and harsh on sensitive skin, try a gentle liquid body cleanser such as Nivea Moisturizing Shower Gel, Dove Nutrium Body Wash, or Olay Daily Renewal Body Wash. Keep the skin moist with lightweight gels that don't trap heat, such as pure aloe vera (found at most health food stores). If the skin becomes dry, use a nonfragranced, nonirritating moisturizer (the fewer plants it contains, the better) such as Lubriderm Seriously Sensitive Moisturizing Lotion. Take tepid or slightly warm showers and baths, and try to enjoy cool baths whenever possible, adding a little bit of light oil, such as safflower or sunflower oil, to the water. Avoid heavy oils such as vitamin E. Despite the fact that vitamin E has a reputation for healing the skin and can help the skin after the radiation and chemotherapy are over (as can other antioxidants), in the midst of treatment keep in mind that vitamin E is a potential allergen, and that its occlusive attributes can trap heat in the skin when it needs to dissipate heat instead.

Many women worry that even washing the skin may increase irritation. It turns out that gentle washing is better for skin than just leaving it alone. According to an article in *Radiotherapy & Oncology* (March 2001, pages 333–339), "Washing the irradiated skin during the course of radiotherapy for breast cancer is not associated with increased skin toxicity [or irritation] and should not be discouraged."

To keep her skin feeling soft and light, one of the first things my sister and I did before she went in for her radiation was to buy silk underwear, including T-shirts, underpants, teddies, and pajamas. She had to give up wearing a bra because the irritation from the straps and the tightness around the breast was just too uncomfortable. The silk was not only soothing, it also helped her feel more feminine and attractive.

Hair care: Some women feel compelled to shave their head in anticipation of losing their hair. That can be the worst possible solution for dealing with the inevitable. Shaving your head may look exotic, but unless you plan to shave every day, it can itch like crazy when it starts to grow back between treatments. It's best to cut your hair very short and consider wearing designer baseball caps or wigs. Scarves always make it look like something is wrong, while baseball caps and wigs are quite normal nowadays.

By the way, the American Cancer Society can provide you with a free wig; call (800) 227-2345. The wigs have been donated and are clean, but use them as a springboard for finding one that is perfect for you. You can buy a wig at a specialty salon or wig shop, but the trick is to find a good one and go to someone who knows how to style it. Wigs almost always need to be cut and styled to match your face. If you live in or near a large metropolitan area, your absolute best option is to find out who styles wigs for the women in the Orthodox Jewish community. For religious reasons, many Orthodox Jewish women cover their own hair with a wig. The shatel-macher (wig maker) is a mainstay of the Orthodox community and knows better than anyone how to make a wig look natural and attractive. Just call the Orthodox synagogue in your area and ask for the number of the woman who styles wigs for the community. The larger the metropolitan area, the more choices there will be.

One woman told me that after she purchased her first quality wig (around $100 to $500), she was a changed woman. "Not only did it fit great, but it looked so real that no one could believe it was a wig. I still wear it now and then, and get the biggest kick out of telling people it's a wig."

When your hair starts growing back, you may find that it grows back in thicker and straighter or curlier than it was. As tempting as it will be to dye your hair or perm it, be patient. Wait for the hair to go through a few normal cycles of growth before using chemicals on it. The skin and hair may still be sensitive or altered by the radiation and chemotherapy, and could react in a way that can cause problems.

Skin care: All of my recommendations for gentle skin care are doubly true during radiation and chemotherapy. And it is even more imperative than usual to avoid the sun, because the skin can become photosensitive. Sunscreen is essential, and the less the body and face are exposed to the sun, the better. That means wearing hats, light, tightly woven cotton pants, and light, long-sleeved blouses whenever possible. Because the skin can become dry, it is important to follow my recommendations for dry-skin care, which include using a gentle cleanser, a skin-softening toner, an emollient moisturizer, and plant oils such as safflower, olive, or sunflower oil over dry patches.

Eyebrows and eyelashes: Accompanying the loss of hair on your head is the probable loss of eyebrows and eyelashes. Avoid the natural tendency to pencil in new brows, which look fake and dated. Instead, try powder shadows to draw on a soft arch of a brow. If you have any eyebrow hair left, consider using the colored brow gels from Bobbi Brown, Origins, or Paula's Select; these can add definition and shape to whatever hair you have left. Another option is to use a waterproof mascara or a waterproof eye pencil that matches your brow color. Although waterproof mascara and waterproof eye pencils can look slightly more artificial, they are worth trying because chemotherapy or other drugs can bring on menopause or menopausal symptoms, and the accompanying hot flashes, followed by profuse sweating, will wash the others away. This one takes some experimenting, so be patient until you find what works for you.

If you do lose your eyelashes, it's best to not use any mascara, even if you have a few lashes left, because gaps in your application will be quite noticeable and mascara can shorten the life of the lashes you still have. Instead, consider lining the eyes with a dark brown shade of powder that you draw on more as shading than as a line. Lining with a pencil or liquid liner and no mascara can look odd, but shading the eye with a dark powder can look smoky and defining without making the lack of lashes more obvious.

Remember that brows and lashes grow back quickly, so that part is the most temporary!

Makeup: When it comes to concealer, foundation, blush, lipstick, and the rest, do whatever you are used to doing. Not only will it make you feel good, it will also normalize much of the process.

One woman wrote me a wonderful e-mail about this issue: "I cannot stress enough the concept that *look good and feel better* really works. I thought I was doing OK and I was, until I found out what it felt like to go out in public with hair and makeup (eyebrows) that looked real. I never lost my sense of humor or my positive outlook; but when I got a great wig and wore makeup (and eyebrows), I felt fantastic."

One of the most powerful things you can do for yourself is to pay attention to your physical appearance and experiment to find what works.

Don't try to pretend that feeling and looking beautiful doesn't matter during this time or that it is a waste of your energy. It may provide some of your most pleasant and uplifting moments until you are on the other side of your treatment.

DOES HAIR DYE CAUSE CANCER?

Problem: I had a nurse tell me not to use any dark brown or black hair coloring because it might cause cancer. I read your book on hair care about this particular subject explaining there is nothing to worry about, but it seems to still be an issue in the medical world. Is *dark* hair color safe, or isn't it?

Solution: I would suggest that few, if any, of the 75 million women who color their hair on a regular basis even know that there is an issue about hair dye and its association with certain types of cancers. However, although the issue is real, what it means isn't settled or conclusive in any regard. The best I can do is to provide you with the information and research available that may help you make a final determination for yourself.

Much of this controversy began when a study conducted by the American Cancer Society found that women who used black hair dye for more than 20 years had a slightly increased risk of dying from non-Hodgkin's lymphoma and multiple myeloma (a bone-marrow tumor that is usually malignant). Researchers surveyed 573,369 women who completed questionnaires about their use of permanent hair dye. However, this same study concluded that women who dyed their hair showed a slightly *reduced* risk overall of dying of cancer than women who never used dyes (sources: *Journal of the National Cancer Institute*, February 2, 1994, pages 210–215; *Environmental Health Perspectives*, June-July 1994, volume 102, number 6–7).

Subsequent studies looking at hair dyes in general found no correlation and did not support any risk of any kind. An article in *FDA Consumer* magazine (January-February 2001) explained that in a " . . . study, published in the October 5, 1994, issue of the *Journal of the National Cancer Institute*, researchers from Brigham and Women's Hospital in Boston followed 99,000 women and found no greater risk of cancers of the blood or lymph systems among women who had ever used permanent hair dyes. Then in 1998, scientists at the University of California at San Francisco questioned 2,544 people about their use of hair-color products. After integrating the results of this study with those of animal and other epidemiological studies, they concluded that there was little convincing evidence linking non-Hodgkin's lymphoma with normal use of hair-color products in humans. The study was published in the December 1998 issue of the *American Journal of Public Health*."

There have also been other subsequent studies showing hair dye to have no association with cancer or other diseases. One noted that: "The lack of an association between exclusive use of a single type of hair coloring application and breast cancer risk argues that hair coloring application does not influence breast cancer risk among reproductive-age women. Thus, the results of the present study, as well as negative ones from most (but not all) prior studies, are most consistent with the conclusion that neither hair coloring application nor hair spray application influences breast cancer risk" (source: *Cancer Causes and Control*, December 1999, pages 551–559). Another stated: "We found no evidence that permanent hair dye use, age at first use, frequency of use, or duration of use is associated with the development of systemic lupus" (source: *Arthritis and Rheumatism*, April 1996, pages 657–662).

This issue was given new life in February 2001 when researchers from the University of Southern California (USC) reported a link between the use of permanent hair coloring and bladder cancer. "They analyzed questionnaires from 897 patients with bladder cancer and compared them to questionnaires from 897 similar individuals without bladder cancer. They found that individuals with bladder cancer were three times as likely to have used permanent hair dyes at least once a month for 15 years or more. In addition, subjects who worked for 10 or more years as hairdressers or barbers were five times more likely to have bladder cancer than people who were not exposed to permanent hair dye" (source: http://www.sciencedaily.com).

It is important to point out that this study was an epidemiological investigation looking at behavior and the possible relationships between products and their effect on health. Epidemiological studies are not definitive in any way. For example, it isn't clear from this study what percentage of this group smoked, what kind of diet they had, or whether or not they had other mitigating illnesses. It also doesn't say that hair dye causes cancer, just that it has a casual relationship (meaning there is no definite or conclusive evidence).

As you can tell the jury is still out on this issue. There truly is not enough information or research to assert with any confidence that you should avoid dark-colored hair dyes.

If you want to be extra cautious you can avoid dark permanent or intermediate hair dyes. In view of the USC study showing that women who dye their hair twelve times or more each year for a period of fifteen years were at a higher risk, you may want to consider dying your hair less frequently, no more than say six or eight times a year. It is also important to keep in mind that although hair dyes may increase the risk of getting bladder cancer, such a risk would represent a relatively small number of cases, since women account for only about 15,000 of the 40,000 new cases of bladder cancer diagnosed each year (source: http://www.webmd.com).

FOUNDATION SETTLING INTO PORES AND LINES

Problem: What causes foundation to settle into the pores and leave tiny little spots, or settle into laugh lines? I do not know whether my moisturizer is too heavy or not heavy enough, whether the foundation is too heavy or too light, or whether I have not waited long enough for the moisturizer to be absorbed.

Solution: Most foundations contain ingredients that allow some amount of movement. If they didn't, they wouldn't blend easily and would feel dry and matte on the skin, making wrinkles look worse. But that also means that those foundations can easily slip into pores, making the skin look mottled. Moisturizing when you don't need it creates even more slippage. Unless you have dry skin, there is no reason to wear a moisturizer under foundation. Most foundations for normal to dry skin have enough emollient ingredients to make an extra moisturizer unnecessary. Too much moisturizer (not too little) or too much foundation can absolutely cause slippage into lines and pores. Once you've blended on a foundation, apply a light dusting of powder to set your makeup. Also, try blending on your foundation with a sponge, not with your fingers. A flat sponge can pick up excess foundation from the skin and blend it on in an even layer. Most important, if you have normal to dry skin, you may want to consider changing to a more matte foundation to avoid slippage. If you have oily skin then you may want to consider an ultra-matte foundation, which won't move throughout the day.

EYELASH DYES

Problem: A friend of mine gets her eyelashes and eyebrows dyed at the hair salon. The effect is really rather impressive and I'm tempted to try this myself. Her blonde lashes look dark and long, even without mascara. What do you think?

Solution: Unfortunately, my solution isn't much of a solution, because all I can do is strongly say, "Don't do it!" The only safe solution for making lashes and brows more visible is to use mascara on the eyelashes and shade your eyebrows, either with an eyeshadow that matches your hair color, an eyebrow pencil, or a brow mascara like Bobbi Brown's Natural Brow Shaper. But first let me give you a little history on why my answer to your question is such an emphatic "no." Back in 1933, a congressional controversy was brewing over the need for new and stronger food, cosmetic, and drug laws. At the time, the FDA had no authority to move against a cosmetic product called Lash Lure that was causing allergic reactions in many women. Two women, in fact, suffered severe reactions to the product; one woman became blind and the other woman died. When the new Food, Drug, and Cosmetic Act was passed in 1938, Lash Lure was the first product seized under its authority. A lot of time has passed since then, but although hair dyes (and that includes lash dyes) have changed a great deal, they are still formulated with peroxide and ammonia or ammonia-like ingredients. If a hair dye doesn't contain those ingredients, it can't affect hair color.

No one should ever dye her eyelashes or eyebrows. An allergic reaction to the dye formulation could prompt swelling, inflammation, and susceptibility to infection in the eye area. These reactions can severely harm the eye and even cause blindness. The FDA absolutely prohibits the use of hair dyes for eyebrow and eyelash tinting or dyeing, even in beauty salons and other establishments. The FDA has also continually warned the public about the use of coal-tar dyes on the eyebrows and eyelashes, stating that such use could cause permanent injury to the eyes, including blindness. (Using eyelash and eyebrow dyes or hair dyes for the eyes or brows should not be confused with using mascaras, eyeshadows, eyebrow pencils, and eyeliners, which contain ingredients that have been approved by the FDA for use in the eye area.)

Be aware that there are no natural or synthetic color additives (or coloring agents) approved by the FDA for dyeing or tinting eyelashes and eyebrows—either in beauty salons or in the home. In fact, the law requires all hair-dye products to include instructions for performing patch tests before use, to identify possible allergic reactions, and to carry warnings about the dangers of applying these products to eyebrows and eyelashes. The health hazards of permanent eyelash and eyebrow dyes have been known for more than 60 years. These dyes have repeatedly been cited in scientific literature as capable of causing serious reactions when placed in direct contact with the eye.

SEASONAL CHANGES

Problem: During the winter I use an emollient moisturizer you recommend and it works great, but during the summer it seems a bit much. Should I change what I do with the seasons?

Solution: Summer can absolutely require a change in skin-care products, particularly moisturizers. Instead of the richer or more emollient moisturizers you were wearing at night to combat the dry heat indoors and the dry cold outdoors, consider using lighter moisturizers that come in gel or gel/lotion consistencies. Keep in mind that the major concept here is to cut back on the amount of moisturizer you use. Moisturizer is for dry skin, so if you don't have dry skin, you really don't need moisturizer. Also, remember that no matter how much moisturizer you wear, and no matter how many antioxidants it contains, it won't change or stop one wrinkle on your face. What a lightweight moisturizer can do is soothe spot dryness and make fine lines less noticeable. Nothing is erased or changed, but wrinkles do look better, and that's great. And this is at night, right? Because during the day you should be using a sunscreen with UVA-protecting ingredients for your face and exposed parts of your body.

Please ignore the fact that many of the products recommended below are labeled "oil-free." This is a meaningless term. What makes these products good for those with minimally dry skin is they contain fewer thickening agents and emollients. Also ignore words and phrases such as "oil-control," "lift," and "firming." None of these products can control oil, lift the skin anywhere, or firm it even a little. These are all good, very lightweight moisturizers, and that's enough.

Here's a list of some of the better lightweight gel moisturizers, regardless of price (remember, price often has no relation to quality): Bio-Medic High Density Gel; Chanel Hydramax Balanced Hydrating Gel; Clinique Moisture Surge Treatment Formula; Estée Lauder Future Perfect Skin Gel and Clear Difference Oil-Control Hydrator; Lancôme Oligo Major Mineral Serum, Vinefit Cool Gel, and Hydra Controle Oil-Free Fresh Gel; L'Oréal Revitalift Night; and Prescriptives Super Line Preventor.

MAKEUP COLOR SELECTIONS FOR REDHEADS

Problem: I am a natural redhead and have problems finding makeup professionals who are trained to advise someone with my coloring (I have bright red hair, pale skin, and freckles). I've had lots of makeovers at department store makeup counters and always walk out looking either overly made up or wearing colors that clash with my hair! What colors do you suggest?

Solution: The answer to your question seems rather simple to me, so I'm not sure what's going wrong when you get your makeup done professionally. For you, the sheerest foundation is best. If a makeup artist is trying to cover up your freckles, he or she should be reprimanded. Neutral golden tan as well as shades of camel and chestnut brown for eyeshadows, blush, and lipsticks are made for your coloring. You can try a golden coral-brown for lipstick or blush if you want a dash more color. Although those colors are considered tried and true for redheads, there really is no color barrier these days when choosing colors. A vibrant red with a soft reddish-brown blush can look wonderful and quite dramatic on someone with your coloring. In the long run, experimenting until you find colors you're comfortable with is the best way to go.

When it comes to mascara, stay with brown and avoid black, which can be too hard a look on fair, freckled skin. Also keep in mind that makeup is not supposed to match hair color. A woman with gray hair doesn't need to wear gray colors, and you have alternatives, too.

WHITER TEETH

Problem: I would so love to have a perfect white smile. I hate my yellowing, stained teeth. What should I do?

Solution: There are many reasons why someone may have yellow or stained teeth. Silver fillings might have grayed the surrounding tooth enamel, so replacing those fillings with the new tooth-colored material dentists use can make a world of difference. Lots of foods such as coffee, tea, and berries can cause stains. You can cut back on the foods causing the problem, but who's going to give up their coffee in the morning, much less fresh berries? Smoking is also a major cause of yellow and brown staining on teeth. And, unfortunately, some people just have natural yellow-colored teeth. Serious staining and discoloration (natural or otherwise) cannot be corrected with toothpaste, but some minimal improvement can be achieved with this kind of product. Colgate Total Plus Whitening Toothpaste is as good a place to start as any (source: *Journal of Clinical Dentistry*, 2002, volume 13, pages 91–94).

Abrasive toothpaste can be a problem because over time the abrasives erode the surface of the tooth, and that can further complicate yellowing. The external part of the tooth is white, but underneath the white enamel is a yellow dentin core. The white part erodes naturally as part of aging, but it's speeded up by using hard toothbrushes or abrasive toothpaste.

For startling results that can make teeth whiter than you ever thought possible, one remarkable solution is to ask your dentist to bleach your teeth. Teeth-bleaching treatments used by dentists come in two forms, one you use at home and the other is done at the dentist's office. The whitening process done at the dentist's office can take several weeks, at about a half-hour per visit, for a cost of $300 to $800. The kit you buy from a dentist and take home uses a similar carbamide peroxide–based bleaching gel. Your dentist will fit a mouth guard to your mouth, and it must be left on for several hours over several days or nights. These at-home kits can cost between $300 and $400. The whitening effect can last up to 47 months in 82% of the patients who use it with no adverse side effects (source: *Journal of Esthetic and Restorative Dentistry*, 2001, volume 13, number 6, pages 357–369). One major drawback of this process is increasing and even painful gum sensitivity.

The teeth-whitening kits with mouthguards that you buy at the drugstore ($15 to $25) use a substantially weaker hydrogen peroxide-based bleach and the mouth guard is not specially fitted to your mouth. If your teeth are even, that's fine, but if they aren't, the mouth guard will not fit correctly and you can get uneven results. The mouth guard the dentist makes for you is created from an impression taken from your mouth and has individual spaces for each tooth. If the teeth do not lighten evenly you can do extra treatments for only the teeth that didn't become light enough.

Bleaching or whitening strips were created to eliminate the problems associated with having to use mouth guards and a bleaching solution (not everyone is comfortable wearing a mouth guard). Whitening strips are available either over-the-counter or from your dentist. Both types of whitening strips use hydrogen peroxide to whiten teeth. The strips that are available from your dentist use a stronger concentration of hydrogen peroxide than those available at the drugstore. Both types of whitening strips can be very effective when applied twice daily for fourteen days, yielding a highly significant improvement in tooth color versus baseline (source: *Compendium of Continuing Education in Dentistry*, June 2000, Supplement, pages S22–S28). Drugstore versions will require more applications to net the same results as those from the dentist. Regardless of your choice there are definite drawbacks to these strips. They can leave a yellow area on the teeth near the gumline. Whitening strips also are limited because they can only cover the front teeth, which means only those will be lightened, leaving all the other teeth unaffected. Perhaps most discouraging is that whitening strips have a short shelf life. This is because whitening strips use hydrogen peroxide as the active agent, and it is an exceptionally unstable ingredient. It can happen that by the time you find, buy, and start using your whitening strips the hydrogen peroxide may have become inactive. The teeth-whitening kits available through dentists have mouth guards that use carbamide peroxide, which is far more stable than hydrogen peroxide and has a very long shelf life.

It is important to keep in mind that none of these treatments is very effective if your teeth are grayed rather than yellowed, or if they are completely yellowed or are brown in color. Teeth-bleaching systems work best for partially yellow or food-stained teeth.

Other than bleaching, if the yellow or dull color of your teeth is from tartar buildup, get your teeth cleaned, and have them cleaned regularly. If you can, avoid foods that can grab onto teeth and make them look darker, such as chocolate, dark-colored berries, red wine, and coffee. Milk and rice can also bond to front teeth and cause a buildup of yellow tartar. Clearly, it is best to brush immediately after eating these foods, but if that isn't possible, rinse your mouth well with water and then chew sugarless gum. Many dentists recommend using the Sonicare electronic toothbrush as a way to prevent tartar or plaque buildup. You definitely cannot manually brush your teeth as well as the Sonicare can, and it is a worthwhile option to check out. And, above all else, don't smoke!

part V

NAVIGATING THE COSMETICS COUNTER

chapter *17*

KNOWLEDGE IS BEAUTIFUL

TERMS YOU NEED TO KNOW

There are wonderful cosmetics on the market these days. But if you don't understand how the industry works, the good, the bad, and the ugly, you will be a victim of its advertising manipulations, and that isn't good for your skin or your budget. We all need some help navigating the cosmetics counter to get the best results and the best buys.

I am often asked, "How do they get away with it?" How do cosmetics companies get away with what appears to be nothing less than misleading and even lying to the public? First, you need to know that, according to the FDA, **cosmetics companies do not have to prove their claims or the efficacy of their products.** What's even more surprising is that the FDA also does not require safety documentation for cosmetics until *after* the product has been brought to market and the FDA starts receiving consumer complaints.

In essence what this lack of regulations means is that cosmetics companies get to say just about anything they want to about their products, and the claims absolutely do not have to be true or have any substantiated proof regarding what is being asserted. What is monitored to some extent are advertising claims, which are evaluated by the Federal Trade Commission (FTC, www.ftc.gov). Although the FTC has frequently cracked down on excessive and false claims made by cosmetics companies, this almost always takes place *after* the ads have run and *after* numerous consumers have fallen prey to another barrage of misleading or false promises.

The only part of the cosmetics industry that is strictly regulated for the consumer is the ingredient list. Since 1978, cosmetics companies have been required to divulge all the contents of their products, listed in the order of concentration from most to least. Unfortunately, the vast majority of consumers don't know how to read a cosmetic's ingredient list, which means they rely on the unregulated claims and assertions the marketing copy boasts about. Yet taking the time to decipher the ingredient lists is the only way to make a rational decision when it comes time to purchase skin-care products.

The following are a few of the more salient points you may not know regarding the marketing jargon, terms, and ingredients that get hyped and over-hyped by the cosmetics industry, yet have little to no meaning when it comes to what you will actually be putting on your skin.

All-Natural: This term denotes that the ingredients in a given product or product line were derived from plants or other organic material as opposed to being produced synthetically. While the "natural" implication resonates with consumers, it is a completely false concept. Natural claims are not regulated by the FDA. Although the FDA has tried to establish official definitions and guidelines for the use of terms such as "natural" and "hypoallergenic," its regulation proposals were overturned in court. Therefore, cosmetics companies can use the "all-natural" term on ingredient lists to mean anything they want, and almost always it means nothing at all. Many companies even claim their products are all-natural when in fact they contain a preponderance of unnatural ingredients. Further, there is no convincing research showing that "natural ingredients" are better for skin than synthetic versions. And finally, when a plant product is added to a cosmetic, and is preserved, stabilized, and mixed with other ingredients, it loses most, if not all, of its natural orientation (source: FDA *Consumer* magazine, May-June 1998; revised May 1998 and August 2000).

Hypoallergenic or Good for Sensitive Skin: These terms suggest to the consumer that the product is less likely to cause allergic reactions or skin sensitivities. However, there are no standard testing restrictions or regulations for determining whether a product qualifies as meeting this claim. A company can label their product as "hypoallergenic" or "good for sensitive skin" with no substantiation for the claim. This is also true for terms such as "dermatologist-tested," "sensitivity tested," "allergy tested," or "nonirritating." None of these terms are required to be based on any proof that they are better for your skin than products without these claims, because there are no standardized guidelines (source: www.fda.gov).

Alcohol-Free: This generally means that a product does not contain denatured alcohol, ethyl alcohol, methanol, benzyl alcohol, isopropyl (rubbing) alcohol, or SD alcohol, all of which are akin to grain alcohol, which is very drying and irritating for skin. However, many cosmetics may contain other "alcohol" compounds, such as cetyl alcohol, stearyl alcohol, cetearyl alcohol, or lanolin alcohol, also known as fatty alcohols, and what these do is completely unrelated to grain alcohol's effect on skin. As is true for any skin irritant, the higher up on the ingredient list the alcohol is, the greater the risk of irritation. Grain-type alcohols that fall after or just before the list of preservatives rarely pose an irritation problem for skin.

Fragrance-Free: This indicates to the consumer that a product contains no perfume or fragrant ingredients. Despite this labeling, many products use fragrant plant extracts that can cause skin irritation or allergic reactions. Furthermore, fragrant ingredients (including fragrant plant oils and extracts) may be added to a "fragrance-free" cosmetic to mask any offensive odor originating from the raw materials used, but in such a small amount that they may not impart a noticeable scent. "Fragrance-free" can mean that a product does not exude a noticeable aroma, but it can still contain those types of ingredients. Either way, because "fragrance-free" is not a term regulated by the FDA, it ends up being meaningless information on a product's label—and one more reason why getting to know ingredients can be extremely helpful (source: www.fda.gov).

Noncomedogenic and Nonacnegenic: These terms are not regulated by the FDA and have no legal meaning. Again, any product can showcase these terms. In real life, the search for products that won't cause breakouts remains a struggle. Wouldn't it be nice if a product could live up to this claim? But given that almost all cosmetic ingredients can trigger breakouts for some people, the term is not only bogus, it can never really be true. Besides, we've all bought products labeled "noncomedogenic" that have made us break out (source: www.fda.gov).

Dermatologist-Tested: No matter how impressive this sounds, as long as there are no published data stating otherwise, all this wording can mean is that a doctor applied the product to his or her skin or watched someone else do that and said they liked the product. It doesn't tell you anything about efficacy or how one product compares to any other product. A similar empty phrase that's often seen is "dermatologist-approved" (source: www.fda.gov).

Laboratory-Tested: A laboratory sounds so scientific—but any place a study is done can be referred to as a "laboratory" setting. Once you're past the scientific impression that term may give you, you realize that the testing issues are rarely logical, and that often the tests are engineered in advance to give the company precisely the results they paid for.

Patented Secrets or Patented Ingredients: There is no such thing as a patented secret. The very concept is an oxymoron. The only way to even obtain a patent is to *divulge* the complete contents of the product and its intended use! There are also no patents that deal with proof of efficacy. All a patent can legally do is attribute to an ingredient or formulation the capability to be used for a specific purpose (such as wrinkles, acne, exfoliation, or skin-lightening). That has nothing to do with whether or not those ingredients can do anything at all. Patents also do not indicate quality, reliability, or usefulness of a product, nor does a patent mean that certain established ingredients can't be used by other companies for other purposes (source: United States Patent and Trademark Office, www.uspto.gov).

I could go on and on, and I will as I explain and cite sources detailing what works and what doesn't when it comes to skin-care products. The information I provide just restates everything the cosmetics industry already knows to be true (it's their information directly from their sources). I simply add what they won't tell you: what you absolutely need to know to make sensible, cost-effective decisions about what you put on your skin.

THE GOLD STANDARD: EXPENSIVE DOESN'T MEAN BETTER

The amount of money you spend on skin care has nothing to do with how your skin looks. And spending more money does not affect the status of your skin. What does affect the status of your skin are the products you use. An expensive soap by Erno Laszlo is no better for your skin than an inexpensive bar soap such as Dove (though I would suggest that both are potentially too irritating and drying for all skin types). On the other hand, an irritant-free toner by Neutrogena can be just as good as, or maybe even better than, an irritant-free toner by Orlane or La Prairie (depending on the formulation), and *any* irritant-free toner is infinitely better than a toner that contains alcohol, peppermint, menthol, essential oils, eucalyptus, lemon, or other irritants, no matter how natural-sounding the ingredients are and regardless of the price or claim. Spending less doesn't hurt your skin, and spending more doesn't necessarily help it. Simple, but true!

THEY'RE CHEATING ON YOU

The concept of brand loyalty is something many consumers feel comfortable with and are seeking. They reason (and this reasoning is reinforced by the cosmetics companies) that using only products from a single brand must be better for their skin, because products from a particular line must be specially formulated to work together. Therefore, mixing one brand of cosmetics with another is supposed to be like trying to fit a square peg into a round hole or mixing oil and water. I understand the reasoning behind this, but more often than not there is no valid reason to use skin-care or makeup products from just one company. Your skin and appearance will not suffer (and may actually improve) if you aren't monogamous with a single cosmetics company. Besides, when you stop to think about the other goods and services you purchase there really isn't much logic behind it. No one buys food products from just one company, and even doctors don't prescribe medications from only one company (and of course there's the fact that generic medications work as well as the brand names). These are cases where it's clear that brand loyalty would not be good for your health. But perhaps an even more convincing reason to ignore the concept of brand loyalty for cosmetics is because the cosmetics companies can't stay loyal to themselves.

The number of mergers and acquisitions that occur in the cosmetics industry is higher than ever before. In fact, over 75% of most department-store cosmetics lines are owned either by Estée Lauder or by L'Oréal. It's the cosmetics-world equivalent of the Hatfields versus the McCoys as these two powerhouse corporations battle for the consumer's attention (and dollars) every day. In an effort to summarize what is revealed about ownership throughout this book, I compiled the list below to show the more notable ownerships, and you may find it quite eye-opening.

Estée Lauder owns Stila, Aramis, Aveda, Clinique, Jane, Tommy Hilfiger Fragrances, Bobbi Brown, Prescriptives, M.A.C., Origins, Donna Karan Cosmetics, Jo Malone Perfumes, Bumble & Bumble, Kate Spade Beauty, and Creme de la Mer (source: www.elcompanies.com).

L'Oréal owns Maybelline, Lancôme, Helena Rubinstein, Kiehl's, BioMedic, Vichy, Biotherm, Giorgio Armani Parfums, Ralph Lauren Parfums, Shu Uemura, Ombrelle, Redken, Matrix, Garnier, and La Roche Posay (source: www.loreal.com).

Procter & Gamble owns Cover Girl, Max Factor, Clairol, Olay, Noxzema, Pantene, and Vidal Sassoon (source: www.pg.com).

Johnson & Johnson, in the realm of cosmetics and skin care–oriented medical products, owns Neutrogena, Aveeno, Clean & Clear, PersaGel, RoC, Retin-A, and Renova (source: www.jnj.com).

Revlon owns Almay and Ultima II (source: www.revlon.com).

Shiseido owns Cle de Peau, Decleor, NARS, and Sea Breeze (source: Shiseido Annual Report, March 31, 2002, www.shiseido.co.jp/e/annual/html/anu92000.htm).

Beiersdorf owns La Prairie, Nivea, Basis, Eucerin, and Juvena of Switzerland (source: www.beiersdorf.com).

chapter *18*
PRODUCT REVIEWS

UNDERSTANDING THE RATING SYSTEM

The following are the rating symbols for the products reviewed in this book. These simple, but succinct (albeit cute), symbols depict approval or disapproval of a specific product.

☺ This smiling face indicates a great product that I recommend highly because of its performance or impressive formulary characteristics. The smiling face means the product is definitely worth checking into and potentially worth buying, especially considering that it is so reasonably priced.

☺ $$$ This symbol designates a great product that meets and/or surpasses the criteria set for that category of product. However, just because the product is well-formulated doesn't mean it is worth the money. Almost without exception there are always reasonably priced versions of a product that meet or exceed the same standards as the more expensive versions.

☺ This neutral face indicates an OK but unimpressive product, or an OK product that can cause problems for certain skin types. I often use this face to portray a dated or old-fashioned product formulation. That doesn't mean it's a bad product, but that it just isn't very interesting or is lacking some of the newer water-binding ingredients, antioxidants, anti-irritants, emollients, or nonirritating ingredients for dry skin. I also use the neutral face to reflect a makeup product that isn't really bad, but that is completely unnecessary, ordinary, or in comparison to other products, not as well-formulated. Depending on your personal preferences, products rated with the neutral face may be worth checking out, but they're nothing to get excited about.

☺ $$$ This symbol indicates an ordinary, boring product whose excessive price makes it ludicrous to consider. For skin-care products, the rating reflects a lack of unique or interesting water-binding agents, anti-irritants, emollients, antioxidants, effective exfoliants, gentle cleansing agents, or combinations of those in a given formulation. For makeup, it reflects a performance that pales in comparison to other far better formulations, but that still can look OK when applied.

☹ For many reasons, this frowning face reflects a product that is truly bad for skin from almost every standpoint, including price, dated formulations, performance, application, and texture, as well as potential for irritation, skin reactions, and breakouts.

No Symbol: For space considerations, if a product earns the same rating symbol as the product above it, no additional symbol is used.

✔☺ *Paula's Pick*

✔☺ **Paula's Pick** When a product exceeds expectations and meets the criteria for a product in its category with minimal to no concerns I indicate that with a checkmark and happy face. Keep in mind that products with only a happy face and no checkmark do have value but are not extraordinary standouts in their category.

GENERAL REVIEW INFORMATION

Prices: Because the cost of drugstore cosmetics often fluctuates from store to store, and because cosmetics companies often change prices every six months, the prices listed in this book may not be up-to-date and may not match what you find when you are shopping. Use the prices as a basis for comparison, but realize that they may not precisely reflect what you find when you go shopping.

Up-to-date information: My staff and I diligently work to make sure all the information we have is accurate and current. However, cosmetics companies frequently and without notice change or reformulate their products, sometimes in a minor way and sometimes extensively. To keep abreast of these changes, which cannot be kept current in a book, I report revisions and new product launches that occurred after this book went to press in my newsletter, *Cosmetics Counter Update* and frequently in my free online *Beauty Bulletin*.

Foreign names: For the most part, I give only the English names of foreign-produced products. The French and Italian names are pretty, but they don't tell you anything about the product if you don't speak the language.

No endorsements: Neither the information nor the evaluations included in any of my works are to be misconstrued as endorsements, nor do they represent a particular company's sponsorship. None of the cosmetics companies paid me for my remarks or critiques. All of the products listed under Paula's Picks are just that, choices and picks, with the final decision left to you.

Order of presentation: The cosmetics products are listed alphabetically by brand name, so the order in which they appear does not represent my preference. There is no implied winner among any of the cosmetics companies included in this book, and no one line has all the answers or the majority of great products. Almost every line has its strong and weak points.

Don't go shopping without me: I encourage you to take this book with you on shopping trips to the cosmetics counters or the drugstore. Then you will have all the information you'll need readily at hand because there is no way you (or anyone) can remember the details of each product, color, and brand. Do try to be discreet at the department-store cosmetics counters—and don't be surprised if you find that using the book in clear view of the salespeople makes them defensive or irritated. There are always risks when a consumer comes prepared with information that disagrees with the salesperson's. I urge you to persevere. Nothing will change at the cosmetics counters if you don't change first.

When we disagree: Please be aware that you may not and need not agree with all my reviews to get some benefit from the information in this book. As you read my comments, you may very well find yourself disagreeing with me. That is perfectly understandable and as it should be, because the criteria you use to evaluate cosmetics may differ from mine. Or, for any one of a dozen reasons (personal preference, different expectations, actual usage such as once a week versus twice a day), a product I dislike may work well for you. Or just the opposite can be true: You may hate a product I rate highly. What I cannot account for is how millions of women will feel or react to a particular product. However, you can learn whether your expectations about a product's efficacy are based on nothing more than a placebo effect, or are based on a worthwhile formulation.

Beauty Note: For updates to this book, please visit my Web site at www.cosmeticscop.com.

The Reviews

What I present in the following pages are reviews of products from some of the most popular and available cosmetics lines. It is impossible in a book of this scope to include reviews for all cosmetics lines available today. These reviews are merely guidelines, based on my extensive research and investigation about what works and what doesn't. If you decide to follow any of my suggestions, be aware that my recommendations are not a guarantee, but instead offer suggestions as to how to narrow down the endless options the cosmetics industry sells. It is my earnest desire to help you choose from this very crowded field so you can make the best choices possible. The final choice, of course, is yours.

BANANA BOAT (SUN CARE ONLY)

The fact that many of Banana Boat's products aimed at sun protection do not contain effective UVA-protecting ingredients means that this sun care line cannot be trusted for sun protection. Over the past two years they have added products that meet the industry standard, yet they've left the poorly formulated ones still on the shelves for unsuspecting consumers to stumble upon. Another problem, even for the sunscreens that do offer state-of-the-art protection, is that none of Banana Boat's products list nonactive ingredients. As a result there is no way to really know what you are putting on the skin. Therefore, the ratings below are strictly about sun protection and not about what other benefits or problems these products may pose for the skin. For more information about Banana Boat, call (800) 723-3786 or visit www.bananaboat.com.

☺ **VitaSkin Lotion Facial Care SPF 30** *($9.99 for 5.7 ounces)* is a good, in-part avobenzone-based sunscreen.

☺ **VitaSkin Lotion SPF 15** *($9.99 for 6 ounces)* is a good, in-part avobenzone-based sunscreen.

☺ **VitaSkin Lotion SPF 30** *($9.99 for 6 ounces)* is a good, in-part avobenzone-based sunscreen.

☺ **VitaSkin Lotion SPF 50** *($9.99 for 6 ounces)* is a good, in-part zinc oxide–based sunscreen.

☺ **Ultra Sunblock Quick Dry Spray SPF 30** *($8.99 for 6 ounces)* is a good, in-part avobenzone-based sunscreen.

☺ **Sunblock Spray Lotion SPF 48** *($8.99 for 6 ounces)* is a good, in-part titanium dioxide–based sunscreen.

☺ **Active Sport Sunblock Gel SPF 30** *($8.99 for 6 ounces)* is a good, in-part avobenzone-based sunscreen.

☺ **Baby Block Sunblock Lotion SPF 50** *($8.99 for 4 ounces)* is a good, in-part titanium dioxide–based sunscreen. There is nothing in this product that makes it preferred for babies. If anything, the synthetic sunscreen agents can be too irritating for a child's skin.

☺ **Kids Sunblock Spray Lotion SPF 48** *($8.99 for 6 ounces)* is similar to the Baby Block above and the same comments apply.

All of the products in the following paragraph either do not contain the UVA-protecting ingredients of titanium dioxide, zinc oxide, or avobenzone, or have an inadequate SPF rating that would give a terribly false sense of protection that could result in serious skin damage.

☹ **Dark Tanning Lotion SPF 4** *($7.99 for 8 ounces)*; **Dark Tanning Oil Spray SPF 4** *($7.99 for 8 ounces)*; **Active Sport Quick Dry Sunscreen Spray SPF 25** *($8.49 for 6 ounces)*; **Faces Plus Sunblock SPF 23, Normal/Combination Skin** *($8.99 for 4 ounces)*; **Kids Sunblock Lotion SPF 30** *($8.99 for 8 ounces)*; **Kids Quik-Blok SPF 25** *($9.99 for 8 ounces)*; **Maximum Sunblock Cream SPF 50** *($8.99 for 4 ounces)*; **Quik Blok Sunblock SPF 25** *($9.59 for 8 ounces)*; **Protective Tanning Oil SPF 8** *($7.99 for 8 ounces)*; **Protective Tanning Oil SPF 15** *($7.99 for 8 ounces)*; **Sport Sunblock Lotion SPF 15** *($8.99 for 6 ounces)*; **Sport Sunblock Lotion SPF 30** *($8.99 for 6 ounces)*; **Sunblock Lotion SPF 15** *($8.99 for 8 ounces)*; **Sunscreen Lotion SPF 8** *($8.99 for 6 ounces)*; **Ultra Sunblock Lotion SPF 30** *($8.99 for 6 ounces)*; and **Aloe Vera Sun Screen Lip Balm SPF 15** *($1.59 for 0.15 ounce)*.

The products in the following paragraph, like all self-tanners, use dihydroxyacetone to affect the color of skin. They would work as well as any.

☺ **Sunless Tanning Creme, Soft Medium** *($7.99 for 3.75 ounces)*; **Sunless Tanning Creme, Deep Dark** *($7.99 for 3.5 ounces)*; and **Sunless Tanning Spray Soft Medium** and **Deep Dark** *($5.99 for 3.75 ounces)*.

☺ **VitaSkin Lotion Daily** *($9.99 for 12 ounces)* is a good, but very standard, moisturizer for dry skin. It contains mostly water, thickeners, silicones, vitamins A and E, film-forming agents, and preservatives.

BOBBI BROWN

Bobbi Brown has been one of the most quoted and referred-to makeup artists in fashion magazines and on television for several years now, and her handiwork has graced the faces of countless models and celebrities. Brown's product line, which was launched over ten years ago with a small collection of brown-based lipsticks, established her reputation as the source of the natural neutral palette. Shortly thereafter, Brown launched foundations and these have become the mainstay of her makeup collection. Although the first round of colors were noticeably yellow, the shades have been tweaked and since then have ranked among some of the more reliable range of foundation shades in the business. In fact, since Estée Lauder purchased Bobbi Brown in 1995, the line has seen tremendous growth. What started out as a small makeup line has evolved into a large line with a diverse array of products.

Lauder's influx of money has allowed Brown to continually expand the line. One growth spurt was the revamping of the entire skin care line in September

2002; out with the old and in with the new. Leaving behind glycolic acid (AHA) and salicylic acid (BHA) products along with some fairly irritating plant extracts in some of the cleansers, Brown's latest offerings do have some improvements, but overall, especially in comparison to the products of other Lauder-owned cosmetics companies, they just aren't as impressive as you would expect. Brown's products aren't bad by any means, it's just that they weren't improved as much as they could have been. While Brown's new products do contain some good water-binding agents, antioxidants, and anti-irritants, they aren't unique in any way. Both Lauder (the more expensive matriarch) and Clinique (the less pricy younger sister) offer far better options with more varied formulations for different skin types and an abundance of state-of-the-art water-binding agents and antioxidants.

A new slant for Brown is the claim that most of the products are "dermatologist-tested," but a quick call to the company revealed that there are no test results to be had. According to the FDA (FDA *Consumer* magazine, May 1995, www.fda.gov) " . . . label claims that a product is 'dermatologist-tested,' . . . carry no guarantee that it won't cause reactions. [The] FDA tried to publish regulations [in 1975] defining hypoallergenic to mean a lower potential for causing an allergic reaction. . . . In addition, we were going to require that companies submit information to FDA establishing that in fact their products were hypoallergenic. . . . However, two cosmetic manufacturers, Almay and Clinique, challenged the proposed regulations in court, claiming that consumers already understood that hypoallergenic products were no panacea against allergic reactions. In July 1975, the U.S. District Court for the District of Columbia upheld FDA's regulations, but the two companies appealed. On Dec. 21, 1977, the U.S. Court of Appeals for the District of Columbia reversed the district court's ruling."

Without regulations and without test results that state why the products deserved the blessings of any dermatologist (or what standards or comparisons were used), the claim of "dermatologist-tested" is meaningless. Aside from the claims, there are some options here to consider, but nothing to get all that excited about. For more information about Bobbi Brown call (212) 572-4200 or visit www.bobbibrowncosmetics.com.

Bobbi Brown Skin Care

☹ **Exfoliating Cream Wash** *($22 for 3.4 ounces)* is an emollient, plant oil–based cleanser that contains several irritating plant extracts including arnica, grapefruit, and eucalyptus. Other than that, it's just a very ordinary cold cream–style cleanser that also contains clay, which makes it more confusing than exfoliating given that clay is best for oily skin and the emollients in here are best for dry skin.

☺ **$$$ One-Step Cleanser and Long-Wear Makeup Remover** *($22 for 3.4 ounces)* contains mostly thickeners, plant oils, glycerin, and preservatives. This basic cold cream–style cleanser is an option for normal to dry skin.

☺ **$$$ Purifying Gel Cleanser** *($22 for 4.2 ounces)* is a standard, detergent-based cleanser that can be an option for someone with normal to oily skin. It does contain fragrance.

☺ **$$$ Rich Cream Cleanser** *($22 for 4.2 ounces)* is a very basic, though emollient, Vaseline-based cleanser. This is little more than cold cream, but it is an option for normal to dry skin. It does contain fragrance.

☺ **$$$ Extra Balm Rinse** *($50 for 6.8 ounces)* is a lot of money for what is essentially just glycerin, olive oil, orange oil, slip agents, and a teeny amount of antioxidant, which adds up to cold cream. There are far less expensive ways to remove the last traces of makeup.

☺ **$$$ Eye Makeup Remover** *($18.50 for 3.4 ounces)* is a very standard detergent-based eye-makeup remover similar to almost every other one of this ilk, and it would work just as well, though there are far cheaper versions. It does contain fragrance.

☺ **$$$ Soothing Face Tonic** *($22 for 6.7 ounces)* is a decent toner that would work well for most skin types. It contains mostly water, slip agents, glycerin, plant extracts, water-binding agents, fragrant plant extract, and preservatives. The plant extracts are a nice mix of anti-irritants.

☹ **$$$ Extra Soothing Balm** *($50 for 0.5 ounce)* is a fairly basic emollient balm containing mostly thickeners, emollient, vitamin E, plant oils, fragrant oils, preservatives, and coloring agents. The plant oils are a nice mix of soothing agents and antioxidants, but hardly unique or worth this inflated price tag.

☺ **$$$ Hydrating Eye Cream** *($32.50 for 0.5 ounce)* is a very good emollient moisturizer for normal to dry skin that contains mostly water, plant oils, silicone, thickeners, water-binding agents, antioxidants, and preservatives. This is nice, but not as interesting as alternatives from Clinique or Lauder that are available for less money and have more state-of-the-art formulations. This is fragrance-free.

☺ **$$$ Hydrating Face Cream** *($38 for 1.7 ounces)* is similar to the Hydrating Eye Cream above only this one contains fragrance. The same basic comments apply.

☺ **$$$ Hydrating Face Lotion SPF 15** *($38 for 1.7 ounces)* is a good, in-part, titanium dioxide–based sunscreen in a lightweight moisturizing base. It contains a good mix of antioxidants and anti-irritants, but only a tiny amount of water-binding agents, which is disappointing. In many ways, this is quite similar to Clinique's Weather Everything Environmental Cream SPF 15 *($18.50 for 1 ounce)* and Lauder's Day Wear Super Anti-Oxidant Complex SPF 15 *($37.50 for 1.7 ounces)*.

☺ **$$$ Intensive Skin Supplement** *($50 for 1 ounce)* is a very good, silicone-based lotion that contains a good mix of antioxidants, anti-irritants, water-binding agents, and preservatives. The small amounts of vitamin C and mulberry root are probably not present in a high enough concentration to have an effect on melanin production.

☺ **$$$ Extra Moisturizing Balm SPF 25** *($75 for 1.7 ounces)*. I had to double-check the price tag on this balm twice to be sure I was seeing clearly; I was. This in-part avobenzone-based sunscreen contains some emollients, plant oils, fragrance, anti-irritants, antioxidants, a tiny amount of a water-binding agent, and preservatives. It is a very good sunscreen for dry skin, but the cost doesn't jive with what you're getting. Keep in mind that sunscreen must be applied liberally if you are going to net any benefit from it. How liberally are you going to apply a $75 sunscreen that won't last more than a couple of weeks if you're applying it correctly? The only extra about this product is the cost, not the benefit for skin.

☺ **$$$ Shine Control Hydrating Face Gel** *($38 for 1.7 ounces)* contains mostly water, silicones, film-forming agent, anti-irritants, water-binding agents, vitamin E, and preservatives. This is a good lightweight moisturizer for normal to slightly dry skin, but there isn't anything in it that will "control" oil, though it does have a matte finish.

☺ **$$$ Sunless Tanning Gel for Face and Body** *($27.50 for 4.2 ounces)* contains dihydroxyacetone, the same ingredient that all self-tanners use to affect the color of skin. This one would work as well as any, and offers no advantage over versions sold at the drugstore, from Coppertone to Bain de Soleil.

☹ **SPF 15 Lip Balm** *($15.50 for 0.12 ounce)* does not contain the UVA-protecting ingredients of titanium dioxide, zinc oxide, or avobenzone, and is not recommended. It also contains menthol and peppermint, which can be skin irritants.

Bobbi Brown Makeup

According to Brown's Web site, a woman's true beauty style is not about following the latest runway trend or creating a cookie-cutter face. Rather, it's about wearing makeup that's self-enhancing. While that statement is indeed admirable and empowering, it neglects the fact that Bobbi Brown *is* a trendsetter, as her anticipated seasonal looks attest. It was trendiness that was the backbone of Brown's now-defunct ColorOptions line.

This line really excels in its original offerings of superior foundations, true matte blushes and eyeshadows, and all of the other basics that are essential to a woman's classic makeup wardrobe. All of these are certainly worth checking out and they win this line high marks.

FOUNDATION: ☹ **$$$ Foundation Stick** *($35)* bills itself as "foundation and concealer in one." It falls short on both counts, especially in comparison with Brown's other foundations. This is fairly emollient and could easily crease into lines around the eyes or mouth. The coverage is light to medium with a creamy finish, making this best for normal to dry skin. Most of the colors are quite neutral and not nearly as yellow as they originally were. The twelve shades present options for light and darker skin, but avoid Walnut (too red) and Warm Natural (too peach). Natural and Golden may be too peach for some skin tones, but are still worth considering.

☺ **$$$ Oil-Free Even Finish Makeup SPF 15** *($35)* is a replacement for Brown's former Oil-Free Foundation. Whether or not you think it is an improvement depends on what you liked or didn't like about the original version. In contrast to the original Oil-Free Foundation (which I preferred), this formula has a sunscreen, although because it lacks the effective UVA-protecting ingredients of titanium dioxide, zinc oxide, or avobenzone it cannot be relied on for adequate protection. This version does have a lighter, slightly smoother texture than its predecessor, but also offers a less substantial matte finish and less initial coverage. Application is easier than before, but if you need more than light coverage you may want to consider other options. There are twelve shades available, including options for darker skin tones, and almost all of them are beautiful. The only ones to consider avoiding are Warm Natural, Golden, and Walnut. This is worth a look if you have normal to slightly dry or slightly oily skin and don't mind wearing a separate effective sunscreen underneath.

☺ **$$$ Moisture-Rich Foundation SPF 15** *($38)* has a wonderfully soft, creamy texture that blends beautifully and dries to a natural finish. Coverage is in the light to medium range and the twelve shades are almost impeccable—the only ones to watch out for are Golden, which is quite yellow, and Walnut, which is slightly red. There are even some excellent dark tones, along with traditional options for light skin tones. The major drawback is the lack of adequate UVA protection from the sunscreen, which is dismaying. Of lesser importance is the fact that this is housed in a pump bottle, which is not the most economical method for dispensing foundation, because you tend to pump out more than you need and there's no getting it back in the bottle. However, if you have normal to dry skin and are willing to wear a separate sunscreen underneath this, it is worth checking out. **Fresh Glow Cream Foundation** *($35)* is best for normal to slightly dry or slightly oily skin. This has a whipped texture and a thicker consistency, but blends on better than you might expect. The coverage is medium to full, with a semi-matte finish, meaning those with very dry skin expecting a rich foundation will not be happy with this one. Avoid these colors: Warm Natural, Golden, and Walnut. The lighter colors are excellent, and Espresso is beautiful on very dark skin.

☺ **$$$ Oil-Free Even Finish Compact Foundation** *($38)* is a silicone-based creamy compact makeup that applies and blends beautifully. Rather than a traditional cream-to-powder finish, this one has a very slightly moist, natural finish that is flattering on normal to dry skin. This sheer to medium coverage formula would be too rich for those with breakout-prone skin. Of the twelve shades, the only ones to consider avoiding are Warm Natural, Golden, and Walnut. This can double as concealer, and its texture is preferable to Brown's Creamy Concealer.

✔☺ **$$$ SPF 15 Tinted Moisturizer** *($35)* has been reformulated because, according to the counter personnel I spoke with, Bobbi Brown wasn't satisfied with the colors. If you were a fan (and there were many) of the previous version, you will notice only minor changes in terms of texture, application, and finish. The SPF 15 still offers UVA protection with an in-part titanium dioxide–based sunscreen, and the formula is now more silicone-based, so it has a lighter feel on the skin. The five colors are mostly exceptional—only Deep is too orange for most skin tones. For effective sun protection, sheer color, and a beautiful finish, this is highly recommended.

CONCEALER: ☹ **$$$ Concealer Kit** *($35)* is a revision of Brown's former Professional Concealer, though it isn't much better than the original. This is now a two-part product, with a creamy, thick, crease-prone concealer nestled on top of a small jar of loose powder. I suppose this will seem handy for some, but it adds little to the appeal of this product. The pros for the concealer are excellent coverage and reliable colors—only Bisque and Beige are too peachy pink to pass muster. The lightest shade, Porcelain, is a great color for very fair skin, but it is coupled with a Pure White powder that can look ghostly on the skin. The rest of the ten shades come paired with Brown's Pale Yellow powder, which can be too yellow for some skin tones. The **Creamy Concealer** *($25)* is also available alone, but it's sobering to realize you're paying an extra ten dollars for a tiny container of loose powder and mini powder puff!?

☺ **$$$ Blemish Cover Stick** *($20)* has a creamy, slightly greasy texture that is not what I would recommend using over a blemish. This stick concealer contains too many ingredients that can be problematic for use on breakout-prone skin. However, its natural finish and good coverage make it a winner for use on dark circles or other discolorations. The six shades nicely represent light to dark skin tones, and the only one to be cautious with is Warm Honey, which is slightly yellow-orange.

☺ **$$$ POWDER:** Bobbi Brown's loose **Face Powder** *($29)* is a standard, talc-based powder that has an airy, silky texture and a dry finish. The colors are a mixed bag: half are just too orange or yellow (sallow) to recommend. If you're considering trying one of these, proceed with caution and double-check the color in natural light. **Pressed Powder** *($26)* is virtually identical to the loose powder, with the same colors and same warnings. For both powders, avoid Sunny Beige, Golden Orange, and carefully consider Pale Yellow. **Sheer Finish Loose Powder** *($30)* is a talc-based powder that has the requisite soft, dry texture and—true to its name—a sheer application, with six mostly attractive colors. What is frustrating and rather shocking about this powder is that it costs more than Brown's regular loose Face Powder and offers 75% less product (0.25 ounce versus 1 ounce)! If you must have Bobbi Brown Powder, there is no reason to choose this one over the regular Face Powder above because both have a similar application and appearance on skin. **Sheer Finish Pressed Powder** *($28)* is also talc-based and has the same basic texture, finish, and color selection as the Loose Powder version above. Although overpriced, it is an option for a soft, matte-finish pressed powder.

☺ **$$$ BLUSH:** The powder **Blush** *($19)* features gorgeous colors that apply and blend evenly with a smooth matte finish. The only colors to think twice about are Rose, Blushed, and Soft Pink, which are all shiny. **Cream Blush Stick** *($25)* is a sheer, slightly greasy cream blush that remains creamy on the skin. Blending takes some time, and this is really best for flawless normal to dry skin, as it is too greasy for oily skin types. The only color to be careful with is Warm Peach, which can be too orange for most skin tones. **Bronzing Stick** *($28)* has the same texture as the Cream Blush Stick, but the Bronzing Stick has great bronze tones that are an option if you want to create a sun-kissed look. All three shades are quite sheer, with no shine to be found. **Bronzing Powder** *($26)* would be a better choice for normal to oily skin types than the Bronzing Stick. The powder is richer in pigment and it is easier to apply it and to control the intensity because you apply it with a brush. All three shades are beautiful and only slightly shiny.

EYESHADOW: Bobbi Brown's ☺ $$$ Eye Shadows *($18)* have a silky, smooth-blending texture and most of the colors are beautifully matte. There are some great choices for darker skin tones, and many of these shades would work well for lining the eyes or defining the eyebrows. The only colors to consider avoiding are Navy and Moss. **Shimmer Eye Shadow** *($18)* is at least named accurately, because there are three very shiny cream-to-powder eye colors. The shine is soft, making these wearable for a special evening look.

☺ $$$ **Shimmer Wash Eye Shadow** *($18)* is a collection of sheer to intense iridescent colors that are set apart from the matte colors on the tester unit, making them easy to avoid. They apply easily, but the shiny particles tend to flake on the skin—not the desired effect, but a reality nonetheless.

☹ **Cream Shadow Stick** *($20)* is a creamy eyeshadow in a roll-up stick form. These may be an option for some, but they tend to go on choppy and are difficult to blend out evenly. Plus, the texture of this starts smooth, but once it has set, it remains sticky!

EYE AND BROW SHAPER: ☺ $$$ **Creamy Eye Pencil** *($20)* is a standard needs-sharpening pencil that definitely has a creamy texture. It tends to have a sticky finish, and is not for someone who dislikes eyeliner smudging. Check out Brown's excellent matte eyeshadows for lining instead.

✔☺ $$$ **Long Wear Gel Eyeliner** *($18)*, which comes in a glass pot and needs to be applied with an eyeliner brush. This is sort of a hybrid between using a powder eyeshadow and liquid liner. The product applies slightly wet, has a fair amount of slip, and then "sets" to a solid powder finish. If you can master the application, you'll find this to be quite a tenacious product. Still, if you're prone to eyeliner fading or smudging, this is a unique product that is a must-try.

✔☺ $$$ **Natural Brow Shaper** *($16.50)* is a great way to groom and shade your eyebrows with natural-looking color. This is truly best for the brows only; it applies well and dries quickly, yet the bristles on the brush aren't long enough to reach down to the roots of any gray hair you may wish to conceal. The colors aren't the best for very dark brown or black hair, but there is a nice range for lighter hair shades, including redheads. A Clear version is also available.

LIPSTICK AND LIP PENCIL: This is where Bobbi Brown began, and although the color palette is exceptional, the formulas are pretty standard. The ☺ $$$ **Lip Color** *($18)* is strictly a cream lipstick with nice opaque coverage and great colors, most of which are brown-based. **Lip Shimmer** *($18)* is basically the same as the Lip Color above, only with iridescence. Besides the shine, the colors include more mauve and plum options. **Lip Stain** *($17)* is more of a gloss in lipstick form than anything else, and these are too sheer to leave any trace of a stain. Nice colors, though. **Cream Lip Gloss** *($18)* features ten beautiful colors (they really are exquisite), but otherwise it's a standard opaque lip gloss that has a traditional thick, sticky texture and the requisite wet, glossy finish. If paying top dollar for lip gloss doesn't bother you, it would be wise to start here! **Shimmer Gloss Stick** *($18)* is heralded as an innovative product that combines the look of gloss and the convenience of lipstick application. Although this very glossy lipstick has a slick texture that's completely non-sticky, it's hardly unique. However, extra points are earned for the beautiful colors, each laced with iridescence.

☺ **$$$ SPF 15 Lip Shine** *($17.50)* is a creamy, shiny lipstick that is overpriced for what you get and the sunscreen has no UVA-protecting ingredients. The **Lip Gloss** and **Shimmer Lip Gloss** *(both $18)* are extremely overpriced, standard, sticky glosses with a poor brush that tends to splay after a few uses; the Shimmer version just adds sparkle. **Crystal Lip Gloss** *($15)* is a very thick, sticky and syrupy gloss that comes in a squeeze tube. This will provide a high shine to the lips, but the thick feel is less than pleasant. **Art Stick** *($25)* is a copycat version of everyone else's jumbo pencils for lips and cheeks. This is too greasy to work well as cheek color because application can be streaky and blending tricky. As a lipstick, it may be OK, but at this price a regular lipstick is far easier and doesn't need to be sharpened. The four available colors are neutral and workable. **Creamy Lip Liner** *($20)* is a standard pencil that comes with a lip brush on one end, which is a nice convenience. This is almost identical in texture and application to the Creamy Eye Pencil on facing page, and that's just fine for lips as long as you don't have a problem with lipstick feathering.

☹ **Lip Balm SPF 15** *($15.50)* does not contain the UVA-protecting ingredients of avobenzone, titanium dioxide, or zinc oxide—but does contain irritating peppermint oil—and is absolutely not recommended.

☹ **Lip Tint SPF 15** *($15).* Given the various lip glosses Brown's line features, this addition without adequate UVA protection was hardly necessary. The sheer, slightly sticky lip gloss has a minty flavor and barely-there colors that just aren't exciting given the price.

MASCARA: ☺ **$$$ Defining Mascara** *($16)* is Bobbi Brown's original mascara that does an excellent job with lengthening and tends not to clump or smear. **Thickening Mascara** *($16)* is not thickening in the least, but could work for a natural, defined lash look if you don't mind the large brush. The Plum shade is quite purple and best avoided. **Lash Lustre Waterproof Mascara** *($16)* is a very good mascara that builds some length but very little thickness. It is indeed waterproof, but the brush tends to stick the lashes together while you're applying it, so be careful. **Lash Glamour Lengthening Mascara** *($19)* is a lightweight, sheer mascara that darkens lashes without adding any length. It doesn't clump, but does add some thickness. This is a repackaged, renamed version of Brown's LashTint Mascara in a Tube.

BRUSHES: ☺ $$$ Brown's **Brushes** *($18.50–$62.50)* are quite nice, with well-tapered edges and dense bristles. The Concealer and Eyeliner brushes are superb. As an added bonus, all of the brushes are available in either a travel (four-inch) or professional (six-inch) length. There are some to carefully consider, and some to ignore altogether. One to ignore is the **Loose Powder Brush** *($62.50)*, which for this amount of money should be perfect, but it's too floppy and soft to apply powder well. The same holds true for the **Blush Brush** *($42.50)*, also too floppy and soft for controlled application. The **Brow Brush** *($18.50)* is very stiff and scratchy, and the **Contour Brush** *($29)* and **Eye Shader Brush** *($26)* are both too big for most women's eye area, again making control and placement of color an issue. The rest of the collection is worth a look for some nice additions or extras for your makeup toolkit. **Conditioning Brush Cleanser** *($16.50 for 3.4 ounces)* is nothing more than standard, gentle shampoo that will nicely clean your brushes, but it can easily be replaced with much less expensive options from L'Oréal, Johnson & Johnson, or Neutrogena.

SPECIALTY ITEMS: The number of accessories available has grown to the point where they certainly deserve a belated mention. From **Professional Brush Cases** *($27.50–$40)* to **Makeup Palettes** *($22.50–$25)*, a variety of **Makeup Bags** *($30–$75)*, and the well-designed **Beauty Kit** *($67.50)*, there are some valid, somewhat pricey, options for organizing and traveling with your cache of makeup.

CLINIQUE

Clinique was Estée Lauder's first attempt to expand its market with a completely separate line and image. Lauder was clearly a mature woman's line and Clinique became known as the indispensable line for the woman under 30 concerned with breakouts, oily skin, and fragrance-free products (meaning less likely to cause allergic or sensitizing skin reactions). Clinique's tremendous success reshaped the way cosmetics lines identified themselves, sending the concept of line loyalty out to pasture. Today, cosmetics companies expand their market either by buying already established companies or by creating new ones. Of course, cosmetics companies keep this multiple-personality identity hidden from the consumer. If the general buying public realized that these apparently different companies were so intertwined with each other, how could the different lines flaunt their independence and claim that their unparalleled formulations are secret? Unless you think Lauder (or any company) would, even if they could, keep secrets from one branch separate from the others.

The niche Clinique built launched the notion of cosmetics being "allergy-tested," "hypoallergenic," "100% fragrance-free," and "dermatologist-tested." Of those marketing claims the only one that has significance is the "100% fragrance-free," which, for the most part, Clinique maintains (it does have some fragrant extracts in a few products). But unless you can see the test results, what difference does it make if a product is "allergy-tested"? What if the test showed 20% of the women who used it had a sensitizing reaction, dryness, or irritation? Moreover, "hypoallergenic" is a term that is not regulated by the FDA, so any product can claim it. "Dermatologist-tested" is also bogus, because without published test results, the term can easily mean nothing more than that a dermatologist picked up the product, looked at the container, and said, "This looks good."

Clinique's products, particularly the skin-care products, are aimed at oily or combination skin types, which is probably why Clinique attracts a younger clientele, but many of these products are exceptionally irritating. Among these disappointing products are the ones that contain a lot of alcohol, which would be drying, or the emollient moisturizers, recommended for oily, acne-prone skin, which could trigger breakouts. The strong points of Clinique products are the lack of fragrance of any kind in many of the products, some great moisturizer formulas, and excellent sunscreens. One thing you can be sure of at most Clinique counters is service. There always seem to be four to five white-jacketed women dashing around behind those cases. (The white jackets are supposed to look medical—how contrived can you get!) One more plus is that the products are far more affordable than those of numerous other lines in department stores. For more information about Clinique, call (212) 572-3800 or visit www.clinique.com.

Clinique Skin Care

☹ **Facial Soap Extra Mild** *($11 for 6 ounces)* is just soap, which means it is too drying and irritating for all skin types. It's not one iota different from other "soaps" at the drugstore.

☹ **Facial Soap Mild** *($11 for 6 ounces)* is similar to the Facial Soap Extra Mild above and the same comments apply.

☹ **Facial Soap Oily Skin Formula** *($11 for 6 ounces)* is similar to the Facial Soap Extra Mild above and the same comments apply.

☺ **Comforting Cream Cleanser** *($16.50 for 5 ounces)* is an excellent emollient cleanser that would be an option for dry skin. It would work just fine, but it is almost identical to Neutrogena's Gentle Skin Cleanser for half the price.

☺ **Extremely Gentle Cleansing Cream** *($22.50 for 10 ounces)* is an exceedingly standard mineral oil– and Vaseline-based wipe-off cleanser that can leave a greasy film on the skin. It is an option for very dry skin, but there is little reason to use this rather than just plain, fragrance-free mineral oil.

☹ **Rinse-Off Foaming Cleanser** *($16.50 for 5 ounces)* is a detergent-based cleanser that uses more drying cleansing agents than most, plus it adds lemon, eucalyptus, pine, and cardamom, and that makes it an irritation waiting to happen.

☹ **Wash-Away Gel Cleanser** *($16.50 for 5 ounces)* is similar to the Rinse-Off Foaming Cleanser above and the same comments apply.

☺ **Extremely Gentle Eye Makeup Remover** *($10 for 2 ounces)* is a basic lotion that will remove makeup—boring, but effective.

☺ **Naturally Gentle Eye Makeup Remover** *($14.50 for 2.5 ounces)* is supposed to be as "gentle to the eyes as tears." Since when were tears made up of hydrogenated polyisobutene, butylene glycol, ammonium acryloyldimethyltaurate/VP copolymer, or acrylates/C10-30 alkyl acrylate crosspolymer? This is a good eye-makeup remover, but it is very basic and no gentler than others. The second ingredient is sesame oil, and if you happen to have that in your kitchen cabinet, it, too, would really be gentle for removing makeup.

☺ **Rinse-Off Eye Makeup Solvent** *($13.50 for 4.2 ounces)* is a standard detergent-based eye-makeup remover that would work as well as any.

☺ **Take the Day Off Makeup Remover, for Lids, Lashes and Lips** *($15.50 for 4.2 ounces)* is a standard, silicone-based makeup remover that would work as well as any.

☺ **7 Day Scrub Cream** *($15 for 3.5 ounces)* is a mineral oil–based scrub that uses polyethylene (ground-up plastic) as the abrasive. This is a fairly unrinseable, heavy, greasy scrub that would only be an option for dry to very dry skin.

☺ **7 Day Scrub Cream Rinse Off Formula** *($15 for 3.4 ounces)* is a very basic, emollient cleanser that uses polyethylene (ground-up plastic) as the abrasive. As a mechanical exfoliant it would be an option for normal to dry skin.

☹ **Exfoliating Scrub** *($15 for 3.4 ounces)* would have been a good option for a scrub in a rinseable, detergent-based cleanser using polyethylene (ground-up plastic) as the abrasive; however, it contains some menthol, and that adds unnecessary irritation to the skin.

☹ **Clarifying Lotion 1** *($10.50 for 6.7 ounces)* is similar to the Lotion 3 on facing page, and the same comments apply.

☹ **Clarifying Lotion 2** *($10.50 for 6.7 ounces)* contains alcohol and menthol, which makes it too irritating and drying for all skin types.

☹ **Clarifying Lotion 3** *($10.50 for 6.7 ounces)* lists alcohol as the second ingredient, and that is too drying and irritating for all skin types, so instead of clarifying it's just a problem for healthy skin.

☹ **Clarifying Lotion 4** *($10.50 for 6.7 ounces)* is similar to, but even more potent than, the Lotion 3 above and the same comments apply.

☺ **Mild Clarifying Lotion** *($10.50 for 6.7 ounces)*. At least this one doesn't have any irritants! It contains about a 0.5% concentration of BHA, and since the pH of this toner is about 4, that makes it effective for some amount of exfoliation. This can be an option for someone with breakouts, but a pH of 3 to 3.5 would make it more effective.

✔☺ **Advanced Stop Signs Visible Antiaging Serum** *($35 for 1.7 ounces)* isn't all that advanced, but it is a very good, silicone-based moisturizer with an excellent blend of antioxidants, water-binding agents, and anti-irritants. However, you will have to wait a very long, long time if you're hoping it will stop you from aging.

✔☺ **All About Eyes** *($26 for 0.5 ounce)* is similar to the Advanced Stop Signs above only with even more silicone, giving it a somewhat silky, slippery feel. It would be a great option for normal to dry skin.

☺ **$$$ Anti-Gravity Firming Lift Cream** *($35 for 1.7 ounces)*. The more than 50 ingredients in this product aren't lifting your skin anywhere, at least not any more than any other moisturizer in Clinique's moisturizing lineup. This is a good moisturizer for normal to dry skin, with a fair to good mix of antioxidants, anti-irritants, and water-binding agents. All in all, the Advanced Stop Signs above has a more impressive formulation.

☺ **$$$ Anti-Gravity Firming Eye Lift Cream** *($28.50 for 0.5 ounce)* is a good emollient moisturizer for dry skin, but there is nothing in it that can fight gravity in any way, shape, or form. The product says it: "Helps erase the look of lines and builds cushion back into time-thinned skin." Except for the "builds cushion back," that would be true for any moisturizer, but there simply are no moisturizers that can put "cushion" back into skin. The cushioning of skin is provided by the fat layer of skin, which becomes depleted as we age, and this product can't build fat into skin. This is a more emollient version of the Firming Lift Cream above and the same comments apply.

☺ **Anti-Gravity Firming Lift Lotion** *($35 for 1.7 ounces)* is indeed a lotion version of the Firming Lift Cream above and the same basic comments apply. This silicone-based version does have a soft matte finish and is good for normal to slightly dry skin.

☺ **Daily Eye Benefits** *($26 for 0.5 ounce)* contains mostly water, slip agent, glycerin, thickeners, plant oil, plant extracts, water-binding agents, a form of vitamin A, Vaseline, and preservatives. This does contain tannin (a plant component found in tea and coffee) that can have potent antioxidant properties, but tannin can also constrict skin and cause irritation, though the amount in this product is so small it probably isn't a problem for skin. This would be an OK moisturizer for normal to dry skin.

☺ **Dramatically Different Moisturizing Lotion** *($20.50 for 4.2 ounces).* The only thing dramatic about this moisturizer is how dated a formulation it is. This contains only water, mineral oil, sesame oil, slip agent, thickeners, Vaseline, preservatives, and the famous coloring agents that impart the product's well-known soft yellow color. It doesn't contain even a minute amount of any of today's state-of-the-art moisturizing ingredients.

✔☺ **Exceptionally Soothing Cream for Upset Skin, Anti-Itch Cream** *($30 for 1.7 ounces)* and **Exceptionally Soothing Lotion for Upset Skin** *($30 for 1.7 ounces)* both contain hydrocortisone acetate, which can indeed soothe irritated skin. What Clinique doesn't warn about is that continuous use of hydrocortisone over time can actually cause skin damage by thinning the skin and breaking down the skin's support structure. If you are aware of this very serious shortcoming and plan only occasional use, there are many reasons why you may prefer Clinique's products to Lanacort or Cortaid. Even though the active ingredient in these products is the same, the moisturizing base in both Clinique products is a far more elegant one, with soothing agents, silicone, and water-binding agents. However, in the long run, the base shouldn't make that much difference, because you should only be using it short-term.

✔☺ **Moisture In Control** *($31 for 1.7 ounces)* won't control anything. There is no way a product can put moisturizing ingredients in a dry area on the face, while at the same time holding them off the face in other areas and instead applying ingredients that absorb oil. It is a lightweight moisturizer that would be ideal for someone with normal to slightly dry skin. It contains good water-binding agents and antioxidants.

✔☺ **Moisture On-Call** *($31 for 1.6 ounces)* is supposed to help skin cells "remember" how to produce their own moisture barrier. This is a physiological impossibility, because you can't change the basic way your skin functions with a moisturizer. Of course, any moisturizer used *daily* will help your skin protect its moisturizer barrier, and this is a very good emollient moisturizer. It contains a very good mix of water-binding agents and antioxidants. The caffeine in it has skin-constricting properties, which can be a skin irritant, but the amount of it is so small that it probably has no effect.

✔☺ **Moisture On Line** *($31 for 1.7 ounces)* is almost identical to Moisture On-Call, and supposedly can "re-educate" the skin. There are no moisturizing ingredients anywhere in the world that can change the nature of skin or make skin remember anything! But skin cells can look better if you faithfully reapply the moisturizer every day, which is exactly what the instructions on this moisturizer tell you to do. Aside from the hype, this is an exceptional moisturizer for someone with normal to dry skin, with excellent water-binding agents and antioxidants.

✔☺ **Moisture Surge Eye Gel** *($26 for 0.5 ounce)* is similar to the Moisture In Control and the same basic comments apply. This would be an option for normal to slightly dry skin.

✔☺ **Moisture Surge Extra Thirsty Skin Relief** *($31 for 1.7 ounces)* is a very good, silicone-based moisturizer that contains a nice complement of antioxidants and water-binding agents. It would work well for normal to slightly dry skin.

☹ **Sheer Matteness T-Zone Shine Control** *($13.50 for 0.5 ounce)* can leave a matte feel on skin, but it offers no other benefit, and with alcohol tops on the list along with clove, this isn't the best option for skin.

☺ **Skin Texture Lotion Oil-Free Formula** *($21 for 1.25 ounces)* is a good, lightweight moisturizer with some good water-binding agents and antioxidants. This would be an option for someone with normal to dry skin.

☺ **Total Turnaround Visible Skin Renewer** *($30 for 1.7 ounces)*. Like all of Clinique's Turnaround products, this one contains a teeny amount of salicylic acid; however, the pH of 5 in these formulations prevents the BHA from being effective as an exfoliant. Other than that, in many ways this product is Clinique's rendition of Lauder's Idealist *($42.50 for 1 ounce)*. While you're trying to decide what to do with all the other Lauder products you own that claim to return your skin to a more youthful state, or whether or not you want your skin renewed with this product or firmed with the one above, keep in mind that Clinique's versions are almost always cheaper. For example, both Idealist and Total Turnaround contain acetyl glucosamine. The limited research establishing this ingredient as being good for wrinkles comes from the company that sells the raw ingredient and from Lauder. But then Lauder feels that lots of ingredients are good for wrinkles, so why this one more than their others is a mystery! Acetyl glucosamine is an amino acid sugar, the primary constituent of mucopolysaccharides and hyaluronic acid, and it's found in all parts of the skin. It has value as a water-binding agent, and is effective (in large concentrations) for wound healing. There is research (source: *Cellular Molecular Life Science*, February 1997, pages 131–140 and *Biomaterials*, June 2001, pages 1667–1673) showing that chitins (also known as chitosan, which is composed of acetyl glucosamine) can help in the complex process of wound healing. However, that's at least a few generations away from what acetyl glucosamine may accomplish in teeny amounts in a skin-care product. This product contains mostly water, silicones, slip agent, water-binding agents, plant extracts, acetyl glucosamine, vitamin E, fragrant plant extract, thickeners, film-forming agent, and preservatives. This is a good, silky-feeling, lightweight moisturizer for normal to dry skin.

☺ $$$ **Total Turnaround Visible Skin Renewer for Oilier Skins** *($30 for 1.7 ounces)* is nearly identical to the original Total Turnaround Cream, although this lotion does have a lighter texture and more of a matte finish on the skin. Again, the pH of 5 and the tiniest amount of salicylic acid make this a poor choice for an exfoliant, but it's still a lightweight, rather elegant moisturizer, and a good option for normal to slightly oily skins with dry areas. Contrary to the claim, this is not capable of "de-shining" the skin, though it is unlikely to make skin look or feel greasy. It is fragrance-free.

☺ **Turnaround Cream** *($26 for 1.7 ounces)* has a great name! It sounds as if this cream can turn your skin back to a younger time, but it can't (anymore than any of the other products in this line, or in the entire Lauder stable of lines can, for that matter). It contains a small amount of salicylic acid (BHA), but the pH of 5 makes it fairly ineffective as an exfoliant. This is an OK, basic moisturizer for normal to slightly dry skin, with very little to offer over many other Clinique moisturizers.

☺ **Turnaround Cream for Dry Skin** *($26 for 1.7 ounces)* is similar to the Turnaround Cream above, but this one is definitely more emollient and has slightly more water-binding agents. That does make it a better option for normal to dry skin, but it still isn't all that interesting for skin.

☺ **Turnaround Lotion Oil Free** *($26 for 1.7 ounces)* is a silicone-based moisturizer with slightly more salicylic acid than the versions above, but the pH is the same, which means that this one is no more effective as an exfoliant than the others. It does contain a good mix of water-binding agents, anti-irritant, and antioxidants, and is a good option for normal to dry skin.

✔☺ **Weather Everything Environmental Cream SPF 15** *($18.50 for 1 ounce)* is a very good, pure titanium dioxide–based sunscreen in a good moisturizing base that has a nice complement of antioxidants and water-binding agents. It would be a great option for someone with normal to dry skin.

☺ **Sun Care Body SPF 15 Sun Block** *($15.50 for 3.4 ounces)* is a very good, in-part titanium dioxide– and zinc oxide–based sunscreen in a rather standard moisturizing base that makes it an option for someone with normal to dry skin. It has a small selection of antioxidants and water-binding agents.

✔☺ **Sun-Care Body SPF 25 Sun Block** *($15.50 for 3.4 ounces)* is a very good, in-part titanium dioxide– and zinc oxide–based sunscreen in an emollient moisturizing base that has some antioxidants and a tiny amount of water-binding agents. This would be very good for someone with normal to dry skin.

✔☺ **Body SPF 30 Sun Block** *($16.50 for 5 ounces)* is similar to the Sun-Care Body SPF 25 Sun Block on facing page and the same comments apply.

☹ **Body Spray SPF 15 Sun Block** *($16.50 for 5 ounces)* doesn't contain the UVA-protecting ingredients of titanium dioxide, zinc oxide, or avobenzone, and is not recommended.

☺ **Body Spray SPF 30 Sun Block** *($16.50 for 5 ounces)* is a good, in-part avobenzone-based sunscreen. Unfortunately, alcohol is the first ingredient, which makes this drying and irritating for skin. That means it's not the best, though the sun protection is excellent.

✔☺ **Face SPF 30 Sun Block** *($16.50 for 2.5 ounces)* is similar to the Sun-Care Body SPF 25 Sun Block above and the same comments apply.

☺ **Lip/Eye SPF 30 Sun Block** *($15.50 for 0.21 ounce)* is very good in-part zinc oxide– and titanium dioxide–based sunscreen in a standard though emollient balm form.

✔☺ **City Block Sheer SPF 15** *($15.50 for 1.4 ounces)* is an excellent, titanium dioxide– and zinc oxide–based sunscreen in a good, emollient moisturizing base. It also contains a small amount of high-quality water-binding agents and antioxidants.

✔☺ **Super City Block SPF 25 Oil-Free Daily Face Protector** *($15.50 for 1.4 ounces)* is an excellent, pure titanium dioxide–based sunscreen in a very good, moisturizing base that includes a great mix of antioxidants and water-binding agents. This is best for someone with normal to dry skin because titanium dioxide can be too occlusive for those with oily or blemish-prone skin.

☺ **City Block Oil-Free Daily Face Protector SPF 15** *($14.50 for 1.4 ounces)* is similar to the Super City Block above, only with a less impressive moisturizing base. Otherwise, the same basic comments apply.

☺ **Face Quick Bronze Tinted Self Tanner** *($15.50 for 1.7 ounces)* uses the same ingredient to affect skin color as all self-tanners do, dihydroxyacetone. This one would work as well as any. It essentially does the exact same thing as the Self Tanning Lotion below with the exact same ingredient; the price difference is sheer caprice.

☺ **Self Tanning Lotion** *($15.50 for 4.2 ounces)* uses the same ingredient to affect skin color as all self-tanners do, dihydroxyacetone. This one would work as well as any.

☺ **Deep Cleansing Emergency Masque** *($18.50 for 3.4 ounces)* is a standard clay mask with some cleansing agents and a mix of irritating and anti-irritant plant extracts. It also contains cornstarch and that can be a problem for those with blemish-prone skin.

☺ **All About Lips** *($20 for 0.5 ounce)* is a good, silicone-based moisturizer that has a matte finish on lips.

☺ **Superbalm Lip Treatment** *($10 for 0.24 ounce)* is a standard, Vaseline-based, emollient lip balm with some antioxidants and water-binding agents. The spearmint is the only thing that gets in the way of this being a very good treatment for dry lips.

☺ **Moisture Stick** *($13.50 for 0.14 ounce)* is a very standard emollient "lipstick" that contains mostly castor oil, thickeners, lanolin oil, plant oil, and a teeny amount of vitamins. This would work well for dry skin.

Clinique Acne Solutions

☺ **Antibacterial Facial Soap** *($9 for 5.2 ounces)* is a standard bar cleanser that contains triclosan, a topical disinfectant. There is no research showing that triclosan is effective against acne bacteria. This also contains menthol, which can be a skin irritant.

☹ **Acne Solutions Body Treatment Spray** *($18.50 for 3.4 ounces)* lists alcohol as the second ingredient, and it also contains peppermint. These add up to irritation and dryness, and that doesn't solve anything when it comes to acne.

☹ **Acne Solutions Night Treatment Gel** *($16 for 1.7 ounces)* is similar to the Body Treatment Spray above and the same comments apply.

☹ **Acne Solutions Daytime Shield** *($16 for 1.7 ounces)* is a lightweight, silicone-based moisturizer that could have been a great soothing option for dry skin, except that it contains peppermint, and that adds unnecessary irritation.

✔☺ **Acne Solutions Emergency Gel Lotion** *($13.50 for 0.5 ounce)* is a very good 5% benzoyl peroxide topical disinfectant for blemishes.

☹ **Acne Solutions Spot Healing Gel** *($12.50 for 0.5 ounce)* lists alcohol as the second ingredient, which is too irritating and drying for all skin types.

Clinique Makeup

Other than the addition of even more shine-infused products and a couple of new lipstick formulas and mascaras, Clinique's makeup has largely remained the same since the previous edition of this book. They still offer a vast palette of colors and textures, especially in their huge, almost imposing, selection of foundations. Most skin tones will be well served here, although the blushes and eyeshadows still lack significant depth to show up on darker skin tones. Even the High Impact Eyeshadows, which boast "intense color coverage," are still too soft and sheer to work well on dark skin. Those with very light to medium skin tones will find almost limitless options, though more than a few products (and shade names) are a bit too cloying to appeal to the sophisticated cosmetics consumer.

Clinique has pumped up its makeup workshops using cleverly designed brochures and the lure of free gifts to guide women through the selection, application, and inevitable purchase of their makeup. Although these workshops can be helpful, especially for the makeup novice, the information you're given is more often than not geared toward improving "The Expert's" (Clinique Consultant's) average unit (in dollars) sale, and the emphasis of the workshops is on stressing that multiple products are needed to enhance your appearance, including an excess of skin-care products. Clinique is also one of the few major cosmetics players that has yet to offer its own makeup brushes. That means the Consultant must use cotton swabs, cotton pads, and disposable sponge-tip applicators to apply makeup, which is about as elegant and useful as eating filet mignon with a plastic fork.

FOUNDATION: Clinique's vast stable of foundations runs the gamut from barely there to ultracoverage, and many of them are wonderful and worth considering. Most skin types will find that at least one of these formulas meets their needs.

✔☺ **Dewy Smooth Antiaging Makeup SPF 15** *($19.50)* is definitely smooth, with a silky, silicone-based texture that feels amazing and blends without a hitch. Titanium dioxide is not only the sunscreen agent, it also lends an opacity that allows this makeup to provide medium to full coverage with a natural matte finish that feels slightly moist. This does not make skin look dewy or drenched in moisture—it's best for normal to slightly dry skin, or dry skin that will wear a moisturizer underneath. Beyond the sunscreen, there is nothing antiaging about the formula. Ignore the marketing hype and you'll be left with a superior foundation that comes in ten gorgeous colors for very light to dark skin.

✔☺ **Almost Makeup SPF 15** *($17.50)* is a very sheer foundation with a good, titanium dioxide–based sunscreen with an SPF 15. The colors have expanded from four to six, and what's available is great, including the darker (but not very dark) shades. This would work well for normal to dry skin for minimal coverage and a beautiful natural finish. ✔☺ **City Stick SPF 15** *($21)* is a very good stick foundation to consider and the SPF is excellent, with pure titanium dioxide as the only active ingredient. The coverage is sheer to medium, with a definite silky powder finish. As is true for any cream-to-powder foundation, the powder element can be drying for someone with dry skin, and the cream part can be greasy for someone with combination to oily skin, so that makes this one best for those with normal to slightly dry or slightly oily skin. Of the eight shades, the only one to watch out for is Beige Twist, which can be too peach for most skin tones. ✔☺ **City Base Compact Foundation SPF 15** *($21)* is similar to the City Stick SPF 15 foundation above only in compact form, but this one leaves a slightly heavier, creamier finish. The finish is still powdery, with a slightly silky feel, but not enough to hold back much shine in oilier areas, making this a best bet for normal to slightly dry skin. Except for Porcelain Beige, the ten shades are excellent and would work for a wide range of skin tones, from light to dark, but not for someone with very light or very dark skin. The SPF 15 is great, containing titanium dioxide as the only active ingredient. ✔☺ **SuperFit Makeup** *($19.50)* is an excellent option for those with oily skin who have been displeased with ultra-matte foundations. This is a great, soft-matte finish foundation that features a featherlight texture, and it also has twelve mostly excellent, neutral color options (though it lacks a shade for very light skin tones). The only colors to avoid are Petal, which can be too peach, and Spicy, which can turn copper. Champagne and Vanilla are just slightly peach, which may be a problem for oily skin types. SuperFit blends on easily, has good staying power, and easily washes off, though it isn't as oil-resistant as the ultra-matte finish products. You will get shine sooner than you would with a product like Almay's Amazing Lasting Foundation or Revlon's ColorStay. ✔☺ **Stay-True Makeup Oil-Free Formula** *($16.50)* is a very good foundation for fairly opaque, semi-matte coverage. This has an initial thick texture that blends easily and should work beautifully on very oily or normal to slightly oily skin that is looking for a soft matte (as opposed to an ultra-matte) finish. There are some great colors for both light and dark skin tones, but of the ten shades, avoid Stay Beige, Stay Porcelain, (too pink), Stay Sunny (rose), True Toffee (slightly orange), and True Bronze (too reddish-pink).

☺ **Balanced Makeup Base** *($15.50)* is one of Clinique's oldest foundations, although the number of shades has dwindled. This is best for those with fair to light skin tones who have dry to very dry skin. The mineral oil–based consistency is emollient and creamy, but it blends on well, leaving a natural finish. The coverage is light to medium, and four of the seven colors are excellent; the ones to avoid are: Creamy Peach (too peach), Warmer (too peach), and Honeyed Beige (very pink). **Soft Finish Makeup** *($19.50)* is quite similar to Clinique's Balanced Makeup Base above in terms of consistency and coverage, but this one has a silicone-enhanced slip and is slightly more sheer than the Balanced. This also claims to contain "optical diffusers" to diminish the appearance of wrinkles, but a quick check in daylight while wearing it will quickly disprove that. This is still a good foundation for normal to very dry skin. Of the nine shades, all are beautifully neutral except Soft Cream and Soft Porcelain, which are both too pink.

☺ **Superbalanced Makeup** *($17.50)* is Clinique's top-selling foundation worldwide, in no small part because it claims to provide moisture and absorb oil when and where needed—a skin-care dream many women share. However, this ends up doing neither job very well. There is no way any product can differentiate between the oily parts of your face and the dry parts. The absorbent ingredients in it will soak up any oil they come in contact with (including the moisturizing ingredients in this product or in the one you applied to your skin) and the moisturizing ingredients will get deposited over areas you don't want to be moisturized. What that adds up to is a light to medium coverage, light-matte finish foundation that is best for someone with normal to slightly dry or slightly oily skin. Someone with any amount of excess oil would not be happy with the finish or with how it wears during the day. Even more disappointing are the colors, which include some astonishingly poor options for fair to light skin. Although the darker shades are actually some of the best around, many of the lighter colors are strongly peach to orange. Of the 24 shades, the following colors are best avoided by most skin tones: Petal, Fair, Cream, Ivory, Nude Beige, Linen, Porcelain Beige, Golden, Sunny, Warmer, and Honeyed Beige. Alabaster, Light, and Breeze are the best neutral shades to consider if you have fair skin. **Clarifying Makeup** *($17.50)* is an updated, vastly improved version of Clinique's Pore Minimizer Makeup. While the Clarifying Makeup still contains alcohol as the third ingredient, the foundation application itself is impressive. It has a soft, ultralight texture, sheer-to-light coverage, and a smooth matte, somewhat transparent, finish. The colors are very nice, with most being neutral to yellow-based. Of the nine shades the only one to avoid is Blushing Buff, although the following three shades are borderline peachy and may turn orange on very oily skin: Perfect Almond, Light Beige, and Neutral Spice. A note of caution: This formula tends to separate, and should be thoroughly shaken before use. **Continuous Coverage SPF 15** *($15.50)* is a very opaque, full-coverage makeup that will certainly not look natural. What it will do is provide substantial camouflage for irregular pigmentation or birthmarks. The sunscreen active ingredient is all titanium dioxide, and this, coupled with the thick, powdery finish, can lend a chalky look to the skin. The four available shades are good, but the pluses and minuses mean that this is definitely a trade-off foundation. **Gentle Light Makeup** *($22.50)* is a sheer liquid foundation that feels light as a feather on the skin and blends wonderfully. It dries to a soft matte finish, but only in feel. The actual appearance on the skin is shiny, almost sparkly, as this makeup contains a good deal of gold iridescence, supposedly to make the skin look luminous. According to Clinique, this makeup contains "mosaic-like mirrored particles equal in size and shape." You can sum up that marketing spin in a one-word translation—glitter—which is exactly what you will see on your face. Perhaps this would work for an evening look or for a special occasion, but for day-to-day wear, an artificially shimmering face is no substitute for the clean, dewy glow you could easily achieve by simply not using any powder. Of the nine shades available, only Cream Light and Beige Glow are a bit too peachy pink, but this product is sheer enough that it's almost not an issue. The remaining (sparkling) colors are all excellent, including options for dark skin. Minus the shine, this would be a superior sheer foundation.

☹ **Workout Makeup All-Day Wear** *($15.50)* is a creamy, water-resistant foundation that provides medium coverage and a rather heavy application. Almost all of the six shades are too peach, orange, pink, or rose to look convincing. **Pore Minimizer Makeup** *($15.50)* is back, apparently by popular demand. I still can't understand the appeal of this watery, alcohol- and talc-based foundation. Yes, it does provide a solid matte finish, but the resulting irritation from the alcohol and the meager, often spotty, coverage are simply not worth the effort. Clearly, there were enough women who liked this makeup to convince Clinique to reinstate it (but only in four shades). However, for the uninitiated, this does not deserve consideration over Clinique's Skin Clarifying or SuperFit Makeups.

CONCEALER: ☺ **Soft Conceal Corrector** *($12.50)* comes in a squeeze tube and offers smooth, even coverage in a great, but small, selection of colors (Light is slightly ash-rose). This has a thick texture and soft powdery finish with only a minimal tendency to crease.

☺ **Advanced Concealer** *($12.50)* comes in a squeeze tube, goes on like a thick cream, but quickly dries to a powder. Coverage is very good without looking heavy. This comes in two shades, Light and Medium, and both are excellent. But beware: This concealer works only if the skin under your eyes is smooth; any dry or rough skin will look worse if you place this over it. **Quick Corrector** *($11.50)* comes in a tube with a wand applicator and has a fluid, slightly moist application. It smooths on easily and covers well with a minimally matte finish, though the unstable matte finish can translate into some creasing around the eyes. Avoid Medium, which is too pink. **City Cover Compact Concealer SPF 15** *($13.50)* is one of the few concealers that has a reliable SPF 15 with UVA protection. With the exception of City Light Pink, the colors are quite workable and capable of almost full coverage. The problem is that this has a creamy consistency that will crease before you're out the door. If the sun protection appeals to you, make sure you try this at the counter first and see how it wears over a period of time—or, for a greatly reduced tendency to crease, consider Lancôme's Photogenic Skin-Illuminating Concealer SPF 15 *($20)* instead. **Line Smoothing Concealer** *($13.50)* has a creamy-smooth, slightly slippery texture that blends on decently and dries to a natural finish with a hint of iridescence. The claim for this concealer is that it can be used over lines and wrinkles to "build a bridge" without settling into them, thus making these "flaws" less noticeable. While the risk of creasing is minimal, there is enough visible shine to draw attention to lines—so much for that bridge-building claim. The three shades are all slightly peach-toned, but may work for some skin tones.

☹ **Acne Solutions Concealing Cream** *($12.50)* is terrible in just about every respect. This is one of the driest, thickest, most opaque and difficult-to-blend concealers I have encountered. It does contain 1% BHA (salicylic acid), but the pH is too high for it to be an effective exfoliant, and it also includes alcohol and sulfur, making the whole thing a troublesome irritation for the skin. **Concealing Stick** *($13.50)* is a lipstick-style concealer available in only one color, which is too peach for most skin tones. Even if the color were more neutral, this is a greasy product that easily slips and doesn't have the best coverage. Still, enough people must be buying this to warrant keeping it around.

POWDER: ✔☺ **Blended Face Powder & Brush** *($16.50)* is one of the best talc-based loose powders available, and in an attractive array of colors. This has a light, supple finish that clings well without caking. Of the eight shades, avoid Transparency 1 (almost pure white), Transparency 2 (pale pink), and Transparency Bronze (nice color, but too shiny). ✔☺ **Stay Matte Sheer Pressed Powder Oil-Free** *($16.50)* is an excellent, talc-based powder with a slightly dry, sheer finish that is great for oilier skin types. The eight shades are beautiful and there are some good options for light and dark skin tones.

☺ **Soft Finish Pressed Powder** *($16.50)* is intended by Clinique to be used for drier skin, and that makes sense, as this talc-based formula has a creamier, silky feel and smooth, even coverage. The light-diffusing claims are bogus, but there are five great neutral colors. **Superpowder Double Face Powder** *($16.50)* is a standard, talc-based pressed powder with a smooth, soft texture. It can be used alone or as a regular finishing powder. There are eight very sheer shades, and most of them are excellent. As a reminder, you may be told this can be used wet, but attempting this method of application can result in a streaked, choppy appearance.

☺ **$$$ Gentle Light Pressed Powder** *($20)* supposedly "turns skin radiant" but that's courtesy of the sparkles interspersed throughout this talc-based powder. The can't-miss-it shine is not for those concerned with keeping a shiny appearance down, but for everyone else the five beautiful colors are all options, and this applies smoothly. **Gentle Light Powder and Brush** *($21)* is a talc-based loose powder that is exceptionally light and soft, yet is infused with enough shine to make a chorus of Las Vegas showgirls sparkle with envy. The five shades are beautiful, but this is one shiny, sparkly powder!

BLUSH: The color products (blushes, eyeshadows, and lipsticks) are arranged into four groupings: Nudes/Naturals (which are not all that nude), Tawnies/Corals/Reds, Pinks/Roses/Fuchsias, and Violets/Blues/Berries. This is definitely a helpful way to organize a large color collection!

☺ **Sheer Powder Blusher** *($16.50)* has a great selection of colors, but they are so soft and sheer as to be almost nonexistent on the skin when applied. Even after layering some of the "deeper" colors, it was hard to notice any intensity. Most of the colors also have a slight amount of shine, but it, too, is barely noticeable on the skin. This would be a goof-proof option for the blush-shy! **Soft Pressed Powder Blusher** *($16.50)* does up the ante a bit in terms of depth of color, but these are still quite sheer, and darker skin tones will have a hard time getting these to show up. The colors are all fine, though several have a minimal to moderate amount of shine. **Gel Blush** *($10.50)* has been reintroduced. This traditional gel blush is available in four colors that are lovely and sheer, but—as with all cheek stains—these work best on smooth, flawless skin and must be blended quickly if they are to look convincing. This can also be used on the lips for a sheer stained effect.

☹ **Blushwear** *($14.50)* is Clinique's version of a cream-to-powder blush and it really isn't worth considering. This tends to "grab" on the skin and look spotty, dotting the pores with color and sparkles—each of the shades has a subtle to glaring shine. Clinique has done much better with this type of product in the past. For a superior, nonshiny cream-to-powder blush option, consider Paula Dorf Cheek Color Creme *($18)*.

☺ **$$$ Rich Texture Blush** *($18.50)* is a pressed powder blush that has a blend of three colors in one compact. These are mixed in a speckled pattern but come off as one slightly shiny color on the skin. I'm not sure what Clinique means by "rich texture" as this is rather dry and unappealing, not to mention almost as sheer as their other blushes.

EYESHADOW: ☺ **Stay the Day Eyeshadow** *($11.50)* is supposed to last all day with no fading. You may not notice whether it fades or not because the few colors that are still available are all quite powdery and go on very sheer. The softness of these and their inability to cling well to the skin makes them difficult to recommend. **Pair of Shades Eyeshadow Duo** *($15.50)* features 24 different duos in a formula virtually identical to the Stay the Day Eyeshadows, and, thus, these tend to have the same problems. Most of the duos have one very shiny shade, and for an everyday look that can be more sparkles than one face needs. **High Impact Eyeshadow** *($11.50)* is the latest powder eyeshadow from Clinique, and it seems poised to eclipse Stay the Day Eyeshadow. This formula has slight improvements over the existing powder eyeshadows, but all of the colors are shiny, and many of them are, well, *too* colorful for an understated look. For those who want stronger colors (compared to what Clinique ordinarily offers) with lots of shine, these are one more option in a growing field of eyeshadow colors that "color" the eye, rather than shade it. These do work well when used wet, but once you opt to do this, reverting to dry application is difficult. **High Impact Eyeshadow Duos** *($16.50)* share the same traits as Clinique's High Impact Eyeshadow above—these are equally bold (but still not too intense) colors, all of which are quite shiny—almost glittery. There are some good shade combinations, but this much all-out shine is best reserved for unwrinkled eyes or the under-25 set.

☺ **Touch Base for Eyes** *($12.50)* is one of the better cream-to-powder eyeshadows. This comes in a compact that must be kept closed tightly or the product will dry out and be useless. However, it might dry out even if you follow that guideline, so recommending this is risky. Take a look and try it out first before buying, as there are a couple of matte colors (Canvas and Nude Rose) that would work as an eyeshadow base if your foundation or concealer is not up to the task. **Touch Tint for Eyes** *($13.50)* are tubes of semisheer, cream-to-powder eyeshadows. These have a creamy, slightly slick texture that makes controlling the color trickier than usual, but they eventually dry down to a soft powder finish. Each of the five colors are shiny, and not the soft, subtle shine seen in many other products. These are an option if you're seeking a departure from powder eyeshadows, but Revlon's Illuminance Cream Eyeshadow *($6.49)* gives you more bang and less glaring shine for your buck. **Smudgesicles** *($12.50)* gets my vote for one of the cutest makeup names ever, but the enthusiasm stops there. These are cream-to-powder eye colors in stick form that go on relatively smoothly and blend out sheer. However, they are tricky to use with other colors, and each shade is iridescent. For a one-color, quick eye design, these can be an option.

EYE AND BROW SHAPER: ☺ **Brow Shaper** *($14.50)* is a powder brow color that comes in four excellent shades. The texture is slightly heavy, but these blend onto the brow quite well, even though the brush that comes packaged with these is too stiff and scratchy. For the money, a matte, brow-toned eyeshadow would work just as well and could also double as an eyeshadow; this version is too heavy for eyeshadow. **Eye Defining Liquid Liner** *($13.50)* is an excellent choice for liquid liner, provided you don't mind the price. This has a great soft-feeling, but firm, brush and applies an intense line of color that can go from thin to thick with precise ease. It stays on well without smearing or flaking, but equally good, less expensive options are available at the drugstore.

☺ **Quickliner for Eyes** *($14.50)* is a standard automatic pencil that provides a smooth, no-tugging application and is very easy to smudge before it sets. It's nearly identical to several less expensive pencils at the drugstore. **Quick Eyes** *($15.50)* is unique—one end is a creamy pencil and the other end houses a powder eyeshadow in the cap that is dispensed onto a smudge tip. While this may seem convenient, the powder shadows are all very shiny and the pencil is too creamy to last the day. **Eye Shading Pencil** *($11)* is a basic pencil with a smooth, creamy feel and some nice colors. Nothing less, nothing more. **Water-Resistant Eyeliner** *($14.50)* is old-fashioned cake liner that you use with a damp brush. The two matte shades (brown and black) are too softly pigmented to make a dramatic line, but if you prefer this type of product, it's worth a look. Otherwise, a deeply pigmented matte eyeshadow would make a brilliant alternative to this.

☹ **Touch Liner** *($12.50)* is a poor liquid liner that comes in one shiny color that takes forever and a day to dry. The brush tip is also poor, making this a total washout. **Brow Keeper** *($14.50)* is a brow pencil that comes in three good shades and has a soft, creamy, but slightly sticky, consistency. These tend to stay creamy, and are prone to smudging or fading.

LIPSTICK AND LIP PENCIL: ☺ **Different Lipstick** *($11.50)* is a standard collection of lipsticks with a semisheer, glossy finish. Don't count on this one for long wear or being any different from any other sheer lipstick. **Lip Shaping Pencil** *($11)* is a standard pencil with a slightly dry texture. These go on nicely, but the formerly large selection of colors has been reduced to just a handful of shades. **Glosswear for Lips Sheer Shimmers** *($12.50)* is a different formula than the original Glosswear (reviewed below), and this one wins out since it is much lighter, smoother, and less sticky. Equipped with the wand applicator, you can dab iridescent, glossy shine and not have to be concerned with lips feeling too goopy. ✔☺ **Long Last Soft Shine Lipstick** *($12.50)* has a luscious feel and smooth, even application with opaque coverage. The color selection is extensive, with equally impressive pale and deep shades. ✔☺ **Long Last Soft Matte Lipstick** *($12.50)* remains my favorite of Clinique's lipstick choices.

This is a creamy, smooth formula with a nice stain and a slightly matte finish that feels great.

☺ **Liquid Lipstick SPF 15** *($12.50)* comes in a tube with a wand applicator and has a glossy, nonsticky finish. These have fairly opaque coverage for a gloss, but the sunscreen offers no UVA protection, making these hard to recommend if sufficient sun protection is your goal. **Moisture Sheer Lipstick SPF 15** *($13.50)* also does not contain adequate UVA protection and remains a sheer, glossy lipstick that comes in a nice selection of "juicy" colors. Continuing this pattern of inadequate UVA-protecting sunscreen is **Moisture Surge Lipstick SPF 15** *($12.50)*. Since we've already seen Clinique's revamped sunscreen formulas that all use avobenzone, titanium dioxide, or zinc oxide, it's obvious that they know better and it's bothersome that two of these lipsticks with inadequate UVA-protecting sunscreens were launched *after* Clinique's retooled sunscreen collection! Moisture Surge is just a standard, slightly greasy lipstick with a pleasant selection of shades and a glossy finish. If your aim is to combine lipstick with sun protection, a far better choice would be Revlon, Cover Girl, or Almay's lipsticks with effective sun protection. **Almost Lipstick** *($13.50)* is a sheer, glossy lipstick that is similar to the Different Lipstick above. Although the formula is nothing special, the colors are beautiful. **Glosswear for Lips** *($12.50)* has a sticky texture and some good colors. This is fine for a standard wand-application gloss, but less expensive options abound. **Quickliner for Lips** *($13.50)* is an automatic, nonretractable pencil that is not preferred over less expensive options, as this one tends to smudge and is quite creamy. **Chubby Stick** *($12.50)* is a collection of short, fat pencils with a creamy lipstick application, but they are so soft they never stay sharp enough to draw a good line, making this just a gimmicky, rather unreliable, choice for lip color.

MASCARA: ✔☺ **Lash Doubling Mascara** *($12.50)* does a very good job of living up to its name, as this quickly builds lots of length and a fair amount of thickness with ease. The formula sweeps on with no clumps or smearing— each lash is well-defined—and from my perspective, this is hands down the best mascara in Clinique's lineup!

☺ **Naturally Glossy Mascara** *($12)* is a basic mascara that builds some length and minimal thickness. It's fine for a natural, light look. **Full Potential Mascara** *($12)* goes on very well, with no smudging or clumping, and builds moderately long, thick lashes with minimal effort. **Long Pretty Lashes Mascara** *($12.50)* has an accurate name, as this mascara produces lots of length and does so without clumping, smearing, or flaking. Be warned, though: The clean, quick application does not produce any thickness. Still, if length is what you're after, this is well worth trying! If any of you remember Clinique's problematic Longstemmed Lashes, this is a revised (and much improved) version of that ill-fated mascara. **Gentle Waterproof Mascara** *($12.50)* is a bit of a misnomer, as waterproof mascara in general is hard on lashes for both wear and removal. Still, this is reliable mascara that builds nice length and some thickness, and it's truly waterproof.

☺ **Supermascara** *($12)* is supposedly better for contact lens wearers because it is fiber-free. Well, so are the rest of Clinique's mascaras! In comparison, this one pales when it comes to lengthening and long, nonsmudging wear.

COPPERTONE (SUN CARE ONLY)

Coppertone makes one of the most woefully disappointing groups of sunscreen products around. Except for a handful of good avobenzone-based sunscreens, all the other sunscreens in its lineup have no UVA protection—there's no titanium dioxide, zinc oxide, or avobenzone in any of them! Clearly, now that the line does include products containing avobenzone, it's not as if the Coppertone people don't know about the issue. Coppertone also boasts that its sunscreens for kids are the ones recommended most by pediatricians. If that's true, be sure you find another pediatrician right away. It would mean your doctor doesn't know about the damage from UVA rays, and I would worry about what else he or she wasn't up to date on. There is something wanton about a corporation so recognized as a sunscreen manufacturer selling such an abundance of pathetically formulated sunscreens. For more information about Coppertone, call (800) 842-4090 or visit www.coppertone.com.

☺ **Sunblock Lotion SPF 30** *($6.99 for 4 ounces)* is a good, in-part avobenzone-based sunscreen in a very standard lightweight moisturizing base that would be OK for someone with normal to slightly dry skin or slightly oily skin.

☺ **Sunblock Lotion Spray SPF 30** *($8.99 for 7 ounces)* is similar to the Sunblock Lotion above and the same comments apply.

☺ **Shade Sunblock Lotion SPF 45, UVA/UVB Protection** *($7.99 for 4 ounces)* is similar to the Sunblock Lotion above and the same comments apply.

☺ **Oil Free Sunblock Lotion for Faces SPF 30** *($7.99 for 3 ounces)* is similar to the Sunblock Lotion above and the same comments apply.

☺ **Shade Sunblock Spray Mist SPF 30** *($7.99 for 4 ounces)* is a good, in-part avobenzone-based sunscreen. Although you will get UVA protection from this one, it also contains about 80% alcohol, which can be drying and irritating for all skin types.

☺ **Shade Oil-Free Gel SPF 30, UVA/UVB Protection** *($6.99 for 4 ounces)* is similar to the Sunblock Spray Mist above and the same comments apply.

☺ **Sport Sunblock Gel SPF 30** *($8.99 for 6 ounces)* is similar to the Sunblock Spray Mist above and the same comments apply.

☺ **Sport Sunblock Gel SPF 15** *($8.99 for 6 ounces)* is similar to the Sunblock Spray Mist above and the same comments apply.

☺ **Endless Summer Sunless Tanning Lotion, Light/Medium or Dark** *($10.99 for 3.7 ounces)* uses the same ingredient to affect skin color as all self-tanners do, dihydroxyacetone. This one would work as well as any.

☺ **Oil-Free Sunless Tanner** *($7.99 for 4 ounces)* is similar to the Sunless Tanning Lotion above, and the same comments apply.

☺ **Cool Gel Aftersun Aloe Light, Summertime Fragrance** *($5.49 for 16 ounces)* is just aloe vera with some slip agents, preservative, fragrance, and coloring agents. There is nothing about this that makes it preferred over pure aloe vera gel from the health food store.

☺ **Cool Gel Aloe Aftersun** *($5.49 for 16 ounces)* is identical to the version above, only with a different fragrance. The same comments apply, just as neither should contain fragrance.

All of the following products are not recommended, either because they do not contain the UVA-protecting ingredients of titanium dioxide, zinc oxide, or avobenzone, or because they have SPF numbers less than 15, which means that they do not provide sufficient protection from sun damage and the subsequent risk of skin cancer and wrinkles. Many of these also contain irritating plant extracts and alcohol. Some make claims of protecting from UVA/UVB radiation; however, the FDA-regulated, mandatory active ingredient list does not list any ingredients capable of protecting from the entire UVA spectrum.

☹ **Waterproof UVA/UVB Protection 4, PABA Free Moisturizing Suntan Lotion** *($4.79 for 4 ounces)*; **Waterproof UVA/UVB Protection 8, Ultra Moisturizing with Aloe & Vitamin E Sunscreen Lotion** *($4.79 for 4 ounces)*; **Bug & Sun Sunscreen with Insect Repellent, Adult Formula SPF 15** *($6.99 for 4 ounces, $8.59 for 8 ounces)*; **Bug & Sun Sunscreen with Insect Repellent, Kids Formula SPF 30** *($6.99 for 4 ounces, $8.59 for 8 ounces)*; **Dry Oil Tanning Spray SPF 4** *($7.49 for 6 ounces)*; **Dry Oil Tanning Spray SPF 8** *($7.39 for 6 ounces)*; **Aloe & Vitamin Lip Balm with Sunscreen SPF 15** *($1.99 for 0.15 ounce)*; **Waterproof UVA/UVB Protection 15, Sunblock Lotion** *($7.99 for 8 ounces)*; **Kids Colorblock Disappearing Wacky Foam, Sunblock SPF 40** *($8.99 for 6 ounces)*; **Kids Colorblock Disappearing Purple Colored Sunblock SPF 40** *($9.29 for 8 ounces)*; **Kids Glitter Sunblock Lotion SPF 30** *($8.99 for 6 ounces)* **Kids Spray & Splash Sunblock Spray SPF 30** *($8.99 for 8 ounces)*;

Kids Sunblock Lotion Trigger Spray SPF 30 *($8.99 for 6 ounces)*; Kids Sunblock Stick SPF 30 *($4.79 for 6 ounces)*; Kids SPF 40, 6 Hour Waterproof Sunblock Lotion *($8.99 for 8 ounces)*; Kids Sport Sunblock Lotion SPF 30 *($8.99 for 6 ounces)*; Natural Fruit Flavor Lip Balm with Sunscreen SPF 15 *($1.99 for 0.15 ounce)*; Oil Free Sunblock Lotion SPF 45 *($8.99 for 8 ounces)*; Oil-Free Waterproof Sunblock SPF 15 *($6.99 for 4 ounces, $8.59 for 8 ounces)*; Oil-Free Waterproof Sunblock Lotion SPF 30 *($9.49 for 8 ounces)*; Oil-Free Waterproof Sunscreen Lotion, SPF 8 *($8.99 for 8 ounces)*; Rub-Free Sunblock Spray SPF 15 *($8.99 for 7 ounces)*; Shade Sunblock Stick SPF 30 *($4.79 for 0.6 ounce)*; Sport Stick SPF 30 *($4.79 for 0.6 ounce)*; Sport Ultra Sweatproof Sunblock SPF 15 *($7.99 for 8 ounces)*; Sport Ultra Sweatproof Sunblock SPF 30 *($7.99 for 8 ounces)*; Sport Ultra Sweatproof UVA/UVB Sunblock SPF 15 *($9.19 for 8 ounces)*; Sport Ultra Sweatproof Sunscreen Spray SPF 4 *($8.99 for 7 ounces)*; Sport All Day Protection SPF 48, UVA/UVB Sunblock *($8.99 for 8 ounces)*; Sport Sunblock Spray SPF 15 *($10.99 for 7 ounces)*; Sport Sunblock Spray SPF 30 *($8.99 for 7 ounces)*; Sunblock Gel SPF 30 *($8.99 for 6 ounces)*; Sunblock Lotion SPF 15 *($6.99 for 4 ounces)*; Sunscreen Lotion SPF 4 *($7.39 for 8 ounces)*; To Go Sunblock Spray SPF 15 *($9.99 for 7 ounces)*; To Go Sunblock Spray SPF 30 *($9.99 for 7 ounces)*; Tropical Blend Dark Tanning Lotion Spray Sunscreen SPF 2 *($5.99 for 8 ounces)*; Tropical Blend Dark Tanning Oil Spray Sunscreen SPF 4 *($5.99 for 8 ounces)*; Water Babies Lotion Spray SPF 30 *($10.99 for 8 ounces)*; Water Babies Lotion Spray SPF 45 *($8.99 for 8 ounces)*; Water Babies UVA/UVB Sunblock Lotion SPF 30 *($10.99 for 8 ounces)*; Water Babies UVA/UVB Sunblock Lotion SPF 45 *($8.99 for 8 ounces)*; Water Babies Sunblock Lotion Single Use Packets SPF 45 *($8.99 for 12 each)*; Water Babies Sunblock Stick SPF 30 *($4.79 for 0.6 ounce)*; Waterproof Ultra-Moisturizing SPF 15, with Aloe & Vitamin E *($10.99 for 8 ounces)*; Waterproof Ultra-Moisturizing SPF 30, with Aloe & Vitamin E *($9.99 for 8 ounces)*; and Waterproof Ultra-Moisturizing SPF 45, with Aloe & Vitamin E *($10.99 for 8 ounces)*.

COVER GIRL (MAKEUP ONLY)

Cover Girl has retained its role as a major contender in the makeup world by continuing to put on a whole new look—and it's an impressive face-lift. They have been busily eliminating most (though not all) of the overly fragranced (meaning malodorous) foundations, blushes, eyeshadows, and pressed powders. Even more significant is the elimination of all of the poor foundation textures, chalky powders, and flaky eyeshadows! Their newest additions are a breath of fresh air, and some of the best prices you will find at the drugstore. Before I get too carried away, I should state that some of the powders still have a wafting, sweet fragrance that is, at best, overpowering. Yet these are now the exception to the rule and are forgivable given the noteworthy improvements Cover Girl has made just over the past few years.

Cover Girl's Web site is extremely easy to navigate and presents a wealth of product information, along with praiseworthy tips and tricks for successful makeup application and for finding the shades that work best for you. Its consumer relations number is consistently helpful if you have any questions or concerns. For example, if some favorite item was among the many products that were discontinued, you may be wondering what new (and pleasantly improved) item has replaced it, and they will let you know. It is clear that Cover Girl is carrying on with the best intentions and an eagerness to provide not only superior products but also superior service. For more information about Cover Girl, call (800) 543-1745 or visit www.covergirl.com.

FOUNDATION: Cover Girl would win even higher marks if they would provide adequate testers for all of their products. While some stores do sell mini-samples of specific formulas, those are few and far between. For now, and even though the colors have gotten remarkably better, without testers the chance of buying the wrong color is fairly high.

☺ **Fresh Complexion Oil Control Makeup** *($6.49)* maintains that it will provide "beautiful coverage that lasts," but they should have inserted the adjective "sheer," as this talc-based pressed-powder foundation barely registers on the skin in terms of coverage. It does have a velvety texture that never looks dry or powdery, but the finish almost leaves a glow on the skin—not something those with oily skin have on their makeup checklist. It's best for normal to dry skin; you won't net any lasting shine control with this product. The eight shades present some visibly pink and peach colors, but the sheerness makes the color almost irrelevant. The ones to use with caution are Buff Beige, Natural Beige, and Classic Beige. Fair to light skin tones have the best chance of finding a perfect shade, but dark skin tones should look elsewhere. **Fresh Look Clear Up Tinted Acne Treatment Cream** *($5.79 for 0.65 ounce)* is a very good, 10% benzoyl peroxide product in a nonirritating, matte finish gel base. It is also supposed to be a slightly tinted concealer, but it does a poor job of concealing anything and it's available in only one very sheer shade. What it does a good job of is disinfecting, and that is an important step in the treatment of breakouts. However, 10% benzoyl peroxide is quite strong and not the best place to start for all skin types. It would be far better to start with a lower concentration of this active ingredient and move up gradually if your acne does not respond to the lower concentrations. **CG Smoothers All Day Hydrating Makeup** *($7.59)* actually has mostly great colors (fifteen in all)— what a shame the color on the container doesn't even vaguely resemble the color inside! Still, of all the Cover Girl foundations, this formula is the one I most often see in mini-sizes, so it's inexpensive to experiment with the shades. The talc content gives this sheer-to-medium coverage foundation a soft matte, slightly powdery finish, which is anything but hydrating (and definitely not for eleven hours, as the package states). It would work well for someone with normal to oily or combination skin. The following colors are too pink, rose, or peach for most skin tones: Natural Ivory (just slightly pink), Natural Beige, Medium Light, Warm Beige, Creamy Beige, and Toasted Almond. Soft Sable is a beautiful color for dark skin tones. This is fragrance-free.

✔☺ **AquaSmooth Makeup SPF 15** *($8.50)* is an ultralight, water-to-powder compact makeup that smooths easily onto the skin and dries to a soft, powdery matte finish. As with similar foundations, quick, deft blending is key— these formulas dry fast, and are not easy to move once they do. The sunscreen is all titanium dioxide, so even sensitive skin should be able to wear this, though the formula and finish are best for normal to slightly oily skin—dry skin will only look more noticeable with this type of foundation. There are fifteen shades, offering light to medium coverage. The ones to avoid due to overtones of pink or peach are Natural Ivory, Medium Light, Warm Beige, Natural Beige, Creamy Beige, and Toasted Almond. The remaining shades feature some excellent options for light and dark skin tones. ✔☺ **Fresh Look Makeup Oil-Free for Combination to Oily Skin SPF 15** *($7.59)* has an incredibly reasonable price, the SPF 15 sunscreen is all titanium dioxide, the finish is nicely matte (though not as matte as Revlon's Shine Control Mattifying Makeup SPF 15), and there is a streamlined assortment of nine colors. This really is a great formula with a smooth, even application and no noticeable fragrance. There are shades for very light skin tones, but nothing suitable for darker skin tones. The following colors are too peach, pink, or rose for most skin tones: Natural Ivory (just slightly pink), Creamy Beige, Natural Beige (very pink), and Tawny. ✔☺ **CG Smoothers SPF 15 Tinted Moisture** *($7.59)*. These are exceptionally sheer moisturizers that impart the smallest amount of color to the skin. The four shades are all worth considering, although if you need significant coverage you will want to use concealer along with it. The reformulated product is completely fragrance-free, the base formula is oil-free and less emollient than before, and the sunscreen is in-part zinc oxide, making this product appropriate for normal to slightly dry or slightly oily skin. **Continuous Wear**

Makeup *($7.79)* has fifteen mostly excellent shades (including colors for darker skin tones) that blend on smoothly and would work well for someone with normal to dry skin seeking sheer to light coverage. Unfortunately, the container is opaque, which makes it next to impossible to identify your possible color—a serious shortcoming I hope will be corrected soon. The following shades are too peach, pink, or rose for most skin tones: Medium Light, Natural Beige, Warm Beige, Creamy Beige, and Toasted Almond.

☺ **Clean Makeup Fragrance Free** *($5.49)* mercifully omits the sickly sweet scent that is present in the Clean Makeup below, as well as the irritating extracts. Unfortunately, almost all of the fifteen shades are just too strongly peach, pink, or rose for most skin tones. The only four shades worth considering are Ivory, Classic Ivory, Soft Honey, and Classic Tan. **Ultimate Finish Liquid Powder Makeup** *($7.29)* features a nice smooth texture, although the aluminum starch (second ingredient) is a skin irritant and the isopropyl myristate in it can aggravate breakouts. It may be OK for normal skin types not prone to blemishes, but drier skin will find that it just exaggerates every dry skin cell. The fifteen shades are a mixed bag; most are too glaringly peach, pink, or rose for most skin tones; avoid Natural Ivory, Creamy Natural, Classic Beige, Medium Light, Warm Beige, Creamy Beige, Natural Beige, and Toasted Almond. Soft Sable and Tawny are worthwhile shades for darker skin tones.

☹ **Clean Makeup** *($5.49)* is one of the original Cover Girl foundations (launched in 1961) that hasn't yet been discontinued—and I doubt it ever will be, because according to Cover Girl, they sell just over 23 million bottles per year! Yet this dated, basic formula contains clove, menthol, camphor, and eucalyptus, which are extremely irritating for skin, plus the colors are largely unusable for any skin tone and the fragrance is intrusive. **Simply Powder Foundation** *($7.99)* goes on thick and heavy, and easily cakes on the skin. It's a lot more than powder; it's a messy layer over the skin and ranks way below the newest excellent products from Cover Girl.

CONCEALER: ✔☺ **Invisible Concealer** *($4.69)* is a surprisingly excellent, affordable concealer. The five colors are mostly great for lighter to medium skin tones, but the Medium shade can be too rose. This applies smoothly and evenly without creasing, and is one to try! ✔☺ **Fresh Complexion Undereye Concealer** *($4.99)* has a wonderful, lightly creamy texture and a soft application that provides almost too much slip. Although blending this concealer takes a bit more time, the natural matte finish and smooth coverage are worth it. This wouldn't be my top choice if your optimum concern is **great coverage**, but those with minor imperfections should check it out. **Of the four colors,** only Natural Beige is too pink to purchase.

☺ **CG Smoothers Concealer** *($5.79)* is a standard, lipstick-style concealer that doesn't go on as greasy as it appears and provides good coverage with minimal creasing. However, four of the six shades are on the peach side, and the coverage is opaque enough for that to be a problem for some skin tones. Neutralizer is OK, but Illuminator is too whitish pink for even very light skin. Whitish pink is not a shade to use over blemishes.

POWDER: ☺ **CG Smoothers Fresh Look Pressed Powder Combination to Oily Skin** *($5.79)*, **CG Smoothers Fresh Look Pressed Powder Normal to Dry Skin** *($5.79)*, and **Clean Pressed Powder Fragrance-Free Normal Skin** *($5.49)* are all talc-based powders that have a similar sheer, smooth, almost invisible finish despite the different names and formulations. The colors are all decent, with only a few having slightly pink or peach tones, but the tones are so slight it's barely worth mentioning. The packaging has been updated for all of these powders, and now the enclosed puff, which used to almost completely hide the powder color, is behind the compact—so the colors are in full view! Though I rarely comment on a product's smell, the scent for the Fresh Look Pressed Powder Normal to Dry Skin is awfully obtrusive. In contrast, the others are mercifully fragrance-free.

☹ **Clean Pressed Powder for Normal Skin** *($5.49)* is almost identical to its fragrance-free counterpart, but this one includes eucalyptus oil and camphor, both of which are very irritating even in small amounts. Do I need to mention the overpowering fragrance this has? **Professional Loose Powder** *($5.69)* comes in six mostly well-conceived shades and a fine texture, but that is cancelled out by the pointless inclusion of eucalyptus, camphor, clove oil, and menthol—four potent irritants—and the sickly sweet fragrance.

☹ **BLUSH:** All of Cover Girl's powder blushes contain menthol, camphor, eucalyptus oil, and clove oil—irritants that have no business being in makeup and serve no positive purpose for the skin. **Instant Cheekbones** *($5.69)* has three colors in one compact—a blush tone, a contour color, and a shiny highlighter. The colors for these and for the single blush version, **Cheekers** *($3.79)*, still haven't been updated, which is strange because most of Cover Girl's drugstore contemporaries have more modern blush hues, while these remain rather pastel and intense. That may be OK for darker skin tones, but for anyone looking for subtle colors, these will be left out of the running. Most of the colors are slightly shiny. **Classic Color Blush** *($5.69)* is a larger-sized powder blush that comes in four single shades that are vivid, but blend on sheer. These are fairly powdery, and the color intensity is too soft for darker skin tones.

EYESHADOW: ☺ **Professional Eye Enhancers** *($4.69 "4 kit"; $4.69 "3 kit"; $2.99 "1 kit")* are labeled as matte or "perle," but most are very shiny to slightly shiny. Some of the matte shades, however, are indeed matte (but be careful) and are worth checking out. The texture and application of these is much better than in years past. Some of the 3-kit and 4-kit compacts have practical color combinations, so you can really use all of the shades!

The following Quads and Trios offer all matte shades: Chilled Grape, Slates, Shades of Suede, and Tranquil Browns. The following Singles are neutral and matte: Toasted Almond, Snow Blossom, Dewy Pink, Grey Suede, Midnight Jazz, and Hazelnut.

☺ **CG Smoothers Gel Eye Color** *($5.79)* are chubby pencils that go on somewhat wet, which means they glide on easily, and then the color dries to a matte finish that doesn't budge or smear all day. By the way, though I love the way these pencils go on, trying to keep a point on the pencil isn't easy, and that makes it difficult to create a thin, controlled line. There are several shades, and many of them are very shiny.

EYE AND BROW SHAPER: ✔☺ **Perfect Blend Eye Pencil** *($4.69)* is a fairly standard, but good, pencil that goes on slightly drier than most others and has decent staying power. There are six shades, all come with a sponge tip to ease blending. Avoid Cobalt Blue. ✔☺ **Liquid Pencil Felt Tip Eyeliner** *($5.69)* is an excellent, gel-based liquid eyeliner that applies easily and stays on without fading or chipping off. It is also very easy to wash off, so if you're a fan of this type of eyeliner, this is a strong contender—and the four shades are all contenders, too. ✔☺ **Perfect Point Plus** *($5.39)* is an automatic eye pencil that glides on easily without being greasy and maintains a consistent, sharp point. Chestnut is a great shade for an auburn eyeliner, but Dusky Blue and Midnight Blue are best avoided.

☺ **CG Smoothers Natural Brow and Lash Mascara** *($5.49)* is an acceptably priced, extremely standard, clear brow gel that leaves a minimal sticky feel. This brush isn't ideal, but it works—just take care that you coat the brows evenly, because any clumps will dry and flake off, an unpleasant side effect of this particular gel formula. **Brow and Eye Makers** *($2.89)* feature two short pencils that are the same color. It seems you're supposed to use one for eyes and one for brows, but the dry, waxy texture of these makes them best suited for brow pencil, and then only if you insist on using pencil over powder. Soft Blonde is a good light beige hue, and Henna Brown is an option for redheads.

LIPSTICK AND LIP PENCIL: Cover Girl has an excellent lipstick collection, and continues to offer impressive textures and a vast array of muted and bright colors. ☺ **CG Smoothers Hydrating Lipstick** *($7.59)* claims to provide just as much moisture for your lips as "the leading lip balm," but the fact is that most creamy, slightly greasy lipsticks (like this one) will do just that. This lipstick wears well and has enough stain to keep the color around for part of the day, which would be a better basis for a catchy claim. **Continuous Color Lipstick** *($5.79)* is available in Cremes, Shimmers, and Sheers. All of these are accurately named and have a smooth, slightly greasy texture. The Sheers are more fleeting, but the Cremes and Shimmers (which aren't too iridescent) have enough stain to go the distance, at least until lunch! **LipSlicks Lip Gloss** *($3.69)* is a basic, emollient gloss with some very shiny shades in packaging that makes getting it on the lips very tricky for anyone with thin lips. **Triple Lipstick SPF 15** *($5.89)* is one of the few lipsticks that offer UVA protection, with an in-part titanium dioxide base. This is a creamy, semiopaque formula with a slightly greasy finish and minimal stain. The color range is impressive. **CG Smoothers Lip Liner** *($5.79)* is as standard a lipliner as they come, in a nice, though limited, range of colors. These do need sharpening, and will work as well as any other pencil.

✔☺ **Outlast All Day Lipcolor** *($10.99)* pretty much lives up to its claim about staying on without coming off on anything. In some cases, you may even find that this has lasted all day, all night, and into the next morning. Other than the price, the only difference between this and Max Factor (Cover Girl's sister company) is that Outlast has slightly more colors (30+ colors!).

MASCARA: ☺ **Super Thick Lash** *($5.49)* is a great mascara, building long, thick lashes with only the slightest tendency to clump. This lasts well without smearing or flaking, and is arguably Cover Girl's most "dramatic" mascara. **Triple Mascara** *($6.29)* is a single mascara that does a good job of lengthening and thickening lashes, plus it doesn't smear or flake and can last all day. While this isn't the cream of the crop of the lengthening and thickening mascaras out there, it is certainly worth a try!

✔☺ **Professional Waterproof Mascara** *($5.49)* has a formula that applies easily and with some effort builds nice length and minimal thickness. Best of all, it really does hold up when wet and it's easy to remove!

☺ **Remarkable Washable Waterproof Mascara** *($5.49)*. Washable, yet waterproof, isn't that an oxymoron? Nonetheless, this applies evenly and builds good length and thickness. It isn't as waterproof as others, withstanding only a little water (such as a light rain) and breaking down underwater—so swimmers and criers will have to look elsewhere. As a plus, this does come off easily without taking your lashes with it!

☹ **Professional Smudgeproof Mascara Classic Look Curved Brush** *($5.49)* builds good length and some thickness, but tends to go on unevenly, an effect that seems to be a hallmark of these awkward curved-brush mascaras. **Professional**

Smudgeproof Mascara Classic Look Straight Brush *($5.49)* has an easier-to-wield wand than the curved version on the facing page, but this builds lengthy lashes unevenly and needs more fine-tuning than a mediocre mascara should. **Marathon Waterproof Mascara** *($5.49)* is back and just as poor as it was in the past. No matter how this is applied, it tends to clump and somehow manages to make lashes seem shorter. You won't see a modicum of thickness, and to top it off it's extremely difficult to remove.

BRUSHES: ☹ **Large Blush Brush** *($5.29)* is a poor option because the bristles are too soft and too sparse to provide much control. The **Powder Brush** *($6.39)* has a flat-cut top, which tends to work against the natural contours of the face and makes it easy to overpowder. The ☺ **Eyeshadow Brush** *($4.69)* is nicely shaped but quite thick. Some women may prefer that, but I find it tends to apply eyeshadow in stripes and is hard to use for blending.

ESTÉE LAUDER

What sets the venerable Estée Lauder company apart from its rivals is that it owns most of the cosmetics lines it competes with. Lauder's formidable reach includes Clinique, Origins, Prescriptives, M.A.C., Bobbi Brown, Stila, Aveda, Jane (a drugstore line aimed at teenagers), and La Mer, among others. That sort of takes the notion of cosmetic secrets and throws it to the winds, doesn't it? Would Estée Lauder keep so-called secrets from its own companies?

Of course, Estée Lauder is still the grande dame of makeup lines, with a loyal following and a plethora, if not endless redundancy, of products. Ask any of the salespeople who work for this seasoned cosmetics company and they will tell you that the products sell themselves. A few years ago, Night Repair and Eyezone were jumping off the shelves; then Estée Lauder's AHA product, Fruition (discontinued in favor of the far better formulated Fruition Extra), caught fire; and now Idealist and LightSource are the flavor du jour. It only takes a cursory look at the stable of Estée Lauder products, from the line itself to its protégés, to notice that there is an overwhelming number of antiwrinkle products (over 300 in all). But the question to ask is this: If just ten of its products could live up to their claims to get rid of wrinkles, why would you need an additional 290 products claiming to do the same thing? The Estée Lauder lineup boasts some wonderful moisturizers, but also some absurd prices for products that can't live up to their more glorious claims. For more information about Estée Lauder, call (212) 572-4200 or visit www.esteelauder.com. **Note:** All Lauder skin-care products contain fragrance unless otherwise noted.

Estée Lauder Skin Care

☺ **Perfectly Clean Solid Cleanser Normal to Dry** *($16.50 for 4.2 ounces)* is a pricey bar cleanser that is almost identical to Cetaphil's Bar Cleanser but at five times the price. This contains fragrance and coloring agents. Despite the Vaseline content, it can still be fairly drying for all skin types, but especially for dry skin.

☺ **Perfectly Clean Solid Cleanser Normal to Oily** *($16.50 for 4.2 ounces)* is similar to the Normal to Dry version above only minus the Vaseline. The same basic comments apply.

☺ **Perfectly Clean Foaming Lotion Cleanser, Normal/Dry and Dry Skin** *($16.50 for 4.2 ounces)* is a standard, detergent-based cleanser that also contains a good amount of plant oil, making it a good option for someone with normal to dry skin.

☺ **Perfectly Clean Foaming Gel Cleanser, Normal/Oily and Oily Skin** *($16.50 for 4.2 ounces)* is an exceptionally standard, detergent-based, water-soluble cleanser for normal to oily skin.

☺ **Soft Clean Milky Lotion Cleanser** *($16.50 for 6.7 ounces)* is a lotion-style cleanser that doesn't contain any detergent cleansing agents, making it an option for normal to dry skin. It doesn't remove makeup very well and may require using a washcloth to get everything off.

☹ **Rich Results Hydrating Cleanser** *($18.50 for 4.2 ounces)* contains menthol, coriander, and sage, which can all be skin irritants.

☺ **Splash Away Foaming Cleanser** *($18.50 for 3.4 ounces)* is a fairly drying, detergent-based, water-soluble cleanser. It can be an option for normal to oily skin.

☺ **Tender Creme Cleanser** *($26 for 8 ounces)* is a standard, lotion-style cleanser with no detergent cleansing agents that can be an option for normal to dry skin. For the money, Neutrogena's Extra Gentle Cleanser is almost identical for a third the price.

☺ **Gentle Eye Makeup Remover** *($13.50 for 3.4 ounces)* is an exceptionally standard, detergent cleanser–based eye-makeup remover and it works the same as most, though this one does not contain fragrance.

☺ **Take It Away Makeup Remover** *($18 for 6.7 ounces)* is a fairly standard, wipe-off makeup remover that would work for most skin types.

☺ **$$$ So Polished Exfoliating Scrub** *($19.50 for 1.7 ounces)* is a detergent-based cleanser that uses pumice as the abrasive. This can be an option for normal to oily skin, but it isn't preferred over using plain baking soda with a gentle cleanser.

☹ **Clear Finish Purifying Toner N/D** *($16.50 for 6.7 ounces)*. This extremely standard toner contains menthol, which can be a skin irritant for most skin types.

☹ **Clean Finish Purifying Toner N/O** *($16.50 for 6.7 ounces)* is similar to the version above, only this one adds grapefruit to the menthol irritation factor.

☺ **$$$ Re-Nutriv Extremely Delicate Skin Cleanser** *($32.50 for 7.5 ounces)* is a very standard, mineral oil–based, cold cream–style cleanser. There is very little reason to spend this amount of money for what is essentially Pond's Cold Cream. This can be an option for very dry skin, though the price is not warranted. The teeny amount of royal jelly in this product has no benefit for skin.

☺ **$$$ Re-Nutriv Moisture-Rich Creme Cleanser** *($27.50 for 3.4 ounces)* is similar to the Delicate Skin Cleanser above, only less greasy, and the same basic comments apply.

☺ **$$$ Re-Nutriv Intensive Hydrating Cream Cleanser** *($35 for 4.2 ounces)* is an emollient, cold cream–style cleanser that is an option for someone with normal to dry skin, but it holds no advantage over far less expensive versions at the drugstore or even other versions in this line!

☹ **Re-Nutriv Gentle Skin Toner** *($30 for 6.7 ounces)* is an exceptionally standard toner whose second ingredient is cetrimonium chloride, a cleansing agent and disinfectant. It isn't bad for the skin, it just isn't all that gentle. It also contains arnica, which is a problem when used repeatedly on skin.

☺ **$$$ Re-Nutriv Creme** *($78 for 1.75 ounces)* is a very emollient, mineral oil–based moisturizer for dry skin. It does contain some good water-binding agents and antioxidants.

☺ **$$$ Re-Nutriv Firming Eye Creme** *($47.50 for 0.5 ounce)*. This won't firm the eye area, and the amino acids, elastin, and collagen cannot get rid of wrinkles, though they are good water-binding agents. What this lacks is the assortment of antioxidants that many of the other Lauder products contain.

☺ **$$$ Re-Nutriv Firming Throat Creme** *($55 for 1.7 ounces)* is a good emollient moisturizer for dry skin that contains a good mix of water-binding agents and a small amount of antioxidants. There is nothing in this formulation that makes it better for the throat than the face.

☺ **$$$ Re-Nutriv Intensive Firming Plus** *($95 for 1.7 ounces)* is a very overpriced, basic moisturizer for dry skin that doesn't begin to compare to lots of other far better formulated Lauder moisturizers. It does contain a small amount of AHAs, but the pH is too high for them to be effective for exfoliation.

✔☺ **$$$ Re-Nutriv Intensive Lifting Creme** *($150 for 1.7 ounces)*. While this is a good moisturizer with lots of good water-binding agents, antioxidants, and anti-irritants, there is nothing in it that will lift skin anywhere, and the price is nothing less than obscene given the ingredient list. Estée Lauder charges a lot less for other moisturizers that have a similar ingredient list.

✔☺ **$$$ Re-Nutriv Intensive Lifting Serum** *($170 for 1 ounce)* contains an impressive array of water-binding agents, anti-irritants, and antioxidants in an emollient, Vaseline-based moisturizing lotion. Everything from retinol to grape extract, mulberry, and a bevy of plant extracts make an appearance here. The concentration of each isn't much and this won't lift skin anywhere, but it is definitely an excellent moisturizer for normal to dry skin.

☺ **$$$ Re-Nutriv Intensive Lifting Series** *($250 for 14 vials, total 0.95 ounce).* Do women really believe that there is anything in this product worth $4,000 for sixteen ounces? Actually, this isn't even as impressive as the Intensive Lifting Serum above, as it lacks many of the unique plant extracts and water-binding agents its sister contains. This one is good for normal to dry skin, but for the money, this just doesn't add up.

✔☺ **$$$ Re-Nutriv Ultimate Lifting Cream** *($250 for 1.7 ounces).* If this is the ultimate cream, it makes you wonder why Lauder needs to sell the other 300 antiwrinkle, antiaging products in their line. Ultimately, this Cream uses the kitchen-sink approach to skin, meaning it contains a little bit of everything. But what if skin needs more than just fractional amounts of a lot of ingredients? No one knows, but here you are playing for a great deal of money, and it's an expensive guessing game. There are lots of water-binding agents, antioxidants, anti-irritants, and emollients in here that are great for skin, but many Lauder products contain similar assortments for a lot less.

☹ **$$$ Re-Nutriv Replenishing Creme** *($78 for 1.7 ounces)* is an emollient moisturizer that contains some good water-binding agents, though it lacks any of the interesting antioxidants typical of many less expensive Lauder moisturizers. This one also contains several plant extracts that are potential skin irritants, including lemon, clove, and cinnamon.

☹ **$$$ Re-Nutriv Lightweight Creme** *($75 for 1.75 ounces)* isn't all that light. It contains lots of thickening agents, plant oils, and a small amount of water-binding agents and antioxidants. It is an OK, though exceedingly overpriced, moisturizer for dry skin.

☺ **$$$ Re-Nutriv Intensive Lifting Mask** *($70 for 1.7 ounces)* is mostly an emollient moisturizer that adds nothing in the way of extra benefit over many of the other Lauder moisturizers. It does contain some very good plant oils, anti-irritants, and some antioxidants.

☹ **$$$ Resilience Elastin Refirming Creme** *($60 for 1.7 ounces)* is a good, but extremely ordinary, moisturizer for someone with normal to dry skin. It does contain some good water-binding agents, but lacks many of the interesting antioxidants found in other Lauder products. Elastin is merely a good water-binding agent; there is no research showing it can affect the quality of elastin in skin.

☺ **$$$ Resilience Elastin Refirming Lotion** *($62.50 for 1.7 ounces)* is similar to the Elastin Refirming Creme on the facing page, only in lotion form, and the same review applies.

☺ **$$$ Resilience Eye Creme Elastin Refirming Complex** *($42.50 for 0.5 ounce)* is an OK moisturizer for normal to dry skin, with several state-of-the-art water-binding agents and emollients like Vaseline and shea butter, but only a teeny amount of vitamin E. However, it won't lift the skin anywhere and there is nothing about it that makes it better for the eye area than the face. There are also minute amounts of plankton, caffeine, and barley, among other extracts. If these ingredients are the answer for wrinkles, then why aren't they in the other products for wrinkles that Lauder sells? Or does everything get rid of wrinkles? Must be, because there is no uniformity among these myriad antiwrinkle products.

☺ **$$$ Resilience Eye Creme** *($42.50 for 0.5 ounce)* is an OK, silicone- and film-forming agent–based moisturizer for normal to dry skin. It does contain a decent assortment of water-binding agents, but lacks the antioxidants and anti-irritants found in many other Lauder products.

☺ **$$$ Resilience Lift Eye Creme** *($42.50 for 0.5 ounce)* is similar to the Resilience Eye Creme above only with more emollient, and the same comments apply.

✔☺ **$$$ Resilience Lift Overnight** *($70 for 1.7 ounces)* is an emollient, Vaseline-based moisturizer that contains a very good assortment of water-binding agents and antioxidants.

✔☺ **$$$ Resilience Lift Face and Throat Cream SPF 15** *($65 for 1.7 ounce)* and **Resilience Lift Face and Throat Lotion SPF 15** *($45 for 1 ounce)* are two good sunscreens with part titanium dioxide to help provide UVA protection. But no one is spending this much money on these two products just for sun protection! Clearly, the word "lift" is meant to imply that these can make a serious difference in the appearance of skin. They can't. They are simply standard sunscreens in good moisturizing bases that contain an array of water-binding agents and antioxidants, and that isn't going to lift the skin anywhere.

☺ **$$$ Verite Light Lotion Cleanser** *($22.50 for 6.7 ounces)* is an emollient, cold cream–style cleanser that is an option for someone with dry skin.

☺ **$$$ Verite Soft Foam Cleanser** *($22.50 for 4.2 ounces)*. One of the detergent cleansing agents in this product, sodium C14-16 olefin sulfonate, is not the best for any skin type, but especially not for sensitive skin. Though the Vaseline does help soften the effect, in the long run it just ends up being confusing for skin.

- ☺ $$$ **Verite Soothing Spray Toner** *($22.50 for 6.7 ounces)* is an OK toner for normal to dry skin that contains mostly water, slip agent, water-binding agents, plant extracts, fragrance, and preservatives.
- ✔☺ $$$ **Verite Calming Fluid** *($60 for 1.7 ounces)* won't calm anything, but it is a very good moisturizer with great water-binding agents and antioxidants for someone with normal to dry skin.
- ☺ $$$ **Verite Moisture Relief Creme** *($50 for 1.75 ounces)* is an OK moisturizer for someone with normal to dry skin.
- ✔☺ $$$ **Verite Special Eye Care** *($50 for 1.7 ounces)* is a very emollient, Vaseline-based moisturizer that contains a good mix of water-binding agents and antioxidants.
- ☺ $$$ **100% Time Release Moisturizer Creme** *($35 for 1.7 ounces)* is a moisturizer with a small amount of water-binding agents and antioxidant that is OK for someone with normal to dry skin. It is one of the more ordinary offerings in the Estée Lauder lineup.
- ☺ $$$ **100% Time Release Moisture Lotion** *($35 for 1.7 ounces)* is similar to the Creme version above and the same basic comments apply.
- ✔☺ $$$ **Advanced Night Repair Protective Recovery Complex** *($70 for 1.7 ounces)* isn't all that advanced, but it is a very good moisturizer with a first-rate mix of antioxidants, water-binding agents, and anti-irritants. One strange twist: It also contains a good amount of sunscreen, which doesn't make sense in a product that's meant to be used at night, although the sunscreen is not rated with an SPF.
- ✔☺ $$$ **Advanced Night Repair Eye Recovery Complex** *($45 for 0.5 ounce)* claims to address pretty much every eye-skin-care woe you can think of, from puffiness to dark circles, wrinkles, and tired skin. It sounds like the ultimate choice for eyes, but we've all heard this song before with countless other Lauder eye products, from Uncircle to Unline to Eyezone, along with a vast selection from the ten other lines under Lauder's ownership. Still, skin-repairing claims aside, this is undeniably a very good, silicone-based moisturizer that would take good care of dry skin anywhere on the face.
- ☺ $$$ **Age Controlling Creme** *($60 for 1.7 ounces)* is a good, lanolin-based, emollient moisturizer for someone with very dry skin that also contains some plant oils, Vaseline, mineral oil, and a small amount of water-binding agents and antioxidants. There is nothing in this product that can control even one minute of aging.

☺ **Clear Difference Oil-Control Hydrator for Oily Normal/Oily and Blemish-Prone Skin** *($27 for 1.7 ounces)* is a silicone-based moisturizer that contains some good water-binding agents and an antioxidant. It also contains salicylic acid, but the pH of the product is about 4, and that is just borderline for allowing it to be effective for exfoliation. There is nothing in it that can control oil production.

✔☺ Estoderme Emulsion *($27.50 for 4 ounces)* is a good emollient moisturizer for dry skin that contains some good water-binding agents and antioxidants.

☺ **$$$ Eyezone Repair Gel** *($35 for 0.5 ounce)* contains mostly water, film-forming agents, algae, slip agent, water-binding agent, vitamin A, and preservatives. The tiny amount of algae and even smaller amount of vitamin A here won't do anything for skin, much less repair it, but this is an OK, ordinary moisturizer for slightly dry skin.

☺ **$$$ Time Zone Eyes Ultra-Hydrating Complex** *($40 for 0.5 ounce)* is a lightweight, ordinary moisturizer for normal to slightly dry skin.

☺ **$$$ Time Zone Moisture Recharging Complex** *($55 for 1.7 ounces)* is similar to the Eyes Ultra-Hydrating Complex above, only with more emollients. It would be good for dry skin.

✔☺ **$$$ Fruition Extra Multi-Action Complex** *($70 for 1.7 ounces)*. The original Fruition was discontinued, and the Extra is now the only version available. The original was supposed to be an exfoliating AHA product, but it didn't contain enough AHA to have any effect; basically it was just a good lightweight moisturizer. Fruition Extra adds salicylic acid to the mix, so this is a BHA product now. It does work well as an exfoliant, but is incredibly overpriced for what you get, which is a good, lightweight moisturizing base with silicones, film-forming agents, water-binding agents, antioxidants, fragrance, coloring agents, and preservatives.

✔☺ **$$$ Future Perfect Micro-Targeted Skin Gel** *($45 for 1.75 ounces)* is not more perfect than any other moisturizer in the Lauder group. It is just a good, silicone-based, emollient moisturizer for normal to dry skin that contains a good mix of water-binding agents and antioxidants.

✔☺ **$$$ Idealist** *($42.50 for 1 ounce)*. The spin on this product is that it's a non-retinol and non-AHA wrinkle remover; it claims to be the best option around for skin. If that's the case, does that mean Estée Lauder's Fruition Extra and Diminish are now history, along with all the other AHA, BHA, and retinol products the other Estée Lauder–owned lines sell? That would never happen, of course, despite Estée Lauder's claim that Idealist is now the answer for your less-than-youthful visage. The two standout ingredients, according to Estée Lauder " . . . are acetyl glucosamine and sodium lactobionate." For some reason, if these two ingredients can banish wrinkles, the only company that knows about it is Estée Lauder.

What we do know about N-acetyl glucosamine is that it's an amino acid sugar, the primary constituent of mucopolysaccharides and hyaluronic acid, and is found in all parts of the skin. It has value as a water-binding agent and is effective (in high concentrations) for wound healing. There is also research (*Cellular and Molecular Life Sciences*, 53(2), February 1997, pages 131–140) showing that chitins (also known as chitosan—which is composed of acetyl glucosamine) can help in the complex process of wound healing.

However, that is a few generations removed from the acetyl glucosamine being included in a skin-care product. Besides, you have to wonder what any of that has to do with exfoliation, especially in the tiny concentration this product contains. And please understand that wound healing isn't related to wrinkles because wrinkles aren't wounds. What about the sodium lactobionate? It seems to be used in solutions as a preservative, but I wasn't able to find any research confirming Estée Lauder's contentions for it. It's a mystery. All told, this is a good, lightweight moisturizer for normal to dry skin—the silicone will leave a silky feel on the skin—and it does have plenty of anti-irritants and antioxidants. Whether or not the acetyl glucosamine and sodium lactobionate do something different is yet to be seen.

☺ **$$$ LightSource Transforming Moisture Creme SPF 15** *($45 for 1.7 ounces)* is a very good emollient moisturizer, containing a reliable SPF 15 using avobenzone as one of the active ingredients. This would work well for someone with normal to dry skin. Now to the claims! Lauder's brochure for this product states that it contains "millions of micro-crystals [emeralds that] convert light into positive energy, giving your skin an amazing brightness and freshness—even without makeup. Skin experiences an upsurge of energy—and is empowered to remain active . . . to do] all the things it's always done, but now with dramatically enhanced levels of performance." Wow! Actually, I'm speechless. I don't know what to say about any of this. Can minuscule amounts of crushed "reflective" stones give skin energy? Not that I've seen. Is there a shred of clinical published research proving any of this to be true (other than what the Lauder company asserts)? Not a one. But at least Lauder had the good sense to add an effective sunscreen, because there will no doubt be women who will believe that sunlight's negative effects can somehow be tamed or converted by this product, and they can't. By the way, about the "millions of micro-crystals"—the amount of emerald in this product is at best described as a trace.

☺ **$$$ LightSource Transforming Lotion SPF 15** *($45 for 1.7 ounces)* is similar to the LightSource Creme version on the facing page only without the Vaseline, which makes it better for normal to slightly dry skin, and the same basic comments apply.

☺ **$$$ Skin Perfecting Creme Firming Nourisher** *($35 for 1.75 ounces)* is a good, lightweight, emollient moisturizer for dry skin. This product does contain arnica, a possible skin irritant with repeated use, but the amount is so small that it probably won't have any impact on skin.

☹ **Skin Perfecting Lotion Lightweight Moisturizer** *($27.50 for 1.7 ounces)* is indeed lightweight, but it's also boring. The Creme version above is far better formulated because it has both more interesting water-binding agents and less fragrance.

✔☺ **Swiss Performing Extract Moisturizer** *($25 for 1.7 ounces)* is a very emollient and very good moisturizer for someone with dry skin. It contains a good mix of antioxidants, plant oils, and water-binding agents. The minor concern about arnica for the Skin Perfecting Creme above applies here as well.

☺ **$$$ Uncircle** *($37.50 for 0.5 ounce)*. There is nothing in this product that will have any greater effect on circles than would any other moisturizer in this line. Vaseline and film-forming agent are not what I or anyone else would call an exotic or excitingly new formulation, and fish cartilage can't affect anything around the eyes. It does contain some good water-binding agents and a small amount of antioxidants, and that's good, just not great.

☹ **Unline Total Eye Care** *($35 for 0.5 ounce)*. Although many aspects of this one make it a good moisturizer, the mint and wintergreen oil are irritants and a particular problem for the eye area.

✔☺ **$$$ Nutritious Bio Protein** *($45 for 1.7 ounces)* is a very good moisturizer for normal to dry skin. However, despite the clever name, you can't feed the skin from the outside in. Still, it does contain some very good antioxidants and water-binding agents.

✔☺ **$$$ Diminish Retinol Treatment** *($70 for 1.7 ounces)* came on the scene with a fanfare of claims about getting rid of lines, evening-out skin tone, improving skin texture, and on and on, much like the claims about several of the other products in this line. It definitely contains retinol, but only about 0.1% or 0.2%. Other than that, the rest of the ingredients are an impressive mix of water-binding agents and antioxidants.

✔☺ **$$$ Day Wear Super Anti-Oxidant Complex SPF 15** *($37.50 for 1.7 ounces)*. The antioxidants are not exactly at the top of the ingredient list, nor are they any more special than those in hundreds of other products, so none of that is all that super. What is good about this day cream is that it contains an SPF 15 sunscreen that is in-part titanium dioxide, one of the better ways to protect against sun damage. In that regard, this product is right on, as are most of Estée Lauder's sunscreens.

☺ **Spotlight Skin Tone Perfector** *($30 for 1.7 ounces)* is a good, silicone-based moisturizer for normal to slightly dry skin. This product is meant to improve skin color, thanks to the presence of some vitamin C and plant extracts that include mulberry root and licorice. There is some research that indicates these ingredients in pure form can inhibit melanin formation, but probably not in the tiny amount present in this product. It also contains shine.

☺ **Enriched Under-Makeup Creme** *($25 for 4 ounces)* is definitely emollient, but also boring. This is a very ordinary moisturizer for someone with very dry skin.

☹ **Counter Blemish Lotion** *($14 for 0.45 ounce)*. Alcohol is listed as the second ingredient, and it also contains zinc phenolsulfonate and cinnamon, which means this ends up causing irritation and dryness, effects that don't counter blemishes in the least.

☺ **Go Bronze Tinted Self Tanner for Face** *($18.50 for 1.7 ounces)* and **Go Bronze Tinted Self Tanner for Body** *($25 for 5 ounces)* are like all other self-tanners in that they use the active ingredient dihydroxyacetone to turn the skin brown. The advantage to the tint is that it lets you see where you've applied it, helping to achieve a more even tan look.

☺ **Stay Bronze Moisturizing Tan Extender for Face** *($19.50 for 1.7 ounces)* is just a self-tanner that uses dihydroxyacetone, the same ingredient in all self-tanners, to affect the color of skin. It would work as well as any other.

☺ **$$$ So Clean Deep Pore Mask** *($19.50 for 3.4 ounces)* is a standard clay mask that also contains some good water-binding agents, though their effectiveness would be negated by the absorbing properties of the clay. This would work as well as any for absorbing oil.

☺ **$$$ So Moist Hydrating Mask** *($19.50 for 3.4 ounces)* is indeed hydrating, but no more so than any other moisturizer in the Estée Lauder family.

☺ **$$$ Stress Relief Eye Mask** *($27.50 for ten 0.4-ounce packets)* is a somewhat sticky mask that doesn't feel great on the skin, although it is a good light-weight moisturizer. Still, there is nothing in it that will give the skin relief from anything.

☺ **$$$ Triple Creme Hydrating Mask** *($27.50 for 2.5 ounces)* contains good moisturizing ingredients, so it would feel good on dry skin, but no more so than any other moisturizer in the Estée Lauder lineup.

✔☺ **Sunblock for Body SPF 25** *($18.50 for 5 ounces)* is a good, in-part titanium dioxide- and zinc oxide-based sunscreen in a good emollient moisturizing base with a small amount of water-binding agents and antioxidants. It would be a good option for normal to dry skin.

✔☺ **Sun Block for Face SPF 15** *($18.50 for 1.7 ounces)* is similar to the Sunblock for Body SPF 25 on facing page and the same basic comments apply.

✔☺ **Sun Block for Face SPF 30** *($18.50 for 1.7 ounces)* is similar to the Sunblock for Body SPF 25 above and the same comments apply.

☹ **Oil Free Sun Spray SPF 15** *($18.50 for 4.2 ounces)* doesn't contain the UVA-protecting ingredients of titanium dioxide, zinc oxide, or avobenzone, and is not recommended.

Estée Lauder WhiteLight Brightening System

☺ **$$$ WhiteLight Brightening Cleansing Foam** *($26 for 4.2 ounces)* is a standard, rather gentle, water-soluble cleanser that has a mild foaming action. It contains a nice assortment of anti-irritants and water-binding agents, which can be helpful for skin, though they would be rinsed off before they had much chance to have any benefit. Like all the WhiteLight products, it does contain fragrance. If left on the skin, the vitamin C, along with the mulberry extract in this product, may inhibit melanin production, but in a cleanser that benefit would be rinsed down the drain.

☺ **$$$ WhiteLight Brightening Cleansing Powder** *($26 for 4.2 ounces)* is a wax- and talc-based cleansing powder that forms a soaplike lather when used with water. This can feel mildly abrasive on the skin as well as be overly drying. It can also leave a soapy film on the skin (the fourth ingredient is sodium hydrogenated tallow glutamate). The comments about the vitamin C and mulberry ingredients in the Cleansing Foam above apply here, too.

☺ **$$$ WhiteLight Brightening Treatment Lotion** *($30 for 4.2 ounces)* claims it is "far more than a toner," but based on the ingredient list this is much closer to a toner than anything else. It contains mostly water, slip agents, vitamin C, antioxidants, tourmaline (a gemstone), clay, fragrance, preservatives, and mica (a shiny earth mineral). This is good, but not great. The vitamin C and mulberry extract can help inhibit melanin production.

☹ **WhiteLight Concentrated Brightening Stick** *($30 for 0.22 ounce)* is essentially a silicone-based cream-to-powder stick concealer that has a strange mauve tint. This does little to conceal brown or tan discolorations, except for giving a somewhat ashen appearance when applied. Even if you are all for the use of color correctors, mauve is traditionally used to neutralize yellow or sallow undertones, not brown ones. It does contain a small amount of mulberry extract, which may help inhibit melanin production.

☺ **$$$ WhiteLight Brightening Moisture Creme** *($37.50 for 1 ounce)* is a good moisturizer for normal to dry skin that contains mostly water, emollient, slip agent, thickeners, silicone, antioxidants, water-binding agents, anti-irritants, fragrance, and preservatives. It does contain a small amount of mulberry extract, which may help inhibit melanin production.

☺ $$$ **WhiteLight Brightening Protective Base SPF 30** (*$30 for 1.7 ounces*). Diligent use of sunscreen with UVA-protecting ingredients is the most important element for reducing skin discolorations, and this moisturizer covers that need nicely. Featuring one of the longest ingredient lists you'll likely ever see for a sunscreen, it contains an impressive group of antioxidants and water-binding agents and includes zinc oxide as one of the active sunscreen ingredients. It is worth considering if you have normal to dry skin that's not prone to breakouts.

☺ $$$ **WhiteLight Concentrated Brightening Serum** (*$65 for 1.3 ounces*) promises to make "the look of porcelain-perfect skin a reality," but the effect is entirely cosmetic, thanks to the lavender opalescent powder it contains, which lends an ethereal soft blue glow to the skin. This silicone-based serum has a good assortment of antioxidants and anti-irritants. But if what you're paying for is the promise of perfect skin and no skin discolorations, this product is incapable of delivering that, despite its otherwise state-of-the-art formula. It is best for normal to slightly dry or slightly oily skin.

Estée Lauder Makeup

If any line has a golden touch when it comes to launching new makeup products, it's Estée Lauder. Season to season, they seem to have a divining rod on the pulse of what women want—or maybe the women who frequent the Lauder counter have simply come to expect their choices to be dictated by this well-heeled company. The cosmetics collection is nothing short of exhaustive, at least when it comes to the sheer number of products available. The tester units have become more accessible, but if you're hoping to compare different foundations, concealers, or powders, you'll need a salesperson's assistance, because it is almost impossible to navigate this line alone.

It is interesting to note that other Lauder-owned companies, from Clinique to Prescriptives, often launch similar, if not identical, products. For example, several months after Lauder's Equalizer foundation debuted, Lauder-owned Origins came out with Stay Tuned Balancing Face Makeup, a nearly identical formula (sans sunscreen) that costs less than half of Lauder's Equalizer. The same thing happened with Lauder's Fresh Air Continuous Moisture Tint SPF 15. Again, a nearly identical Origins product, Nude & Improved Bare-Face Makeup SPF 15, came on the scene, boasting effective sun protection and a significantly smaller price tag. The only real difference among many of these products is the marketing angle and the targeted consumer demographic.

Lauder's selection of makeup excels in their foundation textures and colors (including improved options for darker skin) and their eyeshadows, which are superior to those from most other department-store lines. Other strong points include some reliable concealers and blushes, and an ever-imposing selection of lipsticks. The makeup loses momentum with its uninspired collection of mascaras and merely OK brushes. Given that other lines under the Lauder umbrella (such as Clinique and Stila) are ably producing superior versions of these makeup must-haves, there's no reason to remain loyal to Lauder's namesake line.

FOUNDATION: Estée Lauder's foundations offer something for everyone in terms of texture and formulation. However, several of the formulas are without the recommended UVA-protecting ingredients, and while a couple have the benchmark SPF 15 rating, there are still those that miss the mark. It's even more important to take great care in finding the right shade, as Estée Lauder still likes to sneak in the occasional rosy pink and peach colors. However, foundation samples are readily available for almost all of the formulas reviewed below—so don't hesitate to ask for these if you're uncertain about shade or formula.

✔☺ $$$ So Ingenious Multi-Dimension Makeup SPF 8 ($32.50) is a truly silky liquid makeup. This airy foundation establishes a new benchmark when it comes to an ultrasmooth feel, great application, and a natural, nondrying matte finish. If only the titanium dioxide sunscreen were boosted to a higher number; the SPF 8 is an embarrassment! As is, you'll have to pair this with an effective sunscreen to net a full day's worth of protection. There are sixteen shades available, with options for very light and darker skin tones. Although most of them are admirable, they aren't as across-the-board brilliant as those from Lauder's So Ingenious Powder Makeup are. The following shades are too gray, peach, or pink for most skin tones: Fresco, Auburn, Outdoor Beige, Pebble, and Linen. If you have normal to slightly dry skin and prefer sheer to medium coverage, this one should be on your short list! ✔☺ So Ingenious Multi-Dimension Powder Makeup ($32.50) offers an ultrasmooth, suede-like texture that does not have an overly dry finish. This provides a clean, quick application and blends extraordinarily well over the skin, leaving a soft matte finish. As is typical with powder foundations, coverage is light to medium, and this type of foundation is best suited to all except very oily or very dry skin types. Essentially, talc-based powder foundations like this are middle-of-the-road options for those whose skin is neither too greasy nor too parched. Lauder has set a precedent by introducing sixteen beautiful skin-realistic shades. There are suitable options for light and dark skin tones, and the only colors to view with caution are Cool Champagne (slightly pink) and Cool Praline (very slightly peach), but even these shades may work for some skin tones and should not be altogether ignored. By the way, this product features Lauder's QuadraColor technology, which supposedly allows pigments to self-adjust depending on what type of light you're in. You won't see this powder magically fine-tune itself as you go from sunny outdoors to the fluorescent lighting of your office, but it's natural finish and seamless coverage do keep it from looking too thick or chalky on the skin, regardless of the lighting. This comes with a dual-sided sponge, with one side porous and the other smooth. The smooth side affords a nicer finish and more even coverage, but test both sides to see which one you prefer. ✔☺ **Equalizer Smart Makeup SPF 10** *($32.50)* is similar in concept (and number of shades) to Lauder-owned Origins Stay Tuned Makeup ($15). Both of these foundations make the same improbable claim of being able to moisturize dry areas while absorbing oil from oily areas. How a product could hold back its moisturizing ingredient from one area while absorbing oil or moisture from another is a mystery, and in fact it doesn't work—which you will be able to tell immediately from the first application. All claims aside, Equalizer leapfrogs over Stay Tuned by adding an all titanium dioxide–based sunscreen. (What would have really been smart would have been an SPF 15; an SPF 10 is cheating skin for no good reason.) It also has a very silky, light texture, offering sheer to medium coverage with a soft, slightly powdery finish that would be great for those with normal to slightly oily skin. If you have any dryness, it can feel tight and look flaky soon after it's blended. There are 20 shades, and the majority of them are wonderful. Several colors do shy toward being a bit too peach, but not nearly enough to warrant avoiding them. However, there are two colors that you should steer clear of, Vanilla and Copper, because they are just too peach or pink to come across as natural on almost any skin tone. There are a couple of options for very light skin tones, but darker skin tones have the edge here, as almost all of the deep colors are gorgeous.

☺ **$$$ Futurist Age-Resisting Makeup SPF 15** *($32.50)* leaves out the most important antiaging weapon anyone can have: a sunscreen with UVA-protecting ingredients! How disappointing that a foundation with such a superlative texture and luminous finish has this as its major flaw. If you have normal to dry skin and are prepared to wear a sunscreen underneath, you will get a great medium-coverage foundation, but be careful of the following colors, all of which can be too rose, orange, or copper for most skin tones: Fawn, Pale Almond (slightly pink), Tender Cream, Cool Sand, Golden Petal, Cameo, Sunlit Topaz, and Bare Beige. **Lucidity Light-Diffusing Makeup SPF 8** *($29.50)* claims it has "special light-diffusing pigments" that "actually reflect light away from fine lines and wrinkles so they seem to disappear," but this is just a standard, silicone-based moisturizing foundation with a smooth texture and medium coverage. Any wrinkles will still be plainly visible, if not magnified—but that's true of any foundation. Lucidity's SPF 8 is not only too low for daily protection, it does not contain UVA-protecting ingredients. It's an option if you have normal to dry skin and are willing to wear a separate sunscreen underneath. Of the thirteen shades, the following can be too peach or pink for most skin tones: Outdoor Beige, Cool Beige, Neutral Beige, Sun Beige, Rich Ginger, and Vanilla Beige. Porcelain and Ivory Beige are slightly pink, but still worth considering if you have light skin. **Minute Makeup Creme Stick Foundation SPF 15** *($29.50)* has a light, creamy texture that applies smoothly and dries to a soft, powder finish. But don't let the name fool you—it takes as long to apply as any other makeup, unless you're going for spot application. Consider this one if you have normal to dry skin and prefer sheer to medium adjustable coverage. There are eight mostly excellent shades, and only Maize and Golden tend toward the peachy side, though not irreparably so. One word of warning: Estée Lauder claims this is nonacnegenic. I disagree. Several ingredients in it could trigger breakouts, not the least of which is the active sunscreen ingredient, titanium dioxide, which is great for UVA protection but can be problematic for acne-prone skin. **Double Wear Stay-in-Place Makeup SPF 10** *($29.50)* is great—at least when it comes to a terrific matte texture that doesn't move. Someone with normal to oily skin will be impressed with the application and the way it holds up over a long day, though it can provide too much coverage—this is pretty thick stuff—and, as is true for most ultra-matte foundations, it's hard to remove. Of course, the SPF should be 15 even though it does have a pure titanium dioxide base. As the formula stands, you would require another sunscreen underneath, which can add an oily or layered feel on oily skin. Still, this is one of the last strong contenders in a diminishing selection of ultra-matte, long-wearing makeup. Of the twelve shades available, four can be too peach, pink, or rose for most skin tones: Pebble, Bronze, Spice, and Soft Tan. **Enlighten Skin-Enhancing Makeup SPF 10** *($29.50)* has a wonderful texture, and uses titanium dioxide as the sunscreen agent; what a shame it only has an SPF 10, which leaves the skin in need of more sun protection. The application is smooth and sheer, leaving a beautiful, slightly matte finish. It is best for someone with normal to combination or slightly dry skin. The eight-shade color selection isn't as strong as the selections of Lauder's newer foundations, though there are some options for very light skin tones. The following colors are too pink or peach for most skin tones: Neutral Beige, Gentle Ivory, Outdoor Beige, and Vanilla Beige. **Re-Nutriv Intensive Lifting Makeup** *($65)* is elegantly packaged in a frosted-glass jar complete with golden cap and trim. This is billed as Lauder's ultraluxurious makeup, perfect for dry to very dry skin. Yet this silky, silicone-based formula blends down to a natural matte finish that is not at all emollient or something those with dry skin would enjoy. It's best for those with normal to slightly dry or slightly oily skin seeking medium coverage and a whatever-it-may-cost makeup. The seven shades are impressively neutral, with the exception of the peach-tinged Radiant Wheat and Radiant Tan. Do I need to mention that this won't lift the skin even one millimeter?

☺ **$$$ Maximum Cover Camouflage Makeup for Face & Body SPF 15** *($26)* goes on creamy-smooth and tends to stick to the skin, which can feel uncomfortable. It doesn't provide as much coverage as the name implies (this isn't Dermablend), but it does cover well, provides a titanium dioxide sunscreen, and blends to a solid matte finish. The range of seven shades is commendable, with only Creamy Tan being a bit too peach. There are no options for darker skin tones.

☺ **$$$ Impeccable Protective Compact Makeup SPF 20** *($29.50)* has a texture similar to the Minute Makeup SPF 15 on page 551, only this is slightly creamier and offers heavier coverage and has inadequate UVA protection. If you are willing to wear an adequate sunscreen underneath, this could work well, but there are better options out there, such as Clinique's City Base Compact Foundation SPF 15 *($21)*. Of the eight shades, Vanilla and True Beige can be too pink or rose. **Fresh Air Continuous Moisture Tint SPF 15** *($34)* is an impressive tinted moisturizer in terms of its silky, easy-to-blend texture, radiant finish, and four wonderful shades that offer a sheer veil of color. What's disappointing, not to mention shocking, is the lack of adequate UVA protection from the sunscreen. This would have been an easy one to recommend for normal to dry skin, but with the insufficient sunscreen, there is no reason to consider this over Origins Nude and Improved Bare-Face Makeup SPF 15 *($15)*.

☹ **Double Matte Oil Control Makeup SPF 15** *($29.50)* was launched after the winning Double Wear Makeup, and one would have thought the reliable SPF would carry over since this foundation has a similar theme. Well, the SPF is higher, but it doesn't contain UVA protection. In addition, the texture is thick, five of the nine colors are poor, and the finish is slightly sticky and chalky, making this a bona fide "Why bother?" Oilier skin looking for a foundation with reliable sun protection would do well to consider Revlon's Shine Control Mattifying Makeup SPF 15 instead. **Maximum Cover Color Corrector** *($26)* is the exact same formula as the Maximum Cover Makeup above, but this is a mint green shade. Not only is green an odd color to use on the face, this is too opaque to look anything but obvious. **Polished Performance Liquid**

Makeup *($26)* and **Country Mist Liquid Makeup** *($21)* are holdovers from several years ago, and they're both standard, no-frills, emollient foundations for normal to dry skin that come in disappointing colors and are not worth considering over Lucidity. **Fresh Air Makeup Base** *($21)* is equally disappointing, though it has a lighter texture and a clay-based matte finish that would only please someone with oily skin. If that's you, consider Clinique's superior Stay True Makeup over this one.

CONCEALER: ☺ $$$ **Double Wear Stay in Place Concealer SPF 10** *($17)* is a liquidy, ultra-matte concealer that provides intense coverage and includes a titanium dioxide sunscreen. You must be exact in your blending, as this dries very quickly to a matte finish that won't budge. There are six shades, and the two darkest colors are a bit peach, but they may work for some skin tones. For dark circles, this is preferred to Estée Lauder's **Smoothing Creme Concealer** *($17)*. The Smoothing Creme comes in a squeeze tube, so be cautious of pressing out too much. However, it does have a pleasant, creamy texture and a natural finish that allows for semiopaque coverage with minimal chance of creasing. The three colors are all worthy of consideration, but there is nothing for very light or dark skin tones. **Lucidity Light-Diffusing Concealer SPF 8** *($18)* features a fountain pen–style applicator. You need to turn the base of the concealer to feed the product onto a sponge tip, and then apply. The typical problem with this method is that it often gives you too much concealer, and thus you end up wasting or overapplying product. Still, the texture of this is exceptionally smooth, with a soft matte finish, and the six shades are mostly excellent and provide even coverage. The only color to be cautious with is Light, which is too peach for most fair skin tones. The titanium dioxide–based sunscreen has an SPF 8, which is too low to rely on for significant sun protection, though it's a nice adjunct to a foundation with SPF 15.

☺ $$$ **Uncircle Concealer SPF 20** *($17)* is a thick cream concealer in a pot that offers an excellent sunscreen, but despite this and the one very good color, it can crease into lines, so test it carefully before making the investment.

☹ **Automatic Creme Concealer** *($15)* comes in only two colors and a mauve tint. The mauve is unnecessary and the other shades are too rosy peach to recommend.

POWDER: ☺ $$$ **So Ingenious Multi-Dimension Loose Powder** *($30)* is impressive for the sizable packaging alone! The powder looks like it's suspended in air as you gaze upon the clear container, an entirely impressive presentation from every angle. What's inside is just as impressive—a silky, imperceptibly light talc-based powder. The six colors become peachier as you go from light to dark, but the sheer application prevents that from having any effect on the skin. This powder is so smooth you may not even notice the shiny particles on hand to add a glistening finish, though I did. They're not too intrusive, but still noticeable and diminish this as an option for anyone looking to use powder for a polished matte finish. **Equalizer Smart Loose Powder** *($28)* provides a comparatively small amount of loose powder in a container that is covered with a built-in screen. You take the enclosed thin powder puff and press down, and a sheer veil of powder is forced up onto the sponge. This is supposedly an innovation for those on the go who wish to use loose powder as if it were pressed, but it's still a messy proposition, and you'll end up with excess powder on your fingers no matter how careful you are. This talc-free formula uses nylon-12 as the absorbent, and each of the five peachy, but sheer, shades contains "thirsty micro-sponges" to "intercept oil for all-day shine control." Even if these so-called sponges worked, they would be too exhausted trying to mop up the emollients and lavender wax already in the formula, let alone your skin's oil. Consider this an overpriced, but fine-textured, light-coverage powder that's ideal for normal to dry skin. Anyone seeking serious shine control would fare better with Lauder's Double-Matte powders. **Lucidity Translucent Loose Powder** *($27)* and **Lucidity Translucent Pressed Powder** *($22)* are standard, but good, talc-based powders. Both have six great colors (though Medium Intensity 3 can be too peach) and a wonderful soft, silky finish with a faint hint of shine. Lucidity is supposed to change the way light focuses on your face. It doesn't. Though they feel nice and smooth, neither of these looks any different from dozens and dozens of other powders. **Enlighten Skin-Enhancing Powder** *($22)* is a standard, talc-based powder, available as a pressed powder only. It has a light, dry texture and applies extremely sheer. It is sold with a brush rather than a puff and that makes sense, given the concept of this "no-powder" powder, whose four shades are all excellent. **Double-Matte Oil-Control Loose Powder** *($22)* and **Double-Matte Oil-Control Pressed Powder** *($22)* are talc- and silica-based powders. They both have a great texture, with a dry, slightly chalky finish, which can be a problem for some skin tones; however, someone with very oily skin will appreciate how well these absorb. The pressed version has a thicker texture, but it still provides light coverage. All the colors are good options for very light to medium-dark skin tones. **Bronze Goddess Soft Matte Bronzer** *($27)* has a much smoother texture, downplayed (but still visible) shine, and a beautiful tan color.

☺ **$$$ Re-Nutriv Intensive Smoothing Powder** *($50)* is a very smooth, talc-based loose powder with an outrageous price tag! The "radiant finish" attributed to this silky powder is simply shine—and lots of it. The four colors are mostly excellent, though Medium is just too peach to look natural on the skin. If you fall for the notion that shiny powders will minimize wrinkles, consider the considerably less expensive options from Revlon SkinLights first. **Instant Sun All-Over Bronzing Duo** *($27)* is a dual-sided powder bronzer that applies unevenly and is quite shiny. It's not worth considering, especially over Lauder's Bronze Goddess Soft Matte Bronzer reviewed on facing page.

BLUSH: ☺ $$$ **Blush All Day Natural CheekColor** *($21.50)* has a soft, dry texture that feels slightly grainy and doesn't apply as smoothly as it could. Still, it does the job, goes on color-true, and the varied shade selection has options for very light to medium skin tones. Each blush color has some amount of shine, with the most obvious being Potpourri, Raspberry, Rose Marble, and Pink Sand. **Minute Blush Creme Stick for Cheeks** *($26)* has a light, creamy, slippery texture that dries to a sheer, minimal powder finish. The six colors are gorgeous, with a couple of options for deeper skin tones (Russet and Spice). This type of product works best for normal to dry skin types. **Note:** Each shade tends to go on warmer than it looks from the stick. **BlushLights Creamy CheekColor** *($25)* is a silky-smooth cream-to-powder blush that offers eight sheer, attractive colors, but must be applied with a deft hand because it dries almost immediately to a soft powder finish. Although each shade has a hint of shine, only Honey Shimmer and Pink Shimmer are too shiny for daytime wear.

EYESHADOW: ✔☺ **Color Intensity Microfine Powder Eyeshadow** *($13.50)* has an ultrasmooth texture and applies exceptionally well without being too powdery. These are pressed quite softly, so be cautious of the powder cake breaking apart. As for the color intensity, these are somewhat bolder than what Lauder has offered in the past, but not by much. What's really great is the selection of matte shades. Sand Dollar, Fawn, Brown Sugar, Hazelnut, Dusk, Twilight, and Chocolate are the ones to check out the next time you're near a Lauder counter. Equally impressive are the ✔☺ $$$ **Color Intensity Duos** *($25)* and **Color Intensity Quads** *($35)*. The Duos feature some sensible (though mostly shiny) pairings, with Truffle the sole matte option. The Quads actually provide five colors—three well-coordinated eyeshadows that vary set to set, and two cake eyeliner/brow filler shades that are the same in each set. Although these are predominantly shiny, Vintage, Tulip, and Brunette are great combinations. ✔☺ **Pure Color Eyeshadow** *($20)* are single eyeshadows packaged in weighty, Lucite cubes with a crystal flip cap. The product inside lives up to the ostentatious container, as each shade has a satin-smooth texture and beautiful application that blends well. There are a few matte options to consider, such as Tea Box, Espresso Cup, Plum Pop, and Caramel Square. Each shade is sheer compared to Lauder's Color Intensity Microfine eyeshadows.

☺ **$$$ Go Wink Liquid** and **Go Wink Powder Eyeshadows** *($16)* offer more choices for adding glitz and gleam to your eyes. The liquid version is actually a cream-to-powder formula that comes with a wand applicator. It dries quickly to a reasonably solid powder finish, and the iridescence is visible from across the room. The powder version is a multitextured eyeshadow that is pretty to look at, but it's really just another shiny eyeshadow to embrace or ignore, depending on your preferences.

☹ **Shadow Stay Eyelid Foundation** *($15)* is a silicone- and wax-based stick that has a sheer mauve tint. This goes on a bit thick, does not prevent eyeshadows from creasing, and is absolutely not needed if you have a reliable matte-finish concealer on hand.

EYE AND BROW SHAPER: ☺ **$$$ Automatic Pencil for Eyes** *($22.50, $10 for refill)* is a standard, twist-up, retractable pencil in an elegant container. It is among the more pricey pencils on the market, but the refills are a bargain and then you have the sexy container, if you're into that kind of thing. Some of the colors are too shiny and fairly greasy, so be careful; this can smear under the eye. **Automatic Brow Pencil Duo** *($22.50, $10 for refill)* comes in the same elegant, refillable packaging as the Automatic Pencil for Eyes above. This has a soft, slightly creamy texture that applies evenly without being too thick or greasy. The price is steep, but if you're a dyed-in-the-wool brow pencil fan, it's worth an audition and there are options for blondes and redheads.

☺ **Brow Gel** *($15)* is a standard brow groomer with a good brush and minimal sticky after-feel.

☺ **Eye Defining Pencil/Smudger** *($15)* is a basic pencil that needs sharpening and has a creamy texture that glides on. These claim to have a "nonsmudge" formula, but they are creamy enough so they can definitely smudge by midday. ☺ **$$$ Two-in-One Eyeliner/Browcolor** *($25)* goes on wet or dry, but works best when used wet. It comes in one compact with two colors: Brown and Black. Although it does work to fill in brows or line the eye, the color selection is limited and almost any matte eyeshadow can perform the identical function. These two colors are also represented in Lauder's Color Intensity Quad Eyeshadows.

☹ **Liquid Eyeliner** *($15)* comes in two shades and features a thin brush that applies an even line. As nice as that is, this tends to dry so slowly as to seriously try your patience and risk smearing. **Natural Brow Filler** *($15)* is a fat, one-color eyebrow pencil that isn't by any means a one-size-fits-all product. The broad tip makes it hard to control the color through the brow, and the color isn't in the least natural if you have very light or dark brows.

LIPSTICK AND LIP PENCIL: ☺ $$$ **Pure Color Long-Lasting Lipstick** *($22)* is being called "the most technologically advanced color line on the market" by Lauder executives, but I assume none of them have experimented with as many lipsticks as I have. Although this lavishly packaged lipstick is a comfortable, creamy formula with a smooth texture and opaque coverage, the finish is glossy enough to slip into any lines around the mouth. The mostly splendid colors also have minimal to no stain, which means they won't wear nearly as well as other options from Lauder, such as their True or Go Pout lipsticks. **Pure Color Crystal Lipstick** *($22)* promises "sheer electricity, daring shine," but the only thing that will get a charge out of this slick, glossy lipstick is your credit card. The colors are fine, but fleeting. **Sumptuous Lipstick** *($18)* claims it has a "never-before-seen gel-based formula that glides on, stays on," but after one test drive you'll be ready to dispute the claim for yourself. This creamy, opaque lipstick is silicone-based, so it does glide on with ease and feels light on the lips. Yet aside from having a small amount of stain, these won't redefine anyone's expectations for a long-wearing lipstick (well, except for perhaps Lauder's). **Go Pout Lip Color** *($16)* presumably adds dimension and fullness to the lower lip and shadows the contour of the upper lip. Quite a feat for a standard lipstick! However, all this adds up to is a good creamy lipstick with a fair amount of iridescence. That can indeed affect the way light is reflected off the lips (or anywhere else), just not in the way the marketing language wants to make you think it does. **True Lipstick** *($17.50)* comes in Satin or Matte. Both have a slick feel and are opaque. The Satins have a glossy finish, whereas the Mattes (which are not matte in the least) have a creamy finish. There is enough stain in the products to let these colors go the distance, but the number of shades is dwindling to make room for Lauder's newer formulas.

☺ $$$ **Futurist Lipstick SPF 15** *($17.50)* is a rather standard, creamy lipstick that has enough of a greasy feel to make those with bleeding-lipstick problems cringe. The SPF 15 sounds impressive, but alas, without UVA protection there is no reason to consider this part of your or anyone else's future plans. **All Day Lipstick** *($15)* is extremely creamy, bordering on greasy, with medium coverage and no stain to speak of. Consider yourself lucky if you can get this to last past midmorning! **Lip Blush SPF 15** *($16)* does not have adequate UVA protection, so count on this being nothing more than a very standard, sheer, glossy lipstick. **High Shine Lip Lacquer SPF 15** *($16)* also does not have reliable UVA-protecting ingredients, making this just a sticky, semiopaque "wet" gloss. **Automatic Pencil for Lips** *($22.50; $10 for refill)* is a standard, twist-up, retractable lipliner, but the tip of the pencil comes out of a wider than

normal opening, which makes it too thick to be capable of drawing a thin outline around the mouth.

☺ **$$$ Pure Color Gloss ($20)** carries over the opulent packaging of its lipstick
predecessor, but this costly gloss offers little innovation when it comes to feel,
performance, or finish. It's just minimally sticky lip gloss with sheer, iridescent
colors. **Go Pout Sheer Lip Glaze ($16)** is for those who couldn't get enough
pouting from the original Go Pout lipstick. This smooth, nonsticky iridescent
lip gloss offers sheer colors that leave an alluring, iridescent glossy finish. If
packaging isn't your paramount interest, you'll find that this lasts longer and
is richer than the Pure Color Gloss above.

☺ **Lip Defining Pencil/Brush ($15)** is a standard pencil with a creamy feel and
enough stain to help lip color cling a little longer. The pencil includes a brush
at one end, which is a convenient feature.

MASCARA: ☹ **$$$ More Than Mascara ($18)** is just mascara, plain and simple.
It does little to impress, especially at this price. For decent length without
clumps, this remains an effective, but boring, option. **Illusionist Maximum
Curling Mascara ($19.50)** is a rather disappointing mascara, especially when
you consider the grandiose claims attached to it. Illusionist begs you to "give
your lashes dramatic curl and unprecedented lift in one sweep," but it takes
several sweeps to build average length, minimal thickness, and no discernible
curl. This doesn't clump, smear, or flake and is an option if you need lengthening mascara, but it's no match for less expensive options such as L'Oréal's
Le Grand Curl ($7.49).

☹ **Pure Velvet Dramatic Volume Mascara ($18)**. If length, thickness, and volume
are your goals, this mascara may send you over the edge trying to achieve
them. You will get a clean, sheer application, but it's incredibly slow going.
Lash Primer Plus Full Treatment Formula ($16) is sold as a pre-mascara con-
ditioning base for lashes. It is an unwarranted step, given the industry-wide
availability of superlative one-step mascaras. The formula itself is no more
conditioning than most mascaras, so that promised benefit is easy to dispel.

☺ **$$$ Futurist Lash-Extending Mascara ($18)** is a distinct improvement over
the other Estée Lauder mascaras, building nice length and thickness with no
clumps or smudges. This tends to go on wetter than most, so be extra-cautious
of smearing.

BRUSHES: ☺ Estée Lauder's **Brushes ($15–$35)** were mildly retooled, though
the improvement is still not enough to make these worth considering over the
excellent brushes from Lauder's vast portfolio of brushes from other lines,
from Aveda to Stila. Both the **Powder Brush ($25)** and **Blush Brush ($20)** are
options, but they're almost too soft and are not dense enough to control ap-

plication. There is only one **Eyeshadow Shading Brush** *($15)* and it remains a fine option for a smaller, flat shadow brush. The **Eyelining Brush** *($15)* is the same nylon "push" eyeliner brush made popular by Trish McEvoy. The synthetic **Concealing Brush** *($15)* is versatile, and can double as an eyeshadow brush, while the retractable **Golden Lip Brush** *($15)* and oversized, but stout, **All Over Face and Body Brush** *($35)* are easily passed up in favor of more practical options from other lines.

L'ORÉAL

Does anyone else think that L'Oréal's "Because I'm worth it" tag line is ingenious? Perusing the packages for all of their products, this mantra pops up everywhere, and almost subliminally reinforces not only that L'Oréal products are elite, but also that you *deserve* to use them. You owe it to yourself, you are making the right choice, and you *will* become beautiful as a result. What powerful feelings and images those four words stir! It's too bad that the slogan doesn't carry over to the majority of L'Oréal's skin-care products.

As they stand, there is little about these products that's "worth" your attention. Particularly inexcusable are several sunscreens without UVA-protecting ingredients. (L'Oréal has known for years about the issue of UVA protection. Not only do their products sold outside the United States usually contain UVA-protecting ingredients—titanium dioxide, zinc oxide, and avobenzone—but they also own a patent on Mexoryl SX, a UVA-protecting sunscreen ingredient used only outside the United States.) Their toners are almost all alcohol-based, and the moisturizers are long on fantastical claims and short on fulfillment or state-of-the-art formulations. There are a few shining stars, but you have to search for them amidst a parade of underachievers. Still, the best of L'Oréal's skin care is amazingly similar to what you will find at the Lancôme counter. (L'Oréal is Lancôme's parent company.) I find it amusing that, more often than not, when I compare Lancôme and L'Oréal products by price it is apples to oranges. But when you examine the formulas, you'll see a rose by any other name is still a rose, even though it is being sold at the drugstore. For more information about L'Oréal, call (800) 322-2036 or visit www.lorealparisusa.com. **Note:** All L'Oréal products are highly fragranced unless noted otherwise.

L'Oréal Skin Care

☺ **HydraFresh Deep Cleanser Foaming Gel for Normal to Oily Skin** *($4.99 for 6.5 ounces)* is a very good, very basic, detergent-based, water-soluble cleanser that would work well for someone with normal to oily or slightly dry skin.

☺ **HydraFresh Cleanser Foaming Cream for Normal to Dry Skin** *($4.99 for 6.5 ounces)* is a standard, detergent-based cleanser that can be too drying for someone with normal to dry skin, but is still an option for someone with normal to oily skin.

☺ **Shine Control Foaming Face Wash with Pro-Vitamin B₅** *($5 for 6 ounces)* is virtually identical to the Hydra Fresh Cleanser Foaming Cream above, minus the plant oil. That is helpful for oily skin, but other than that, this is just a cleanser and it doesn't control shine in the least. The tiny amount of vitamin B_5 in this cleanser is barely detectable.

☺ **RevitaClean Cold Cream for Dry or Maturing Skin** *($5.29 for 5 ounces)* is a mineral oil– and Vaseline-based cleanser that can be an option for dry skin, but it can leave a greasy feel on the skin. The teensy amount of retinyl palmitate (a form of vitamin A) has no effect on skin.

☺ **RevitaClean Gentle Foaming Cleanser** *($5 for 6 ounces)* is a very good, very basic, detergent-based, water-soluble cleanser that would work well for someone with normal to oily or slightly dry skin. The teeny amounts of vitamin A and sunflower oil can have little to no impact on skin.

☺ **Refreshing Eye Makeup Remover** *($4.99 for 4.2 ounces)* contains mostly water, slip agent, detergent cleansers, preservatives, and fragrance. This is a standard eye-makeup remover, though it can be more drying than most.

☺ **Turning Point Instant Facial Scrub** *($8.99 for 1.7 ounces)* is a basic scrub that uses a synthetic abrasive in a fairly emollient gel base that includes thickeners, silicone, and mineral oil. This does contain salicylic acid, but the pH is too high to let it be effective for exfoliation. This would work just fine for someone with normal to dry skin.

☹ **HydraFresh Toner** *($4.99 for 8.5 ounces)* is an alcohol-based toner with a small amount of salicylic acid (BHA). There is never a reason to use alcohol on the skin, and the pH of this toner is too high for the salicylic acid to be effective for exfoliation.

☹ **Shine Control Double-Action Toner Oil Free** *($4.99 for 8.5 ounces)* is an alcohol-based toner, and that can be drying and irritating for all skin types.

☹ **Shine Control Oil-Free Toner** *($5.99 for 4 ounces)* is similar to the Double-Action Toner above and the same comments apply.

☹ **Active Daily Moisture Lotion SPF 15, with UVA/UVB Sunscreen, for All Skin Types** *($7.39 for 4 ounces)* doesn't contain the UVA-protecting ingredients of titanium dioxide, zinc oxide, or avobenzone, and is absolutely not recommended.

☺ **Active Daily Moisture Lotion for Normal to Dry Skin** *($5.99 for 4 ounces)* is an exceptionally mediocre emollient moisturizer for dry skin.

☹ **Age Perfect Day Anti-Sagging & Rehydrating Cream SPF 15** *($15.99 for 2.5 ounces)* doesn't contain the UVA-protecting ingredients of titanium dioxide, zinc oxide, or avobenzone, and is absolutely not recommended.

☺ **Age Perfect Night Cream Anti-Sagging & Rehydrating Cream** *($15.99 for 2.5 ounces)*. While this is an OK moisturizer for dry skin there is nothing in it that can keep the skin from sagging. The skin's sagging is a function of the fat content of skin (and this isn't going to add fat to the skin), the fact that skin keeps growing (is any cream going to claim it will stop skin from growing?), and that the face muscles shift position downward (no cream can affect the position of muscles). This does contain BHA, but the pH of this product makes it ineffective for exfoliation. This also contains niacinamide, the same B-vitamin ingredient that shows up in Olay's Total Effects moisturizer and that can be a good ingredient for skin. Given how much more of the showcased niacinamide that is present in Olay's version, you would be better off with it than with this L'Oréal version.

☺ **Age Perfect Skin Illuminator & Age Spot Diffuser** *($15.99 for 2 ounces)* has a pH of 5, and that means that the exfoliating properties of the salicylic acid in this product will be ineffective. Other than that, it is just a standard moisturizer with some mica that gives it a subtle iridescent finish, but it does nothing to change the brown discolorations you may see on the back of the hand. The same comments made about niacinamide for the Anti-Sagging version above also apply here.

✔☺ **Age Perfect Anti-Sagging and Ultra-Hydrating Cream Eye** *($13.99 for 0.5 ounces)* is an emollient moisturizer for dry skin that has some interesting water-binding agents and antioxidants. It also contains wild yam extract, but that does not have any hormonal benefit for skin.

☹ **Excell A3 Alpha Hydroxy Cream SPF 8 with Triple Fruit Acid** *($11.99 for 1.7 ounces)* has an SPF that is far below the standard SPF of 15 set by the American Academy of Dermatology and the Skin Cancer Foundation. It also doesn't contain the UVA-protecting ingredients of titanium dioxide, zinc oxide, or avobenzone, and is absolutely not recommended.

☺ **Eye Defense with Liposomes** *($9.99 for 0.5 ounce)*. Liposomes are a delivery system (not an ingredient) and are capable of holding other ingredients and releasing them once the liposome is absorbed into the skin (source: *Journal of Pharmaceutical Sciences*, March 2002, pages 615–622). However, it is helpful for there to be worthwhile ingredients like antioxidants and water-binding agents for the liposomes to deliver into the skin, elements this moisturizer doesn't contain much of.

☺ **Future E Moisture + A Daily Dose of Pure Vitamin E Normal to Dry Skin**

($8.99 for 4 ounces) is just an OK moisturizer with small amounts of vitamin E and water-binding agent. The pH of this product is too high for the salicylic acid to be effective for exfoliation.

☺ **Future E Moisture + A Daily Dose of Pure Vitamin E Oil Free** *($9.99 for 4 ounces)* is similar to the Vitamin E Normal to Dry version above and the same basic comments apply.

☹ **Future E Moisture + A Daily Dose of Pure Vitamin E for Your Skin SPF 15 Normal to Dry Skin** *($9.99 for 4 ounces)* doesn't contain the UVA-protecting ingredients of avobenzone, titanium dioxide, or zinc oxide, and is not recommended.

☹ **Future E Moisture + A Daily Dose of Pure Vitamin E Oil Free SPF 15** *($9.99 for 4 ounces)* doesn't contain the UVA-protecting ingredients of avobenzone, titanium dioxide, or zinc oxide, and is not recommended.

☹ **HydraFresh Moisturizer for Normal to Oily Skin SPF 15** *($8.99 for 2.5 ounces)* doesn't contain the UVA-protecting ingredients of avobenzone, titanium dioxide, or zinc oxide, and is not recommended.

☹ **Hydra Fresh Mineral Charged Moisturizer for Normal to Dry Skin SPF 15** *($9.99 for 2.5 ounces)* doesn't contain the UVA-protecting ingredients of avobenzone, titanium dioxide, or zinc oxide, and is not recommended.

☺ **Hydra Fresh Circle Eraser** *($9.99 for 0.5 ounce)* is supposed to eliminate puffy circles under the eyes, but there is nothing in here (or anywhere) that can do that. The tiny amount of caffeine can't reduce swelling from overnight fluid retention or fat deposits. This is a standard emollient moisturizer with tiny amounts of water-binding agents and antioxidants.

☹ **Hydra Renewal Daily Dry Skin Cream with Pro-Vitamin B$_5$** *($5.99 for 1.7 ounces)* is an extremely standard, emollient moisturizer for dry skin. It contains tiny amounts of vitamin E and vitamin B$_5$, but too little to have much effect. The urea can have exfoliating and water-binding properties similar to those of an AHA product. It contains the preservative Kathon CG, which is not recommended for use in leave-on products.

☺ **Line Eraser Pure Retinol Concentrate** *($14.99 for 1 ounce)* is another product joining others on the retinol bandwagon. This one from L'Oréal is in a rather simple, but good, moisturizing base and contains about 0.25% retinol, which is the same amount as most retinol products being sold. It is good for someone with normal to dry skin. The packaging is the kind that ensures the retinol will be stable.

☹ **Line Eraser Pure Retinol Concentrate SPF 15** *($16.99 for 1.2 ounces)* doesn't contain the UVA-protecting ingredients of avobenzone, titanium dioxide, or zinc oxide, and is not recommended.

☺ **Overnight Defense** *($11.99 for 1.7 ounces)* is an OK emollient, but standard, moisturizer for dry skin.

☺ **Wrinkle Defense** *($11.99 for 1.4 ounces)* contains nothing that has any chance of defending against wrinkles. It is a simple moisturizer for dry skin, with minimal amounts of water-binding agents and antioxidants. It also contains UVB sunscreen ingredients, but is not rated with an SPF.

☺ **Revitalift Anti-Wrinkle Firming Cream with Pro-Retinol A & Par-Elastyl, for Face and Neck** *($9.99 for 1.7 ounces).* This product does not contain retinol; rather, it contains retinyl palmitate, which is a form of vitamin A that can be an effective antioxidant, only there isn't very much of it in here. There is no such chemical or compound as par-elastyl, that is merely a marketing term L'Oréal created to make a rather basic moisturizing formula sound more exotic. It does contain sunscreen ingredients (UVB only), but is not rated with an SPF.

☺ **Revitalift Eye Anti-Wrinkle and Firming Cream** *($9.99 for 0.5 ounce)* is similar to the Face and Neck version above, and the same comments apply.

☺ **Revitalift Oil-Free Anti-Wrinkle + Firming Lotion** *($10.69 for 1.7 ounces)* is just an OK moisturizer with a rather ordinary formulation for normal to slightly dry skin.

☹ **Revitalift Complete Multi-Action Treatment SPF 18** *($11.99 for 1.7 ounces)* doesn't contain the UVA-protecting ingredients of avobenzone, titanium dioxide, or zinc oxide, and is not recommended.

☺ **Revitalift Slim Face Contouring and Toning Solution** *($10.49 for 1.7 ounces)* has a name that should at least raise your eyebrows (if not your skin), with a formulation that has mostly water and alcohol plus some silicone, glycerin, slip agents, caffeine, water-binding agent, and film-forming agent. This is one to leave on the shelf, though I suspect it will be hard to pass up given the claims that Revitalift Slim is supposed to "combat the numerous factors that affect the look and feel of aging skin. For many women over 40, that means sagging, slackening, or puffiness around the jawline and neck." The truth is that caffeine can't undo that and neither can L'Oréal's other showcased ingredient, par-elastyl. It is interesting to note that there is nothing in this product called "par-elastyl," though I suspect it refers to the soybean protein, because the L'Oréal Web site defines "par-elastyl" as being derived from vegetable protein. Any form of protein makes for a good water-binding agent, but it doesn't have special properties that make it capable of altering the shape of skin.

☺ **Visible Results Skin Renewing Moisture Treatment SPF 15 Fragrance Free** *($18.96 for 1.6 ounces).* Finally L'Oréal has a sunscreen with UVA protection! This is a good, in-part titanium dioxide–based sunscreen in a standard emollient base that would be an option for normal to dry skin. However, this is absolutely not fragrance-free; it contains lavender oil, and without question that ingredient adds fragrance.

☺ **Plenitude Turning Point Instant Facial Cream** *($11.99 for 1.7 ounces)* is similar to many moisturizers in the L'Oréal product group, yet is even more mediocre. The pH of this product isn't low enough to allow the salicylic acid to act as an effective exfoliant.

☺ **Plenitude Visible Results Skin Renewing Treatment Eye** *($16.96 for 0.42 ounces)* is a silicone-based, very mundane moisturizer that contains a bit of shimmer and little else. It contains a tiny amount of Vitamin C but nothing else of particular interest for the eye area or anywhere else on the face.

L'Oréal Pure Zone

☺ **Pure Zone Anti-Breakout Cleanser Cream** *($7.99 for 5 ounces)* is a 2% salicylic acid cleanser in a lotion form that isn't the best for normal to oily skin, but that may possibly work for dry skin. However, the pH (over 5) is too high for the BHA to be effective as an exfoliant. It also contains menthol, and though it's probably not enough to be a problem for skin, it is a waste to have it in here at all. It does contain fragrance.

☺ **Pure Zone Anti-Breakout Cleanser Foaming** *($7.99 for 5 ounces)* is a standard, detergent-based cleanser that contains 2% salicylic acid, though the pH (over 5) isn't low enough for it to be effective as an exfoliant. It does contain small amounts of menthol and fragrance.

☺ **Pure Zone Anti-Breakout Cleanser Scrub** *($7.99 for 6.7 ounces)*, with alcohol and menthol in the mix, adds up to being more irritating than your skin bargained for. The pH of this product makes the salicylic acid ineffective. It does contain fragrance.

☺ **Pure Zone Skin Relief Oil Free Moisturizer** *($7.99 for 2.5 ounces)* is an interesting option for a "moisturizer." This silicone-based, 0.6% salicylic acid lotion is mostly water, silicone, glycerin, clay, thickeners, preservatives, and fragrance. It will leave a matte feel on skin and the 0.6% solution would be suitable for someone with normal to dry skin and minimal problems with breakouts. However, the pH of 5 makes the salicylic acid ineffective for exfoliation.

☹ **Pure Zone Pore Tightening Astringent** *($7.99 for 6.7 ounces)* lists alcohol as the second ingredient, which makes it too irritating and drying for all skin types. That is unfortunate as this is the only salicylic acid product in the Pure Zone group (all of these contain it) that has a pH of 3.5 and is, therefore, an effective exfoliant.

☻ **Pure Zone Spot Check** *($7.99 for 0.5 ounce)* is similar to the Tightening Astringent on the facing page and the same comments apply.

L'Oréal Makeup

L'Oréal's extensive makeup collection has evolved into something spectacular. The foundations have not only shown improved textures and smoother-than-ever applications, but the color range is also (slowly) improving. There are still a fair number of peach and pink shades to watch out for (Lancôme's foundations still offer superior colors), but the effort is being made. The rest of the makeup offers a series of pleasant surprises, from superior concealers to silky powder blushes, superior eyelining options, and some of the best-performing mascaras available at the drugstore or anywhere else for that matter. You will also find L'Oréal's lipsticks are competing every step of the way with Lancôme's lip formulas, for only one-third the price. Turning this line around was no short order, but category for category L'Oréal's makeup has now become the most reliable line at the drugstore. If their foundations followed Revlon's lead and featured effective sunscreens, and the eyeshadows were improved, it would be almost impossible to resist.

FOUNDATION: ☺ **Ideal Balance Balancing Foundation for Combination Skin** *($11.99)* is another foundation claiming to moisturize dry areas while keeping shine in check over oily ones. Considering the number of women who readily identify with the combination skin profile, it's not surprising that products with promises to reconcile the demands of that two-part condition keep appearing. Despite the name, this makeup is not capable of balancing anything, though the slightly thick, noticeably silky texture glides on and feels smooth. This has a soft matte finish that won't hold back excess oil for long—you can almost sense the moisture in the formula at war with an army of dry-finish ingredients. Overall, this formula is best for someone with normal to slightly oily skin, because it's matte enough to look unflattering over any dry or flaky patches. If you decide to try this, the best almost-neutral shades from the assortment of twelve colors are Soft Beige, Beige, Buff, Tan, Caramel, and Cappuccino (the last two are excellent for dark skin tones). The remaining colors are unabashedly pink or peach. **AirWear Breathable Long-Wearing Foundation SPF 14** *($11.99)* has a wonderfully light, ultrasilky texture and a soft powdery finish that would make it a good choice for someone with normal to oily skin seeking light to medium coverage. Regrettably, the sunscreen does not contain any UVA-protecting agents, but if you're willing to wear a sunscreen underneath this, it is worth considering. The range of nine shades is mostly impressive, with choices for light to dark (but not very dark) skin tones. The only shades to consider avoiding are Cream (pink) and Caramel (may be too golden orange for some skin tones). By the way, there is absolutely nothing in this formula that provides oxygen to the skin, which is actually good news, because oxygen triggers free-radical damage and that's why "antioxidants" (think anti-oxygen) are good for skin. **AirWear Breathable Long-Wearing Powder Foundation SPF 17** *($11.69)* is a soft, smooth-textured, talc-based powder foundation that applies and blends nicely, affording sheer to light coverage. Typically of L'Oréal, this pressed-powder foundation doesn't contain the UVA-protecting ingredients of titanium dioxide, zinc oxide, or avobenzone. But, sun-protection gripes aside, the six available colors are all very good, especially Tan and Caramel, which are good shades for darker skin tones. **Quick Stick Long Wearing Foundation SPF 14** *($10.99)* is a reasonably smooth stick foundation that includes a titanium dioxide sunscreen, and an SPF that's almost to the benchmark of SPF 15. The smooth application dries to a solid, unmovable, difficult-to-remove matte base. If matte, full coverage is what you're after, this one would be an option. One caution: This has a strong silicone base that absolutely does not blend over a silicone-based moisturizer or especially over a silicone serum. The formula works best for normal to oily skin. There are twelve shades to consider, but five are a problem for most skin tones: Soft Ivory, Nude Beige, Buff, Golden Beige, and Cocoa are all too pink or peach. There are, however, some good choices for dark skin tones. **Visible Lift Line Minimizing Makeup SPF 12** *($10.29)* has made a dismaying switch to octyl methoxycinnamate as its only active sun-protecting ingredient—so this is no longer a sufficient option as a foundation with sunscreen. However, it does have a silky texture that melds with the skin and dries to a soft matte finish. Coverage runs from light to medium and despite the fact that the target market for this is women with dry skin, the nonemollient formula is best for normal to oily skin. The antiwrinkle claims surrounding this one are dubious. It can help to smooth out skin to some degree, but that is the nature of most foundation applications. There are fifteen shades to consider, including options for very light skin tones. The following shades should be avoided by most skin tones: Pale, Buff, Creamy Natural, Golden Beige, Sand Beige, Sun Beige (just slightly peach), Cocoa, and Cappuccino. The other shades are worth testing, but what a shame the sunscreen has been downgraded. **Feel Naturale Compact Light Softening One-Step Makeup SPF 15** *($11.29)* is a very good cream-to-powder makeup that has a wonderfully smooth, creamy application and a soft, slightly matte finish along with phony claims that it can manipulate light to create flawless skin. The duality of this type of makeup is that it's creamy enough to slip into any lines on the face and at the same time powdery enough to exaggerate any dry, flaky skin. Normal to slightly dry skin would fare best with this. Although the label makes the ubiquitous "oil-free" claim, this does have waxes that will likely aggravate the situation for those prone to breakouts. If you thought the sunscreen had adequate UVA protection, you don't know L'Oréal. Strangely, a few of the darkest shades do not list *any* SPF or active ingredients.

The twelve shades feature some remarkably neutral choices; the ones to avoid are Sand Beige, Golden Beige, Buff (can be too peach), Soft Ivory (slightly pink), Sun Beige (too peach), and Cocoa (ashy red).

☺ **Translucide Naturally Luminous Makeup SPF 18** *($11.99)* has a fantastic texture that's easy to blend to a soft matte finish with light to medium coverage, and contains the smallest amount of vitamin C imaginable. The nine shades available (with nothing for very light or dark skin tones) weigh in a bit too heavily on the peach or pink side, although they may still work for some skin tones. The following shades should be considered with caution: Soft Ivory, Nude Beige, Natural Beige, Caramel Beige, and Cappuccino. As expected, the sunscreen is incomplete when it comes to UVA protection. **Visible Lift Extra Coverage Line Minimizing Makeup SPF 12** *($10.29)* does not contain adequate UVA protection, though you may notice that titanium dioxide is listed as the third ingredient on the regular ingredient listing. However, if it is not listed as "active ingredient," that doesn't count for UVA protection. Despite the sun-protection problems, this silky, creamy formula lives up to its extra-coverage claim. The finish is natural matte, making this a good choice for someone with normal to slightly dry skin who is willing to wear a separate sunscreen underneath. There are nine shades available, but almost all of them are too peach or pink and they look incredibly artificial given the opaque nature of this foundation. The only contenders are Nude Beige, Natural Beige, and Golden Beige. **Feel Naturale Makeup SPF 15** *($10.99)* has no reliable UVA protection and the application might make you want to sing Paul Simon's "Slip Slidin' Away," but the sheer-coverage, light-matte finish and improved selection of colors make this a possibility for normal skin willing to pair this with an effective sunscreen. Oily skin won't enjoy the slickness of this product. Of the twelve shades, the ones to leave on the shelf include Pale, Nude Beige, Sand Beige, Buff, and Cappuccino.

☹ **Mattique Oil-Free Matte Makeup** *($8.79)* is L'Oréal's oldest foundation, and compared to their latest creations this is subpar. The fairly matte texture is accompanied by a slightly sticky feel, which someone with oily skin might not like. As for the nine colors, with the possible exception of Nude Beige, all are too peach or pink to recommend.

CONCEALER: ✔☺ **AirWear Long-Wearing Concealer** *($9.89)* is a smooth, silicone-based concealer that glides on and covers well without looking heavy or thick. It has a crease-free matte finish that is a pleasure to blend, and it layers beautifully for areas that need more intense camouflage. Of the six colors, avoid Corrector (too yellow), Brightener (too pink), and Deep (may turn ash on some darker skin tones). ✔☺ **Visible Lift Line Minimizing Concealer** *($9.99)* has an elegant, creamy application that dries to a soft matte finish and it doesn't crease into the lines around the eyes. It is very similar to Lancôme's ever-popular Effacernes Concealer *($21)*; check it out for yourself. The four skin-tone shades are beautiful, though Medium-Deep won't work very well for darker skin tones. Avoid the overly yellow Neutralizer and white Lightener shades. If you want to test the line-minimizing claim, use this concealer around one eye and leave the other bare. Now tell me which side has fewer apparent lines; the one with the concealer has more lines, right?

☺ **Feel Naturale Concealer** *($7.69)* has a lot of initial slip, so keeping the coverage where you want it can be a challenge. This dries to a soft matte finish and provides decent sheer-to-medium coverage without creasing. The three shades are workable, but Deep may be too peach for some skin tones. **Cover Expert Exact Match Concealer** *($8.99)* features two cream-to-powder concealers in one pot. You can use the light or dark shade as needed, or blend them to create the closest match. The color combinations are very good, but there are only two duos available, with nothing for light or dark skin tones. Those who fall in the happy medium will be pleased with the colors and will find that this one has a smooth, silky texture reminiscent of Lancôme's Photogenic Concealer. The formula is easy to apply, blends very well, and provides excellent coverage for dark circles or other imperfections.

POWDER: ☺ **Visible Lift Line Minimizing Powder** *($11.99)* is a translucent, talc-based powder with a silky, very sheer finish that has a hint of sparkling shine. It won't diminish one line on your face, but it nicely sets makeup and could work for all skin types. All but one of the shades are excellent, just avoid Colour Lift, a pink tone that no one should be dusting all over their face. **Feel Naturale Ultrafine Light Softening Powder SPF 15** *($11.59)* has been reformulated numerous times, and this latest version provides an undeniably silky texture and superior application. Sunscreen-wise, this misses the mark for UVA protection, but is still a great pressed-powder option. Of the three shades, Deep is the only dud. **On the Loose Shimmering Powder** *($5.99)* comes in small pots and creates an intense, though smooth, application of shiny powder. This wins major points for its superior ability to cling to the skin. For evening, it's an option, and will give you the appropriate glittering shine everyone else seems to be wearing. I would suggest avoiding the orange Five Alarm and blue Diva Down unless your music video is in heavy rotation on MTV. ✔☺ **Translucide Naturally Luminous Powder** *($9.89)* is a talc-free loose powder that has a marvelous, powdered-sugar texture and a smooth, even finish. It feels like silk on the skin and comes in four shades, of which only Deep is a bit too coppery for most darker skin tones. This fragranced powder is perfect for those who hate to look powdered but want to look polished.

BLUSH: ✔☺ **Feel Naturale Light Softening Blush** *($10.99)* is a great collection of blushes with beautiful colors, textures, and an application that is strikingly similar to Lancôme's Blush Subtil *($25.50)*. It should suit all skin types very well. The following shades are quite shiny, and best for evening, if at all: Charmed Peach, Mauvelous, Mocha Rose, and Plume. ☺ **Translucide Luminous Gel Blush** *($9.49)* is an interesting option for a sheer, tinted-gel blush. The six shades range from barely to moderately shiny finishes, but each blends out exceptionally sheer to almost no color at all. The application is wet-feeling and then dries to a matte (in feel) finish. It would be hard to make a mistake with this one, since the color is so soft, yet it takes patience to blend it on and wait for it to dry; and if you want noticeable color, it can take a lot of trouble to build up much intensity. Still, this minimalist blush does have its purposes. ☺ **Cheek to Cheek Sculpting Blush Duet** *($9.89)* is a dual-sided powder blush that offers a light and medium blush tone for highlighting and "sculpting" the face. This has a smooth, but slightly too-thick, texture. Application can be spotty or it can go on too sheer, requiring repeated applications to build anything close to sculpture! Besides, the best way to sculpt (read: contour) the face is with a matte, tan-brown or golden brown color. The Blissful Bronzes shade comes close, but is too soft to adequately contour. **Blush Delice Sheer Powder Blush** *($7.99)* may be sheer when it comes to color impact, but not when it comes to shine. This is one of the shiniest blushes at the drugstore! Wearing any one of the five shades is more about adding iridescence over color, but if that's your goal or you have a disco night planned, this smooth blush won't disappoint. **Touch-On Colour Lips, Eyes, Cheeks** *($9.89)* shares the same general comments as the Blush Delice above, only this has a slightly grainy cream-to-powder texture and softer (but still quite shiny) colors. This does not feel great over the lips, and the colors are a bit too harsh for the eye.

EYESHADOW: ☺ **Wear Infinite Long-Wearing Silky Powder Eyeshadow** *($3.79 singles, $4.69 duos, $6.59 quads)* are a reformulation of L'Oréal's former Soft Effects eyeshadows. The colors are still divided into perle (noticeably shiny) and matte (true matte to subtle shine) finishes, but the color selection has improved. For example, there are a number of viable options among the quads, though (with the exception of Wood Rose) each one has at least one shiny shade. The formula is very silky, but also very sheer and almost waxy-feeling. Don't count on anything close to infinite wear from these, but for very soft color and easy application, they'll do. The best matte Singles to consider are Sable, Bark, Chocolat, Raven, and Sand. From the Duos, only Classic Khakis is matte. **Colour Fresco Refreshing Creme Eyeshadow** *($6.59)* is a twist-up, cream-to-powder eyeshadow that has a cool, wet feel and glides on almost too well. It dries to a powder finish and tends not to smudge, which is nice. Application can be tricky because these colors are all shiny and tend to go on strong, which can make blending an even trickier proposition. They will need to be softened quickly unless a bold stripe of shimmery color is your goal.

EYE AND BROW SHAPER: ✔☺ **Line Intensifique Extreme Wear Liquid Liner** *($7.89)* is an outstanding liquid liner that is relatively easy to apply (for liquid liner) and it holds up well—no smearing, chipping, or flaking all day long. The brush is almost too flexible, but it does work well. Give this a try if you're a fan of Lancôme's Artliner *($25)*.

☺ **Super Liner Perfect Tip Eyelining Pen** *($7.19)* must have been tweaked, because now it is almost as good as the newer Line Intensifique. This has an identical brush and equally good application, but doesn't quite have the latter's extra long wear. **Wear Infinite Silky Powder Eye Liner** *($6.89)* is a standard pencil that has a swift, smooth application and a reliable powder finish. If you prefer pencils, this is one to consider, as it is less likely to smudge or fade than many others. However, the color selection is mostly shiny, and there are several hues that are inappropriate for lining the eyes, unless you're going for all-out techno-glamour or are auditioning for the role of Cleopatra. **Le Grande Kohl Line and Define Pencil** *($6.79)* is an extra-long standard pencil very reminiscent of Lancôme's Le Crayon Kohl *($18)*. This applies smoothly without being greasy and blends well without streaking. Many of the colors have shine, but Black Sable and Onyx are safe bets. **Brow Stylist Sculpting Brow Mascara** *($7.49)* is a very good, sheer brow tint that features a dual-sided brush with long and short bristles, a feature that makes this type of product useful in grooming and defining both full (think Brooke Shields) and sparse or thin (Bette Davis) brows. There are two colors plus a Clear version, and all are options for subtle brow enhancement.

☺ **Pencil Perfect Automatic Eye Liner** *($6.79)* isn't what I would call perfect; if anything, it tends to go on creamier than most, and that means a greater risk of smearing. As a plus, it doesn't need sharpening. **Eye Smoker Line and Shadow Crayon** *($8.39)* is a chubby pencil that goes on creamy, and also features shiny colors. It has the odd quality of smudging in place rather than smearing, but I suppose that's the intended effect. **Brow Colourist Colour and Highlighting Pencil** *($8.39)* is a standard, slightly creamy brow pencil that is not preferred to the Brow Powderist described below. There is a shiny highlighting powder eyeshadow at the other end of the pencil that isn't really necessary, but I suppose it adds some appeal to this otherwise ho-hum pencil. **Brow Powderist Redefining Powder** *($7.29)* is a sheer, dry-textured brow powder that includes two coordinating colors in one compact. The colors are suitable and allow for a custom match, though each has an understated shine. The powder has a tendency to flake unless you are diligent about knocking all of the excess off the brush before applying. That means the final result will take longer, but the flaking should be minimal. The brush that comes with this is terrible and should be discarded immediately.

☹ **Lineur Intense Defining Liquid Liner** *($7.19)* is a traditional liquid liner that goes on like the name says—intense—but compared to the Line Intensifique on the facing page, this takes too long to dry and smudges before the day is done.

LIPSTICK AND LIP PENCIL: ☺ **Endless Comfortable 8-Hour LipColour** *($7.89)* is remarkably similar to Lancôme's Rouge Attraction Lipcolour *($20)*. Both share the same lightweight, creamy-smooth texture and selection of opaque, mostly iridescent colors. Perhaps most telling is that both use the same technology. L'Oréal refers to theirs as "Soft-Seal," while Lancôme calls it "StayPut." Either way, if you're curious to test the long-wear claims, your financial bottom line will be better if you start with L'Oréal's version, and don't count on either the long-wear or stay-put claim working out. It's just a lightweight, softly creamy lipstick with more marketing finesse than technological flair. **Endless Comfortable 8-Hour Liquid LipColour** *($7.89)* is a semi-opaque liquid lip gloss that feels extra light and has a glossy, smooth finish. This silicone-based product has a good stain, but will last eight hours only if you refrain from eating, drinking, or speaking too much! Otherwise, expect to touch this up about as often as a creamy lipstick. **Shine Delice Sheer Shimmering LipColour** *($6.99)* is a slick, glossy lipstick that comes in a marvelous selection of colors that aren't all that sheer. This is perfect for subdued lipstick, but the fragrance is intense. **Colour Endure Stay On LipColour** *($9.39)* is similar to Revlon's ColorStay, except L'Oréal's tends to wear better without chipping. Both go on matte and stay in place. However, regardless of the claims about not feeling dry there is no emollient feel to this at all. The color selection has been reduced somewhat, but the choices are still numerous for fans of ultra-matte lipsticks. **HydraSoft Deeply Softening LipColour SPF 12** *($10.39)* doesn't contain UVA protection, but it is a very good, standard, glossy lipstick in a slim container. This one has no distinct advantage over dozens of other creamy, sheer lipsticks. If anything, Revlon and Almay have the edge when it comes to lipsticks with effective sunscreens.

✔☺ **Colour Riche Rich Creamy LipColour** *($7.19)* is rich in every way except price, which is a boon for you! This decadently creamy lipstick offers intense colors that have admirable staying power, though it is creamy enough to slip into lines around the mouth. You will find this to be almost identical to Lancôme's Rouge Sensation LipColour *($19.50)*, right down to the fragrance.

✔☺ **Colour Riche Crystal Shine LipColour** *($7.19)* is identical to the Colour Riche lipstick above, only these shades are infused with loads of iridescence for ultrasparkly lips. ✔☺ **Rouge Pulp Anti-Feathering Lip Liner** *($8.49)* is an automatic, nonretractable pencil that comes in six very good shades and really is impressive at keeping lipstick in place. This is a keeper! ✔☺ **Glass Shine High Shine Lip Gloss** *($7.99)* is a standard, nonsticky lip gloss that comes in an aluminum tube reminiscent of Stila's popular Lip Gloss *($17)*. Most of the gorgeous shades offer semiopaque color and a slight stain, but it's still gloss, so be prepared for frequent touch-ups.

☺ **Rouge Pulp Liquid Lipcolour** *($8.39)* is the precursor to Glass Shine, and remains a fine, nonsticky, wand-type lip gloss that includes some vivid, splashy colors. This is not as glossy as the High Shine Lip Gloss above. **Colour Riche Rich Creamy Lipliner** *($7.19)* is a standard, twist-up, retractable pencil that has a built-in sharpener. The sharpener part isn't necessary given the finer point that most twist-up pencils like this one already have, plus after one use the shavings clog in the sharpener and that's that. The application is smooth and creamy, and the available colors are versatile. **Crayon Petite Automatic Lip Liner** *($6.89)* is a standard twist-up lip pencil that is definitely creamier than most and offers some good colors, including a Clear version. **Lip Duet Lip Liner and Colour Crayon** *($8.89)* gives you a standard lipliner and lip color in one thick, dual-sided pencil. This has the edge over other crayon-type lipsticks due to its smooth application, well-coordinated colors, and nongreasy finish. If this concept appeals to you, this version won't disappoint.

MASCARA: ✔☺ **Lash Intensifique Lash by Lash Body Building Mascara** *($6.69)* is indeed intense, and is dramatically similar to Lancôme's Amplicils *($20)*. Both go on quite heavily, and build admirable length and copious thickness. Clumping can be a problem if this is applied too eagerly, and the large brush may be a problem for getting to those hard-to-reach lashes—yet for lash impact, this should be on your short list of contenders! ✔☺ **Lash Intensifique Curved Brush Mascara** *($6.69)* is identical to the Lash by Lash Body Building Mascara above, only the curved brush allows you to create maximum impact a bit faster. ✔☺ **Lash Intensifique Waterproof Mascara** *($6.69)* is way above average for waterproof mascara. This builds remarkable length, lift, and curl while keeping your lashes at their best through tears or a swim. ✔☺ **Lash Architect 3-D Dramatic Mascara** *($7.49, straight or curved brush)* is amazing mascara! Talk about long, thick lashes. With just a few strokes you can actually look like you're wearing false eyelashes. As enthusiastic as I am about this one, there is one downside: It can be clumpy and uneven, and has a tendency to flake (though not smear) during the day, especially if you overapply, which is easy to do because it builds length so fast. If your goal is ample length with thickness, then the Lash Intensifique above is the way to go. ✔☺ **Le Grand Curl** *($7.39)* is still one of the best mascaras that goes on well without clumping, holds up through the entire day, remains smear-free, and, oh yes, lengthens and thickens with ease. It will lift and curl as you apply it, but that is the nature of any good mascara, and this is no exception. ✔☺ **Le Grand Curl Waterproof Mascara** *($5.99)* builds fantastic length, lift, and curl. You lose some thickness, but that's the sacrifice with most waterproof mascaras, and this one does not give in when lashes get wet.

☺ **Superior Longitude Extreme Lengthening Mascara** *($9.29)* isn't what I would consider extreme, especially after trying the cream of L'Oréal's mascara crop above. However, this does lengthen without much effort and builds subtle thickness. It lasts all day without flaking, but can smear slightly during application. **Lash Out Curved Brush** *($5.99)* has a better brush than the original Lash Out mascara below, and that enables you to build a touch more length with a softer, cleaner separation. Thickness is not in this mascara's bag of tricks, but if that's not what you need or prefer, this is fine. **Voluminous Volume Building Mascara** *($6.69, straight or curved brush)* remains a superior lengthening mascara, but it doesn't build the same thickness or create the same all-out drama that it did before. It doesn't clump or smear, however, and it does hold up beautifully throughout the day. **Voluminous Mascara Curved Brush** *($5.99)* is nearly identical to the Volume Building version above, only this goes to great lengths faster, thanks to a longer-bristled brush.

☺ **Lash Out Lengthening and Separating Mascara** *($5.99)*. Given the enticing name, this isn't too impressive. It's OK, but not on a par with L'Oréal's best. Lash Out does lengthen well, but as it separates the lashes it also tends to stick them together, which can create long lashes with sparse body. **Longitude Lash Out Extra Lengthening Waterproof Mascara** *($5.99)* is just a very mediocre mascara that can take up to fifteen coats before you see much length or thickness, and even then the results are mediocre. It does hold up underwater, but unless you're willing to settle for less, skip this one in favor of Le Grand Curl

Waterproof above for best results. **FeatherLash Softly Sweeping Mascara** *($6.19)* ends up being a patchy application of mascara that builds uneven length and minimal thickness. It won't smear and doesn't clump, which is great, but the payoff is not what I have come to expect from a L'Oréal mascara. Still, for minimal lash enhancement, it works. **FeatherLash Mascara Curved Brush** *($6.19)* has the same traits as the original FeatherLash, but the brush makes it easier to apply an even, sheer layer for barely defined lashes. **FeatherLash Water Resistant Mascara** *($6.19)* is marginally adept at lengthening, but gets a thumbs-down for thickness. It goes on easily, with no globs or clumps, but be prepared to work for anything more than a subtle effect. What's best about this mascara is that lashes stay soft to the touch and the formula nicely resists water, yet is easily removed with a water-soluble cleanser. **Voluminous Waterproof Mascara** *($5.99)* is rather lackluster when compared to the waterproof Le Grand Curl and (especially) Lash Intensifique mascaras, but it does the job with noticeable length and definition, plus it holds up underwater.

LANCÔME

This very French line maintains a more casual ambience when compared to the other French lines sold at department stores such as Yves St. Laurent, Orlane, Givenchy, Guerlain, and Chanel, whose elitist airs are so thick you can cut them with a knife. Over the years, Lancôme has done a noteworthy job of making sure its image and products radiate a contemporary elegance. Owned by L'Oréal, one of the top cosmetics companies in the world, Lancôme has the advertising dollars to keep its "high-end" image in consumer's minds as one of the standards for beauty products. In tandem with the air of European style that Lancôme exudes, its products have always been aimed at baby boomers and anyone else concerned with the "ravages of time."

Lancôme's skin-care line includes a vast group of products, yet in the area of interesting water-binding agents, antioxidants, and anti-irritants they fall astoundingly short. Cosmetics companies such as Estée Lauder are so far ahead of Lancôme it is almost shocking. Another fact that is likely to be of some interest to the consumer is that Lancôme is owned by L'Oréal, and you can often find L'Oréal products that are virtually identical to the Lancôme products—the products are first launched at the L'Oréal shelves and then turn up at the Lancôme counters a month or two later. In terms of quality, both L'Oréal and Lancôme lag behind, though if you think Lancôme has the answers for you, try L'Oréal first. Just be warned: Their products are highly fragranced, a very French thing to do. For more information about Lancôme, call (800)-LANCÔME or visit www.lancome.com. **Note:** All Lancôme products contain fragrance.

Lancôme Skin Care

☺ **Ablutia Fraicheur Purifying Foam Cleanser** *($21.50 for 6.4 ounces)* is a very standard, detergent-based, water-soluble cleanser that can be drying for some skin types, but it's appropriate for someone with normal to oily skin.

☺ **Clarifiance Oil-Free Gel Cleanser** *($21.50 for 6.8 ounces)* is a standard, detergent-based, water-soluble cleanser that would work well for most skin types except for dry skin.

☺ **Vinefit Cleansing Bar** *($13 for 4 ounces)* is an extremely standard bar cleanser that contains the tiniest amount of grape extract and oil. It can be drying for most skin types.

☺ **Clarifiance Oil-Free Gel Cleanser** *($21.50 for 6.8 ounces)* is a very basic, though good, detergent-based cleanser that would work well for most skin types except for dry skin.

☺ **$$$ Gel Controle** *($19.50 for 4.2 ounces)* is a standard, detergent-based cleanser that would work well for normal to oily skin. It contains a tiny amount of salicylic acid, but the high pH of this cleanser makes it ineffective for exfoliation.

☺ **$$$ Mousse Controle** *($19.50 for 4.2 ounces)* is a detergent-based cleanser that dispenses like a mousse hair-styling product. The clay in it has some oil-absorbing properties. Of interest is the arginine, an amino acid, listed as the third ingredient. Arginine can be effective in wound healing, but in a cleanser it would just be rinsed away before it had much of a chance to be of help. This product also contains salicylic acid, but the pH of the mousse isn't low enough for it to be effective as an exfoliant.

☺ **Galatée Confort Milky Creme Cleanser** *($37.50 for 13.5 ounces)* is supposed to be a splash-off or tissue-off cleanser for all skin types, but it ends up being a standard, mineral oil–based, wipe-off cleanser that can leave a greasy film on the skin. It may be good for extremely dry skin, although it needs to be wiped off to remove both the makeup and the cleanser.

☺ **$$$ Gel Clarté** *($19.50 for 4.2 ounces)* is a standard, detergent-based cleanser that can be an option for normal to oily skin. The papaya and pineapple extracts have no exfoliating properties.

☺ **Mousse Clarté** *($25 for 6.8 ounces)* is similar to the Gel Clarté above, only in a mousse dispenser, and the same basic comments apply.

☺ **$$$ Mousse Confort** *($19.50 for 4.2 ounces)* is a standard, detergent-based cleanser that can be an option for normal to oily skin. It would be too drying for dry skin.

☺ **$$$ Bi-Facil Double-Action Eye Makeup Remover** *($20 for 4 ounces)* is a very standard, silicone-based, wipe-off cleanser, nothing more. It would work as well as any.

☺ **$$$ Effacile Gentle Eye Makeup Remover** *($17.50 for 4 ounces)* is a detergent-based eye-makeup remover that isn't all that gentle, but it will take off eye makeup.

☺ **Eau de Bienfait Cleanser Water with Vitamins for Face and Eyes** *($23.50 for 6.8 ounces)* is a standard, detergent-based makeup remover that would be gentler than the Effacile above, except that the pineapple and papaya extracts are inappropriate for the eye area.

☺ **$$$ Exfoliance Delicate Exfoliating Gel** *($21 for 3.5 ounces)* is a standard, detergent-based scrub that uses ground-up plastic (polyethylene) as the abrasive, which is fairly gentle for normal to oily skin. This does contain a tiny amount of salicylic acid (BHA), but the pH is too high for it to have any benefit for exfoliation.

☺ **$$$ Exfoliance Confort** *($21 for 3.4 ounces)* is similar to the Exfoliance Delicate Exfoliating Gel above only in a far more emollient base and without the BHA, which means this is far better for normal to dry skin.

☺ **$$$ Exfoliance Clarté Clarifying Exfoliating Gel** *($21 for 3.4 ounces)* is similar to the Exfoliance Delicate Exfoliating Gel above only with more detergent cleansing agents, which does make it better for normal to oily skin. The same comments apply about the BHA.

☹ **Tonique Controle Toner for Oily and Normal to Oily Skin** *($19.50 for 6.8 ounces)* is basically just alcohol, and that is too irritating and drying for all skin types.

☹ **Tonique Clarté** *($19.50 for 6.8 ounces)* is similar to the Tonique Controle above and the same comments apply.

☺ **Tonique Douceur Alcoholic-Free Freshener for Dry/Sensitive Skin** *($27.50 for 13.5 ounces)* is indeed alcohol-free, but it's also little more than applying fragrant water to your skin. This is a very average, do-nothing toner with almost nonexistent antioxidants and water-binding agents, and way too pricey for such a mundane formulation.

☹ **Vitabolic Clarifier Radiance Boosting Tonic** *($27.50 for 3.4 ounces)* is basically just alcohol, along with some potentially irritating plant extracts that only boost the risk of skin irritation and dryness. The pH is too high for the BHA it contains to be effective for exfoliation.

☺ **Tonique Confort** *($19.50 for 6.8 ounces)* is an OK toner with a small, but OK, amount of water-binding agents and an antioxidant. It is an option for normal to dry skin.

☺ **$$$ Absolue Absolute Replenishing Cream SPF 15** *($90 for 1.7 ounces)*. Considering that this is one of Lancôme's most expensive skin-care products they had to put some effort into explaining why paying $90 for a 1.7-ounce product made it better for skin than the other products they sell to produce the same benefit—namely, getting rid of wrinkles. It does contain an in-part avobenzone sunscreen, but this is merely a good, largely silicone-based moisturizer that contains a small amount of antioxidants and even less water-binding agent. It will work well for normal to dry skin. This cream claims it "replenishes skin's appearance that has changed as a result of chronological aging, sun exposure, and hormonal fluctuations" by addressing three primary concerns: dryness, diminished radiance, and loss of elasticity. However, claiming that these concerns can be remedied by the teeny amount of wild yam, soy extract, and sea algae this contains is sheer fantasy. Wild yam does not behave like progesterone in the skin. (It also doesn't appear to do so when eaten or taken in supplements, either. As Dr. Andrew Weil states on his Web site, www.drweil.com, "All sorts of claims have been made about wild yam because it contains a precursor of steroid hormones called diosgenin, which was used as the starting material for the first birth-control pill. But diosgenin itself has no hormonal activity. Nor can the human body convert it into something that does.") Soy does have antioxidant properties, but its documented effects on estrogen, when taken orally, do not give the same results as when it is applied topically to skin, or at least there is no research establishing that to be the case.

What about the sea algae? Is this Lancôme's attempt to compete with Lauder's Creme de La Mer skin care? Sea algae (seaweed) can function as an antioxidant and water-binding agent, and it costs only pennies to include it in a cosmetic product. For the money, a product brimming with antioxidants and water-binding agents would have been far more impressive.

Finally, remember that sunscreens must be applied liberally if you are to obtain the SPF benefit on the label. At this price you may be reluctant to do that.

☺ **$$$ Absolue Absolute Replenishing Lotion SPF 15** *($90 for 1.7 ounces)* is virtually identical to the Cream version above, only in lotion form, and the same basic comments apply.

☺ **$$$ Absolue Eye** *($60 for 0.5 ounce)* is just an OK, emollient, silicone-based moisturizer that would work well for normal to dry skin. It contains mostly water, glycerin, silicones, plant oil, emollient, thickeners, mica (shine particles), algae, preservative, wild yam, more preservatives, and soybean extract.

See the comments for the Absolue Replenishing Cream SPF 15, page 577, concerning those ingredients.

☺ **$$$ Bienfait Total Fluide SPF 15** *($55 for 3.4 ounces)* is a very good, in-part avobenzone-based sunscreen. So why the neutral face rating? Now that so many products contain UVA-protecting ingredients, you can be more picky about what you choose, and this formulation lists alcohol as the third ingredient. That can be drying and irritating for most skin types—not to mention that the price is completely unwarranted.

☺ **$$$ Bienfait Total UV Eye SPF 15** *($28.50 for 0.5 ounce)* is a good, in-part titanium dioxide–based sunscreen that contains a small amount of antioxidants, but lacks water-binding agents. For the price you would expect full benefits. However, the sun protection is very good.

☹ **Bienfait Total Day Creme SPF 15** *($36 for 1.7 ounces)* does not contain the UVA-protecting ingredients of titanium dioxide, zinc oxide, or avobenzone, and is not recommended.

☺ **$$$ Impactive Multi Performance Silkening Moisturizer** *($38 for 1.7 ounces)* is a silicone-based moisturizer that does leave a silky feel on the skin and that contains some good antioxidants and water-binding agents. It is a good option for someone with normal to dry skin.

☹ **Hydra Controle Oil-Free Hydrating Gel** *($35 for 1.7 ounces)* lists alcohol as the fourth ingredient, which can be a problem for skin. It contains only negligible amounts of water-binding agents, antioxidants, and anti-irritants. The triclosan in this product is a topical disinfectant, but there is no research showing it to be effective for controlling blemishes.

☺ **$$$ Hydra zen for Normal/Combination Skin** *($44 for 1.7 ounces)* is supposed to be relaxation in a jar, or at least that's what the name and ad copy suggest. It's "stress relief for your skin" and contains something called "Acticalm." Even if you could apply something to the face to make it calmer, according to Hydra zen that would only take a moisturizer, because that's all this product is. The only unique thing about Hydra zen is the name. If mind over matter works, then you will feel calmer, but it probably isn't from applying this good, but rather ordinary, ho-hum, silicone-based, lightweight moisturizer that contains minimal water-binding agents and antioxidants. Some of the plant extracts can be irritants.

☺ **$$$ Hydra Zen Cream for Normal to Dry Skin** *($44 for 1.7 ounces)* is similar to the Hydra zen for Normal/Combination Skin above except that this one contains several plant oils, which does make it better for dry skin. Still, it lacks the amounts of antioxidants and water-binding agents that would have warranted a better rating.

☺ **$$$ Hydra Zen Cream for Very Dry Skin** *($44 for 1.7 ounces)* is similar to the Hydra Zen Cream on the facing page and the same basic comments apply.

☺ **$$$ Hydra Zen Skin De-Stressing Anti-Puffiness Eye Treatment** *($36 for 0.5 ounce)* is an OK, emollient, silicone-based moisturizer that contains a decent amount of antioxidants and water-binding agent, though it's not exactly brimming over with them. The caffeine it contains can't depuff the eye and the plant extracts are a mix of irritants and anti-irritants.

☺ **$$$ Niosome + Perfected Age Treatment** *($68 for 2.5 ounces)* is a good basic moisturizer for dry skin. There are some antioxidants, but such negligible amounts that they don't count for much.

☺ **$$$ Nutribel Nourishing Hydrating Emulsion** *($40 for 2.5 ounces)* is a very emollient moisturizer for dry skin that contains mostly water, plant oils, glycerin, mineral oil, thickeners, urea, water-binding agents, and preservatives. This isn't exciting, but it is good.

☺ **Nutrix Soothing Treatment Creme** *($32 for 1.9 ounces)* costs a lot of money for what you get, which is primarily mineral oil, Vaseline, lanolin, waxes, and tiny amounts of water-binding agents. It is an option for very dry skin. However, lines from Lubriderm to Eucerin offer similar formulas for far less money.

☺ **Trans-Hydrix Multi-Action Hydrating Creme** *($36.50 for 1.9 ounces)* is a very basic, ordinary, emollient moisturizer for dry skin.

☹ **Progres Counter des Yeux Eye Creme** *($37.50 for 1.5 ounces)* is a thick, heavy eye cream of mostly thickeners, Vaseline, and emollient. It also contains preservatives that are recommended for use in rinse-off products only, and, as such, is not recommended.

☺ **$$$ Primordiale Intense Creme** *($74 for 1.7 ounces)*. There is simply nothing intense about this silicone-based moisturizer for dry skin except the price. The plant extracts it contains are meant to sound like they can perform like AHAs, but they have no exfoliating properties. The teeny amount of vitamin E is barely detectable, and there are no water-binding agents of any consequence.

☺ **$$$ Primordiale Intense Eye** *($46 for 0.5 ounce)* contains mostly water, silicones, glycerin, film-forming agent, plant oils, slip agent, vitamin E, preservatives, caffeine, wound-healing agent, algae, fragrance, and water-binding agent. The teeny amounts of vitamin E and plant extracts can't provide much benefit and caffeine can be a skin irritant, though when present in such a small amount that's unlikely. This would have been better if it had much larger amounts of antioxidants and water-binding agents.

☺ **$$$ Primordiale Lip** *($29 for 0.5 ounce)* is an emollient, clear, somewhat glossy lipstick—period. It isn't concentrated in the least.

☺ **$$$ Primordiale Intense Night Renewing Age Defense Treatment** *($63 for 1.7* *ounces)* is virtually identical to Lancôme's former Primordiale Nuit; the only noticeable difference on the ingredient list is a different form of silicone. Despite the fantastic claims, this remains a rather ordinary moisturizer for dry to very dry skin.

☹ **Renergie Lift Contour Skin Firming and Conditioning Complex** *($54 for 1 ounce)* is, with only minor differences (and I mean really minor differences), virtually identical to L'Oréal's Revitalift Slim Face Contouring and Toning Solution. The major difference? L'Oréal's is $10.49 for 1.7 ounces, which means a possible savings to you of more than $60 if you give the L'Oréal version a try instead of this one from Lancôme. That is, if you really want to buy into the claim that these two primarily alcohol-based products can reduce facial puffiness and firm and lift skin. Not only is that unlikely, but the alcohol when present in this amount can be drying, and the *Terminalia sericea* plant extract can be a skin irritant. This one is up to you, but there are better products than this from both Lancôme and L'Oréal to consider.

☺ **$$$ Renergie Double Performance Treatment Anti-Wrinkle and Firmness** *($80 for 2.5 ounces)* contains nothing that can firm or have any impact on stopping wrinkles. This very basic moisturizer includes mostly water, thickeners, silicone, Vaseline, water-binding agents, sunscreen ingredient, fragrance, vitamin E, caffeine, preservatives, and coloring agents. This is mediocre and repetitive, just like many of the Lancôme moisturizers.

☺ **$$$ Renergie Emulsion Oil-Free Lotion, Double Performance, Anti-Wrinkle, Firming** *($65 for 1.7 ounces)* is even more empty of beneficial skin-care ingredients than the Renergie Double Performance above. This version takes out the Vaseline, which makes it better for oily skin, and adds a tiny amount of cornstarch, but even the trace amount of vitamin E is gone, replaced with a minuscule amount of vitamin A. Otherwise, the same basic comments apply, but for the money this is truly a serious disappointment for any skin type.

☺ **$$$ Renergie Eye** *($46 for 0.5 ounce)* is similar to the Renergie Double Performance Treatment above and the same basic comments apply.

☺ **$$$ Re-Surface** *($52.50 for 1 ounce)* is Lancôme's contribution to the retinol bandwagon, only L'Oréal beat Lancôme to the punch a few months earlier with its Line Eraser Pure Retinol *($12.89 for 1 ounce)*. These products are virtually the same, with the same retinol, the same small amount, the same lightweight lotion formulation, and the same airtight packaging (which is necessary to keep the retinol stable). If you're thinking of retinol, despite the meager evidence that there is any reason to use it, why would you choose the Lancôme version over the L'Oréal version? Keep in mind that the only benefit to using this product *is* retinol, because it comes up short for any other worthwhile skin-care ingredients.

☺ **$$$ Re-Surface Eye** *($44 for 0.5 ounce)*. If you thought Lancôme's Re-Surface retinol moisturizer was a necessity, then of course the eye version would be part of the package. At least that's what Lancôme is hoping you believe about this moisturizer with retinol. However, if retinol is the ingredient you're after, the original Re-Surface above, at $52.50 for 1 ounce, could absolutely be used around the eyes and be a significant savings. However, you do remember, don't you, that L'Oréal's version, Line Eraser Pure Retinol *($12.89 for 1 ounce)*, is an equally good option for a retinol product?

☺ **$$$ Vinefit Complete Energizing Lotion SPF 15** *($37.50 for 1 ounce)*. The best part of this overpriced sunscreen is the sunscreen, which is an appropriate SPF 15 with an in-part titanium dioxide–based sunscreen. Other than the touted grape seed oil and grape extract, which are good antioxidants, this product does contain niacinamide. There is research showing that niacinamide is effective in the production of ceramides (a vital component of skin) and in reducing the negative effects of sun exposure (which suppresses the skin's immune response). Whether or not niacinamide can do that when applied topically is unknown, but it is still an intriguing ingredient to consider using on skin. However, Olay has far better products that include this ingredient than Lancôme. Overall, the moisturizing base, for normal to dry skin, is exceptionally ordinary.

☺ **$$$ Vinefit Cream SPF 15** *($37.50 for 1.7 ounces)* is a cream version of the Vinefit Complete version above and the same basic comments apply.

☺ **Vinefit Cool Gel** *($26 for 1.7 ounces)* has grape extract and a tiny amount of vitamin E and niacinamide, but it also lists alcohol as the fourth ingredient, and that's not cooling, that's irritating for skin.

☹ **Vinefit Lip SPF 8** *($14.50 for 0.5 ounce)* is a poorly formulated sunscreen with no UVA-protecting ingredients and an abysmally low SPF 8, far below the standard of SPF 15 set by the Skin Cancer Foundation and the American Academy of Dermatology. This is just embarrassing.

☺ **$$$ Vitabolic Dark Eye Circle Treatment** *($46 for 0.5 ounce)* is yet another addition to the world of vitamin C skin-care products. Vitabolic uses ascorbic acid. Refer to Chapter 2, Miracles, Frauds, & Facts: An A to Z Guide, for more details about ascorbic acid and vitamin C. Basically, with only ascorbic acid, and no other antioxidants or water-binding agents, this is a one-note product. All in all, Avon's vitamin C product is far more interesting (it even has the same form of vitamin C) for less money.

☺ **$$$ Vitabolic Deep Radiance Booster** *($45 for 1 ounce)* is almost identical to the Vitabolic Dark Eye Circle version on page 581 and the same basic comments apply.

☺ **$$$ Vitabolic Oil Free** *($49 for 1 ounce)* is almost identical to the Vitabolic Dark Circle Eye version on page 581, except that they took out the plant oil, though the same basic comments still apply.

☺ **$$$ Complexion Expert** *($46 for 1 ounce)* is supposed to lighten skin discoloration. This very standard, extremely ordinary emollient moisturizer may just do that because it does contain kojic acid, along with the exceptionally standard emollients and plant oil and teeny amounts of vitamins E and C. There is definitely convincing research, both in vitro and in vivo, and in animal studies, showing that kojic acid is effective for inhibiting melanin production (sources: *Biological and Pharmaceutical Bulletin*, August 2002, pages 1045–1048; *Analytical Biochemistry*, June 2002, pages 260–268; *Cellular Signaling*, September 2002, pages 779–785; *American Journal of Clinical Dermatology*, September-October 2000, pages 261–268; and *Archives of Pharmacal Research*, August 2001, pages 307–311). So why doesn't this ingredient show up in more skin-lightening products (most use hydroquinone, or plant extracts that have arbutin as one of their components)? It's because kojic acid is an extremely unstable ingredient in cosmetic formulations. Upon exposure to air or sunlight it turns a strange shade of brown and loses its efficacy, and it is also considered extremely irritating as well (source: www.emedicine.com, "Skin Lightening/Depigmenting Agents," November 5, 2001).

☹ **Pure Empriente Masque Purifying Mineral Mask with White Clay** *($24 for 3.4 ounces)* is a standard clay mask that contains camphor, making it too irritating for all skin types.

☹ **Hydra Intense Masque** *($24 for 3.4 ounces)* lists alcohol as the second ingredient, and that makes it completely hydra un-intense and not recommended.

☹ **Pore Controle Masque** *($24 for 3.4 ounces)* is a standard clay mask with some salicylic acid, but the pH of the base is too high for it to be an effective exfoliant. It also contains menthol, which won't help skin in the least; it is just irritating and a problem for all skin types.

☺ **$$$ T. Controle Oil-Free Powder Gel Instant T-Zone Matifier** *($22.50 for 1 ounce)* is an interesting product made of silicone and film-forming agent, period—there is no powder in here. It will put a silky film over the skin, but don't count on this helping your oily skin because there is nothing in this product that can hold back oil. It is a decent lightweight silicone moisturizer, but that's about it. Definitely test it before you even consider purchasing this misleading product. If anything, it will make someone with oily skin feel somewhat oilier!

Lancôme Oligo Mineral

Lancôme has been quietly selling this small collection of products exclusively at Neiman Marcus, and no wonder! Neiman's is known for carrying upscale (read: very expensive) cosmetics, and they pride themselves on their select menagerie of skin-care and makeup lines. I suspect that one of the reasons the Oligo Mineral line is not available in "mainstream" department stores is because the products are almost identical to Lancôme's other products; the major difference is that these carry lofty, needlessly marked-up price tags. Naturally, the hook that supposedly justifies the hefty price is the inclusion of several minerals, from copper to zinc. Yet even if such an assortment of minerals had some extraordinary benefit for topical use on the skin, Lancôme adds them in such small amounts that their impact (if any) would be nominal. Leaving aside the illusion of affluence that purchasing these products may convey, there is no reason to stop by the Neiman Marcus Lancôme counter to check these out. If Lancôme is where you want to spend your cosmetics dollars, your skin won't notice the difference if you ignore this subline and focus on their Nordstrom or Macy's department-store offerings. The only difference you will notice is in your budget.

☺ **$$$ Oligo Mineral Cleanser** *($48.50 for 4 ounces)* is an extremely standard foaming cleanser that can be quite drying for most skin types, though it certainly does clean well. The fragrance comes way before the fountain-of-youth minerals, which means their presence is more for show than effect.

☹ **Oligo Mineral Toner** *($40 for 6.8 ounces)* is an embarrassing formulation that lists alcohol as the second ingredient. That makes it too drying and irritating for all skin types, and Lancôme knows better (at least they do in their less expensive toners). What a shame, because sans alcohol, this would have been a very good moisturizing toner for dry skin.

☺ **$$$ Oligo Mineral Fortifying Cream** *($125 for 2.6 ounces)* is a silky, emollient moisturizer that would be a fine option for normal to dry skin, but there is nothing especially unique in this that makes it worth the investment. It does contain some good antioxidants, but the amounts are minuscule, and for this price, it should be overflowing with them.

☺ **$$$ Oligo Mineral Eye Cream** *($75 for 0.5 ounce)* is almost identical to, but less elegant than, the Fortifying Cream above, and the same basic comments apply. This does have a tiny amount of caffeine, but it's not enough to be a significant problem for irritation, and it won't wake up the eye area, either.

☺ **$$$ Oligo Mineral Lotion** *($95 for 1.7 ounces)* is a very good lightweight lotion for normal to slightly dry skin, featuring an effective blend of water, silicones, slip agent, mineral oil, anti-irritant, vitamins E, C, and A (antioxidants), minerals, preservatives, and fragrance. But save your money. Lancôme's Vinefit Complete Energizing Lotion SPF 15 *($37.50 for 1.7 ounces)* offers an even silkier formula with equally good antioxidants and effective sun protection to boot, yet costs almost two-thirds less.

Lancôme Sun Products

☺ **SPF 15 Face and Body Lotion with Pure Vitamin E** *($25 for 5 ounces)* is a very good, avobenzone-based sunscreen in a lightweight lotion base for someone with normal to dry or slightly oily skin. It is a very basic moisturizer with a minuscule amount of vitamin E.

☺ **$$$ UV Expert SPF 15 Water Light Fluid** *($31 for 1 ounce)* is similar to the SPF 15 Face and Body Lotion above, only in a matte finish, lotion base, and the same basic comments apply.

☺ **SPF 25 Face and Body Lotion with Pure Vitamin E** *($25 for 5 ounces)* is similar to the SPF 15 Face and Body Lotion above and the same review applies.

☺ **Water-Light Spray SPF 15 with Pure Vitamin E** *($25 for 5 ounces)* is a very good avobenzone-based sunscreen that is mostly slip agents, film-forming agent, and plant oil. It should work well for someone with normal to dry skin.

☺ **$$$ High Protection SPF 30 Face Creme with Pure Vitamin E** *($24 for 1.7 ounces)* is similar to the lotions above, but there is nothing unique or special about this one that warrants the far smaller amount of sunscreen product for the same price.

☺ **$$$ Soleil Expert Sun Care SPF 30 High Protection Sun Stick** *($19.50 for 0.26 ounce)* is an avobenzone-based sunscreen, and the amount you get for the price is ludicrous given that this is simply a good sunscreen in an ordinary emollient lipstick-type base.

☺ **$$$ Soleil Ultra Eye Protection SPF 40** *($25 for 0.5 ounce)* is a good, but extremely overpriced, sunscreen that includes titanium dioxide and zinc oxide as two of the active sunscreen ingredients. This combination is not unique to Lancôme and the use of an SPF 40 sounds like you are getting "more" protection, but all you would be getting is longer protection, and there just isn't that much sunlight in a day. (SPF ratings over 30 are not going to be around after the FDA's new sunscreen regulations take effect.) Nothing about this sunscreen makes it preferred for the eye area; if anything, the talc and other active ingredients (octyl methoxycinnamate and oxybenzone) can be irritating if they get in the eye. This is an ordinary moisturizer for normal to dry skin.

☺ **$$$ Soleil Ultra Face and Body Lotion SPF 40** *($25 for 0.5 ounce)* is similar to the Soleil Ultra Eye Protection on the facing page minus the talc, and the same comments apply. Actually, these two products are so similar there is no reason to spend more money on the earlier version.

☺ **$$$ Soleil Cool Comfort After Sun Rehydrating Face and Body Lotion** *($25 for 5 ounces)* is a very basic, ordinary moisturizer for normal to dry skin with tiny amounts of antioxidants and fractional amounts of anti-irritants. Mica adds a small touch of shine to the skin.

☺ **$$$ Flash Bronzer Self Tanning Face Gel with Pure Vitamin E**, available in **Medium, Deep, and Extra Deep** *($24 for 1.7 ounces)*; **Flash Bronzer Oil Free Tinted Self Tanning Face Lotion for the Face with Vitamin E** available in **Medium** or **Dark** *($24 for 1.7 ounces)*; and **Flash Bronzer Tinted Self Tanning Mousse** *($27 for 5 ounces)* all contain dihydroxyacetone, the same ingredient all self-tanners use to affect the color of skin. These would work as well as any, but there is nothing in these formulations that makes them preferred over far less expensive versions available in drugstores.

☹ **Flash Bronzer Instant Self Tanning Body Spray with SPF 15 and Pure Vitamin E** *($27 for 4.2 ounces)* doesn't contain the UVA-protecting ingredients of titanium dioxide, zinc oxide, or avobenzone, and is not recommended.

Lancôme Makeup

In contrast to their rather lackluster skin-care products, Lancôme's French-bred, American-made makeup is a stellar collection that, in some categories, continues to set precedents as new technology evolves. Their selection of everything from foundations to lipsticks is enormous—and there are prime picks in every category. I don't know how the counter personnel keep track of everything, but for the most part Lancôme's sales force is adept at navigating through the products. In contrast to the staff at Estée Lauder, Lancôme's representatives maintain a more passive-aggressive, casual approach, which can still be unnerving but is definitely less intense. Although the makeup tester units still do not divide colors into logical groups (such as pinks and plums), the specific products are distinguished and grouped together, so you're not left to guess which lipstick formula you're sampling or which concealer you're blending.

If you're looking for a force to reckon with for foundations, Lancôme is a must-see. They continue to offer some of the most elegant, silky formulas anywhere and in a color range that is overwhelmingly neutral, whether your skin is porcelain or ebony. The only troubling aspect is that most of Lancôme's foundations with sunscreen do not contain adequate UVA protection. Considering that Lancôme obviously knows about the risks with this issue, I recommend these foundations with mixed emotions. The fact that they continually launch new foundations with incomplete sun protection is tantamount to a company like Ford knowingly selling new cars without air bags. Beyond this major gripe, you will discover that Lancôme has a well-deserved reputation for their fantastic mascaras, and their latest powder-based products apply with a silkiness that makes them gratifying to work with. The rest of the makeup comprises some completely valid options, but before you commit to Lancôme, consider the similar options available for less from sister companies L'Oréal and Maybelline. Striking a balance between the best of each of these lines will give you first-class makeup that beautifies without breaking the bank.

FOUNDATION: ✔☺ $$$ **Dual Finish Versatile Powder Makeup** *($31)* is a talc-based wet/dry powder foundation that offers a soft matte finish and a beautiful selection of colors. The application, especially when used dry, is smooth and even, although this type of foundation is best for normal skin; dry skin may find this too dry and oily skin may find it too cakey after it is applied. I would avoid wet application since this type of product tends to go on choppy and streak. The only disappointing color among the sixteen is Matte Miel Fonce IV, which may turn orange on some skin tones. Matte Porcelaine Delicate and Matte Rose Clair are slightly pink, but not enough to show on lighter skin. ✔☺ **Maquicontrole Oil-Free Liquid Makeup** *($32.50)* is Lancôme's original ultra-matte foundation (launched over seventeen years ago, well ahead of its time) and it has remained an exceptional oil-free foundation that offers medium to full coverage and a true matte finish. It has incredible staying power and is ideal for oily to very oily skin. Of the ten shades, avoid Beige Natural III and Beige Bisque III. ✔☺ **Teint Idole Enduringly Divine Makeup** *($32.50)* is one of the best (and last) ultra-matte makeups. It has a decent slip, but blending must still be precise because it dries quickly and doesn't budge. The smooth texture offers medium to full coverage, and this wears beautifully. Of the fifteen shades, only Bisque 0, Suede 0, and Suede 2 are problematic. Suede 10 is perfect for dark skin, while Ivoire 0 would work for the fairest complexion. ✔☺ **Bienfait Total UV Tinted SPF 15** *($36)* is an excellent option for a lightweight, sheer, tinted moisturizer for normal to oily skin types. The texture has a soft, creamy slip that blends beautifully on the skin and it sets to a soft matte finish. Of course, any shine-prone areas will show through relatively quickly, but for those who prefer a light wash of color with an in-part titanium dioxide sunscreen, this is brilliant. The four shades are mostly winners—only Tawny may be too peach for some skin tones, but just barely. ☺ $$$ **Photogenic Skin-Illuminating Makeup SPF 15** *($32.50)* is divine, with a light, fluid texture that blends to a soft, natural finish with light to medium coverage. The nineteen shades are mostly wonderful, and this blends with ease. If Lancôme would just add some UVA protection, Photogenic would be a great recommendation for normal to slightly dry or slightly oily skin types. If you're willing to wear sun protection underneath this, there are some superior colors to consider for both light and dark skin tones (but not for very dark skin). The following shades are too pink, peach, or copper for most skin tones: Bisque 2 (slightly pink), Bisque 4, Bisque 8, Suede 4 (slightly copper), and Suede 6. **Photogenic Ultra-Comfort Skin Illuminating Makeup SPF 15** *($32.50)* is a marvelous-feeling foundation that is piggybacking off the success of Lancôme's original Photogenic makeup. This version is designed for normal to dry skin and it shows. The silicone-based formula feels silky and airy on the skin while imparting light coverage and a soft, natural finish that blends easily. Of the ten shades available, only Ultra Bisque 2 and Ultra Bisque 4 (both slightly peach) should be considered with caution. The other eight colors are true to Lancôme's usually excellent neutral foundation palette. The only drawback that keeps this from being a Paula's Pick is the sunscreen, which does not contain UVA-protecting ingredients. If you're willing to wear an effective sunscreen underneath this, it is wholeheartedly recommended! **Maqui-Libre Skin-Liberating Makeup SPF 15** *($32.50)* offers sheer coverage and a natural finish with its lightweight, fluid texture that blends easily. If only the sunscreen contained effective UVA protection, this would be a slam-dunk for casual weekend makeup for those with normal to dry skin. If you're willing to pair this with a reliable sunscreen, you will find most of the seven shades are superior. Rose Clair II and Beige Bisque III are too pink and rose, respectively. **Teint Optim'age Minimizing Makeup SPF 15** *($32.50)* claims it is "makeup for a new age," yet it contains no UVA-protecting ingredients, which borders on archaic. If sun protection isn't your goal, this enviably smooth makeup blends on superbly, offering sheer to light coverage with a soft matte finish. It is best for normal to dry skin. The claims about "age minimizing" are bogus—there is nothing in here to support that and it won't make one wrinkle on your face look less noticeable—but it is still an excellent foundation. Be careful with the following shades: Beige Bisque III (may turn slightly pink) and Beige Dore III (just slightly peach). **Maquivelours Hydrating Foundation** *($32.50)* is an emollient, demi-matte–finish formula that is best for normal to dry or very dry skin seeking medium coverage. Of the nine shades, the ones to avoid are Rose Clair II, Beige Rose III (both too pink), and Beige Bisque III (peachy).

☺ **$$$ Imanance Tinted Day Creme SPF 15** *($36)* is an in-part titanium dioxide–based SPF 15 tinted moisturizer. The coverage is sheer and the emolliency makes it suitable for normal to dry skin only. The only useful skin-tone color is Bisque; the three remaining shades are all orange or red, though Tawny may work for some medium skin tones.

CONCEALER: ✓☺ $$$ **Effacernes Waterproof Protective Undereye Concealer** *($21)* has a lush, creamy texture that provides superior coverage and allows smooth blending. The squeeze tube takes some getting used to (it's easy to squeeze out too much product), but once you acclimate, this concealer is an ace in the hole, and it doesn't crease! The four shades are quite nice, though Porcelaine I is slightly pink. Contrary to the name, this concealer is not waterproof. ✓☺ $$$ **Photogenic Skin-Illuminating Concealer SPF 15** *($21)* is one of the best concealers available. First, it has an all titanium dioxide–based sunscreen, which makes this a wonderful counterpart to your regular sun protection, whether from a moisturizer or your foundation. Second, it has an incredibly soft, ultralight texture that blends beautifully—almost melting into the skin—yet covers quite well. The finish is soft matte, and it has only a slight tendency to crease into lines. The six colors are mostly superb. Only Correcteur (slightly yellow) and Camee (too peach) should be avoided, and bronze may be too copper for very dark skin tones.

☺ $$$ **Maquicomplet Complete Coverage Concealer** *($21)* has taken a turn for the worse. This smooth, liquidy concealer with excellent, crease-free coverage now features seven shine-laden shades. How maddening! With all of the other shiny products in the Lancôme lineup, why adulterate a perfectly good concealer? This is still worth considering, but please realize that the shiny finish does nothing to minimize wrinkles, nor does it look good over blemishes. **Palette Mix Complexion Kit** *($30)* is a compact with three different flesh-toned shades that you use in combination to get just the right color for your skin. Although this cream-to-powder formula has a superbly smooth finish, most women will have difficulty combining colors like this on their face. It isn't a bad idea, just more time-consuming than a makeup application should be.

POWDER: ✓☺ $$$ **Photogenic Sheer Loose Powder** *($30)* and ✓☺ $$$ **Photogenic Sheer Pressed Powder** *($25)*. These talc-based powders have replaced Lancôme's Poudre Majeur, and claim to contain the "Photo-Flex Complex of 2-D reflecting powders and 3-D diffusing powders." I guess when you're charging upwards of $25 for something as basic as powder you need a good hook. Admittedly, both of these powders have a soft, finely milled, sumptuous texture and a smooth, dry finish (the Pressed Powder version is slightly drier), but the special effects are nothing more than subtle iridescence, plain and simple. Although the shine is barely discernible, those hoping to reduce shine may want to look elsewhere. Both powders offer seven shades, and almost all of them are beautifully soft and neutral, including options for darker (but not very dark) skin tones. Only Soft Bronze stands out as too orange for dark skin, and Deep Bronze would make a great bronzing powder. **Note:** A major plus for the Loose Powder version is its packaging, which adds a powder screen to prevent flyaway loose powder from getting all over everything. ✔☺ **Matte Finish Shine Control Sheer Pressed Powder** *($22)* has a stunningly smooth texture and an even application that does not look powdery or thick on the skin. This talc-based powder comes in six gorgeous colors (though Suede may be too copper for dark skin) and is best for normal to oily skin looking to tame shine without a powdered appearance.

☺ **$$$ Poudre Blanc Neige Light-Reflecting Compact Powder** *($30)* is a standard pressed powder with a smooth, silky finish and a truly soft shine. For a subtle amount of shine, which is a welcome change of pace from the glitter in most products, this is an option. The one shade is a sheer, very pale yellow.

☹ **$$$ Poudre Soleil Sun-Kissed Bronzing Powder** *($30)* is a pressed-powder bronzer with an OK, sheer application and three overly shiny, unnaturally copper colors. This is far from a natural-looking bronzer, and at this price, you can confidently ignore it. **Star Bronzer Bronzing Powder for Face & Body SPF 8** *($35)* is similar to the Bronzing Powder above, except this comes in an oversized compact and features a paltry sunscreen that lacks UVA protection. Both shades are shiny, and a bit too peach (Dore) or copper (Intense) to be considered a top choice.

BLUSH: ✔☺ **$$$ Blush Subtil Delicate Oil-Free Powder Blush** *($25.50)* is a talc-free powder blush that has an enviably soft texture and even application. The color selection is beautiful, but each one has at least some shine. The prime offenders in regard to shine are the ultrasparkly Miel Glace, Bronze Glow, Pink Parfait, Pink Pool, and Soiree. Rouge Glow is a great shade for darker skin, while Bronze Brule is excellent for contouring. ☺ **Couleur Flash Blush Stick** *($28.50)* is a twist-up, cream-to-powder blush with a creamy slip-on application that quickly dries to a soft, sheer powder finish. This has been pared down to a single shade, a pale plum that would work for light skin tones.

☹ **Blush Focus Exceptional Wear Sheer Cheek Color** *($19.50)* is meant to combine the one-touch application of a cream blush with the long wear and soft finish of a powder blush, but it fails to perform well in either category. The texture is hard to explain, but I'll do my best. It's semicreamy with the dryness of a powder, yet tends to flake and chip right out of the container. What's more confounding is that while it is difficult to pick up color with a brush, using your finger picks up too much color and makes it hard to apply with a light touch. It also applies unevenly, looking sheer in spots and intense in others. Perhaps what's most distressing about this blush is that it took the place of Lancôme's far superior cream-to-powder blush Pommette. Lancôme, what were you thinking?

EYESHADOW: ☺ **$$$ Colour Focus Exceptional Wear EyeColour ($16.50)** at last allows Lancôme to offer single powder eyeshadows instead of just duos. In comparison to their MaquiRiche eyeshadows, this formula is undeniably silkier and not nearly as powdery. It applies evenly and easily, with just enough color saturation so that successive applications are not necessary before you can build any intensity. What is frustrating is that almost all of the 35+ shades have either a soft shimmer or a traffic-stopping shine! Couldn't just a few matte shades exist for those who aren't interested in the trend? Consider the following colors almost matte due to their extremely soft shine: Daylight, Positive, Peep, Scene, and Horizon. By the way, the flying saucer–style compact houses a tiny curved eyeshadow applicator that is truly bizarre and unusable, though it does look cool!

☺ **$$$ MaquiRiche CremePowder EyeColour Duo** (*$26 for duo with compact*) are Lancôme's powder eyeshadow selections, and you get to create your own compact by selecting two eyeshadow colors of your choice. It's a great concept, but it would be better if there were some basic matte choices. As is, every color is noticeably shiny. This formula has a creamier, more powdery feel than the Colour Focus above, and has a greater tendency to flake during application. **Ombre Couture Multi-Effect EyeColour Trio ($31.50)** provides two eyeshadows and a powder eyeliner in one sleek compact. The trios are well-coordinated and blend beautifully, though the texture is a bit slippery and several strokes are required for color intensity. Two of the three shades in every set are exceedingly shiny, so these are best ignored if you have any lines or sagging around the eye area. **Aquatique Waterproof EyeColour Base ($19)** is billed as "foundation for eyes." You're supposed to believe you need a separate product (beyond foundation or concealer) to even out the skin tone on the eyelid and to prevent eyeshadows from creasing. This offers an opaque, thick formula that most certainly can crease, and what's worse is that the single color is strongly peach, not exactly what all women need or want. **Ombre Perfecteur Perfecting EyeShadow Base ($20)** is a waterproof concealer for the eyelid area that is also supposed to extend the wear of eyeshadows. The nude, matte color is applied from a pen outfitted with an angled sponge tip. It tends to go on thick, but does blend evenly. It's OK, but not really necessary if you already use a matte-finish concealer. **L'Ombre Style Duo Eye-Powder Pen** (*$25 for applicator pen with two colors*) is a unique concept: This is a dual-ended pen with each end holding a sponge-tip applicator that is "fed" with powder color from the base. However, several shades labeled as matte have obvious shine. Only Matte Fumee (charcoal gray) and Matte Brun (chocolate brown) are truly matte. For a simple eye design, this could work—but the delivery system is not for everyone.

EYE AND BROW SHAPER: ☺ **$$$ Le Crayon Kohl** *($18)* is a standard eye pencil in a nice range of colors. This one is longer than most, so it may seem clumsy at first. These are no better than many others that go for far less money (particularly those from L'Oréal). **Brow Artiste** *($28)* offers two matte-finish, powder-type brow colors in a compact. While most women need only one brow color and mixing takes time, these are still a viable option and have a nice dry texture and matte finish.

✔☺ **$$$ Artliner Precision Point EyeLiner** *($25)* is excellent for a liquid eyeliner that maintains an easy-to-apply, quick-drying, long-lasting formula and has a good brush. For considerably less money, you can get the same results (sans some of the funkier colors) from L'Oréal's Line Intensifique. ✔☺ **Le Crayon Poudre for the Brows** *($19.50)* is one of the best needs-sharpening brow pencils. It goes on easily, if a bit creamy, and the colors are matte and soft. There's even a good brush at one end for softening and blending the color.

☺ **$$$ Le Stylo Waterproof Long Lasting EyeLiner** *($19.50)* is a smooth-textured, twist-up eye pencil with mostly shiny colors that all tend to smudge, though no more so than most creamy pencils. This is fine for a smoky look, and it is reasonably waterproof. **Modele Sourcils Brow Groomer** *($17.50)* is a rather sticky brow gel available in clear or tinted versions. This has a thick, bushy brush that can coat the brows with too much product, which only increases the unpleasant stickiness. This remains an option for full, unruly brows.

☹ **Maquiglace Lumineuse Automatic Eyeliner** *($20)* is no match for the Artliner Precision Point Eyeliner above. The salesperson steered me away from this, commenting that it is very difficult to apply evenly. She was right, plus the two shades are intensely shiny.

LIPSTICK AND LIP PENCIL: ☺ **$$$ Rouge Attraction Lasting Impact Lip-Colour** *($20)* boasts about the StayPut technology it uses to keep the color on the lips as long as possible, but I'll wager you will find this doesn't make it until lunchtime before needing a touch-up. Although it does have a beautifully smooth, silky texture and the shades are richly pigmented, the finish is too slippery and creamy to make most women's expectations of long wear a reality. The colors offer some striking choices—including glitter, metallic, and hologram finishes, in case you're feeling impetuous the next time you're visiting a Lancôme counter. **Rouge Sensation Multi-Sensation LipColour** *($19.50)* has a supremely creamy texture and soft glossy finish. This isn't as greasy as it used to be, though it will still travel into lines around the mouth. The opaque colors are simply stunning. **Rouge Absolu Creme Absolute Comfort Moisturizing LipColour ($19.50)** is about as creamy as Rouge Sensation above, but with a noticeably slicker feel that easily slips off the lips and into lines around the mouth. If feathering is not an issue for you, this is as comfortable as a cream lipstick gets. **Sheer Magnetic Extra Shine Weightless LipColour ($19.50)** is a relatively standard, semisheer lipstick that has a lot of slip and maintains a glossy finish while imparting subtle (often iridescent) color. **Lip Dimension Lasting Liquid Lip-Shaping Colour ($20).** If it weren't for the high price, I would wholeheartedly recommend this lipstick/lip gloss hybrid. It has a silky-smooth, lightweight texture, easy application, and a brilliant selection of sophisticated, opaque colors. For those of you looking for a less expensive alternative, check out L'Oréal's Glass Shine High Shine Lip Gloss ($7.99). **Lip Brio Lastingly Brilliant Lip Lacquer ($20)** is assuredly overpriced, but this smooth gloss has been around for years, so someone must be buying it! For light-coverage colors and a lower-wattage glossy finish, this wand-applicator gloss wins high marks to match its high price. **Le Crayon Lip Contour ($18.50)** is a standard automatic, retractable lip pencil with good colors and a smooth application. You will notice little difference between this and L'Oréal's Colour Riche Rich Creamy Lipliner ($7.19). **Le Lipstique LipColouring Stick with Brush ($19.50)** is a standard pencil with a blending brush at the other end. That's convenient, but not worth the price. This does have some staying power, leaving a slight stain on the lips. The texture is drier than the Le Crayon version above, and that can reasonably help prevent feathering.

☺ **Juicy Tubes Ultra Shiny Lip Gloss ($14.50)** has a thick, viscous application and a sticky, high-gloss finish. It comes in a squeeze tube and offers a range of sheer, trendy colors, but putting up with stickiness and intense fragrance may not be your cup of tea.

MASCARA: Lancôme calls itself "the world's mascara leader," and if you take into account their superior options along with those from sister companies L'Oréal, Maybelline, and Helena Rubinstein, it's hard to dispute this claim!

✔☺ **$$$ Definicils High Definition Mascara ($20)** is Lancôme's perennial top seller, and it is easy to see why. This is an excellent lengthening mascara that builds some thickness with minimal to no chance of clumping. ✔☺ **$$$ Intencils Full Intensity Mascara ($20)** builds extremely thick, full lashes, but also has a slight tendency to clump. If you have a lash comb handy, this mascara is great for all-out drama. ✔☺ **$$$ Magnificils Full Lash Precision Mascara ($20)** builds magnificent length and definition without a clump or smear. I once recommended passing on this mascara, but not anymore. This wears all day and keeps lashes incredibly soft, too! Lancôme insists this is the original formula, but I'm skeptical.

☺ **$$$ Flextencils Full Extension Curving Mascara** *($20)* claims that its "ultra-curving PowerSHAPE formula with patented brush gives lashes up to 30% more visible length with an eye-opening 30° curve." They then go on to say the claim is based on an in vitro (test tube) study, which is curious since one wonders whose eyelashes were used in this manner! Flextencils ends up being less impressive than most of Lancôme's mascaras. It lengthens moderately and does add a soft curl, but it doesn't have the same "wow factor" as the ones above. **Amplicils Panoramic Volume Mascara** *($20)* has a name that probably sounds more intriguing to an audiophile than to a cosmetics customer, but the communication is clearly about making lashes more than they are. This is a respectable mascara, but it's not Lancôme's best (for that, Definicils and Intencils are still preferred). Amplicils doesn't achieve quite the length the others do and it can clump if you're not careful. Yet if you use restraint and carefully wipe down the wand a bit, you'll find you can create relatively long lashes with thickness to spare. For a more refined, Paula's Pick version of this mascara, L'Oréal's Lash Intensifique Mascara *($6.69)* is a must-try.

☺ **$$$ Eternicils Enduring Mascara Waterproof** *($20)* works very well (almost *too* well!) as a waterproof mascara, and it provides decent length and thickness. However, this is unusually difficult to remove, and is best reserved for occasional use. **Aquacils Waterproof Mascara with Keratine** *($20)* is currently not sold at Lancôme counters, but it can be special-ordered and is available on their Web site. This remains a fine waterproof mascara that lasts whether you're caught in a drizzle or a downpour.

☺ **$$$ Forticils Fortifying Lash Conditioner** *($16.50)* is a lash primer that is supposed to be applied before mascara. This will not condition the lashes at all, but it will add an extra layer, which may help; but if you need this product, it just means you bought an inferior mascara to start with.

☺ **$$$ BRUSHES:** Lancôme offers a decent assortment of **Brushes** *($13–$52.50)* with a gorgeous feel and softness, though they are truly overpriced for what you get. Although the bristles may feel great, the shapes and sizes of many of the brushes are not the best for most face shapes and they can be awkward to work with. When you're considering spending $25 and up on an eyeshadow brush, it should be perfect. For the money, you would be far better off shopping at Bobbi Brown, Trish McEvoy, Laura Mercier, or Stila for brushes. If you wish to remain Lancôme-loyal, the best brushes to consider are the **Le Bronzer Bronzing Powder Brush** *($35)*, **Le Lip, Lip Brush** *($20)*, and **La Brosse Precise Eye Makeup Brush** *($16.50)*. Avoid the **Pinceau Lustrage Face**

Fiber Optic Brush *($25)*, which looks cool but serves little purpose and, according to the Lancôme consultants I spoke to, doesn't last long. **Star Bronzer Magic Bronzing Brush** *($29.50)* is a soft, tapered powder brush whose handle is a reservoir for a sheer, shiny golden bronze powder. A push button at the base of the handle shoots powder into the brush, and from there it can be dusted over the face or body. A clever execution to be sure, but this pricey product has little impact other than the sparkling shine it leaves.

MARY KAY

In the winter of 2001, at the age of 83, Mary Kay Ash passed away, leaving behind a cosmetics empire bearing her name. Hers was one of the original home-sales cosmetics companies. It began in 1963, when Mary Kay Ash (with her son's help) created a company that evolved to include more than 300,000 salespeople. Ash's trademark style, as has also happened with the other grande dames of cosmetics (Helena Rubinstein, Marcella Borghese, and Elizabeth Arden), has become infused with her memory and is now part of her company.

With all due respect to Ash's fortitude and rallying presence, and as impressive as her business acumen proved to be, the average Mary Kay salesperson's income is only about $5,000 to $10,000 a year. Obviously, the ability to sell does not come naturally to every member of the sales force.

In regard to the products, much of the Mary Kay lineup is a mixed bag of strong and weak points and the weak points are really weak. Skin Revival has been discontinued, though it was heralded by the company initially as a skin-care miracle; but miracles in the cosmetics industry do tend to come and go. TimeWise is now supposed to be the answer to speedy skin care, with only two steps that clean, tone, and fight aging. But TimeWise doesn't include a sunscreen, which makes this pair of products time-foolish. The basic Mary Kay skin-care routine is a dated mix of greasy cleansers, irritating toners, and daytime moisturizers with poorly formulated SPFs. Wading through this mix of products is cumbersome, but there are a few new state-of-the-art formulations worth checking out. For the most part, though, this is a line in need of fresh air and a fresh face. For more information about Mary Kay, call (800) 627-9529 or visit www.marykay.com.

Mary Kay Skin Care

☺ **Gentle Cleansing Cream Formula 1** *($10 for 4 ounces)* is a traditional, greasy, mineral oil- and Vaseline-based cold cream. It might be gentle, but it is also quite heavy, and can leave a greasy film on the skin. It is an option for very dry skin.

☺ **Creamy Cleanser Formula 2** *($10 for 6.5 ounces)* is a mineral oil–based, wipe-off cleanser that can leave a greasy film on the skin. It is less heavy than the Gentle version on the facing page and is an option for someone with dry skin.

☺ **Deep Cleanser Formula 3** *($10 for 6.5 ounces)* is an extremely standard, but good, detergent-based, water-soluble cleanser that is an option for most skin types except dry skin.

☹ **Velocity Facial Cleanser** *($10 for 5 ounces)* lists TEA-lauryl sulfate as the second ingredient, which makes this potentially too irritating and drying for all skin types.

☹ **Purifying Bar** *($12 for 4.2 ounces, $10 for refill)* is a standard bar cleanser that won't purify anything, at least not any better than Dove bar cleanser. Mary Kay's version contains eucalyptus, which is a skin irritant.

☺ **Oil-Free Eye Makeup Remover** *($14 for 3.75 ounces)* is a standard, silicone-based eye-makeup remover that will work as well as any reviewed in this book.

☹ **Hydrating Freshener Formula 1** *($11 for 6.5 ounces)* contains a small amount of menthol, arnica, and peppermint, which can all seriously irritate the skin.

☹ **Purifying Freshener Formula 2** *($11 for 6.5 ounces)* contains mostly water and alcohol, which can irritate and dry skin.

☹ **Blemish Control Toner Formula 3** *($11 for 6.5 ounces)* lists alcohol as the second ingredient, and it also contains eucalyptus, making this too irritating for words regardless of your skin type.

☺ **Moisture Rich Mask Formula 1** *($12 for 4 ounces)* is a very emollient, very or-dinary cream for dry skin. It contains an insignificant amount of antioxidants, but it also contains a small amount of menthol, which can be a skin irritant.

☺ **Revitalizing Mask Formula 2** *($12 for 4 ounces)* is a standard clay mask that also contains ground-up walnut shells. It can be a good exfoliant, but the waxes in this product (carnauba wax, in particular) can be a problem for blemish-prone skin. It is also hard to rinse off.

☺ **Clarifying Mask Formula 3** *($12 for 4 ounces)* is a standard clay mask that can be an option to absorb oil for normal to oily skin.

☺ **Indulging Soothing Eye Mask** *($15 for 4 ounces)* is a decent mask with some good anti-irritants and a tiny amount of a water-binding agent.

☺ **Enriched Moisturizer Formula 1** *($16 for 4 ounces)* isn't all that enriched or all that different from the Balancing and Oil-Control versions below. This is an extremely standard, mundane moisturizer for normal to dry skin.

☺ **Balancing Moisturizer Formula 2** *($16 for 4 ounces)* is a very boring, basic, mineral oil–based moisturizer. This is OK for normal to dry skin, but there are far better options for skin than this humdrum choice.

☺ **Oil-Control Lotion Formula 3** *($16 for 4 ounces)* is a lightweight, silicone-based moisturizer. Nothing in this product can control, change, or affect the amount of oil your skin produces. It is just an OK moisturizer for slightly dry skin with a matte finish and that's about it.

☺ **Oil Mattifier** *($15 for 1 ounce)* is similar to the Oil-Control Lotion above and the same comments apply.

✔☺ **Acne Treatment Gel** *($7 for 1.25 ounces)* contains 5% benzoyl peroxide in a nonirritating gel formulation. This would work fine as a disinfectant for acne-prone skin.

☹ **Velocity Lightweight Moisturizer** *($12 for 4 ounces)*. With alcohol listed as the third ingredient and some plant extracts that can be irritating for skin, this moisturizer can be a heavyweight problem for skin.

☹ **Daily Protection Moisturizer with Sunscreen SPF 15** *($16 for 4 ounces)* doesn't contain the UVA-protecting ingredients of avobenzone, zinc oxide, or titanium dioxide, and is not recommended.

☺ **$$$ Day Solutions SPF 15** *($30 for 1 ounce)* is a good, in-part avobenzone-based sunscreen in an emollient base that includes a long list of antioxidants and water-binding agents, and it would work well for normal to dry skin. However, the antioxidants and water-binding agents are listed so far after the preservatives that they barely amount to more than a dusting. This also contains some plant extracts that are potentially irritating, but thankfully, there are not a lot of those in here, either.

☹ **Night Solution** *($30 for 1 ounce)* lists alcohol as the second ingredient and also contains several plant extracts that are potential skin irritants, and though this gel-based moisturizer with AHA and BHA has a good concentration of each and a relatively low pH of 3.5 to 4, the alcohol is no solution for any skin type.

☺ **Nighttime Recovery System** *($25 for 2.8 ounces)* is a rather unimpressive lightweight moisturizer for normal to slightly dry skin.

☺ **Advanced Moisture Renewal Treatment Cream** *($19 for 2.5 ounces)* is an emollient, mineral oil– and Vaseline-based moisturizer that contains tiny amounts of antioxidants and water-binding agents. It is an OK option for dry skin.

☺ **Calming Influence** *($20 for 1 ounce)* contains the most minute amounts of anti-irritants and even less than that of water-binding agents. This also contains some plant extracts that can be skin irritants, making this a poor influence for everyone.

☺ **Extra Emollient Night Cream** *($11 for 2.5 ounces)* is a very standard, very emollient moisturizer that contains mostly Vaseline, mineral oil, waxes, fragrance, and preservatives. It does contain menthol, which can be a skin irritant, though the amount is so small it probably doesn't affect skin in the least.

☺ **Instant Action Eye Cream** *($15 for 0.65 ounce)* is an emollient moisturizer for dry skin that contains a good mix of antioxidants, water-binding agents, and anti-irritants, but there is nothing about it that is special for the eye area or that will do anything but moisturize skin.

☺ **$$$ Lumineyes Dark Circle Diminisher** *($28 for 0.5 ounce)* is an emollient moisturizer that contains vitamin K and retinol. There is no research showing that retinol can affect dark circles. The only information showing that vitamin K may affect dark circles is from the company selling the ingredient. This is as good a moisturizer as any if you are interested in a retinol product, and there's even some vitamin E and C in here as well, so this may be considered a grand slam.

☹ **$$$ Spot Solution Skin Lightening Cream** *($28 for 0.5 ounce)* is a hydroquinone-based skin lightener, but there is no information as to how much of it this product contains. Hydroquinone is effective for skin lightening and a 2% concentration is best, but there is no way to tell if that's what you are getting. This may be a good option and the formulation is a good one (including retinol), but there is no way to know for sure, hence the neutral face.

☹ **Triple-Action Eye Enhancer** *($15 for 0.65 ounce)* claims to have more benefits in one little product than almost any other I've ever seen. According to the company's magazine, it has much more than just triple action; I lost count after six benefits. It has free-radical scavengers, AHAs, and light-diffusing ingredients; it can be used as an eyeshadow base or as an under-eye concealer; it reduces puffiness and increases skin firmness; and, finally, it reduces the appearance of wrinkles. What's in this little miracle? Mostly silicone, film-forming agent, clay, several thickeners, and preservatives. There are tiny amounts of vitamins E and A, but they appear at the end of the ingredient list and so are completely insignificant. Then what about those benefits? Well, there aren't enough AHAs in this product to exfoliate skin (less than 2% lactic acid). It doesn't have light-diffusing properties, unless you consider a little shimmer a camouflage. The film-forming agents can form a tight layer over the skin, giving the illusion of smoother skin. This product is a poor under-eye concealer. And as an eyeshadow base it's too emollient, which would just help makeup settle into creases.

☺ **Triple Action Lip Enhancer** *($15 for 0.5 ounce)* is a very good emollient moisturizer for the lips, but the amount of AHA in it is minimal, and the triple benefit it should have contained, but doesn't, is sunscreen.

☹ **Satin Lips** *($18 for 0.15 ounce of Lip Mask and 0.15 ounce of Lip Balm).* **This** could have been a great topical exfoliant and emollient balm for lips, but both the Lip Mask and Lip Balm contain menthol and that can make chapped lips worse, not better.

☹ **Sun Essentials Ultimate Protection Sunblock SPF 30** *($9.50 for 4.5 ounces)* doesn't contain the UVA-protecting ingredients of avobenzone, zinc oxide, or titanium dioxide, and is not recommended.

☹ **Sun Essentials Sensible Protection Sunblock SPF 15** *($9.50 for 4.5 ounces)* doesn't contain the UVA-protecting ingredients of avobenzone, zinc oxide, or titanium dioxide, and is not recommended.

☹ **Sun Essentials Lip Protector Sunblock SPF 15** *($6.50 for 0.16 ounce)* doesn't contain the UVA-protecting ingredients of avobenzone, zinc oxide, or titanium dioxide, and is not recommended.

☺ **Sunless Tanning Lotion** *($10 for 4.5 ounces)* uses dihydroxyacetone, the same ingredient in all self-tanners, which affects the color of skin. This would work as well as any.

Mary Kay TimeWise

☺ **$$$ TimeWise 3-in-1 Cleanser** *($18 for 4.5 ounces)* is a standard, mineral oil–based cleanser with a small amount of detergent cleansing agents. It is an option for dry skin. The plant extracts are a mix of anti-irritants and irritants.

☺ **TimeWise Age Fighting Moisturizer** *($20 for 3.3 ounces)*. While there are some good water-binding agents in here, they are present in the smallest amounts imaginable. This is a good basic moisturizer for someone with normal to dry skin, but that's about it.

Mary Kay Makeup

Mary Kay's makeup products have been renamed MK Signature, and along with the name change, there have been several improvements in a few categories. Accompanying the positives, however, are many familiar negatives, including foundations that still have embarrassingly low levels of sun protection, not to mention more than a handful of unacceptable colors. The concealers have markedly improved, and the blushes and eyeshadows offer more elegant textures and fashion-forward colors than before (though you still need to watch out for way too much shine and some truly dated shade couplings). The remaining color products reflect Mary Kay's history of providing OK to very good makeup that rarely completes that last lap to superiority—a feat that a select few companies routinely accomplish. Mary Kay claims, "We're a company that knows what women want . . ." and they are clearly doing something right, especially when you consider the entire line generated sales of $1.4 billion in 2001 (source: *The*

Rose Sheet, August 26, 2002). However, impressive sales figures do not necessarily equate to the best products or mean that this is *the* cosmetics line for you. MK Signature shows promise, but still has a way to go before it is a line that makes it worth calling a Mary Kay representative.

FOUNDATION: ☺ Day Radiance Cream Foundation with Sunscreen SPF 8 Dry Skin *($14)* is only for those with dry skin who prefer a thick, creamy, full-coverage foundation. This blends decently, but lacks the smoothness of foundations from Estée Lauder, Origins, Bobbi Brown, and Lancôme, to name a few. The SPF 8 is too low (SPF 15 is the minimum recommended by the American Academy of Dermatology and the Skin Cancer Foundation), but it is a titanium dioxide–based sunscreen. The following colors are too peach, pink, ash, yellow, or copper for most skin tones: Blush Ivory, Delicate Beige, Mocha Bronze, Bittersweet Bronze, Rich Bronze, Toasted Beige, and Cocoa Beige.

☺ Day Radiance Liquid Foundation with Sunscreen SPF 8 Normal/Combination Skin *($14)* feels light and moist and blends easily to a light-coverage, natural finish. The SPF is identical to that of the foundation above, and the same comments apply. The following colors are too peach, pink, ash, yellow, or copper for most skin tones: Soft Ivory, Blush Ivory, Delicate Beige, Toasted Beige, Mocha Bronze, Rich Bronze, Walnut Bronze, Bittersweet Bronze, and Mahogany Bronze. **Day Radiance Oil-Free Foundation** *($14)* is a very good, matte-finish foundation that has adequate slip for easy blending. This is ideal for those with oily skin who are looking for sheer to light coverage, though the finish is a bit sticky. The following colors are too peach, pink, ash, yellow, or copper for most skin tones: Delicate Beige, Toasted Beige, Blush Ivory, Mocha Bronze, Bittersweet Bronze, Walnut Bronze, and Rich Bronze. **Creme-to-Powder Foundation** *($14 for foundation, $9 for refillable compact)* has a great, smooth, soft finish without feeling greasy or too thick, and provides medium coverage with an effect that's not too powdery or too creamy. There are eleven shades, and among them Ivory 2, Beige 2, Bronze 1, Bronze 1.5, and Bronze 2 are best avoided.

☹ $$$ TimeWise Dual Coverage Powder Foundation *($14 for foundation, $9 for refillable compact, $4 for powder brush)* has the requisite smooth, dry texture that characterizes most pressed-powder foundations, but this goes on sheer and blends exceptionally well, leaving a satin finish. The nine shades aren't the most neutral around, but the majority pass muster and they're really too sheer to be problematic. The only significant drawback is the shiny particles added to this powder. They are clearly visible on the skin, especially in daylight, which may not be the result you want.

CONCEALER: ✔☺ MK Signature Concealer *($9.50)* comes in a squeeze tube and is very concentrated. This has an improved, silicone-enhanced texture that blends without slip-sliding all over your face, which is a huge plus. It provides almost full coverage without looking thick or creasing, so it's a top choice if you have very dark circles. The six colors are fairly good, with the best ones being Light Ivory, Ivory, and Beige. Avoid Yellow—the name says it all.

POWDER: ☺ **MK Signature Loose Powder** *($12.50)* is a talc-based powder with a soft, dry consistency. This goes on sheer, and four of the five colors are quite good—only Bronze can be too peach for most skin tones.

☺ **$$$ Highlighters Bronzing Beads** *($18, $10 for Retractable Powder Brush)* are iridescent powder beads that provide a soft wash of shiny bronze color. For the money, this doesn't hold any advantage over The Body Shop's Brush-On Bronze *($16.50)*.

☺ BLUSH: **MK Signature Cheek Color** *($9 for blush tablet, $8 for refillable compact)* has a smooth, dry texture and an application that begins sheer, but builds nicely for color that is more vibrant. However, many of the shades are quite sparkly, and that's too distracting for daytime wear. The matte options include Nutmeg, Desert Bloom, Maple Walnut, Just Peachy, and Cranberry Bold.

EYESHADOW: ☺ **MK Signature Eye Color** *($6.50 for each eyeshadow, $8–$38 for the various compacts)* are utterly silky, and these apply beautifully without flaking or streaking. They are pigment-rich, too, so it only takes a tiny amount to shape and shade the eye. How disappointing that almost all of the single shades are inordinately shiny. The **Eye Color Duets** *($6.50)* are all shiny and feature a few of the most unattractive, dated color selections ever. The sole matte options are White Sand and Hazelnut.

☺ **MK Signature Eyesicles Eye Color** *($10)* are slick, cream-to-powder eyeshadows that leave more of a sheen than a shine. They are quite easy to blend, though a bit hard to control when it comes to placement. Still, they're one of the better options for fans of this type of eye makeup.

EYE AND BROW SHAPER: ☺ **MK Signature Eyeliner** *($9.50)* is a standard, twist-up, nonretractable pencil that has a smooth finish and a reasonable price. This product makes waterproof and smudgeproof claims and although it does hold up underwater, it will eventually smudge. Avoid Indigo and Violet unless you want people to notice your eyeliner more than your eyes. **MK Signature Brow Liner** *($9.50)* is a very good automatic, nonretractable brow pencil that comes in four great colors and is relatively easy to apply, though it's still not preferred to a brow powder or brow mascara.

☺ **Brow Definer Pencil** *($7.50)* is a standard pencil that must be a holdover, as this rather slick pencil only comes in one color, best for blonde brows.

☹ **MK Signature Liquid Eyeliner** *($10.50)* isn't something I'd want to put *my* signature on. This takes longer than usual to dry, tends to smear, and can ball up and roll off as it's worn. On top of all that, the brush is difficult to control.

LIPSTICK AND LIP PENCIL: ☺ **MK Signature Creme Lipstick** *($12)* leans heavily toward the greasy side of creamy, and has a semiopaque, soft gloss finish. The range of over 35 shades has been modernized and is now handily divided into Berries, Reds, Neutrals (which are not neutral at all—they are popular cool tones), Metals (which are largely unattractive), Pinks, and Chocolates. **MK Signature Lip Liner** *($9.50)* is a good, automatic, non-retractable lip pencil that does not distinguish itself from most other pencils, except for a preponderance of drab or deep brown tones.

✔☺ **MK Signature Lip Gloss** *($12)* is a semifluid, syrupy lip gloss that is barely sticky and leaves an ultrawet glossy finish. The striking shades aren't for the sheer-and-soft crowd, but those who appreciate a kick of color won't be disappointed. A colorless version is also available.

MASCARA: ☹ **Flawless Mascara** *($8.50)* is only flawless if you have minimal expectations from mascara. This goes on sheer and thin, so building any thickness is impossible, but you will get meager length with no clumps or smearing. **Waterproof Mascara** *($8.50)* takes several sweeps before you get anything close to a noticeable difference, and that's a generous comment. At least this is waterproof and tends not to clump.

☺ **Endless Performance Mascara** *($8.50)* has been improved and is now recommended as an acceptable lengthening mascara that defines lashes quickly without clumps or flaking. It's not on a par with the best lengthening mascaras at the drugstore or department store, but it's still worth considering if your lashes do best with modest enhancement.

MAX FACTOR (MAKEUP ONLY)

Max Factor earned his place in cosmetics history as *the* makeup artist for movie stars and the rich and famous of the 1920s and beyond. Among his many credits, Max Factor developed innovative makeup colors and textures that were unheard of (and sorely needed) at the dawn of cinema's Technicolor era. Movie studios and Hollywood's elite relied on his expertise to create all manner of makeup, from the line's still-available Pan-Cake Makeup and Erace Secret Cover Up to the very first lip gloss, circa 1930. (I don't recommend Pan-Cake foundation for anyone, but it's nice to recognize the roots of the makeup we are all wearing.) Another little-known, but monumentally important, contribution made by Factor was his Theory of Color Harmony. This theory referred to the art of selecting and blending colors based on a woman's skin tone, eye color, and hair color, and today you would be hard-pressed to find a cosmetics company that doesn't use some incarnation of this idea to coordinate makeup palettes.

Although this line's namesake is highly regarded, most of today's Max Factor products are either decades out of date or modern-day blunders. This line was close to drowning until parent company Procter & Gamble resuscitated it with the launch of the remarkable Lipfinity. For the first time in a long time, lipstick lovers everywhere found themselves clamoring for this innovation, or at least were curious about its claim of "lasts all day" color. As you will see in the review below, this momentous product really does live up to the hype, although not without a few caveats. Other than Lipfinity, however, and a few nice mascaras, I cannot come up with a convincing reason to shop this line. The prices are reasonable, but Factor's competition at the drugstore is eons ahead of this once-groundbreaking line. For more information about Max Factor, call (800) 526-8787 or visit www.maxfactor.com.

MAKEUP REMOVER: ☺ **Remover for Long Lasting Makeup** *($3.99 for 2 ounces)* is a very standard, mineral oil–based lotion that will definitely remove just about any makeup, but plain, fragrance-free mineral oil will, too, and for mere pennies.

FOUNDATION: ☺ **Facefinity Long Lasting Makeup with PermaWear SPF 15** *($8.99)* is an intriguing option for an ultra-matte foundation, and one that leaves me ambivalent. On the one hand, it does have a smooth texture that spreads evenly and allows enough time for careful blending, which is essential (but not always a reality) for an ultra-matte makeup. Facefinity provides medium to full coverage and offers a solid, slightly powdery matte finish, and the sunscreen is pure titanium dioxide, which is great. What's not appealing is how obvious this looks on the skin—no matter how little you use, this tends to create a "made-up" look that is not flattering, and it often looks pasty or chalky on the skin. And there are just too many superior foundations available that match Facefinity's best qualities without announcing their presence on the skin. If you decide to audition this one, be aware that it is strictly for normal to oily skin—the slightest hint of dry skin will be magnified by this makeup. This does indeed hold up well throughout the day, while still being easy to remove with a water-soluble cleanser. As far as the nine colors go, they are mostly quite good, which is almost surprising from Max Factor, whose foundations typically tend to lean toward the peach and pink side. What's odd is that the three lightest colors are all extremely light—almost white, and appropriate only for very fair skin. The remaining six colors are best for fair to medium skin tones; only Cool Bronze and Cream Beige are too pink or peach for most skin tones. Rose Beige is slightly pink, but may work for some light skin tones.

⊗ **Pan-Cake Makeup** *($6.99)* and **Panstik Makeup** *($6.99)* are both packaged in sealed plastic wrap that prevents you from viewing the colors (and testers are routinely absent). For that reason alone, these are difficult for me to recommend, but in addition, the textures of both foundations are too heavy, thick, or greasy, and almost all of the colors are strongly peach or pink. **Whipped Creme Makeup** *($6.79)* is hands down the worst foundation at the drugstore. No other makeup comes close to offering such shockingly awful colors, and with a rather inelegant texture to boot. **Lasting Performance Stay Put Makeup** *($7.99)* served as the precursor to Facefinity, and although it does stay put, the unpleasantly dry texture and stiff, chalky finish make this a weak entry in the ultra-matte foundation category. If you decide to try it anyway, avoid Cream Beige and Natural Honey. **Powdered Foundation** *($7.44)* works better as a talc-based pressed powder than as a foundation. Although the colors are reasonably good, this tends to be too powdery and cakey on the skin. **Silk Perfection Liquid to Powder Makeup** *($6.99)* desperately needs the axe or a reformulation. This old-fashioned cream-to-powder makeup is too waxy, looks artificial on the skin, and comes in only one salvageable color, Light Champagne.

CONCEALER: ⊗ **Erace Secret Cover Up** *($4.49)* was the staple of my first makeup experiences. The coverage with this one was and still is good, with a creamy consistency that doesn't get greasy, but the strong fragrance and turn-for-the-worse color selection is not what I would choose today.

POWDER: ⊗ **Lasting Performance Pressed Powder** *($6.99)*. The texture of this is silky, yet it's a strangely waxy powder that takes forever to show anything on the skin, and the four talc-based colors are strongly peach or pink.

BLUSH: ☺ **Natural Brush-On Satin Blush** *($6.49)* is a soft, exceedingly smooth blush in a subtle range of pastel and earth tones, each with its share of obvious shine. This is an option, though far from the best.

EYESHADOW: ☺ **Lasting Color Eyeshadows** *($3.79)* are single pressed-powder eyeshadows that have a great texture and blend well, but watch out for flaking. The color mix is primarily pale pastels alongside bright shades, and all of them have shine.

EYE AND BROW SHAPER: ☺ **PenSilks Glide On Eye Pencil** *($5.49)* is an automatic, nonretractable eye pencil and one end is a sponge tip to soften the line after you apply it. While this does glide on easily it stays relatively creamy, which means it will also smear easily. There is a sponge tip at one end to smudge the line before that happens naturally. **Eyebrow and Eyeliner** *($5.39)* are just standard pencils that are a tad too greasy to choose over those from Revlon, L'Oréal, or Cover Girl.

☹ **Linemaker Eyeliner** *($5.39)* is a liquid eyeliner that is applied with a felt-tip pen applicator, which works well, but it takes a bit too long to dry and is prone to some initial chipping.

LIPSTICK AND LIP PENCIL: ✔☺ **Lipfinity** *($8.99)* may be the biggest lipstick launch ever. It is one of two lipstick products (the other is Cover Girl's Outlast) that uses PermaTone technology. What's PermaTone? According to Max Factor's Web site, it is a "revolutionary new color bond complex which provides semipermanent color by gently attaching color pigments to lips in a 'flexible mesh' effect." The formula, researched and developed by Procter & Gamble, consists of complex pigments and silicone-based polymers that resist normal wear and tear and will not come off while you are eating, drinking, or even kissing. In fact, according to Max Factor, Lipfinity gives you "perfect, nonbudge color for an amazing eight hours!" Sounds too good to be true doesn't it? Well, for the most part, Max Factor, in this case, is not stretching the truth. This really is a breakthrough lipstick in terms of long and comfortable wear, though you need to remember a few important tips, because this isn't traditional lipstick you just put on and go. Lipfinity consists of a lip gloss–like product that puts a layer of opaque color over the lips accompanied by a top coat that's similar to Chap Stick (but more emollient-feeling). The colored portion of the product is applied separately to the lips with a sponge-tip applicator and then the color needs about a minute or two to dry completely. Once dry, you can slick on the top coat, and voilà—you get the long wear and coverage of an ultra-matte lipstick and the familiar feel of a traditional creamy lipstick.

However (you knew that was coming, didn't you?), along with the pros, there are some considerable cons to keep in mind before trying Lipfinity. First, application of the "paint" layer can be tricky. The color goes on thick and opaque and must be smoothed out immediately or you will be left with an uneven layer. Application needs to be almost perfect, as any irregularity can quickly turn into a permanent mistake, though mistakes and the entire lip color can be removed with pure mineral oil or plain Vaseline. Finally, your lips must be absolutely clean, smooth (any flaking, no matter how minor, will be greatly exaggerated), and dry before you use this. The moisturizing top coat does indeed make this feel great, and for the most part the color stays on and stays true, even through meals (as long as they aren't greasy or oily meals). You may notice some color fading toward the inner part of the lips, but you weren't expecting perfection were you? A few more minor drawbacks include the lack of testers, coupled with the fact that the color swatch on the box (and the product itself) does not provide an accurate indication of what the actual color will look like once applied. Although you should not need to touch up the color for most of the day (really!), the top coat does need to be reapplied at regular intervals to avoid dry lips. If you can find a color you like and you're not prone to dry, chapped lips, this is definitely worth a try! The **Lipfinity Moisturizing Top Coat** *($5.99)* is now sold separately, which is convenient, as you will likely go through this long before the partnered lip color is gone. For a touch of pizzazz, you may want to consider the glistening **Lipfinity Top Coat Shimmer Finish** *($6.39)*.

☺ **Lasting Color Lipstick** *($6.49)* has a lush, creamy finish, but it's doubtful you'll find it lasting longer than any other creamy lipstick, and the strong fragrance can be off-putting.

MASCARA: ✔☺ **2000 Calorie Mascara** *($3.97)* is a masterful, all-purpose mascara that provides equal amounts of length and thickness, with only a minor tendency to clump if you overdo it.

☺ **S-T-R-E-T-C-H Mascara** *($3.97)* is the diet version of 2000 Calorie Mascara. You can add clump-free length with this one, but it's lean on thickness and drama. **Lash Enhancer No. 1 Mascara** *($3.97)* is a no-frills mascara that works well for a natural look, and it lasts all day without incident. **2000 Calorie Aqualash Mascara** *($3.97)* builds enough length and thickness to be satisfactory for those occasions that call for reliable waterproof mascara. ✔☺ **Lashfinity Mascara** *($5.99)* is above-average waterproof mascara that applies cleanly and evenly, building nice length and a touch of thickness. It stays on beautifully throughout the day, looking perfect from morning until nighttime removal, which is quite easy using a water-soluble cleanser. Keep in mind that waterproof mascaras are not the best choice for everyday mascara. Max Factor does not claim that this is waterproof, but it definitely is, and the ingredient list is nearly identical to that of most other mascaras that are labeled as waterproof.

☺ **No Color Mascara** *($3.99)* is identical to Cover Girl's CG Smoothers Natural Brow & Lash Mascara *($5.49)*, and the same review applies—but notice the lower cost for this one.

☹ **BRUSHES:** There is only one option here, and it's the paltry, might-work-in-a-pinch **Blush Brush** *($4.49)*, if you don't mind a brush that splays and isn't all that soft.

MAYBELLINE (MAKEUP ONLY)

Maybelline is one of the best-known and most recognized mass-market makeup lines in the world—it's available in 90 countries. Throughout its long history, which began in 1915 when T. L. Wilson founded the company and named it after his sister, Mabel, the company has prided itself on bringing innovative products to cosmetics consumers. Today, Maybelline is still going strong and has shown a marked improvement in its products since it was bought by L'Oréal in early 1996. With improved product selection and modern textures, it is getting harder to tell the difference between L'Oréal and Maybelline products, though Maybelline has a lower price point and offers more glittery, teen-appeal products. Both specialize in offering a large selection of lipsticks, nail polishes, and mascaras, and their foundations share the same strengths and weaknesses (smooth textures and finishes, but often-poor colors, plus the inclusion of sunscreens that are often without much-needed UVA-protecting ingredients). The pressed powders, mascaras, pencils, and matte-finish concealers are impressive and inexpensive. With a little caution, there's no reason you can't come away from Maybelline with some great bargains and a beautiful look. For more information about Maybelline, call (800) 944-0730 or visit their interactive Web site at www.maybelline.com.

MAKEUP REMOVER: ☹ **Expert Eyes 100% Oil-Free Eye Makeup Remover** *($3.99 for 2.3 ounces)* is a very standard, liquid eye-makeup remover that contains boric acid as one of the main ingredients, which is a problematic antiseptic that should be kept away from the eyes.

☺ **Expert Touch Moisturizing Mascara Remover** *($3.69 for 2.3 ounces)* is an incredibly simple concoction of mineral oil, emollient thickener, lanolin oil, and preservative. This greasy liquid will indeed remove mascara and most other makeup as well—but the greasy film it leaves behind is not something most women would want to put up with.

FOUNDATION: Typically, no testers are available for any of Maybelline's foundations, making it difficult to recommend even the ones I liked a lot, which have good textures and color choices. Without being able to test the color first, you can easily end up with the wrong color and with makeup that looks unnatural and masklike. Your best bet when shopping for foundation at a drugstore or mass-market store is to make sure you can return the makeup if it is not exactly right. Otherwise, it can become a costly venture.

☺ **EverFresh Makeup SPF 14** *($7.49)* is a replacement for Maybelline's Nonstop All Day Makeup. In contrast to that formula, this foundation has more of a liquid texture, but feels slightly heavier on the skin. It blends quite well for an ultra-matte foundation, and provides natural-looking medium coverage. Unfortunately, the sunscreen lacks adequate UVA protection, so this would need to be used with a separate sunscreen, which is not the best option for those with oily skin. There are twelve shades, including some excellent options for dark skin tones. The fair to light shades have a faint to objectionable peach cast, and the ones to pass on include Natural Beige, Soft Cameo, Fawn, and Sand. **True Illusion Makeup SPF 10** *($8.49)* is attractively packaged and closely resembles a Lancôme foundation bottle. Although this has a smooth, sheer application, it lacks reliable UVA-protecting ingredients and the SPF 10 is meager for a full day of protection. If you're willing to wear an SPF 15 lotion with UVA-protecting ingredients underneath, this may be an option, because several of the colors are great, the texture is impressive for someone with normal to dry skin, and the price is almost a steal. Of the ten mostly neutral shades, the following are too orange or peach for most skin tones: True Buff, True Beige, True Golden, and True Sand. **PureStay Powder Plus Foundation SPF 15** *($7.19)* is a standard pressed powder with slightly heavier coverage so it can double as a foundation. It has a superior, smooth texture, an even application, and a soft matte finish that can go from sheer to medium coverage. The expanded range of twelve shades is a mixed bag, with seven of them (Buff, Cream, Soft Cameo, Natural Beige, Fawn, Sand, and Caramel) being a bit too peach or pink on the skin. If the sunscreen provided adequate UVA protection, this would be an across-the-board winner for normal to oily skin. If you're willing to wear a separate sunscreen or foundation with sunscreen underneath (which is a problem for those with oily skin), this is worth looking into, but watch out for those peachy pink shades. **3 in 1 Express Makeup SPF 15** *($8.39)* is the one to choose if you want a stick foundation that goes on creamy and dries to a soft powder finish with a reliable, all titanium dioxide–based SPF 15. This would work well for normal to slightly oily or slightly dry skin that needs sheer to medium coverage. As with most stick foundations, the waxes that keep this in stick form are not great for oily skin that is prone to breakouts. There are twelve shades, but the best ones are strictly for light to medium skin tones—all of the darker shades, from Tan on down, are just too peach or copper for most women of color. **Express Makeup Shine Control SPF 15** *($8.39)* is another stick foundation with a creamy application that blends out to a powder finish. It's quite similar to the 3 in 1 Express Makeup above. This spin-off foundation has an equally smooth application and provides the same light to medium coverage, but it has a more solid matte finish that can feel somewhat drying on all but oily skin. The sunscreen is pure titanium dioxide, which is great, though it is not the best for breakout-prone skin. Still, this is worth a test run, and the nine colors present options for all but very light and deep skin tones. The only colors to consider avoiding due to peach or pink overtones are Buff, Soft Cameo, and Natural Beige. **Shine Free Oil Control Makeup** *($6.49)* has a very smooth, liquidy, silicone-based texture that blends easily and dries to a solid matte finish. For normal to slightly oily skin types, this could work well, although the all-day shine control claim won't hold for those with very oily skin. The ten shades present some viable options for light to medium skin tones that prefer light to medium coverage. Avoid Light Ivory/Buff—it is too peach for most skin tones. The other fair to light shades have a soft peach cast, but not enough to make you pass this up if your skin type and preferences match this foundation's capabilities.

☺ **Smooth Result Age Minimizing Makeup SPF 18** *($6.99)* is yet another foundation that does not contain adequate UVA protection. Smooth Result is indeed smooth, and provides light to medium coverage. What's not so smooth is that among the twelve shades, the lighter colors have a slight peach or pink tint that shows up on the skin. Nude is an excellent neutral color, and the darker shades are striking—but Soft Cameo, Fawn, and Sand are not the shades you want to take home. This foundation is best for normal to dry skin, but must be worn with an effective sunscreen for daytime protection.

CONCEALER: ✔☺ **Great Wear Concealer** *($5.19)* is an excellent, noncreasing concealer that goes on matte, but smoothly, without looking dry or heavy. It comes in four superb shades and is best for someone with normal to oily skin.

☺ **True Illusion Undetectable Concealer SPF 10** *($5.19)* has no UVA-protecting ingredients and the SPF 10 is too low for all-day protection, so it is unreliable for sunscreen; but it is a very good concealer with a smooth texture and a semiopaque, natural matte finish. It blends easily and does not crease; however, the bad news is that only two of the six shades look like skin. Those are Ivory/True Ivory and Light Beige, both of which are great options for light skin tones. **Coverstick** *($4.19)* is an OK, lipstick-style concealer that is now packaged so that you can see the colors. Although most of the shades are workable, this dated formula is too greasy to stay put for long, and it creases easily. This is only recommended for those who prefer this type of concealer to all others and are willing to put up with the drawbacks inherent to the formula.

☹ **Shine Free Blemish Control Concealer** *($5.19)* lists salicylic acid as its active ingredient, and while that certainly has its place in the battle against blemishes, it takes more than a 0.65% concentration to have an effect, plus the pH is too high to allow exfoliation. Besides, all four shades of this tube concealer are glaringly peachy pink, and would only draw attention to what you're trying to hide. **Smooth Result Age Minimizing Concealer SPF 18** *($5.99)* is an undeniably smooth, cream-to-powder textured concealer packaged in a lipstick-style tube. Despite the texture, this has a slightly dry, pasty finish and offers no effective UVA protection. All of the four shades have a pink to peach tinge, with Light Beige and Medium Beige being the most obvious. **Corrector Concealer Cover Stick** *($5.29)* is a creamy, opaque stick concealer in yellow or green. As a whole, color-correcting products such as this just add another step to makeup application and rarely look convincing or natural.

POWDER: ☺ **True Illusion Pressed Powder SPF 10** *($6.99)* has a disappointing SPF number, but it does have a great titanium dioxide–based sunscreen. It can make a nice addition to an effective sunscreen or foundation with sunscreen, but should not be used alone during the day. This talc-free powder has a soft, silky feel and some lovely colors for very light to medium/dark skin tones; avoid True Beige, which is too pink for most complexions. **Shine Free Translucent Pressed Powder** *($5.19)* can't control shine any more than most powders can, but it is a wonderfully soft, dry powder that applies smooth and sheer and is indeed oil-free. It's talc-and-kaolin (clay)–based, and comes in five colors. Deep Beige/Caramel and Natural Beige are too orange, especially for those battling excess oil, but the other three shades are fine. **Finish Matte Pressed Powder** *($5.89)* is an exceptional talc-based powder with three beautiful colors and a silky, even texture. It does contain a tiny bit of mineral oil, but not enough for your skin to notice one way or another. This is best for normal to slightly dry skin that is fair to light.

☺ **Shine Free Oil Control Loose Powder** *($5.89)* comes in two shades, but it is impossible to see them through the unopened package, and that makes this talc-based, dry-finish powder hard to recommend. **Smooth Result Age-Minimizing Pressed Powder** *($6.99)* claims to "smooth away the appearance of first lines" while "providing natural coverage that creates younger looking skin." I suppose if this ordinary talc-based powder can make such enticing claims, then all other pressed powders should be in everyone's antiaging arsenal! This does have a fairly soft, almost creamy feel, but can go on a bit too powdery and tends to settle into, rather than "float" over, lines and wrinkles. The six shades present some attractive options, though Beige and Medium Beige are too peach. Smooth Result is best for normal to slightly oily skin, but is in no way a superior powder to consider for camouflaging wrinkles, be they your first or fiftieth line.

☹ **Corrector Powder** *($6.29)* is a dry-textured pressed powder in pale pink or yellow, and neither shade will serve to correct anything—though they will lend a chalky, pastel look to the skin.

BLUSH: ☺ **Brush/Blush** *($5.19)* is a standard powder blush that comes in an enticing array of colors and has a silky-soft texture that provides a sheer color application with a bit of sheen. The sparkly shades to watch out for are

Mocha Velvet, Pink Tangerine, Mambo Mauve, Plushed Plum, and Beach Club. **Express Blush** *($7.29)* is a nice partner to Maybelline's 3 in 1 Express Makeup. This is a cream-to-powder stick blush that goes on sheer and soft, creating a gentle wash of blendable color. There are eight beautiful shades, of which three have a slight amount of shine. The colors are nicely grouped into warms and cools. This would work for those with normal to slightly dry skin who have the patience to blend this on evenly.

☺ **Cool Effect Blush** *($5.99)* is a shimmery liquid blush that comes in a nail polish–style bottle replete with a brush applicator. It applies easily enough without the brush, which is the preferred method of application, rather than the strange blush-that-looks-like-it's-a-nail-polish gimmick. When used with a sponge or fingertips, this imparts sheer color that's heavy on the sparkling shine but dries to a matte (in feel) finish. This would do the trick for an evening that calls for sparkling cheeks.

EYESHADOW: ☹ **Expert Eyes Eyeshadow Singles** *($3.39)*, **Duos** *($4.09)*, **Trios** *($4.89)*, **Quads** *($5.59)*, and **8-Pans** *($7.29)* are mostly shiny shades or dreadful color combinations, with a texture that clings unreliably and is just all-around messy. To top that off, these have almost no staying power to speak of. There are a few attractive color combinations, but the flaky eyeshadow formula leaves much to be desired.

☺ **Cool Effect Cooling Cream Eyecolor** *($5.59)* has no cooling effect whatsoever, but what it does have is opaque, intense shine that can go on as thick as gold lamé or just sheer, but intensely shiny. For an evening look, it has possibilities, but the mood has to be right. **Cool Effect Cooling Eyeshadow/Liner** *($5.59)* is a chubby eyeshadow pencil that goes on somewhat wet, which means it glides easily, and then dries to a matte finish that doesn't smear or move all day. I only wish the mostly pastel colors were more varied and that you could actually see the color before purchasing it; you have to judge this one by a color swatch on the end of the needs-sharpening pencil. **Crystal Glitters Shadow Pencil** *($5.99)* is another standard, chubby pencil that has a creamy texture that borders on greasy. These have a shiny finish, but none of the colors are glittery, just a soft shimmer that should be set with powder if you want them to last. **Roller Color Loose Powder Eye Shadow** *($5.49)* comes in a small vial and has a roller-ball applicator, so despite the name, this is not a messy way to apply eyeshadow. However, it is an extremely shiny way, and as you roll the color on it does not blend at all, so you're stuck with a sheer stripe of glitter.

EYE AND BROW SHAPER: ✔☺ **Expert Eyes Defining Liner** *($5.09)* is a great automatic, retractable eye pencil that comes in appropriate black and brown shades. The dry finish isn't as smudge-prone as most eye pencils, though it's not quite as worry-free as lining with a matte powder eyeshadow. Definitely worth a look for pencil lovers! ☺ **Expert Eyes Brow and Liner Pencil** *($5.09)* is an automatic pencil that can be sharpened (the sharpener is built into the pencil) to a finer tip than most. Other than that, it's just a standard pencil with a dry texture, which means less smudging. **Smoked Kohl Liner** *($5.59)* is a standard pencil that has a smudge tip at one end, and is as reliable as anything you'll find at the department store, right down to the plethora of colors. **Ultra-Brow Brush-On Brow Color** *($5.59)* is a standard, matte brow powder that comes packaged with the standard hard brush that you should toss away and replace with a good soft professional brush. There are two shades, which is limited to say the least, but what's available works if it matches your brow color. **Brow Styling Gel** *($5.59)* is a standard brow gel that is very easy to apply and feels light and nonsticky. There are two sheer colors, which would work for dark blondes and brunettes, as well as a clear shade for just holding unruly brows in place. It's a good inexpensive option if you're looking to tame your brows or add a soft sheen. **Expert Eyes Twin Brow and Eye Pencil** *($3.09)* is much less greasy than the last time I reviewed it, and although Maybelline claims it has not changed the formula, I suspect something was tweaked along the way. This is still a standard small pencil whose dry, stiff texture is best for brows—this would hurt if you used it for eyelining. There are ample colors for all brow colors, from blonde to black, and the dry finish really stays put.

☹ **Lineworks Washable Liquid Liner** *($6.19)* is a basic liquid liner that dries to a smooth, flat finish. Unfortunately, it applies a bit unevenly and mistakes are hard to correct. For those who can ace the application, it does wear well during the day. **Lineworks Felt-Tip Eyeliner** *($6.19)* is just like a felt-tip pen, and it delivers a liquid liner that dries to a smooth, matte finish that doesn't budge once it's in place—so applying this is serious and it can be unforgiving. However, the end result is a dramatic line that doesn't chip or flake during the day. **Expert Eyes Softlining Pencil** *($4.09)* is a standard "sharpen me again" pencil that goes on creamy and stays that way. It smudges and smears easily. **Great Wear Waterproof Eyeliner** *($6.29)* is a standard, twist-up pencil that glides easily over the skin and draws a thick line. The texture is creamy, but the tacky finish it has doesn't feel great. This does hold up really well, and resists smudging, but it is no more waterproof than most pencils. **Eye Duets Liner/Shadow** *($6.29)* is an exceptionally standard dual-sided pencil. I would love to say these are in some way an improvement over the numerous other dual-sided pencils out there, but they are just mediocre. The eyeliner end is creamy and prone to smudging, and the eyeshadow end, while sheer and powdery, is extremely shiny and tends to flake.

☹ **Eye Express Easy Eyelining Pen *($6.19)*** does go on easily, and it takes a while to dry. Actually, it never quite set itself the way I was expecting, and it stayed tacky to the touch for quite a while. If you accidentally touch it later in the day, it can come off in pieces—so it may be best to pass up this Express. **Lineworks Ultra-Liner Waterproof Liquid Liner *($6.19)*** is just a standard liquid liner that has good staying power underwater, but it tends to peel or smudge if accidentally rubbed. **Line Works Waterproof Liquid Eye Liner *($6.29)*** claims to offer all-day smudgeproof wear, and fails on both counts. This standard liquid liner has a large brush tip, so creating a fine line is difficult. If you prefer thicker lines, it does the job, but the slightest hint of water or moisture around the eye will lead to an early, unbecoming demise of your design. L'Oréal's Line Intensifique Extreme Wear Liquid Liner is a much better option in the same price range as this one.

LIPSTICK AND LIP PENCIL: ☺ **Moisture Whip Lipstick *($6.39)*** has been around for decades and remains a rich, creamy, slightly glossy lipstick that's not for those prone to lip color feathering or bleeding. **Wet Shine Wet Look Lipcolor *($5.19)*** is extremely similar to L'Oréal's So Delice lipstick, as both share the same slick, light texture, soft colors, and high-gloss finish. This version is slightly more sheer than L'Oréal's, but, unlike So Delice, it is fragrance-free! **Wet Shine Diamonds *($5.19)*** is identical to the original Wet Shine Lipstick, only this is infused with loads of sparkles, which can lend a slight grainy feel to the lips. **Wear 'n Go Long Wearing Lipcolor *($6.99)*** offers a beautiful palette of 36 shades that claim to "go on with lip liner precision," yet it takes only one application to see that they go on like almost every other lipstick, and the precision part has to come from your application technique! With that said, this is a basic, creamy lipstick with a slick finish that can be fleeting. Most of the colors go on opaque, and a few have a slight frost, which, for some women, can be an attractive finishing touch. **Gloss Twist Lip Shine *($5.99)*** is another gloss pen that requires you to click up the color into the brush tip. This formula feels great on the lips and imparts sheer, glossy color that's slightly sticky. I doubt you will be able to tell the difference between this one and those from the Stila line, which sell for three times the price.

☺ **Moisture Whip Lip Liner *($5.19)*** is a standard lip pencil that has a thick, creamy texture and strong colors. This applies easily, but the pencil's soft consistency makes it difficult to draw a thin line. **Lip Express Lipstick 'n Liner in One *($5.49)*** is an oversize (width-wise) lip pencil that is supposed to do double duty as lipstick and lipliner. To some extent, that's exactly what it does, just not very well. Like all chubby pencils, this is difficult to sharpen, and the creamy color part is so soft it's impossible to keep a decent tip on the end without perpetual sharpening, which causes you to go through the product much faster than you would with an ordinary lipstick. **Lip Polish Hi-Shine Color** *($5.49)* provides a somewhat creamy, but also powdery, texture that spreads sheer, colored glitter over the lips. It isn't as greasy or messy as some glosses, but it also isn't as smooth—it just has lots of sparkle. **Wear 'n Go Long Wearing Lip Liner** *($5.49)* is an automatic lip pencil that has a soft texture and provides sheer, short-lived color. Funny that the Wear 'n Go Lipstick has a lipliner partner, as that lipstick is supposed to apply with "lip liner precision." Wouldn't that mean no lipliner is necessary?

MASCARA: ☺ **Lash Expansion Mascara** *($5.59)* has a "lash-wrapping" brush that supposedly covers every lash for thicker, longer lashes—but so does any good mascara, and this is no exception. Lash Expansion lengthens and provides moderate thickness without clumping or smearing. It's an in-between option if Maybelline's Illegal Lengths makes your lashes too long (is that possible?) or Volum' Express makes them too thick. **Illegal Lengths Mascara** *($5.09)* has been reformulated and still comes in as one of the better lengthening mascaras around. What you'll notice with this latest version is a bit more thickness and a slightly greater tendency to smear while applying, as this formula is quite "wet." Overall, this remains an excellent lengthening mascara. **Illegal Lengths Waterproof Mascara** *($5.09)* is still a good choice for nicely waterproof mascara that lengthens lashes with ease and that wears well through several laps around the pool. ✔☺ **Full 'n Soft Mascara** *($6.39; regular or curved brush)* is a very good mascara. It doesn't build much thickness, but it does quickly build long lashes without clumping or smearing. ✔☺ **Lash Discovery Mascara** *($5.99; regular or curved brush)*. They say that good things come in small packages, and although this mascara's very small brush made me skeptical initially, I was surprised at how adept it let me be at not only getting to each and every lash but also expertly lengthening, separating, and providing appreciable thickness without clumping or smearing. For those of you still hooked on Maybelline's substandard Great Lash mascara, try this one instead. ✔☺ **Volum' Express Mascara** *($4.69; regular or curved brush)* is the Maybelline mascara to choose if thick, dramatic lashes are your goal. The full brush builds thickness and some length quickly, and without clumping. It lasts throughout the day and removes easily, but overzealous application can cause some smearing. ✔☺ **Wonder Curl Waterproof Mascara** *($5.09; regular or curved brush)* provides excellent length and a soft, fringed curl, all while being remarkably waterproof. This will require a silicone- or oil-based product for removal, but for those times when a long-wearing, waterproof mascara is called for, this shines! ✔☺ **Volum' Express Waterproof Mascara** *($4.69)* builds quickly and thickens well for a waterproof mascara without clumping. It stays on underwater, too!

☺ **Wonder Curl Mascara** *($5.09; regular or curved brush)* doesn't perform any better than others in the arena of making lashes curl more. This is an OK, almost boring mascara in terms of length and overall performance, and isn't as impressive as the L'Oréal or Lancôme versions. **Full 'n Soft Waterproof Mascara** *($6.39)* builds excellent length and noticeable thickness, but be prepared to work at it. This is a rather wet formula, and will smear during application if you're not very careful. It is waterproof and a bit more stubborn to remove than most. **Lash Discovery Mascara Waterproof** *($5.99; regular or curved brush)* isn't as exciting as its nonwaterproof counterpart, but it's still worthwhile if you're looking for a good lengthening mascara that lasts all day and holds up nicely if your lashes get wet. As is true for most waterproof mascaras, thickness is minimal at best.

☹ **Great Lash Mascara** *($3.59; regular or curved brush)* builds some length, though it takes a good deal of effort to get anywhere. The big drawbacks are that it does not build any thickness and it has a tendency to smear. Its continual mention in beauty magazines' "best-of" lists astonishes me, as it does every makeup artist I've ever interviewed. It may (shockingly) be the #1-selling mascara, but that doesn't mean it's the best. **Great Lash Waterproof Mascara** *($3.59)* is an utterly boring mascara that takes lots of effort for an "is that all there is?" result. It stays on in the rain or pool, but so do Maybelline's other waterproof mascaras—all of which are preferred to this one.

☺ **BRUSHES:** Maybelline's name may not be synonymous with brushes, but if you're on a budget and are ready to toss out your miniature sponge applicators and other inferior tools, you'll find the **Eyeshadow Brush** *($4.39)*, **Blush Brush** *($4.89)*, and **Face Brush** *($7.99)* are extremely soft, but firm, and work surprisingly well. The **Eye Contour Brush** *($4.99)* is an option for brows or eyelining, but it's too small for eyeshadow, and the **Retractable Lip Brush** *($4.99)* is a standard lip brush that travels well. Last, the **Brush 'n Comb** *($3.89)* is a standard, feasible brow and lash comb that's affordably priced.

REVLON

As one of the leading mass-market cosmetics lines in the world, Revlon has done an excellent job with product innovation as well as with keeping abreast of the industry when it comes to makeup products. When it comes to skin care, however, Revlon's products are not well-diversified or particularly creative. Revlon's Eterna '27' is still around and remains unchanged after decades on the market. In an attempt to improve their skin-care line Revlon launched Age-Defying products, but those never took off. Now they have Vitamin C Absolutes, which are less about vitamin C and more about wafting fragrance that smells like oranges. Hopefully, consumers are aware that the fragrance is not indicative of how much vitamin C a product contains. There are some well-formulated sunscreens, but the limited choices aren't the best for a range of skin care needs. When it comes to skin care, Revlon-owned Almay has far more effective options. For more information about Revlon, call (800) 4-REVLON or visit www.revlon.com.

Revlon Skin Care

☺ **Age Defying Performance Skin Care Face Cream SPF 15** *($12.61 for 1.75 ounces)* and **Age Defying Performance Skin Care Oil-Free Face Lotion SPF 15** *($12.61 for 1.7 ounces)* are very good, in-part avobenzone-based sunscreens in ordinary moisturizing bases that contain a small amount of antioxidants. These do contain a tiny amount of salicylic acid, but not enough for it to be effective for exfoliation.

☺ **Eterna '27' All Day Moisture Lotion** *($12.99 for 2 ounces)* is an emollient moisturizer for normal to dry skin that contains some good water-binding agents.

☺ **Eterna '27' All Day Moisture Cream** *($12.99 for 1 ounce)* is very similar to the Lotion above, but with still more thickeners and mineral oil. It would be good for dry to very dry skin.

☺ **Eterna '27' with Exclusive Progenitin** *($13.99 for 2 ounces)* contains pregnenolone acetate, often derived from animal urine. Pregnenolone acetate is a precursor to other hormones and can, when taken orally, affect levels of progesterone and estrogen in the body. When applied topically to skin it may work as a water-binding agent. There is no information on whether absorption through skin is possible.

Revlon Vitamin C Absolutes

The orange-colored products and the color of the packaging speak volumes about these skin-care products. The name and color, along with a wafting citrus aroma, are the clinchers for getting across the marketing message these products want you to hear. This is about vitamin C being great for skin. But for skin care, ignore the orange fruit water, which is useless for skin and, if anything, can be a skin irritant (ever get real orange juice on a cut?). What these products do contain is magnesium ascorbyl phosphate (MAP), a very stable and good form of vitamin C. While MAP is a good skin-care ingredient, acting as an antioxidant and potential melanin inhibitor, the amount of it in these products is minuscule and not of much benefit for skin. If they didn't have such a pungent aroma, I would be more excited about recommending what appear to be some well-formulated products. As far as formulation is concerned, there are some very good water-binding agents, anti-irritants, and antioxidants in this group, along with reliable sunscreens, and that is what really feels good for skin.

☺ **Vitamin C Reviving Cleanser** *($7.69 for 6.6 ounces)* is a standard, detergent-based cleanser that would actually work well for most skin types, that is if you can get beyond the smell and coloring agents.

☹ **Vitamin C Absolutes Refreshing Tonic** *($7.69 for 6.7 ounces)*. Between the alcohol and orange water, this is far more irritating than refreshing. It does contain magnesium ascorbyl phosphate, a stable form of vitamin C, but the alcohol makes this formula more of a problem than a benefit.

☹ **Vitamin C Absolutes Radiant Skin Scrub** *($7.69 for 3.2 ounces)* is a standard scrub that uses ground-up plastic (polyethylene) as the abrasive agent. This also contains sodium lauryl sulfate as one of the main ingredients, which would make this otherwise OK scrub a problem for most skin types due to the risk of irritation and dryness.

✔☺ **Vitamin C Absolutes Overnight Renewal Cream** *($14.89 for 1.6 ounces)* is a very good moisturizer for dry skin that contains an incredibly long list of ingredients—the "everything but the kitchen sink" approach is used here, including vitamins A, E, C, and several other antioxidants, as well as water-binding agents. None of these will firm the skin, but they can certainly make dry skin look and feel smoother and softer. This does contain fragrance.

✔☺ **Eye Contour Radiance Cream** *($14.89 for 0.45 ounce)* is far more emollient than the Renewal Cream above, although it contains many of the same other assets that warrant a good rating.

✔☺ **Daily Radiance Cream SPF 15** *($12.99 for 1.6 ounces)* is a good, avobenzone-based sunscreen with several antioxidants that would work well for normal to dry skin. The fragrance can be overpowering, but the formulation is still good for dry skin. The radiance comes from the slight bit of shimmer that the mica imparts.

✔☺ **Oil-Free Radiance Lotion SPF 15** *($14.89 for 1.6 ounces)* is similar to the Cream version above, only in lotion form, and the same basic comments apply.

Revlon Makeup

The mainstay of Revlon's makeup over the past several years has been its two major color lines, Age Defying (for the 35 and over crowd) and ColorStay (for the under-35, oily-skin crowd). Both age groups are served well, as these lines offer excellent options. Age Defying is best for normal to very dry skin, while ColorStay, whose namesake lip color spawned a new generation of lipstick consistency that is both ultra-matte and dry, is great for oily to very oily skin. New Complexion is more for normal to oily skin, and is sort of a go-between for those too oily (or young) for Age Defying and too dry for ColorStay. Recent additions that have caused a resurgence of interest in Revlon are the shine-all-the-time Skinlights and High Dimension lines. The weakest spot in this enormous line are the mascaras, most of which just aren't in the same league (or even the same sport) when measured against L'Oréal and Maybelline mascaras. Still, Revlon has earned its reputation for its superior products, and that helps offset these deficiencies. You can't go wrong if you pay attention to their mostly awesome foundations, concealers, Absolutely Fabulous LipCream SPF 15, and many of the eye pencils. Until the new management team accomplishes their lofty goals, Revlon, for all its strong points, will have to concede as runner-up to L'Oréal when it comes to the best makeup line at the drugstore. But stay tuned, because the competition will undoubtedly become more heated as the perpetual one-up-manship continues.

FOUNDATION: Revlon seldom has testers for its foundations, but many stores do sell sample packs with three shades so you can try the colors for a minimal investment.

☺ **Age Defying Makeup with SPF 10** *($11.49)* is best for someone with normal to dry skin (the formula contains oil) and provides light to almost medium coverage. The SPF is titanium dioxide–based, although the number is marginally low. However, if you're willing to wear an SPF 15 underneath, the makeup's texture, soft matte finish, and twelve shades are quite good. The only shades to view with caution are Cool Beige, Medium Beige, and Sand Beige.

✔☺ **Age Defying Makeup and Concealer Compact SPF 20** *($13.89)* is an excellent option for foundation and sunscreen in one product. The active ingredients are titanium dioxide and zinc oxide, which provide the required broad-spectrum protection. The foundation portion is a cream-to-powder makeup that has a smooth, even finish and some great colors, though nothing for very light or very dark skin tones. The concealer portion has the same SPF, but is fairly greasy and can easily crease into lines under the eyes. Medium skin tones may find that some of the concealer colors are too dark to cover circles under the eye, yet these shortcomings are minor compared to the strong positives, and this would work well for normal to dry skin. There are eight shades, but Honey Beige and Medium Beige are too peachy pink, while Natural Beige is borderline peach. ✔☺ **Age Defying All Day Lifting Foundation SPF 20** *($12.49)* won't lift your skin anywhere. However, it is a luxurious, emollient foundation for normal to dry skin that blends impeccably and can provide medium to almost full coverage. It also has a brilliant SPF, with titanium dioxide and zinc oxide as the active ingredients. There are ten shades to consider, but none for very light or very dark skin tones, which is disappointing. Avoid Honey Beige, Cool Beige, and Natural Beige, which are too pink or peach for most skin tones. ✔☺ **ColorStay Lite Makeup SPF 15** *($11.29)* is simply the best ultra-matte foundation with sunscreen available. Before I delve into a description, let me say that (as of this writing) this foundation *has not* been discontinued. Revlon has done away with the six darkest colors, and some drugstores have stopped carrying it in favor of Revlon's Skin Mattifying Makeup, but Revlon repeatedly confirmed that it is still available. The six remaining shades are great for fair to medium skin, and only Ivory is slightly pink, though it can still work for some fair skin tones. These shades apply lighter than they look, which can make choosing the right one even trickier. ColorStay Lite has a smooth, fluid texture and provides medium to full coverage that dries quickly to a solid, long-wearing ultra-matte finish. It is best to blend this systematically, because any mistakes that dry will require removal and reapplication—this isn't a makeup you can easily smooth out if it's not applied right the first time. Yet if you have oily to very oily skin, the trade-offs and shine control are worth it. The SPF is pure titanium dioxide, and some women may find that exacerbates breakouts, yet that's the paradox and agony of using sunscreen when you have oily skin. The packaging isn't the smartest choice for this liquidy formula, but if you're cautious, it shouldn't be too much of a problem. ✔☺ **ColorStay Stick Makeup SPF 15** *($11.29)* glides on smooth and slightly creamy, and then dries to a soft, translucent finish. It can have light to medium coverage, comes in ten mostly great colors, and the SPF is part titanium dioxide and part zinc oxide. The noncomedogenic claim is bogus, but this is absolutely worth a try if you want a soft, matte, slightly powdery finish. However, please be aware that while this can be great for someone with normal to slightly dry or slightly oily skin, it doesn't have the staying power of the other ColorStay foundations. It can slip and let oil show through like most stick foundations do. Avoid Natural Beige, and be careful with Caramel, which may be too orange for darker skin tones. ✔☺ **New Complexion One Step Compact Makeup SPF 15** *($12.79)* is a cream-to-powder foundation with titanium dioxide as the only sunscreen agent. This one is surprisingly similar to Clinique's City Base Compact Foundation SPF 15 *($20)*. I simply could not tell the difference in a side-by-side face test of the two products. They applied, felt, looked, and wore the same. Revlon has twelve shades (Clinique has ten), and they are, for the most part, fairly neutral, although the range of tones is strange. The selection of lighter shades is extremely limited for Revlon, and the darker colors are all a bit coppery. If you have a more medium skin tone, you're in luck, and if you have normal to slightly dry skin you'll do well if you prefer this type of product. Avoid Natural Beige, Cool Beige, Warm Beige, and Sun Beige. Tender Peach is fairly true to its name, but may work for some light skin tones.

☺ **ColorStay Makeup SPF 6** *($11.29)* is beyond matte, beyond no shine, and far beyond the claim of "It won't rub off." In fact, it won't rub (or wash) off even when you want it to! This is one of the most stubborn makeups I have ever tested. Get it on right the first time, because once it dries, it won't budge. If you get even the slightest wrong color it can look like a chalky mask, and removing it at night takes a great deal of effort, including several attempts with your cleanser and washcloth. Therefore, this is only appropriate for someone with truly oily skin and a deft hand at blending who is looking for medium to heavy coverage. Revlon has expanded the number of shades to sixteen, but all of the deeper shades, from Rich Tan through Mocha, are way too copper, orange, or red for darker skin tones. Also, the deeper colors are without sun protection, but the SPF 6 (titanium dioxide–based) is really far too low to count on anyway. The remaining shades for light to medium skin tones fare better, but watch out for Ivory and Natural Beige—both are slightly pink. Medium skin tones have the best selection of neutral colors with this one. **New Complexion Makeup SPF 4** *($11.79)* has an embarrassingly low titanium dioxide–based SPF, but it does have a very light texture that blends evenly and dries to a natural, light-coverage finish. Of the nine shades, the only good options are Sand Beige, Medium Beige, and Sun Beige. The rest are too pink, orange, or peach. **Shine Control Mattifying Makeup SPF 15** *($10.99)* definitely wins points for having an excellent titanium dioxide– and zinc oxide–based sunscreen, along with a fluid, light texture that applies quite well and dries (almost instantly) to a sheer, solid-matte finish. What's disappointing is the addition of SD-alcohol (it's the third ingredient), which makes this unnecessarily irritating for all skin types, not to mention the subtle alcohol odor. In addition, the twelve colors are a mixed bag. The lighter shades all lean toward being too peach to work well for most skin tones. The darker shades fare better, and the ones to consider are Honey Beige, Natural Tan, Caramel, and Cappuccino. So how does this compare to ColorStay Lite? It's assuredly lighter in texture, and has an even thinner consistency that offers less coverage. It's also not transfer-resistant, but it does stay on well, and although it is not being billed as an ultra-matte foundation, its extremely matte finish may make you think otherwise! **New Complexion Even Out Makeup Oil-Free SPF 20** *($11.79)* is an amalgam of traits that tries to be a little bit of everything and comes up far too short in most departments and way ahead in others. The sunscreen is excellent, containing both zinc oxide and titanium dioxide. Yet the color selection, with many of the nine shades being too peach, pink, or ash, is disappointing. The consistency is rather light and moist, which is great for a sheer finish if you have dry skin. However, this also contains salicylic acid (BHA), which is a waste in a foundation, where the pH is too high for it to be effective. All in all, there are more problems than positives with this one, and I wouldn't choose it over Revlon's New Complexion One Step Compact Makeup, reviewed on page 618. If you want to brave the odds, the only colors that look like skin are Sand Beige, Caramel, Nude Beige, and Natural Tan. **Wet/Dry Foundation SPF 10** *($13.89)* is not an impressive foundation in the least, especially when weighed against Revlon's topnotch foundations. This is a basic pressed powder–type foundation, and includes an in-part titanium dioxide sunscreen whose SPF number is far below the recommended standard of SPF 15. The talc-based texture is not as silky-smooth as many powder foundations, the finish is slightly chalky, and, when used dry, it is hard to blend into the skin. Ironically, this tends to go on better when used wet, though like all wet/dry powders, streaking will be apparent unless you blend very well. What's more, six of the nine shades are too peach or pink for most skin tones. The only colors worth considering are Ivory Beige (slight pink), Sand Beige, and Natural Tan.

CONCEALER: ✔☺ **ColorStay Concealer SPF 6** *($9.69)* is awesome and ranks up there with the best of them. It absolutely doesn't crease, stays on very well, isn't nearly as heavy or thick as the ColorStay original foundation, and comes in three very good neutral colors. It does provide opaque coverage and can be a problem if you want to hide, instead of accentuate, lines under the eyes, but it takes good care of dark circles all day long. If the finish seems too matte, try mixing it with a drop of moisturizer.

☺ **Age Defying All Day Lifting Concealer SPF 20** *($8.89)* is an ideal, creamy, compact-type concealer that covers well and blends evenly without being too slippery. True to the nature of cream concealers, this will crease unless it is set with powder. Unfortunately, that's not the best look if you have prominent lines around the eye. However, for facial discolorations in wrinkle-free zones, this works well, and the titanium dioxide/zinc oxide sunscreen is gravy!

POWDER: ☹ **Love Pat Moisturizing Powder** *($9.49)* is still around and all the colors are still too pink or peach for most skin tones.

☺ **New Complexion Powder Normal to Oily Skin** *($11.69)* is a standard, talc-based powder with a decent color selection, but nothing about this powder will control oil—it's just a good, standard, dry-finish powder. It blends on smooth and soft and comes in a decent assortment of shades. Avoid Warm Beige and Even Out, which is a color-correcting shade of yellow. **New Complexion Bronzing Powder** *($11.99)* is a talc-based, pressed-powder bronzer that comes in a very natural-looking tan shade with minimal shine. It would work best on light to medium skin tones.

☺ **Age Defying Pressed Loose Powder** *($12.59)* is a puzzle. Pressed loose powder is a contradiction in terms, isn't it? This is a lightweight, talc-based pressed powder that applies rather sheer but also slightly chalky. It feels silky and the three colors are fine, but I wouldn't choose this over pressed powders from L'Oréal or Clinique. **Age Defying Smoothing Powder** *($12.59)* is also talc-based and leaves a slightly chalky finish, but it's OK if dusted on with a brush. The six shades offer some good colors, but you'll want to steer clear of Medium Beige and Honey Beige. **New Complexion Shine Control Mattifying Powder SPF 8** *($8.19)* is a talc-based pressed powder that has a somewhat thick, dry texture and a slightly heavy-feeling, but sheer, matte finish. The sunscreen is in-part titanium dioxide, and although the SPF is too low, this can still be a good addition if used with a reliable foundation with adequate sunscreen. Of the six shades, half are worth a look if you have light to medium skin. The colors to avoid are Sheer Mattifyer (too yellow) and Light-Medium and Medium (both too peach, especially for oily skin).

BLUSH: ☺ **Sleek Cheeks Creme Blush Duo** *($9.49)* offers a sheer, shiny cream-to-powder blush along with a luminescent highlighter. These apply moist and are surprisingly easy to blend to a soft powder finish. Each of the six duos has a subtle amount of shine, but it's not really enough to be distracting. The highlighter shade is shinier, and this would be more appropriate for an evening look. Overall, the colors are beautiful and this is worth checking out if you prefer this type of blush and want it to shine. Because it contains waxes, this is not recommended for blemish-prone skin. **Smooth-On Blush** *($8.89)* is a powder blush with a luscious, silky texture and a soft, sheer finish. The original colors weren't much for depth or brightness, and they're deceptively shiny, but this has since been merged with Revlon's former Naturally Glamorous Blush-On, and it now offers some beautiful matte options. Check out Wine with Everything, Berry Rich, and Tawny Blush.

EYESHADOW: ☹ **Wet/Dry Eyeshadows** *($4.19 singles; $4.49 duos; $5.89 quads)* are all shiny and have a texture that just doesn't wear well, wet or dry. The notion of applying eyeshadows wet for a more intense, opaque effect is interesting, but opaque shine often leads to flaking, and this formula doesn't rise above that common side effect. As an option, there is one matte quad set, called In the Buff, as well as a matte duo, Raisin Rage, whose colors are nicely coordinated. The rest just have too much shine and won't look as foolproof and elegant as they do in Revlon's ads. **ColorStay Powder Shadow** *($7.69)* comes in a tube, which is not my favorite way of applying eyeshadow, since blendability is essential and that isn't easy with such a dry, unmovable eye color. All of these colors are about as stubborn as they come; they "grab" onto the skin before you can blend them. And forget about adding more than one color or applying it again, because once this formula sets, any efforts to blend result in clumps and eyeshadow fingerprints! The only positive is that they will definitely last throughout the day without fading. **ColorStay Powder Shadow** *($7.69)* comes in a tube and offers two shiny colors in one stick. Try this if you're one of the few people who might possibly want a stubborn, difficult-to-blend eyeshadow that grabs onto the skin, sets far too soon, and then won't budge. The only plus is that it lasts and lasts—but with the way it looks, do you really want that?

✔☺ **Illuminance Creme Eyeshadow** *($6.29)* offers four shades of cream-to-powder eyeshadow in a sleek compact. Although I am not a fan of cream eyeshadows, as they tend to crease and can be troublesome to blend with other colors, these hold up quite well and go on softly. The color palette is limited, especially if you prefer neutral tones, but those who enjoy cream eyeshadows should strongly consider these. The best sets are Not Just Nudes, Pink Petals, and Wild Orchids (although Wild Orchids can be too purple for some of those with fair skin tones).

EYE AND BROW SHAPER: ✔☺ **Softstroke Powderliner** *($6.79)* has a great powdery texture and a matte finish that has great staying power, and it glides on effortlessly. The only drawback is the frequent sharpening that it needs.

☺ **TimeLiner for Eyes** *($6.79)* is a very good, standard pencil that applies and blends easily. These have a very soft tip, so be wary of applying too much pressure. **Wet/Dry Eyeliner** *($6.49)* is a standard pencil that is slightly creamy and that can smudge if used dry. Wet application dries to a more solid finish, but also gives a more dramatic look. Pure Pearl is a shiny white that can look too stark against most skin colors. **ColorStay Brow Color** *($8.19)* is a two-ended product: One end is a mascara-like wand with color to stroke on the brow, and the other end is a pencil. In some ways, this is the best of both worlds—particularly if you already use a brow pencil and a brow groomer to thicken and tint the brow. This one's tinted brow gel goes on easily and stays well, while the pencil is just a pencil, nothing special, and it doesn't stay around any better than other pencils.

☺ **ColorStay Eyeliner** *($7.19)* is a standard pencil that comes in a twist-up container. It eventually sets and stays put, but it may still smear and go on somewhat choppy. **Brow Maker** *($5.99)* presents a matte brow powder along with a clear, lightweight brow wax. The accompanying (very small) brush is used to apply the slightly waxy powder, and then you simply add a dab of the clear wax to hold brows in place. The concept is fine, but this can feel somewhat sticky and is really no substitute for the mascara-type brow tints available from Bobbi Brown, Origins, and my own line, to name a few. Still, if your brows are annoyingly unruly, this is worth a look.

☹ **ColorStay Liquid Liner** *($7.19)* still has a strange, hard applicator that scratches at the eyelid as you put it on. Why Revlon hasn't changed this yet is beyond me. It does stay well, but applying it is a less-than-ideal process. **High Dimension Eyeliner** *($7.49)* is nothing more than a standard, creamy pencil that is infused with sparkle and applies easily. It tends to smear, and the sparkles can separate and fall onto surrounding skin, making this even more frustrating to use than the average pencil!

LIPSTICK AND LIP PENCIL: ☺ Most of the **Moon Drops Moisture Cremes** and **Frosts** *($8.69)* and **Super Lustrous Cremes** and **Frosts** *($8.69)* have great colors (including some one-of-a-kind vivids) and an emollient, creamy texture. When it comes to lipstick, it doesn't get any more traditional than this, and the latest colors are fragrance-free. **Lip Conditioner** *($8.69)* is your everyday colorless lipstick designed as a lip balm. It works as well as any, and the price is realistic. **ColorStay Lip Liner** *($7.89)* is undeniably tenacious and far less greasy than most. This retractable, twist-up pencil really holds up against greasy lipsticks! **TimeLiner for Lips** *($6.79)* is as standard a lip pencil as it gets, but the price is right. **Line and Shine** *($9.69)* is a two-in-one product that has a standard lip pencil on one end and a liquid lip color on the other. The Shine portion is just semiopaque lip gloss, and in the end you get a little convenience in exchange for a tiny amount of each product.

✔☺ **Absolutely Fabulous Lip Cream SPF 15** *($6.99)* is pretty close to fabulous in every sense of the word! This has a luscious, creamy, opaque texture and an in-part avobenzone sunscreen, so the lips will be beautifully protected from the sun. This is highly recommended as one of the better creamy lipsticks available, with reliable sunscreen to boot, and the color selection is superb.

✔☺ **LipGlide Color Gloss** *($9.49)* is an innovative combination of deeply pigmented gloss and packaging. By turning the base at its midpoint, the lip color is slowly fed onto an angled sponge tip, which allows you to easily control how much product comes up. This is actually easier to work with than most of the click-pen/lip-brush products sold by other companies. It applies smoothly and evenly, though the texture is sticky. However, if that doesn't bother you, LipGlide is something you should check out.

☺ **ColorStay Lipstick** *($9.69)* is slightly less ultra-matte than the original version, but still peels off from the inside out, and that's not a pretty picture. There have been numerous knockoffs of this ultra-matte finish, but without adding extra oils or emollients (the very things that make lipstick fleeting) to prevent the peeling, the ultra-matte paradox lived on—until Max Factor shook up the lipstick world with their almost-perfect Lipfinity, which all but solves the problems inherent to ultra-matte lipsticks. **ColorStay Liquid Lip** *($8.99)* is supposed to be a transfer-resistant lip gloss that comes in a tube with a wand applicator. It applies fairly emolliently and then, after what seems like several minutes, it slightly—"sets." However, the finish stays moist, is not transfer-resistant in the least, and can tend to roll off. Do not expect this to be the sheer, moist stain the ads proclaim. **ColorStay Lip Shine** *($10.19)* is a dual-ended product with one end being a liquid lipstick and the other a silicone-based gloss. You're supposed to apply the lipcolor, wait three minutes for it to set, and then apply the wet-looking gloss. You could wait an hour for this creamy lipstick to set, and miss getting to work on time, and it still feels creamy. It lasts well by itself and isn't anywhere near as greasy as true lip gloss, but once you apply the glossy component, the color tends to slip and bleed and you're right back with the same old problem. That's progress?

MASCARA: ☺ **ColorStay Lash Color** *($6.49)* quickly lengthens, and with repeated effort will add some thickness. This has a slight tendency to clump, but not nearly as much as it had in the past. And it really does stay—removing it will take more than a once-over with a water-soluble cleanser. **ColorStay Extra Thick Lashes Mascara** *($6.49)* takes awhile to build any length, but with patience you do get relatively long, thick, separated lashes without clumping or smearing. The jumbo brush isn't an advantage and has a tendency to feel scratchy if you get it too close to the rim of the eye. **ColorStay Extra Thick Lashes Mascara Waterproof** *($6.49)* is far and away Revlon's best waterproof mascara. It adds enough length, thickness, and clean definition to make it a top choice for those times when you need waterproof mascara. The oversized brush poses the same concern as the brush that comes with the original Extra Thick Lashes Mascara above.

☺ **Everylash Mascara** *($6.49)* is virtually identical in look and performance to Almay's Stay Smooth Mascara, and remains just an OK lengthening mascara with a gimmicky, built-in comb you're unlikely to use more than once. **Everylash Mascara Curling** *($6.49)* does little as far as adding curl, and is otherwise identical to the original Everylash Mascara, though the curved brush lends itself to minor clumping. **Everylash Mascara Waterproof** *($6.49)* meets basic expectations in terms of length, but it takes some effort for this to just be a standard, sufficiently waterproof mascara. Again, you'll have little use for the built-in lash comb. **ColorStay Waterproof Mascara** *($6.49)* is waterproof, but that's about all this ordinary mascara has up its sleeve. Length and thickness are slow-going, and not nearly as impressive as many of Maybelline's waterproof mascaras.

☹ **High Dimension Lash-Lengthening Mascara** *($7.49)* supposedly contains "new light interplay technology for soft-lit lashes" that "goes beyond basic black" to "spark a subtle glint with every flutter of your lashes." I can guarantee you will be doing lots of lash-fluttering, but that's not because of any new technology. Rather, this mascara contains lots of iridescent particles that tend to flake off and end up getting into your eye—not exactly the image this product's description begs you to conjure up. This mascara also builds no length or thickness. In fact, it takes a lot of effort just to look like you have any on. **ColorStay Overtime Lash Tint** *($8.99)* is horrible. I need to say that again: this is *horrible*. This is not mascara per se, but a lash tint that goes on a bit too wet and tends to stick lashes together. Carefully working the wand through will net you adequate lash separation, but once (and whichever way) this dries, you're stuck with that result for three days. That's right, the supposed benefit of this product is it gives you "up to 3 days of dark, defined lashes with no smudges, flakes, or clumps." I wore this for two days and had had enough. There was mild flaking, but otherwise this did not budge, even after a full night's sleep and shower. The major problem with this formula is how it tends to stick lashes together and becomes increasingly uncomfortable the longer it's worn. And removing it is akin to sandblasting your lashes—nothing gets through this (not even oil, as Revlon suggests), and you end up chipping the tint off lash by lash.

BRUSHES: ☺ **Beauty Shapers Brushes** *($5.99–$7.99)* are a small collection of decent, workable brushes. The **Shadow Brush Plus** *($5.99)* is a reliable, soft, eye-contouring brush, and one end has a pointed rubber tip for blending eyeliner. The **Powder Brush** and **Travel Face Brush** *($7.99 each)* are options as well. Both are soft, reasonably full, and have a good shape. The only "maybe" in the bunch is the **Blush Brush** *($5.99)*, which tends to flare out a bit too much for a controlled application of powder blush.

Revlon Skinlights Makeup

Skinlights is designed to "instantly brighten skin, boost luminosity, and soften flaws." But aside from the addition of some trace minerals, all of these products use the same standard, shiny pigments the rest of the industry uses, namely, mica, ultramarines (mineral-based coloring agents), and iron oxides. Still, the Skinlights product line was Revlon's most successful launch of 2001, with sales of over $20 million in the United States alone (source: *The Rose Sheet*, November 5, 2001). Not surprisingly, Revlon quickly added more products to keep the sales momentum going and inspire even more women to "Come play with the power of light . . ." which you can read as "add as much shine to your makeup routine as possible!" The majority of the Skinlights products offer a subtle, low-wattage shine (glow), but in natural light you can still plainly see bits of sparkles wherever the product was used—and also wherever it has migrated. Yet if you do want to incorporate shine into your makeup routine, the majority of these products have a contemporary edge that competes strongly with similar offerings from department-store lines.

☺ **Skinlights Face Illuminator SPF 15** *($10.99)* is a sheer tint for the skin that offers reliable UVA-protecting ingredients, and the SPF was wisely bumped up from a 10 to the standard SPF 15. The formula has a lightweight, softly creamy texture that does not feel heavy or greasy, though the illuminating effect you may have been hoping for is achieved with iridescent particles that are hard to blend away, soften, or control, and they can spread to places where you didn't intend them to go. Seven tints are available and, as sheer colors, all are acceptable except Golden Light, which is too orange for most skin tones. Bronze Light is quite dark, and will look too coppery over fair or light skin tones. If you're a fan of shiny, sheer foundations like M.A.C.'s HyperReal *($24)*, you may want to check this out—you'll get the same effect, but Revlon's offers great sun protection and a better price point. Otherwise, this type of product is best as an adjunct to foundation or used alone for an evening look. **Skinlights Diffusing Tint SPF 15** *($12.29)* has an excellent, in-part titanium dioxide– and zinc oxide–based sunscreen and a soft, slightly creamy texture that can feel somewhat thick when applied, though it blends down to a smooth, natural finish. Of all the Skinlights products, this one has the least amount of visible shine, and it's a decent, sheer-coverage option for daytime wear. There are six colors, with no choices for very light or very dark skin tones. Only Nude is a bit too peach to work for most skin tones—the other colors are beautiful. It does contain rather strong fragrance. **Skinlights Color Lighting for Eyes/Cheeks** *($7.89)* is a collection of five sheer, iridescent cream-to-powder compacts with colors that are a breeze to apply and blend. However, the shine is intense enough to be distracting, and while these are options for nighttime eye makeup, you may want to reconsider applying this much shine to your cheeks. The colors, though limited, are great. **Skinlights**

Illusion Wand SPF 12 *($7.89)* is a very good concealer that comes in a pen-style container with a brush tip. Like others of its ilk, you need to click the base of the container to feed product into the brush tip. This sounds better than it really is because it's quite easy to click up too much product, and then there's no putting it back. Nevertheless, this has a light, smooth texture that is easy to work with, and the finish (at least in "feel") is matte, with only the faintest hint of shine. The two flesh-toned shades are fine, but are best for light to medium skin tones. Luminous Touch is a pale pink highlighting shade that's not as attractive as the others. Finally, although the sunscreen is a winning combination of titanium dioxide and zinc oxide, Revlon knows better than to stop at SPF 12. **Skinlights Glosslights for Lips** *($7.89)* are standard tube glosses that are a bit slicker than most, thanks to the inclusion of mineral oil as one of the main ingredients. Don't expect much longevity from them, but for an emollient, very sparkly lip gloss, these work well.

☺ **Skinlights Face Illuminator Loose Powder** *($10.99)* is a standard, talc-based powder with a silicone-enhanced silky feel and a fair amount of shine. Why anyone would want to dust this much iridescence onto their skin is beyond me, but if that floats your boat, the five available colors are all fine, though Bronze Light is too coppery for all but dark skin. A nice change of pace with this product is the packaging—the cap has a flip-top that houses a small, but workable, brush, a clever touch that eliminates the mess of storing a puff or brush inside the powder itself. **Skinlights Face Illuminator Stick SPF 10** *($10.99)* is a sheer highlighter/cream blush that goes on cool and slightly wet, then dries to a slightly moist finish as you blend. The sunscreen is all titanium dioxide, but SPF 15 would have really been illuminating. The colors are a bit more vibrant than those for the other Skinlights items, and the shine is at its most intense here, too. There are some great options for creating a warm, sun-kissed look, but the shine is almost intrusive, and is about as natural-looking as Styrofoam.

ROC (SKIN CARE ONLY)

Johnson & Johnson, owner of Purpose, Neutrogena, Clean & Clear, and the prescription-only drugs Retin-A and Renova, also owns RoC, a line whose image is designed to align itself with the notion of pharmaceutical-oriented skin care. The mortar and pestle in the logo are meant to convey the idea that these are more than just the usual cosmetic products, and hold to a higher medical standard. But image is not fact; you are not buying anything even remotely medical by investing in this relatively pricey drugstore line of skin-care products.

What you would be purchasing are relatively gentle skin-care products that have some decent formulations. Although there are a handful of exceptions, RoC products generally contain far fewer irritating ingredients than many cosmetics lines, and for the most part RoC's simple formulations are distinctive for their concern about preventing skin irritation or skin sensitivity. The product line as a whole is definitely a consideration for sensitive and dry skin types, though if you have oily or blemish-prone skin there are few, if any, options among RoC products.

Note: RoC in the United States makes some products that are available only in Canada; the reviews of these products follow the first section of reviews, which includes products available in both the United States and Canada. For more information about RoC in Canada, call (519) 836-6500; in the United States, call (800) 526-3967 or visit www.roc.com.

☺ **Cleanser + Toner in One** *($7.99 for 6.76 ounces)* isn't much of a toner or cleanser. It is more of a wipe-off cleanser and it doesn't tone a thing. It could be good for someone with dry skin, but it doesn't take off makeup very well without a lot of wiping. [In Canada this product is called **Cleanser and Refresher for Face and Eyes 2 in 1** *($16 for 200 ml)*.]

☺ **Deep Action Facial Wash with Beta Hydroxy** *($6.99 for 5.07 ounces)* is a standard, detergent-based cleanser that contains a small amount of salicylic acid (BHA), but the pH of the cleanser makes the BHA ineffective for exfoliation. This is an option for someone with normal to oily skin.

☺ **Protient Lift Daily Firming Cleanser** *($7.79 for 5 ounces)* won't lift skin anywhere; it's just an extremely standard, detergent-based cleanser that is an option for normal to oily skin. Protient is supposed to be "a natural firming nutrient, which helps support the skin's natural ability to fight the appearance of sagging skin." Yet there is not one unique or unusual ingredient in this product, and there is no ingredient called "Protient" in it, either.

☺ **Retinol Actif Pur Anti-Wrinkle Cleansing Lotion** *($8.99 for 4.2 ounces)* is an emollient cleanser that is an option for normal to dry skin, though it doesn't rinse off very well without the aid of a washcloth. It contains a minute amount of retinol, but in a product like this any efficacy it would have is rinsed down the drain before it has a chance to be of benefit for skin.

☺ **$$$ Hydra + Effet Reservoir for Normal Skin SPF 15** *($13.99 for 1.35 ounces)* is a very good, in-part avobenzone-based sunscreen in an emollient, though fairly standard, moisturizer for normal to slightly dry skin. [In Canada this is called **Hydra + Effet Réservoir Light Texture** *($24.50 for 40 ml)*.]

☺ **$$$ Hydra + Effet Reservoir for Dry Skin SPF 15** *($13.99 for 1.35 ounces)* is almost identical to the Normal Skin version above and the same basic comments apply. [In Canada this is called **Hydra + Effet Réservoir Enriched Texture** *($24.50 for 40 ml)*.]

☺ **Melibiose Active Firming Treatment for Dry Skin** *($13.99 for 1.35 ounces)* does contain melibiose, a sugar that has a small amount of research (all done in a test tube) showing that it protects other skin substances from breaking down (source: *Mechanisms of Ageing and Development*, January 1999, pages 241–260). That's nice, but it's not enough to rely on as the only way to take care of skin. Especially because, aside from its basic emollient formula, that's the only special ingredient in this product. [In Canada this is called **Melibiose Anti-Ageing Action-Enriched Texture** *($30 for 40 ml)*.]

✔☺ **Retinol Actif Pur Anti-Wrinkle Treatment, Day, SPF 15** *($16.99 for 1.01 ounces)* is a very good, in-part avobenzone-based sunscreen in a standard moisturizing base with a matte finish. It has a small quantity of water-binding agents and an antioxidant. There is a negligible amount of retinol as well. [In Canada this is called **Rétinol Actif Pur Jour, Moisturizing Anti-Wrinkle Day Care** *($32.75 for 30 ml)*.]

☺ **Retinol Actif Pur Skin Refining Treatment** *($17.99 for 1.35 ounces)* is a basic, though good, retinol product that is an option if you are looking for retinol in your moisturizer.

☺ **Retinol Actif Pur Anti-Wrinkle Treatment, for Night** *($18.69 for 1.01 ounces)* does contain retinol (about 0.1%), with water and thickening agents. This also contains about 3% to 4% AHA, though the product's pH of 5 means it will be ineffective for exfoliation.

☺ **$$$ Retinol Actif Pur, Eye Contour Cream** *($16.99 for 0.51 ounce)*. If you are looking for a retinol product, this one contains it, but that's about it, as there is no other special benefit to buying this basic moisturizing formula. [In Canada this is called **Rétinol Actif Pur Eye and Lip Contour** *($28.75 for 15 ml)*.]

RoC in Canada

Note: The following RoC products are available only in Canada. Refer to the above RoC reviews for products that are available in both the United States and Canada. All prices listed below are in Canadian dollars.

☺ **Endrial Dermo Calming Cleanser** *($14.50 for 200 ml)* is a basic emollient cleanser that is an option for normal to dry skin.

☺ **Cleansing Milk Normal to Combination Skin** *($14.50 for 200 ml)*. Despite the claim that this can unblock pores, it contains problematic ingredients that are known for blocking pores. This product is not recommended for combination skin, though it is an option as a cleanser for normal to dry skin.

☺ **Cleansing Milk Dry Skin, Extra Gentle** *($14.50 for 200 ml)* is an emollient cleanser containing lanolin oil, and that does make it appropriate for dry to very dry skin, although it can leave a slight greasy film.

☹ **Foaming Facial Cleanser** *($14.50 for 150 ml)* lists the second ingredient as sodium lauryl sulfate, a cleansing agent that is a potent irritant and also extremely drying and sensitizing. This is not recommended.

☺ **Eye Makeup Remover Lotion** *($14.50 for 125 ml)* is a standard, detergent-based, water-soluble, wipe-off cleanser; it would work as well as any.

☺ **Gentle Exfoliating Cream** *($14 for 50 ml)* is a mineral oil–based scrub that can leave a greasy film on the skin, although it is an option for dry skin.

☹ **Skin Toner Normal to Combination Skin** *($14.50 for 200 ml)* lists alcohol as the second ingredient, and that's a skin irritant. This is not recommended for any skin type.

☺ **Skin Toner, Dry Skin** *($14.50 for 200 ml)* is a standard, detergent-based toner that contains a teeny amount of water-binding agent. It has little benefit for skin other than as an extra step to remove traces of makeup.

☺ **Nutri + Protect, Amino Moisturizing Cream, Dry Skin** *($23 for 50 ml)* is a very emollient, though ordinary, moisturizer for dry skin that contains only water, plant oil, mineral oil, thickeners, lanolin, and preservatives.

☺ **ChronoBlock Daily Moisturizing Care SPF 15** *($32 for 40 ml)* is a very good, in-part avobenzone-based sunscreen in a very ordinary, moisturizing base that is good for normal to dry skin.

☺ **$$$ ChronoBlock Yeux (for Eyes) SPF 15** *($25 for 15 ml)* is almost identical to the Moisturizing Care SPF 15 version above, only RoC gives you less product and charges more.

☺ **Protient Lift Jour (day)** *($38 for 40 ml)*. Without sunscreen this should not be worn for daytime, though regardless of the time of day it won't lift skin anywhere. This is just a basic moisturizer with about 2% AHA, which isn't enough for it to be effective as an exfoliant. Protient is supposed to be "a natural firming nutrient, which helps support the skin's natural ability to fight the appearance of sagging skin." Yet there is not one unique or unusual ingredient in this product and no ingredient called "Protient" is listed, either. It does contain tyrosine, an amino acid that is supposed to stimulate melanin production, but according to the FDA and Health Canada, it can't do that when applied topically on skin.

☺ **$$$ Protient Lift Eye** *($30 for 15 ml)* is similar to the Protient Lift Jour version above except that it contains more tyrosine. Even if that ingredient could stimulate melanin production, why would anyone want more dark color in the area under their eyes?

☺ **$$$ Melibiose Anti-Ageing Action Eye Contour** *($24 for 15 ml)* is almost identical to the Melibiose Active Firming Treatment for Dry Skin reviewed in the RoC section above.

☺ **Revitalizing Night Cream** *($30 for 40 ml)* is a good moisturizer for someone with dry skin; it has a small amount of water-binding agents and antioxidant.

☺ **Retinol A+C+E Triple Action Day/Night** *($38 for 30 ml)* is an emollient moisturizer with some good antioxidants and a small amount of water-binding agents.

☺ **Hydra + Mat, for Combination Skins** *($24.50 for 40 ml)* is a simple, matte-finish moisturizer that includes sunscreen ingredients on the label but does not make any SPF claims. Therefore, it cannot be relied on for sun protection.

☹ **Hydra + Teint Tinted Moisturizing Cream: Clair, Hale, Dore** *($24.50 for 40 ml)* comes in colors that are all a strange shade of peach and are not recommended.

☺ **Hydra + Masque Moisturizing Mask** *($20 for 40 ml)* is just some emollient and a tiny amount of clay, making it a boring, do-nothing mask for someone with normal to dry skin.

☺ **Rétinol Actif Pur Radiance Anti-Wrinkle Mask** *($25 for 40 ml)* contains only a negligible amount of retinol, so even if retinol could make a difference in the skin, it couldn't do so here. This is just glycerin, thickeners, and a small amount of a water-binding agent; boring, but OK for normal to dry skin.

☺ **$$$ Nutri + Lips, Lip Protector** *($7.25 for 3 grams)* is a good, but basic, emollient for dry skin. The teeny amount of vitamin E has no impact on skin.

☺ **Minesol High Protection Sun Cream SPF 25** *($16 for 118 ml)* is a titanium dioxide–based sunscreen, but because it doesn't list any other ingredients there is no way to know what else you might be putting on your face. As a sunscreen, this is a very good option for dry or sensitive skin.

☺ **Minesol Mineral Sunblock Cream Very High Protection SPF 40** *($16 for 50 ml)* is similar to the SPF 25 version above only with zinc oxide and titanium dioxide, and the same basic comments apply.

☺ **$$$ Minesol High Protection Lipstick SPF 20** *($10 for 3 grams)* is an avobenzone-based sunscreen for the lips, but because it doesn't list any other ingredients there is no way to know what else you might be applying. As a sunscreen, this is a good option.

☺ **Minesol Tan Prolonging Lotion** *($18 for 200 ml)* is a good moisturizer for dry skin, although the tiny amount of tyrosine cannot encourage melanin production.

☺ **Auto Bronzant Self-Tanner** *($18 for 100 ml)* contains dihydroxyacetone, the same ingredient all self-tanners use to affect the color of skin. This one would work as well as any.

chapter *19*

HOW THE PRODUCTS ARE RATED

Rating a wide variety of cosmetic products is a rigorous, complex process. Setting up guidelines to distinguish and differentiate a terrible product from a great one, or a good product from one that's just mediocre, requires exact and consistently applied guidelines, and moreover guidelines that must be substantiated with published research and clear criteria. This is exactly what I've created for each product type that I review in this book.

First and above all, you need to know that I do not base any rating decision on my own personal experience with a product. In other words, just because I like the way a cleanser or a moisturizer feels on my skin doesn't mean that thousands of others will feel the same way about it. Personal feelings won't help you evaluate whether a product may hurt your skin or live up to any part of the claims showcased on the label. There are lots of online beauty chat rooms and bulletin boards, fashion magazines, and friends who love to share their personal experiences about the products they use. That might be interesting and entertaining, but it's important to recognize that lots of people like things that aren't good for them. Some people may like sun tanning or using a product that contains irritating ingredients because they think it feels like it's "working." Most people have no idea what kinds of ingredients can damage skin. Even more to the point, these friendly sources of recommendations don't know that other products may perform equally as well if not better for a lot less money. If you're going to spend money on a product, why not find out first whether or not it can live up to its claims and what you can expect in regard to how it may or may not work for you based on formulary or comparison performance issues? That is what you will find out from the reviews in this book.

All of the ratings for the skin-care products in this book are based primarily on an individual product's formulation, using published, peer-reviewed studies about the ingredients in the product, and taking into consideration their possible resulting interaction with the skin. I also evaluate these formulas based on published cosmetics chemistry data about ingredient performance and consistency. From that I can assess a product's potential for causing irritation, dryness, breakouts, sensitivities, greasiness, and other issues of texture and performance.

Makeup products are evaluated more subjectively than skin-care products in regard to application, color selection, texture, and comparison to similar types of products from myriad other lines. Formulation is also a consideration for makeup products, predominantly for claims made in regard to skin care.

This rating process is more challenging than I can describe, because even if I think a company is absurdly overcharging for its products or is exceedingly dishonest in its claims and advertising, and no matter how unethical it seems to me, it does not prevent me from saying that a product of theirs is good for a particular skin type (though I do often say, "This is a good product, but what a shame the price has to be so absurd and the claims so offensive!").

Each cosmetics line is reviewed for several different elements. The first consideration is overall presentation and how user-friendly the displays or company literature are. For lines available at retail locations, I consider it an asset if their display units are set up with convenient color groupings, such as colors divided into warm (yellow) and cool (blue) tones, and are easily accessible. Skin-care and makeup products that are convenient to sample without the help of a salesperson are also rated highly. For drugstore lines, colors must be easy to see, and samples or tester units are considered a bonus.

The fundamental determination for each individual product's rating is based on specific criteria established for each product category. For every category, from blushes to eyeshadows, concealers, foundations, cleansers, toners, scrubs, moisturizers, facial masks, AHA products, brushes, and wrinkle creams, I've created specific standards that the products must meet to garner a happy, unhappy, or neutral (meaning unimpressive but not bad) face.

Makeup products are assessed mostly on texture (Was it silky-smooth or grainy and hard?), color (Was a wide range of colors available, and was there an adequate selection for women of color?), application (Could it be applied easily or was it difficult to spread or blend?), ease of use (Was the container poorly designed, were colors placed too close together in an eyeshadow set, was foundation put in a pump container that squirted too much product or didn't reach to the bottom of the jar?), and, finally, price.

Skin-care products are evaluated almost exclusively on the basis of content versus claim. If a product claims to be good for sensitive skin, it cannot contain irritants, skin sensitizers, drying ingredients, and so on.

I also asked the following questions to see if a product can measure up to its claims, based on established and published research.

1. Given the ingredient list, and based on published research—not just what the cosmetics company wants you to believe—can the product really do what it promises?
2. How does the product differ from similar types of products?
3. If a special ingredient or ingredients are showcased, how much of them are actually in the product, and is there independent research verifying the claims for them?
4. Does the product contain problematic fragrances, plants, topical irritants, or other questionable ingredients that could cause problems for skin?
5. How farfetched are the product's claims?
6. Is the product safe? Are there risks such as allergic reactions, increased sun sensitivity, or poor sunscreen formulations, or potentially toxic ingredients?

WHAT CONSTITUTES LEGITIMATE RESEARCH?

The research quoted and cited in this book is taken almost exclusively from published and peer-reviewed medical and scientific journals, most of which are available online or in medical libraries. As important as this documentation is for the information I provide, perhaps even more significant is the "research" that I was not able to include in my assessments. When any cosmetics company claimed they had research demonstrating the effectiveness of their product, but the study was either not published, was proprietary (meaning it is not available to the public), or was otherwise not obtainable for review, the research was considered unacceptable. Just because a company says it has a "study" or did "laboratory testing" doesn't mean the results are scientifically valid, or have any relevance to overall efficacy. More often than not, the research conducted by cosmetics companies is little more than mere claim substantiation and not truly scientific evaluations.

While the FDA (at www.fda.gov) does not have regulations regarding cosmetics claim substantiation, there is nevertheless an entire industry of claim substantiation at work in the world of cosmetics. Some of this is due to the efforts of the Federal Trade Commission (www.ftc.gov) to crack down on misleading advertising, although budgetary limitations restrict much of their work. However, claim substantiation is growing in response to new European Union cosmetics legislation regarding animal testing, general substantiation of claims, and product safety (source: 6th Amendment to the European Union Cosmetics Directive). This is because the EU guidelines call for more enforcement of product standards than guidelines in the United States. That means the U.S. cosmetics industry is fast and furiously establishing standards that basically meet regulatory rules, but give you no information that is helpful for evaluating how a product will affect your skin. Creative claim substantiation is fast becoming big business.

Very few consumers, or reporters for that matter, are aware of the large number of skin-care "research" laboratories whose only clients are cosmetics companies that want to use enticing statistics or want to validate incredible claims they can use as a marketing strategy. These research labs exist solely to provide pseudoscientific material for the cosmetics industry and these "studies" are never published. That way, if the marketing copy claims that a moisturizer provides an 82% increase in moisturization or a 90% increase in the skin's water content, the company may very well be able to point to a study that says this is true. Quoting these inconclusive, vague studies in a news story or ad can make them sound significant and meaningful, but in truth they are more often than not just hype and exaggeration generated exclusively to sell products. One of these claim-substantiation companies actually advertises its ability to deliver "creative claim generation/substantiation."

Such features are typical of these types of studies. At first glance, the study sounds impressive, yet it is virtually meaningless. It doesn't tell you anything about the product's effectiveness, or even whether that product is good for the skin (it turns out that a high moisture content isn't!), but it gives the cosmetics company statistics it can show off in its press releases.

I've seen this process at work firsthand, and it is disturbing. Whoever is paying the bill hires the research lab. The lab is handed the products and told what to look for and what kind of results are needed—for example, proof of moisturization, exfoliation, smoothness, reduction of wrinkles, or some other parameter. Then the lab goes about setting up a study to prove that position. Rarely are these studies done double-blind, nor do they use a large group of women or show long-term results, and rarely (actually never) are the results negative. More to the point, these studies are never published. Yet consumers are led to believe this unverified information is factual when they read about it in editorials in magazines or newspapers.

(**Note:** Double-blind refers to a testing procedure designed to eliminate biased results, in which the identity of those receiving a test treatment is concealed from both the test administrators and the subjects until after the study is completed.)

This same sleight of hand is used quite effectively in brochures and ads. Many cosmetics counters hand out impressively designed, scientific-looking brochures showing how well a product works on the skin. You might see, for example, a microscopic close-up of a patch of skin paired with an explanation of why it looks bad. Beside it is another close-up of the same patch of skin after the product is applied. See how wonderfully the product worked? The deception here is that you are not given enough "before" information. For example, if the woman had acne, what was she doing before to take care of her skin? Was she using products that clogged pores or aggravated breakouts? Had she never used any effective skin-care products for acne? In that case, any basic skin-care routine for acne could make a difference. And was this the single best result of the lot? Were there perhaps others who still had breakouts despite treatment? Or were the results just improved with computer-savvy finesse (digitally retouched and changed) and have nothing whatsoever to do with the product? Just because information looks scientific doesn't mean it is.

I could go on and on about this kind of inadequate claim-substantiation business that takes place in the world of skin care and I do so numerous times throughout this book. What's important to remember is that phrases like "our studies show" or "our research establishes" or "our test results demonstrate" aren't worth the paper they are printed on unless you can see the entire study and can judge exactly how the research was carried out and whether or not the results are significant or senseless.

DUE DILIGENCE

I can't stress enough how much time and effort my staff and I put into gathering our information. We are diligent about making sure we incorporate accurate and precise information or research for all of the products we review. To accomplish this, the first order of business was to contact every cosmetics company whose products I review and ask them to please send whatever they could about their data or facts regarding their products and claims. Many companies were forthcoming with information, including ingredient and product listings. Yet there were a number of them who weren't willing to send us anything about their company or products, let alone details about the research or studies they use to substantiate their claims.

Let me state clearly that I am more than open to presenting any documented research that substantiates information contradicting something I've stated. I am more than willing to alter previously stated opinions and positions as new research comes to light showing that earlier information is no longer correct. For example, over the years I have changed my opinion on sunscreens with regard to the new research on UVA protection. I have modified my attitude toward antioxidants, too, given the growing body of literature establishing the positive effects of these ingredients for skin care. I have been more open to layering products when different active ingredients are needed, ranging from skin-lightening products to sunscreens to acne products. I want to be explicit about my desire to present the most up-to-date, currently published research that exists when it comes to skin-care formulations and makeup products.

I also want to thank the companies that did send me their information. While I may not agree with them on the quality of all their products or their advertising claims, their willingness to be forthcoming about their formulations and claims is appreciated.

JUDGING A PRODUCT BY ITS LABEL

Many people wonder whether I can judge a skin-care product by its label. You may be thinking, "Wouldn't that be like judging a food just by the ingredients in it? What about tasting it for yourself?" Taste is necessary information, but it is also prudent to judge food by its ingredient list. It is no longer wise for any of us to consume any food without a clear understanding of how much fat, sodium, preservatives, coloring agents, or calories it contains, along with many other details pertinent to our health.

Just as food labels are incredibly important, so are skin-care and makeup ingredient labels. If a skin-care product says it is good for sensitive skin or won't cause breakouts, but contains ingredients known to cause irritation or breakouts; that is essential information. If a skin-care product sells for $100 but contains the same ingredients as a product that costs $20, that is, to say the least, very important information. Perhaps even more significant, if a $100 product contains fewer or less effective ingredients than a $10 version, I think that is crucial consumer information. If a product claims to protect skin from the sun but it doesn't have an SPF 15 or greater and doesn't contain UVA-protecting ingredients, that is vital information regardless of price.

The ingredient list helps you sort through the jungle of choices. Besides, it is a far better starting point than basing decisions strictly on advertising mumbo jumbo or promises that are never delivered.

YOU WOULD BE SHOCKED

I wish there were some way I could teach every cosmetics consumer how to read an ingredient label. Once you became familiar with the chemical and Latin names of the ingredients listed and how they function, you would be stunned at how similar products in a particular category truly are. It's not that there aren't differences between products, but it's astounding how alike many products are. And I mean astounding. It is truly a marketing phenomenon when the cosmetics industry can convince women that there is a qualitative difference between a $10 cleanser and a $50 cleanser, or that a $60 sunscreen is far more advanced than one selling for $20, and so on for each product type. Even Dr. N.V. Perricone, author of *The Wrinkle Cure* (a book describing Perricone's own unsubstantiated, nonscientific data regarding the treatment of wrinkles) and owner of the product line bearing his name, was quoted in the *New York Times* (Nov. 18, 2001, "The Skin Game with New Wrinkles") as saying, "Promise them an unlined face, and you can sell them anything." This is exactly what he and hundreds of other companies are doing, selling empty promises that women fall for every time an ad proclaims the next answer for wrinkles.

What I hope my book brings to light is that there are truly an amazing number of brilliant skin-care products being sold. However, if you are going to take truly beautiful care of your skin, you must also be aware that an alarming amount of misleading, overrated, and erroneous claims are being tossed about by companies who have no legal restrictions encouraging them to do otherwise. If you are seduced by price and advertising rhetoric, your skin and budget run the risk of being damaged, or, at the very least, being poorly taken care of. If you're not, you can gain some real benefits.

IRRITANTS AND COUNTER-IRRITANTS

I am now much more cautious than ever before about products that contain any amount of irritating ingredients, particularly those containing any form of grain alcohol (ethyl, ethanol, methanol, benzyl, or SD alcohol), as well as lemon, grapefruit, mint, peppermint, menthol, camphor, eucalyptus, ivy, fragrant oils, and overly drying or irritating detergent cleansing agents. My more exacting criteria in this area reflect the growing body of research indicating that irritation damages skin and hurts the skin's healing process (sources: *Skin Research and Technology*, November 2001, pages 227–237; and *Microscopy Research and Technique*, volume 37, issue 3, pages 193–199). In the midst of our daily battle against sun damage, wrinkles, and the causes of breakouts, there is never a reason to unnecessarily irritate the skin with ingredients like these, which provide no benefit whatsoever for the face or body and can prevent the skin from healing. See Chapter 3 for more information on the importance of treating your skin gently.

What about counter-irritants? There is a misperception among many in the cosmetics industry, as well as among consumers, that ingredients considered to be counter-irritants, such as menthol, peppermint, camphor, eucalyptus, and mint, have anti-inflammatory or anti-irritant properties, and that is absolutely not true (sources: *Archives of Dermatologic Research*, May 1996, pages 245–248; and Code of Federal Regulations Title 21—Food and Drugs, revised April 1, 2001, at 21CFR310.545, www.fda.gov). In fact, counter-irritants induce local inflammation as a way to relieve inflammation in deeper or adjacent tissues. In other words, they substitute one kind of inflammation for another. That is never good for skin. Both irritation and inflammation, no matter what causes them or how it happens, impair the skin's immune and healing response (source: *Skin Pharmacology and Applied Skin Physiology*, November-December 2000, pages 358–371). And although your skin may not show it, or may not react in an irritated fashion, if you apply irritants to your skin the damage is still taking place and the effects are ongoing and add up over time (source: *Skin Research and Technology*, November 2001, pages 227–237).

EVALUATING SKIN-CARE PRODUCTS

My reviews of skin-care products in each line are, with some exceptions, organized in the following categories: cleansers, eye-makeup removers, scrubs, toners, moisturizers (all kinds, regardless of the claim or type, such as eye or neck creams), alpha hydroxy acid or beta hydroxy acid exfoliants, specialty products, sunscreens, acne products, and facial masks. The criteria I used to evaluate the quality of the products in each of the different categories of skin-care products are explained below.

Cleansers: In reviewing facial cleansers, I am primarily interested in how genuinely water-soluble they are. See Chapter 5 for more in-depth information about cleansers.

I do not recommend cleansers that contain concentrations of alpha or beta hydroxy acids (AHAs or BHA) or topical disinfectants such as benzoyl peroxide or triclosan. While these ingredients can be quite helpful in other skin-care products, in a cleanser they are rinsed down the drain before they have a chance to have a real effect on skin. It is also a concern that these ingredients can inadvertently get into the eye when rinsing the cleanser off the face.

Eye-Makeup Removers: It's not necessary to use a separate eye-makeup remover as an extra step. An effective but gentle, water-soluble cleanser should take off all your makeup, including eye makeup, without irritating the eyes. Unless you are wearing waterproof mascara or can't get the knack of removing your eye makeup with a water-soluble cleanser, there are many reasons to avoid adding this step. See Chapter 5 for more details.

It is important to note that the vast majority of eye-makeup removers use many of the exact same ingredients found in water-soluble cleansers! Other eye-makeup removers use either oils (plant or mineral) or silicones. These can help remove makeup without causing dryness, and for some skin types or personal preferences that can be beneficial.

Eye-makeup removers are one of the categories in which the products are nearly indistinguishable from one another. They are formulated so similarly that there are no surprises or real cautions needed.

Exfoliants and Scrubs: With the advent of alpha hydroxy acids (AHAs) and the increased use of beta hydroxy acid (BHA; technical name, salicylic acid), there is less reason than ever before to use a mechanical exfoliant on the skin. Mechanical exfoliants are scrubs that remove skin cells as you rub particles over the skin. Even when the scrub particles are small and uniform in size, this procedure can still abrade the skin and be harsher than necessary, causing damage and affecting the skin's healing process. That means the major consideration for any topical scrub is that it has to be gentle on the skin and not rough or overly abrasive. It is also important that it rinses off easily without leaving any residue or greasy feel on the skin. Some women prefer the feeling of a scrub on their skin, but there aren't many scrubs that are any better than using plain baking soda mixed with Cetaphil Gentle Skin Cleanser for those with oily skin, or just a plain washcloth for that matter.

Alpha/Beta Hydroxy Acid Products: I expect products containing AHAs or BHA to be effective exfoliants. Though AHAs and BHA can also be effective as moisturizing ingredients, this is not what they do best for skin. Above all else, AHAs and BHA excel in exfoliating skin.

I use very specific criteria to determine if an AHA or BHA product will be an effective exfoliant. I wish you could tell if it would be effective by reading the label, but that just isn't possible. When it comes to AHAs and BHA, the crucial information comes in two parts. One is the type of ingredient and its concentration in the product, and the other is the pH of the product. AHAs work best at concentrations of 5% to 8% in a base with a pH of 3 to 4 (this is more acid than alkaline or neutral), and their effectiveness diminishes as the pH increases beyond 4.5. BHA works best at concentrations of between 1% and 2% at an optimal pH of 3, diminishing in effectiveness as the pH increases beyond 4. The effectiveness of both AHAs and BHA decreases as a product's pH increases and as the concentration of the ingredient decreases.

As a general rule I do not recommend products that use both AHAs and BHA together because each has its specialized action, and that does not translate to all skin types. AHAs work on the surface of the skin and are best for sundamaged skin that has developed a thickened outer layer, or for someone with dry skin who has a buildup of layers of skin that make the skin look dull and impede cell turnover. If you have breakouts, AHAs may help to some extent, but the penetration of BHA into the pore can be more effective.

One word of caution: Anytime you use a well-formulated AHA product that contains more than 5% AHAs, some stinging can occur, though this can diminish as the skin gets used to it. You should not let AHAs or BHA products come in contact with the eyes or any mucous membranes. It is also possible that you may have an irritation reaction or sensitivity to AHAs or BHA. Slight stinging is expected, but continued stinging is not; if the stinging continues, stop using it. See Chapter 3 for more information.

Facial Masks: Many facial masks contain claylike ingredients that absorb oil and, to some degree, exfoliate the skin, which can be beneficial for someone with oily skin. The problem with many masks is that they often contain additional ingredients that are irritating or that can clog pores. There are also a range of masks that contain plasticizing (hairspray-like) ingredients that peel off the face like a layer of plastic. These take a layer of skin off when removed, and that can make skin feel temporarily smoother, but there is no long-term benefit to be gained.

Another type of facial mask that shows up is the kind with strictly moisturizing ingredients. These basically don't differ from other moisturizers except that they are thicker formulations. Calling the product a mask seems to make women feel like they are doing something special for their skin when, in actuality, they aren't. Despite all these shortcomings, which I point out in the individual reviews, there are masks in this book that did get happy faces, either because of their potential benefit for dry skin (if they contained reliable ingredients for this condition) or because of their absorbency for oily skin.

Overall, facial masks did not have any standout formulary considerations or miracles to offer. Therefore, masks are rated based on compatibility for each skin type. For dry skin the mask must have emollient properties and for oily skin absorbent ingredients. See Chapter 5 for more information about masks.

Toners: Toners, astringents, fresheners, tonics, and other liquids meant to refresh the skin or remove the last traces of makeup after a cleanser is rinsed off should not contain any irritants whatsoever. I evaluated these products primarily on that basis. Claims that toners can close pores or refine the skin are un-achievable, so I ignore such language and look for toners that leave the face feeling smooth and soft, are able to remove the last traces of makeup, and do not irritate the skin. Toners that contain a good assortment of water-binding agents, anti-irritants, and antioxidants are rated as being optimal for all skin types. Toners that add plant oils to those preferred ingredients are rated best for normal to dry skin. Toners that add mild detergent cleansing agents with no emollients, but that also have water-binding agents, anti-irritants, and antioxi-dants are rated best for normal to oily skin.

Toners are always considered an optional step for most skin types. See Chapter 5 for more information on toners.

Moisturizers: Despite all the fuss, assertions, and price differences among anti-wrinkle, firming, antiaging, and "renewing" supplements and treatments that claim to restore youth to skin, in truth these products are nothing more than moisturizers.

As a general category, "moisturizers" were quite easy to review. Basically, de-spite the claims, moisturizers in one form or another keep the skin from looking and feeling dry—so I expect the same thing from all of them: They must contain ingredients that can smooth and soothe dry skin, keep water in the skin cell, and help maintain or reinforce the skin's protective barrier. Almost all other claims for this immense group of products are exaggerated and misleading, not to men-tion never-ending. Every month a new assortment is launched with new mar-keting copy to catch your attention.

Apart from the redundant claims moisturizers make in regard to getting rid of wrinkles or firming skin, there are still significant distinct qualitative differ-ences between products. Research on the function of antioxidants, anti-irritants, and water-binding agents that mimic the actual substances comprising the skin's intercellular matrix (the skin's own composition that binds skin cells together) shows that all these ingredients can potentially have a fundamental positive ef-fect on skin. I rate favorably those moisturizers that have a preponderance of these ingredients. However, while these types of ingredients show incredible promise for preserving the health and balance of skin, there is no direct evidence or research showing that any specific antioxidant, anti-irritant, or water-binding agent is better than another, and there's also no research showing that they can get rid of wrinkles. The only "studies" that state otherwise are paid for or con-cocted by the companies showcasing those ingredients.

It is interesting to note that regardless of the claim, none of these products contain unique ingredients. Rather, they all share a range of overlapping, similar ingredients, so the "exclusive" claims become even more unbelievable.

Next, while there are multitudes of ingredients that are potentially helpful for skin, there are also a number that are a waste of time, or worse. These range from bee pollen to gold, plus animal extracts from thymus, spleen, and placenta, as well as many plant extracts that can be potential skin irritants, and I point out as many of these as I can in my reviews. If there is no research showing any of these are helpful for skin, then they are there for marketing purposes only and that doesn't help your skin.

Additionally, I was interested in the order the "good" or "hyped" ingredients were listed on the container. Just as with food labels, the ingredients present in the largest amounts are listed first. Often, the most interesting or the most extolled ingredients are so far down the list that the amounts of them in the product are practically nonexistent. Just because an ingredient appears on an ingredient label doesn't mean there's enough of it to have any impact on skin or to make a difference of any kind.

There are also moisturizers that claim to be great for combination skin because they are able to release moisturizing ingredients over dry areas and oil-absorbing ingredients over oily areas. This is categorically impossible. A product cannot hold certain ingredients back from the skin—where would they go? Imagine a lotion touching your skin and separating out so the ingredients for the oily parts get up and run over here and the ones for the dry area get up and head over there. It just isn't feasible in any way, shape, or form.

Note: Packaging can play a vital role when it comes to a product's efficacy and stability, particularly for products that contain antioxidants, plant extracts, skin-lightening agents, benzoyl peroxide, and vitamins. All of these active ingredients are negatively affected by air and light, and inappropriate packaging leaves the contents vulnerable to decomposition and deterioration. That means you should avoid containers that expose a product to light (via see-through or non-opaque material) or to air (such as a container with a large opening, especially jar containers with screw-off lids) because they allow maximum exposure to light and air every time they are opened (source: FDA *Consumer* magazine, revised May 1995). I did not evaluate packaging for this edition of the book. However, it is something you should unconditionally take into consideration the next time you are thinking of spending money on any product, because if it is packaged in a see-through container or a jar it is unlikely that any of the "active" ingredients still retain any potency or efficacy. Instead, look for opaque or single-use units.

Moisturizers for Oily Skin: The only time to use a moisturizer is when you have dry skin; if you don't have dry skin, you don't need a moisturizer. For many with oily or combination skin the only moisturizer they may need is a toner with good water-binding agents, antioxidants, and anti-irritants. When a product, particularly a moisturizer, claims to be oil-free, noncomedogenic, or nonacnegenic, it often misleads consumers into thinking they are buying a product that won't clog pores. But those terms are not regulated by the FDA and have no legal meaning. A cosmetics company can use any or all of those terms without any qualifying ingredient listing or substantiation.

Here are a few ideas to at least point you in the right direction. Because a thicker formulation is more likely to contain problematic ingredients, just as a highly emollient product can, it is far better for normal to oily skin types to use gel or "serum"-type products that leave out most if not all thickening agents. Moisturizers for oily skin are judged as being preferred for that skin type if they are lightweight and have minimal to no waxy or emollient ingredients of any kind listed near the beginning of the ingredient list (because these can theoretically clog pores).

Moisturizers marketed to those with oily or combination skin must meet similar standards, but in addition to a lack of thickening agents and emollients, I consider it beneficial if they do contain substantial amounts of antioxidants, water-binding agents, and anti-irritants because these types of ingredients are rarely problematic for skin. For more information on moisturizers, see Chapter 3.

Day Creams versus Night Creams: There is no difference between what the skin needs during the day versus what it needs at night. The one big exception is that the daytime product should have an effective SPF (sunscreen) with UVA-protecting ingredients. Other than that, there are no formulation variances that make one preferable over the other. Many moisturizing formulations now have great sun protection, and that is the only way you should differentiate a daytime product from a nighttime version. All other claims on the label are rhetoric you should ignore.

Eye, Throat, Chest, Neck, and Other Specialty Creams, Serums, or Gels: Buying a separate product for a special area of the face or body, whether it is in the form of a cream, gel, lotion, or serum, is altogether unnecessary. Almost without exception, the ingredient lists and formulations for these products are identical to other creams, gels, lotions, or serums identified as being only for the face. That doesn't mean there aren't some great specialty products out there for different skin types, but why buy a second moisturizer for the eye area when the one you are already using on the rest of your face is virtually identical?

Even more bothersome is the fact that most cosmetics companies give you a tiny amount of the so-called specialty products but charge you much more for them than for an equal amount of the face creams, despite the similarities. Paradoxically, what does show up frequently in eye-care products are irritating ingredients such as witch hazel, caffeine, and fragrance. So much for the eye area having special needs that special products can address! Moreover, many eye products don't contain sunscreen. If your well-formulated face moisturizer contains sunscreen but your eye product doesn't, then you would actually be damaging the skin around the eye by not using your face moisturizer on it, because the eye product wouldn't protect from sun damage.

Sunscreens: Valid scientific research abounds demonstrating that wrinkles, skin damage, many skin discolorations, and possibly skin cancer are primarily a result of unprotected sun exposure (source: *Mechanisms of Ageing and Development*, April 2002, pages 801–810). Clearly this subject has to do not only with cosmetics, but also with serious health issues. It is well-established that the only true, first-line-of-defense antiwrinkle product is a well-formulated and carefully applied sunscreen. Please refer to Chapter 4 for more specific information.

The main criterion I use to evaluate sun-care products is the SPF rating, with SPF 15 being the standard. Also, because of the difference between UVA damage and UVB damage, and because there is still no UVA rating system, to be assured that you are getting adequate UVA protection, your sunscreen must contain one of three UVA-protecting ingredients listed as an active ingredient on the label. These active ingredients are avobenzone (also called Parsol 1789 or butyl methoxydibenzoylmethane), titanium dioxide, or zinc oxide (outside of the United States Mexoryl SX may also be used) (sources: *Photodermatology, Photoimmunology, & Photomedicine*, December 2000, pages 250–255; and *Photochemistry and Photobiology*, March 2000, pages 314–320).

No sunscreen receives a happy face unless one of those UVA-protecting ingredients is listed on the active ingredient part of the ingredient list, and it has an SPF of 15 or greater.

Because applying sunscreen liberally is indispensable for the health of skin, all expensive sunscreens are potentially dangerous for skin because their cost could discourage liberal application. After all, how liberally would you apply a $50-for-1-ounce sunscreen to your face or body versus a product costing $20 for two, four, or six ounces?

Sunscreens for Oily or Combination Skin: Sunscreens are a very tricky category for someone with oily or combination skin. It takes experimentation to find the one that will work best for you. The problem is that the ingredients used to suspend the active ingredients are not necessarily the best for oily skin. What I generally recommend is that someone with oily or combination skin select a foundation containing a well-formulated sunscreen. Then they can apply an appropriate lightweight moisturizer over dry areas or just use a well-formulated toner all over, which can be enough "moisturizing" for that skin type.

Water-Resistant Sunscreens: The FDA's December 2002 regulations regarding sunscreen require companies to eliminate the use of the word "waterproof" as a valid claim. In truth, no sunscreen can really be "waterproof" because it must be reapplied if you have been sweating or immersed in water for a period of time. See Chapter 4 for more information on this.

Self-Tanners: All self-tanning products, whether you choose one made by Bain de Soleil, Clarins, Decleor Paris, or Estée Lauder, are created equal. The active ingredient in every one of these products is dihydroxyacetone, which is what turns the surface layer of skin brown.

Where self-tanners do differ is in the amount of dihydroxyacetone present, although there is no surefire way to judge that from the ingredient list. However, you can assume that those self-tanners rated as light, medium, and dark have the correct corresponding amount of dihydroxyacetone. You can also assume that self-tanners without any stated level have a low to moderate concentration of dihydroxyacetone. See Chapter 4 for more information on applying self-tanners.

For more specific critiques of self-tanning products, you'll find the Web site www. sunless.com incredibly helpful, and I strongly recommend a visit.

Acne Products: From all the research I've seen, particularly in dermatological journals and literature from the American Academy of Dermatology, acne products need to deliver four categories of performance to deal with breakouts: (1) gentle cleansing (to reduce inflammation), (2) effective exfoliation, (3) disinfection, and (4) absorption of excess oil (source: *American Journal of Clinical Dermatology*, 2001, volume 2, number 3, pages 135–141). I delve into this subject at length in Chapter 9. I base my reviews for these types of products according to how they respond to these four important skin-care needs.

Skin-Lightening Products: The surge in skin-care products making claims about lightening skin and depigmenting skin discolorations caused by sun exposure or hormonal changes is nothing less than astounding. Now that baby boomers are aging and brown patches are beginning to turn up on hands and faces (caused primarily by sun damage—they are not liver spots or age related at all), skin-lightening products are showing up in all sorts of skin-care lines. Please see Chapter 5 for information on how skin lightening products work.

INGREDIENTS FOR SKIN CARE

While I want to emphasize how extensive the misleading portrayals of skin-care products made by the cosmetics industry are, I also want to underscore that there are hundreds of great products for all skin types. When I describe my elation or enthusiasm about any product, I am also always careful to let you know what can really be expected and how out-of-line the price often is for what you are getting. So just because I think a formula can be amazing for dry skin, that doesn't mean I concur with its claims about firming, lifting, undoing or preventing wrinkling, reducing lines, fighting stress, erasing cellulite, and on and on and on. . . .

Every skin-care product is evaluated on the basis of what ingredients it contains because its ingredients (and their potential effects) are the basis for whether a claim can be verified. I often comment about how a product compares to similar or better versions that cost much less. Of course, you will have to test for yourself how a specific product feels on your skin and how you react to its fragrance or lack thereof.

When I list a product's ingredients in the product reviews, I frequently use the phrase "contains mostly," often followed by one or all of the following terms: thickener or thickening agent, slip agent, water-binding agent, film-forming agent, scrub agent, absorbent, detergent cleansing agent or standard detergent cleanser, disinfectant, preservative, fragrance, plant extract or plant oil, vitamin, antioxidant, and anti-irritant. It was easiest to summarize groups of ingredients by using these general terms, but please read the following explanations of the terms.

Beauty Note: When reading ingredient lists, remember that the closer a specific ingredient is to a **preservative** (such as methylparaben, propylparaben, ethylparaben, imidazolidinyl urea, or quaternium-15) or a **fragrance** (listed as fragrance or often as an individual essential oil like lavender or bergamot oil), or the closer it is to the end of the ingredient list, the less likely it is that there is a significant amount of it in the product. That means its impact, for better or worse, is negligible.

When I use the term **"thickeners"** to describe an ingredient, I'm referring to those components that add texture, thickness, viscosity, spreadability, and stability to a product. Thickeners are also vital for helping to keep other ingredients mixed together. **Thickening agents** often have a waxlike texture or a creamy, emollient feel and can be great lubricants. There are literally thousands of ingredients in this category, and they are the staples of every skin-care product out there, regardless of the product's price or claims about "natural" ingredients.

Slip agents help other ingredients spread over or penetrate the skin and they also have humectant properties. Slip agents include propylene glycol, butylene glycol, hexylene glycol, methyl gluceth-10, polysorbates, and glycerin, to name only a few. They are as basic to the world of skin care as water.

Water-binding agents (also known as **natural moisturizing factors or NMFs**) are ingredients that help skin retain water and maintain its structural integrity. Skin is not in need of water so much as it is in need of substances that support the skin's own structure. **Humectants,** for example, attract water to skin and are one component of a moisturizer. But what good is getting water to the skin if the structure isn't there to keep the water from leaving? It turns out that skin cells usually have plenty of water if they don't become degraded or damaged. Once skin is irritated, overcleansed, exposed to the sun, dehydrated from air conditioning or heaters, and so on, the integrity of the skin surface is compromised. That means the substances that keep the skin cells bound together to create the surface structure we see as skin (the intercellular matrix) are depleted. This intercellular structure is made up of many different components, ranging from ceramides to lecithin, glycerin, polysaccharides, hyaluronic acid, sodium hyaluronate, sodium PCA, collagen, elastin, proteins, amino acids (of which there are dozens), cholesterol, glucose, sucrose, fructose, glycogen, phospholipids, glycosphingolipids, and glycosaminoglycans, to name just a few. All of these give the skin what it needs to keep skin cells intact. Just adding water is meaningless if the intercellular matrix is damaged or impaired. When a moisturizer does contain a combination of NMFs (water-binding agents), it reinforces the skin's natural ability to function normally and that temporarily reduces the presence of dry skin and allows the skin to create healthier skin cells and to repair itself from environmental onslaughts. I rate a moisturizer highly if it has a high number or a high concentration of NMFs.

There is no point in searching for one single mixture or "best" ingredient. Just like there isn't one "best" chocolate cake recipe, there isn't one best anything in the world of moisturizers. I wish there were, but the brilliance of cosmetics chemists and ingredient manufacturers lies in their ability to create and combine a profusion of ingredients to produce lots and lots of wonderful products. There are just too many great options to sum it up in any one ingredient or product. But I assure you, when a product lacks a good combination of important ingredients such as water-binding agents, antioxidants, or anti-irritants, I let you know!

Abrasive or **scrub** ingredients are found in cleansing scrubs or in some facial masks meant to remove dead skin cells. The most typical scrub particles used are polyethylene, almond meal, cornmeal, ground apricot kernels, and almond pits. Polyethylene is the most common form of plastic used in the world and the most popular scrub agent. It is flexible and has a smooth, waxy feel. When ground up, the small particles are used in scrubs as a fairly gentle abrasive. Seashells (listed as diatomaceous earth on the ingredient label) are also used as abrasive substances in scrubs, but they can be extremely rough on skin.

Aluminum oxide (also listed as alumina), the same substance used in microderm-abrasion treatments, is also starting to show up in scrub products. This substance can be extremely gritty and irritating for skin and is not recommended for regular use.

Absorbents are ingredients used in skin-care and makeup products designed to create a matte finish or oil-absorbing film layer on the skin. These absorbent materials are typically talc, silicates (such as magnesium aluminum silicate), clays, dry-finish silicones (usually cyclomethicone or phenyl trimethicone), nylon-12, and film-forming agents (hairspray-like ingredients), which can all absorb oil effectively. Some have drier finishes than others, but that depends on the specific formulation and the amount of the ingredient used. As I often point out, my concern about ingredients like rice starch, cornstarch, and other food products is that they are typically considered problematic for breakouts. Food substances can get into pores and encourage bacteria production, which is not the best when fighting off bacteria is the goal.

Film-forming agents are ingredients such as PVP (polyvinyl pyrrolidone), methylacrylate, and the polyglycerylacrylates presently being used in a vast number of moisturizers, wrinkle creams, and eye gels to help the skin look smoother. Film-forming agents are usually found in hairsprays and hairstyling products like gels and mousses because they place a thin, transparent, plastic-like layer over the hair (and skin). In the past, the kinds of film-forming agents used were problematic for some skin types; today, with the advent of new polymers, these ingredients do a good job of keeping moisture in the skin and are generally used in such tiny amounts that they are unlikely to be a problem for most skin types. They can also work to absorb oil in some formulations. When these film-forming agents are listed higher up on a product's ingredient list, they might be present at an amount that can leave a slightly tacky feeling on the skin.

Most skin cleansers include ingredients known as surfactants. Surfactant is a technical term that refers to a large number of ingredients that can cleanse as well as degrease. When cleansers contain surfactants as the primary cleansing agent, I use the phrases **"detergent-based," "detergent cleansing agent,"** or **"standard detergent cleanser."** Ingredients in this category include cocoamidopropyl betaine, sodium laureth sulfate, TEA-lauryl sulfate, cocamide DEA, ammonium laureth sulfate, and ammonium lauryl sulfate, to name a few (though these tend to be the most typical). Because sodium lauryl sulfate, TEA-lauryl sulfate, and sodium C14-16 olefin sulfate are very strong detergent cleansing agents and are known for their irritation potential (sources: *British Journal of Dermatology*, May 2002, pages 792–800 and *Toxicology in Vitro*, August-October 2001, pages 597–600), I warn against using a product that contains these ingredients when they appear in the first part of the ingredient list.

Preservatives, which are a fundamental component of every cosmetic product, are used in cosmetics to prevent bacterial and microbial contamination of the product. While there is definitely a risk of irritation from the inclusion of preservatives, the risk to skin and eyes from using a contaminated product is considered by many scientists to be even greater.

A group of preservatives known as formaldehyde donors or formaldehyde-releasing preservatives have garnered a reputation for being more problematic than other types of preservatives. Formaldehyde-releasing preservatives are commonly found in cosmetics (source: *Contact Dermatitis*, December 2000, pages 339–343) and include quaternium-15, 2-bromo-2-nitropane-1, 3-diol (trade name Bronopol), methyldibromo glutaronitrile, diazolidinyl urea, imidazolidinyl urea, and dmdm hydantoin. However, there is no research indicating that these ingredients pose a higher potential for irritation than other preservatives. In fact, studies have found no greater increase in skin reactions to formaldehyde-releasing preservatives than to other preservatives (source: *British Journal of Dermatology*, March 1998, pages 467–476). In fact, there is a far greater risk to skin from a product without preservatives due to the potential for contamination and unchecked growth of bacteria, fungus, and mold.

There is a concern that formaldehyde-releasing preservatives, when present in a formulation with amines (such as triethanalomine—TEA; diethanalomine—DEA, or monoethanalomine—MEA), can form nitrosamines, which are carcinogenic substances that can potentially penetrate skin (source: *Fundamentals and Applied Toxicology*, August 1993, pages 213–221). Whether or not that poses a health risk has not been established, and there is substantial disagreement among cosmetics chemists as to whether or not this is really a problem for skin. Many chemists suggest that going out of the house without a sunscreen or sitting in a bar exposing yourself to secondhand cigarette smoke poses more risk to the skin than any combination of skin-care ingredients ever could. However, you should be aware that there are those who consider this nonchalant attitude to be mere apologetics for and sidestepping around a very serious question. As a person who has looked at this issue for some time, I actually understand both viewpoints and have no definitive position to share. To that end, I leave the final decision to you. All you need to do is check the ingredient list of any product you are considering to determine whether it includes amines as well as the formaldehyde-releasing preservatives mentioned above.

When **fragrances** or **fragrant plant extracts** are listed among the ingredients, I indicate this clearly in the review. Fragrance and fragrant plant extracts are used in cosmetics either to mask the smell of a product's ingredients or to add a specific fragrance. My strong recommendation is that skin-care products not contain fragrance. Fragrances of all kinds, including essential oils, are irritants or skin sensitizers and serve little to no function for skin (source: *Contact Dermatitis*, June 1999, pages 310–315).

The cosmetics industry knows that most women emotionally and psychologically prefer cosmetics that smell nice, even if they say they want to avoid fragrance. This is why, in order to kill two marketing birds with one cosmetic stone, companies often list the fragrance components as essential oils or plant extracts rather than as fragrance or perfume on the label. So while you may not see the word "fragrance" on the list, and you may approvingly think wintergreen oil, lemon oil, cardamom oil, ylang-ylang oil, or other oils sound pleasant and healthy, your skin may still respond disapprovingly.

Because of the risk of irritation, sensitivity, or allergic reaction to fragrant or volatile plant extracts, I would prefer that all skin-care products be fragrance-free. Nevertheless, women like their products to smell nice, and it's up to every woman to make her own decision on this matter.

A profusion of **plant extracts** are used in cosmetics, so many that it's impossible to list them all individually and explain their purpose or lack of purpose. According to the various cosmetics companies, the plants they use have the most astonishing merits. When plants are an issue in a skin-care product, I point out the known benefits of those plants, such as antioxidant, anti-irritant, or antibacterial properties. I also explain when plants are a problem in cosmetics owing to their potential for causing irritation or a sensitizing reaction. There are times when plants have the attribute of being potential irritants but also have antioxidant properties. In these instances I generally cite the irritation potential because there are so many plant extracts that have antioxidant properties without being irritating to skin.

Some plant oils, often referred to as **essential oils**, are highly fragrant, volatile oils and are almost always irritants or photosensitizers, and I indicate when this is the case. However, I attribute no superiority to one over another, because there is none. Essential oils are nothing more than a way to get fragrance into a skin-care product.

Nonfragrant plant oils or nonvolatile oils are almost always beneficial as emollients and lubricants. The debate whether or not emu, mink, sunflower, olive, canola, or any of myriad other oils or blends of oils is superior is a marketing game to showcase a product. There is research showing that some plant oils have antioxidant properties. But as more research is done in this field, especially over the past two years, it turns out that many plants have antioxidant properties of one kind or another.

I often list the exact name of any **vitamin** included in a product. Regardless of the individual vitamin—whether it is vitamin A, C, or E—vitamins in skin-care products can't feed the skin. However, many of them can work as antioxidants and theoretically that can benefit the skin.

Antioxidants are a fascinating part of many skin-care formulations. What makes antioxidants so intriguing is that they seem to have the ability to reduce and heal some effects of sun exposure and overall help skin heal. All of that is incredibly beneficial for cell turnover, maintenance, and reducing dehydration. I suspect that antioxidant research for skin will end up being even more fascinating over the next decade as we learn more about how these substances work and how their efficacy can best be applied to skin. In the meantime, even with all the research about antioxidants and their impact on skin, it's still not known how that relates to wrinkles.

Lots of antioxidants, such as selenium, superoxide dismutase, vitamin A (retinyl palmitate and retinol), vitamin C (ascorbyl palmitate and magnesium ascorbyl palmitate), beta-glucan, and vitamin E (tocopherol and tocotrienols), grape extract, green tea, curcumin, coenzyme Q10, and honey, to name the most common ones, are showing up in skin-care products these days. All of these and many, many more are excellent additions to skin-care products and moisturizers of all sorts.

Keep in mind that while antioxidants do have definite benefits, no basic amounts have been set for their effective use. Is 0.25% enough or 3% too much? *Is* there such a thing as too much? How long do they last on skin? When do you need to reapply? There are no answers anywhere to these questions. Until there is more information, it is safe to assume that antioxidants are a crucial aspect when it comes to skin care because the research in that regard is so overwhelming. A search for "antioxidants" on the National Library of Medicine Web site (www.ncbi.nlm.nih.gov/entrez/query.fcgi) produced over 80,000 published studies!

Anti-irritants are gaining more and more recognition and attention in skin-care formulations because of the mounting research showing that any kind of irritation and inflammation of the skin is damaging. Regardless of the source, sun exposure, pollution, stress, irritating skin-care ingredients, or environmental conditions, irritation and inflammation hurt skin. An abundance of research proves this, particularly in regard to inflammation and irritation impeding healing and repair of skin (sources: *Skin Pharmacology and Applied Skin Physiology*, January-February 2001, Supplement 1, pages 87–91; and 2000, volume 13, number 6, pages 358–371). It would follow that anything you can do to reduce inflammation and irritation would be of great benefit to skin. Actually, a great deal of what we know about the effect of antioxidants on skin is due to their ability to reduce inflammation and irritation. Anti-irritants are impressive ingredients that are able to do just that: reduce inflammation and irritation on skin. An ever-increasing number of ingredients can perform this function and they do so quite nicely. When these types of ingredients—such as bisabolol, allantoin, burdock root, aloe, licorice root, green tea, or willow herb—are present in a product, I refer to them by the term "anti-irritant(s)."

Even plain **water** gets overhyped in skin-care products. Many products use an assortment of exclusive-sounding adjectives—deionized, purified, triple-purified, demineralized, fossilized—to describe what is nothing more than just plain water. These terms indicate that the water has gone through some kind of purification process or was taken from a specific water source, but that is standard for cosmetics. You will also find phrases such as "infusions of" or "aqueous extracts of" followed by the name of one or more plants. That means you're getting what I call "plant tea," or plant juice and water. Though descriptions like this indicate that you are getting mostly water and a hint of plant extract, they sound so pure and natural that they create the impression that they must be better for the skin. It turns out water is water. The kind of water used does not affect the skin or the final product. After the water is combined with other ingredients, its original status is unimportant.

Silicones are a remarkable, diverse, and ubiquitous group of ingredients that show up in over 80% of all cosmetic products being sold. Silicones may look, act, and have a feel reminiscent of oil, but these ingredients are not oils. Technically speaking, silicone as a chemical compound is related to fluid technology. Either way, regardless of the precise name, silicone is an elegant skin-care ingredient that has an exquisite, silky, somewhat slippery feel; it also has an affinity to skin and "dries" to an almost imperceptible finish. Its popularity in formulations reflects its versatility and the finish it gives products. For someone with oily or acne-prone skin, silicone is not necessarily a problem, because there are new silicone polymers that have oil-absorbing properties and can leave a soft matte finish on skin.

The daily use of **antibacterial ingredients** for purposes of general cleansing, as opposed to using them to treat acne or in other wound care, poses some problems for skin and for society. While cleanliness has merit, there are limitations to how clean a person can be. In the battle against germs and other loathsome microorganisms floating about our environment, the desire to wash with zest is valid (do not take that as a plug for Zest bar soap; I just couldn't resist the pun). We are also greatly influenced by news programs that ballyhoo the horror of bacteria being spread through less-than-scrupulous washing habits. It isn't surprising, then, to hear that sales of antibacterial soaps have increased dramatically over the past several years.

For the consumer, the problem for skin is that antibacterial soaps and cleansers contain **triclosan** or **triclocarban** (the most typical antibacterial agents used), and there is little to no independent scientific data published to suggest that using these products prevents infection. In addition, and even more problematic, is a finding that triclosan-resistant bacteria have recently been identified (source: *American Journal of Infection Control*, October 2001, pages 281–283). Similar concerns were discussed in *Emerging Infectious Diseases* (2001, volume 7, issue 3, Supplemental pages 512–515). The article stated that "the recent entry of products containing antibacterial agents into healthy households has escalated from a few dozen products in the mid-1990s to more than 700 today. Antibacterial products were developed and have been successfully used to prevent transmission of disease-causing microorganisms among patients, particularly in hospitals. They are now being added to products used in healthy households, even though an added health benefit has not been demonstrated. Scientists are concerned that the antibacterial agents will select bacteria resistant to them and cross-resistant to antibiotics. Moreover, if they alter a person's microflora [the body's useful and functional bacteria], they may negatively affect the normal maturation of the T helper cell response of the immune system to commensal flora antigens; this change could lead to a greater chance of allergies in children." In other words, if we are too clean we actually prevent our bodies from developing healthy and natural immunities to many "germs" in our environment.

The April 19, 1999, issue of the *Journal of Biological Chemistry* concluded that the ability of *E. coli* bacteria "to acquire genetic resistance to triclosan [the antibacterial agent found in many antibacterial hand creams and toothpastes] . . . suggests that the widespread use of this drug will lead to the appearance of resistant organisms that will compromise the usefulness of triclosan."

Because of the limited research demonstrating the need for antibacterial products in daily skin care, these products are not recommended.

Benzoyl peroxide is considered the primary over-the-counter ingredient when a topical **antibacterial agent for acne** is needed in the treatment of blemishes (source: *Skin Pharmacology and Applied Skin Physiology*, September-October 2000, pages 292–296). The amount of research demonstrating the effectiveness of benzoyl peroxide is exhaustive and conclusive (source: *Journal of the American Academy of Dermatology*, November 1999, pages 710–716). Among benzoyl peroxide's attributes is its ability to penetrate into the hair follicle to reach the bacteria causing the problem (propiobacterium), and then killing them—with a low risk of irritation as long as no other irritating ingredients such as alcohol, menthol, peppermint, or citrus are added. It also doesn't pose the problem of bacterial resistance that some prescription topical antibacterials (antibiotics) do (source: *Dermatology*, 1998, volume 196, issue 1, pages 119–125 and *Cutis*, February 2001, pages 25–27).

Benzoyl peroxide solutions range from 2.5% to 10%. For the sake of your skin, start with the less potent concentrations. A 2.5% benzoyl peroxide product is much less irritating than a 5% or 10% concentration, and it can be just as effective. It completely depends on how stubborn the strain of bacteria in your pores happens to be.

Despite benzoyl peroxide's superior disinfecting and penetrating properties, some bacteria just won't give up easily, and in those situations a different weapon may be necessary. That's when you should consider prescription topical disinfectants (topical antibiotics).

Alpha hydroxy acids and *beta hydroxy acid*: Please see Chapter 3 for information on these.

PLANTS: A GROWING QUESTION

Survey after survey indicates that women want products that are all natural. To appease the demands of the consumer, cosmetics companies profess that their products are indeed all natural. Yet, to the chagrin of cosmetics buyers everywhere, it turns out that there is no such thing as an "all-natural" product. The term is not regulated by the FDA (www.fda.gov) and it only takes a cursory look at an ingredient label to notice that the preponderance of ingredients are decidedly unnatural.

Not all plants that show up in cosmetics are beneficial for skin. There are many plant extracts that sound harmless, but the research indicates otherwise. For example, St. John's wort contains several components that are toxic on skin in the presence of sunlight (sources: *Planta Medica*, February 2002, pages 171–173 and *International Journal of Biochemistry and Cell Biology*, March 2002, pages 221–241). *Ephedra sinica* is an extract from a Chinese herb also known as Ma huang that has a high tannin and volatile oil content and has been shown to have toxic properties (source: *Toxicological Sciences*, August 2000, pages 424–430). Or take camphor, an aromatic substance obtained from the wood of a southeast Asian tree *Cinnamomum camphora*, which, when applied to the skin produces a cooling effect and dilates blood vessels, which in turn can cause skin irritation and dermatitis with repeated use (sources: *British Journal of Dermatology*, November 2000, pages 923–929 and *Clinical Toxicology*, December 1981, pages 1485–1498). So much for all plants being harmless and good for skin. There are literally hundreds and hundreds of plant extracts being used in cosmetics and most consumers blindly assume that all of these must hold some special benefit for their skin, when in truth that is not always the case.

The issue of natural versus synthetic is one I've written about extensively over the years. To sum it up succinctly, "natural" does not mean good and "synthetic" does not mean bad. Each group has its shortcomings and strengths, but I would no sooner accept any plant as automatically being good for my skin than I would walk naked through a patch of poison ivy assuming that because it's a plant, it must be OK.

None of this should be taken to suggest that plants have no benefits in skin-care products, because they do. But the notion that any plant, from grape to green tea and on and on, has any antiaging properties for skin is yet to be substantiated. Depending on the plant, it can have both a positive and negative effect on skin. Meanwhile, to imply that a pure tincture of a plant (or an extracted component of it) of the kind used in reported research can have the same effect on skin when mixed into a cosmetic in teeny, fractional amounts is, more times than not, a stretch of the imagination.

Having scoured the research regarding plant extracts, here's what I can report unequivocally.

1. Most plant extracts in products have either minimal or no research establishing their efficacy for skin care when used in a cosmetic formulation.
2. When research does exist, it is usually for the pure plant extract, not for a watered-down version used in fractional amounts mixed into a cosmetic of some kind.
3. Most research that establishes a plant's efficacy doesn't take into consideration that plant extracts are highly unstable. Think about it: How long does a head of lettuce last in your refrigerator? The notion that a plant extract can last and remain effective long term in a skin-care product is most likely sheer fantasy.
4. While plants are unquestionably loaded with all kinds of substances that may be great when taken internally, the notion that all (or any) of those internal benefits can be achieved by application to the skin is unknown. There is either limited or no research establishing that rubbing a plant substance over skin is helpful for wrinkles or any other aspect of skin care (though many

plants do have antioxidant properties). When taken orally, there are many reasons to consider plants or plant extracts for regular use.

But for skin care their benefit is mostly theory, and in a skin-care product, the theory is a lot more diluted.

5. Almost without exception I rate the extracted active substance of the plant as having more efficacy potential than the plant. For example, bisabolol is the active anti-inflammatory component in chamomile (specifically *Matricaria recutita*). While chamomile in a pure concentration can have that type of effectiveness, the likelihood is that this effectiveness is lost when the plant extract is used in teeny amounts in skin-care products. However, when bisabolol is listed on the label, it means the product uses the isolated active ingredient in chamomile that has anti-inflammatory benefits, and that the skin has a better shot at gaining benefit.

EVALUATION OF MAKEUP PRODUCTS

For each product category, I use a specific list of guidelines, considerations, and other factors to determine a product's performance, reliability, or value to skin.

Foundations: My fundamental expectation for any foundation, regardless of type (liquid, pressed powder, loose powder, stick, or cream-to-powder), is that it not be any shade or tone of orange, peach, pink, rose, green, or ash—because there are no people with skin that color. Consistency, coverage, and feel are also important. All foundations, regardless of texture, must go on smoothly and evenly, not separate or turn color, and be easy to blend. Foundations that claim to be matte or ultra-matte must be truly matte, meaning no shine or dewy finish, and they must have the potential to last most of the day. Foundations that claim to moisturize must contain ingredients that can do that.

There is a new generation of shiny, iridescent foundations on the market today from many cosmetics lines. They come either in a sheer, moisturizing-type formula or with a slight amount of tint. What they provide is some iridescence or sparkle on the face. While I generally do not care for sparkly makeup, especially for daytime, these products are rated on ease of use, how well they last, how much they flake (controlling where the shine is placed is important—you don't want sparkles falling on your clothes), and how sheer and easy they are to blend.

Foundations with Sunscreens: Foundations with sunscreens are held to the same standards as any other sunscreen, which means they must have at least an SPF 15 and must include a UVA-protecting ingredient as one of the active ingredients on the label. The only acceptable UVA-protecting ingredients are titanium dioxide, zinc oxide, and avobenzone (also called Parsol 1789 or butyl methoxydibenzoylmethane). In the reviews, you will notice that foundations with poor or inadequate sunscreens are criticized severely, but may still receive a happy face rating. In these situations, the performance of the foundations was considered excellent, but the foundation could not be relied on for sun protection and would require a well-formulated sunscreen to be worn underneath. For more details, see the information on sunscreens presented in Chapter 4.

Beauty Note: Color suggestions for all makeup products are often based on tester units available at the cosmetics counter or on samples (including gifts with a purchase or discounted promotions), but mainly from products that were purchased. The color, shade, or tone of a particular product can fluctuate for a number of reasons. If I refer to a particular foundation as being too peach and you find that it's just right, it may be that we simply disagree, or it may be that the product I tested or bought was different from the one you ended up buying.

Concealers: Concealers should never be any shade of orange, peach, pink, rose, green, or ash, and they should not slip into the lines around the eye. I look for creamy, smooth textures that go on easily without pulling the skin, don't look dry and pasty, and, perhaps most important, do not crease into lines. I generally do not recommend using concealers over blemishes, but there is rarely a problem with using most concealers on other parts of the face if they match the skin.

I don't recommend medicated concealers because they are rarely, if ever, "medicated" with ingredients or formulations that can affect breakouts. For medicated concealers to work, they would need to contain an effective exfoliant or an effective disinfectant, and I have yet to test one that meets those criteria and has a color that anyone would dare put on their face.

Despite claims a product may make for oily skin versus dry skin, please keep in mind that companies can make these claims regardless of what ingredients the product contains. In general, the thicker and greasier the product, the more likely it is to be problematic for oily, acne-prone skin. However, anything you apply over skin can cause problems. Just because a product does or doesn't contain oil is no guarantee one way or the other that it won't cause problems for the skin. There are also lots of ingredients that don't sound like oil that can cause problems for skin. Generally, a matte-finish product is best for oily skin, but that still won't ensure a lack of breakouts.

Color Correctors: I am not a fan of color correctors in any form. Color correctors are marketed as a way to change skin color, so that if your skin has pink undertones, a yellow color corrector is supposed to even that out. The only thing these products do is give the skin a strange hue. See "Less Is Best!" on page 371 of Chapter 15 for more information about color correctors.

Face Powders: Face powders come in two basic forms: pressed and loose. I evaluate them on the basis of whether they go on sheer, shiny, chalky, or heavy and whether they are too pink, peach, ash, or rose. I consistently give higher marks to powders that go on sheer and have a silky-soft texture with a natural beige, tan, or rich brown finish and that have no overtones of red, peach, orange, yellow, or green.

Talc is the most frequently used ingredient in powders in all price ranges, and it is one of the best for absorbing oil and giving a smooth finish to the face. Some companies make claims about their grade of talc being better than another company's. The issue of a grade difference cannot be proven and is irrelevant unless the product's feel and performance are affected.

Other minerals are used for the same purpose as talc, and though they may sound more exotic, they are not any better for the skin. Cornstarch or rice starch in powders do help create a beautiful texture and these are interesting substitutes for talc, but they can also be a skin concern because there is evidence that they can clog pores and cause breakouts. I try to screen for these in that regard.

When it comes to bronzing powders, I generally suggest using them as a contour color and not as an all-over face color. Darkening the face almost always makes for an overdone look. After all, if a foundation is supposed to match the skin, how can the use of a powder that darkens the skin be rationalized? The face will be a color decidedly different from the neck, and there will be a line of demarcation where the color starts and stops. Also, most bronzing powders are iridescent. Dusting a color over the face that is darker than your skin tone is bad enough, but why make it more obvious with particles of shine all over, particularly in daylight? The few bronzing powders without any hint of shine are rated highest.

There are numerous shiny powders being sold today, and I rate these products on ease of use, how well they last, how much they flake, and how sheer and easy they are to blend. Shiny powder as an oil-absorbent is never deemed a good idea because if the idea is to powder down shine, then applying more shine doesn't make sense. These products are an option for those who want to add sparkle to their all-over makeup appearance.

Powders are often designated by the cosmetics companies as being for dry or oily skin. Those designations are often bogus, however, with little if any real differences between the formulations. I rate a face powder as being good for oily skin if it contains minimal waxy or oily ingredients and has good absorbency without being heavy or thick on the skin.

There is absolutely no reason to spend a lot of money on powders. Regardless of formulation, there is nothing about price that differentiates one from the other. Some of the best powders, including those with sun protection, are also available at the drugstore.

Beauty Note: Talc is often criticized as an awful cosmetic ingredient that should be avoided. The concern about talc is not about how it is used in makeup, but, rather, when it is used in pure, large concentrations in the form of talcum powder. Part of the story dates back to several studies published in the 1990s that found a significant increase in the risk of ovarian cancer from vaginal (perineal) application of talcum powder (sources: *American Journal of Epidemiology*, March 1997, pages 459–465; *International Journal of Cancer*, May 1999, pages 351–356; *Seminars in Oncology*, June 1998, pages 255–264; and *Cancer*, June 1997, pages 2396–2401). However, subsequent and concurrent studies cast doubt on the way these studies were conducted and on the conclusions they reached (sources: *Journal of the National Cancer Institute*, February 2000, pages 249–252; *American Journal of Obstetrics and Gynecology*, March 2000, pages 720–724; and *Obstetrics and Gynecology*, March 1999, pages 372–376).

While more research in this area is being carried out to clear up the confusion, none of the research about the use of talc is related to the way women use makeup. There is no indication anywhere that there is any risk for the face when using products that contain talc. That means you need not avoid using eyeshadows, blushes, or face powders that contain talc. But it does mean you should consider not using talcum powder on your children or on yourself vaginally. If you still wish to avoid talc in makeup, it is easy enough to do by just checking the ingredient list.

Face Powders with Sunscreen: There are a few pressed powders available that have a reliable SPF 15 or greater and that contain UVA-protecting ingredients. That is great news. However, I am concerned about the way women may use these products. While I don't doubt the validity of the SPF number, I worry that most women won't apply pressed-powder foundations liberally enough to get the amount of protection indicated on the label. If you lightly dust the powder over the skin, you will not be getting the SPF protection indicated on the label. You must be sure you apply the pressed powder in a manner that liberally, completely, and evenly covers the face. I feel that pressed powders are an iffy choice if they are the only product used for sun protection, though they are a great way to touch up your makeup during the day and reapply sunscreen at the same time!

Blushes: I consider it essential for blushes to have a smooth texture, to blend on easily, and to have a silky feel on the skin. Overall, I don't recommend shiny blushes. Although they don't make cheeks look as crepey or wrinkly as shiny eyeshadows do the eyes, sparkling cheeks look out of place during the day. Blushes that go on with a sheen or shine but do not sparkle I describe with a warning, but they receive a good rating if they go on evenly and smoothly and don't flake. This is more a matter of personal preference than a problem.

Cream blushes, cream-to-powder blushes, and liquid or gel blushes are rated on their blendability, whether they streak, how greasy or dry they feel, and how well they last. I also describe which cream blushes tend to work better over foundation and which ones perform better if applied directly on the skin.

Eyeshadows: It won't surprise most of you who have read any of my previous books or newsletters to find out that I don't recommend eyeshadows of any intense shade of blue, violet, green, or red, whether they shine or not. Intense hues may be a personal preference, but I don't encourage anyone to use them. Makeup that speaks louder than you do may be kicky and fun, but it doesn't help empower a woman or help her be taken more seriously. If that's not your goal in life, ignore my color or shine recommendations.

Regardless of color or shine, I evaluate all eyeshadows on the basis of texture and ease of application. I point out which colors have heavy or grainy textures because they can be hard to blend and can easily crease. Eyeshadows that are too sheer or powdery are also a problem because the color tends to fade as the day wears on, and they can also be difficult to apply, flaking all over the place. I am also leery of eyeshadow sets that include difficult-to-use color combinations. Many lines have duo, trio, and quad sets of eyeshadows, with the most bizarre color combinations imaginable. Sets of colors must be usable as a set and coordinated in complementary colors; they should never paint a rainbow or kaleidoscope of color across the eye. However, if you are looking for a kaleidoscope, I've pointed them out; they just have an unhappy face next to them. Generally, it is best to buy eyeshadow colors singly, not in sets. That way you can be assured of liking all the colors you buy, not just two out of three or four.

Specialty eyeshadow products such as liquids, creams, powdery or creamy pencils, and loose-powder eyeshadows are evaluated on ease of use, blendability, staying power, and how well they work over and with other products. My reviews indicate a clear bias toward matte eyeshadow powders as opposed to any other type of eyeshadow. I find liquids and creams hard to control and even more difficult to blend with other colors. Most of them also tend to crease easily and almost always lose intensity throughout the day.

Eye and Brow Shapers: Basically, all pencils, regardless of brand, have more similarities than differences. Most eye pencils, lip pencils, and eyebrow pencils are manufactured by the same company (meaning the same manufacturing plant) and then sold to hundreds of different cosmetics lines. Whether they cost $30 from Chanel or $7 from Almay, they are likely to be exactly the same product. Some pencils are greasier or drier than others, but for the most part there are few marked differences among them. Eye pencils that smudge and smear and eyebrow pencils that go on like a crayon—meaning thick and greasy—are always rated as ineffective, because they can get very messy as the day goes by. (Keep in mind that whether an eye pencil smears along the lower eyelashes depends to a large extent on the number of lines around your eye, how much moisturizer you use around the eye area, the type of under-eye concealer you use, and how greasy the pencil is. The greasier the moisturizer or the under-eye concealer, the more likely any pencil will smear, and you can't blame that on the pencil.)

Liquid eyeliners are rated on how easy they are to apply and on how quickly they dry. The way these types of liners last throughout the day is also a consideration due to the fact that many liquid liners tend to flake and peel.

Lipsticks and Lip Pencils: Every woman has her own needs and preferences when it comes to lipstick. Some women like sheer applications; others prefer glossy or matte finishes. Colors are also difficult to recommend because of the wide variation in taste. Given those limitations, I primarily review the range of colors and textures available, commenting on texture rather than critiquing it, because personal preference is vital to a final decision. The general groupings are glossy or sheer, creamy, creamy with shine or iridescence, matte, and ultra-matte. As a matter of preference, because of staying power and coverage, I give the highest marks to creamy or semi-matte lipsticks that go on evenly and aren't glossy, sticky, thick, or drying. The ultra-matte lipsticks (introduced first by Ultima II with its LipSexxxy and then made overwhelmingly popular by Revlon's ColorStay, which is virtually identical to the former) are unique because of their dry, flat finish and because they don't come off easily on coffee cups or teeth. They have since fallen out of favor for the very problems I originally commented on when they were first launched—they can chip and peel, and actually cause lips to feel drier and become more chapped.

I evaluate lip pencils according to whether they go on smoothly without being greasy or dry. Lip glosses are also evaluated based on their texture, application, and longevity.

Mascaras: Mascaras should go on easily and quickly while building length and thickness. Mascara brush shapes have improved phenomenally over the years, although there are those that can still be awkward to use if they are too big or too small. Mascara should never smear or flake, regardless of price.

Whether or not mascaras smear is difficult to assess. No matter how well-formulated it is, no mascara can hold up to a heavy layer of moisturizer around the eyes. If you wear an extremely emollient moisturizer around the eyes and a lot of it, your mascara will smear.

I don't recommend waterproof mascaras except for swimming and for special occasions that likely will involve tears. All the pulling and wiping that is necessary to get waterproof mascara off isn't good for the skin and tends to pull lashes out. There are hundreds of waterproof mascaras out there, but only a few capture the best traits of nonwaterproof mascaras while still being waterproof. Keep in mind that waterproof mascaras do not stay on any better than water-soluble ones, given that both break down in contact with emollients from moisturizers, sunscreens, under-eye creams, foundations, creamy under-eye concealers, and other specialty products applied around the eye.

Beauty Note: I should mention that I have a personal preference for mascaras that produce long, thick lashes. I admit that my own preference in this regard can get in the way of my evaluations, so understand that I get particularly excited about mascaras such as L'Oréal 3-D Lash Architect that builds thick, long lashes fast and easily without smearing or flaking, though with some clumping.

ANIMAL TESTING

The National Anti-Vivisection Society (NAVS) is a not-for-profit educational group that opposes the use of animals for any purpose, whether in product testing, research, education, or food. While I find some of their policies and agendas rather extreme and radical, I still support many of their efforts to stop unnecessary animal testing and prevent animal cruelty in all forms. NAVS and I differ in that I do not oppose the use of animal testing for health-care research of afflictions such as breast cancer, Alzheimer's, and heart disease, and I am not vegan (NAVS and PETA, People for the Ethical Treatment of Animals, are both opposed to the use of animals for any medical or food use). However, I do oppose the inhumane treatment of animals (no animal should suffer in the effort to help humankind), as well as the testing of standard cosmetic formulations and ingredients on animals. In this regard, NAVS and I agree.

The definitive book on the issue is NAVS's *Personal Care for People Who Care*, now in its tenth edition. This 200-page book lists which cosmetics companies do and do not test on animals, and is a must-read source for any consumer interested in purchasing products that have not been tested on animals. You can obtain the book by calling NAVS at (800) 888-NAVS, by communicating via e-mail at navs@navs.org, or by writing them at P.O. Box 94020, Palatine, IL 60094-9834. The cost is $10 per book plus shipping and handling. Visit their Web site at www.navs.org.

Please note: When a product's label states that the company that made it doesn't test on animals, and the company reports this information to NAVS for the listing they ultimately use in their book *Personal Care for People Who Care*, there is every reason to believe that the information is correct. However, it is naïve to assume that this general information means animal testing information was not an integral part of creating the product. For example, all sunscreen ingredients and almost all of the new antioxidant ingredients currently used in cosmetics, including vitamin C, vitamin A, and most plant extracts, have all been tested on animals. In reality, what we know about the efficacy of these ingredients was first obtained from animal testing. I have broached this apparent double standard with NAVS several times but they refuse to acknowledge the challenge to their criteria. So, while the label on a skin-care product may indeed be accurate in regard to the particular product and the company's policy of animal testing, what it does not represent is the vast group of ingredient manufacturers and university research facilities that use animal testing to determine the basic efficacy of cosmetic ingredients that we all use.

The August 1999 issue of *Cosmetics & Toiletries* magazine reported on a new in vitro testing alternative that can further reduce the need for animal testing. It was approved by the Inter-Agency Coordinating Committee for the Validation of Alternative Methods (ICCVAM). The new "Corrositex assay [test] determines skin corrosivity of a chemical by placing it on a layer of collagen, the same material that holds skin together. As the chemical penetrates the collagen barrier, a material underneath changes color. Corrosivity is rated according to the time it takes the chemical to penetrate and by the color change of the material beneath the barrier."

I am proud to say that my skin-care company, Paula's Choice, does not test any aspect of its products on animals, and I donate a portion of my company's earnings to The Humane Society of the United States (HSUS) every year, particularly during the month of April, which is officially Prevention of Cruelty to Animals month. Please check out HSUS's Web site at www.hsus.org. Their mailing address is: The Humane Society of the United States, 2100 L Street NW, Washington, DC 20037 (they can use your financial help as well). HSUS's approach to the issue of animal rights and animal testing is one I agree with most strongly. The spring 1998 issue of *HSUS News* stated that "The HSUS shares with these scientists [the many who are opposed to or are uncomfortable with animal testing] the desire to eliminate the harmful use of animals in laboratories. In the meantime The HSUS is planning a campaign to urge the scientific community to adopt, as a priority goal, the elimination of all animal pain and distress in the laboratory. The HSUS believes that an emphasis on humane issues will lead to good science and will benefit, rather than harm, the advance of human knowledge."

Companies That Do Not Use Animal Testing on Their Finished Products

Aesop
Almay
Aramis Lab Series
Arbonne
Astara
Aubrey Organics
Aveda
Avon
Bath & Body Works
BeautiControl
Beauty Without Cruelty
BeneFit
Bioelements
Biore
BioTherm
Bobbi Brown
Burt's Bees
California Baby
Chanel
Christian Dior
Clarins
Clinique
Decleor Paris
Dermalogica
DHC
Dr. Hauschka

Elizabeth Arden
Estée Lauder
Exuviance by Neostrata
Giorgio Armani
H₂O+ Skin Care
Helena Rubinstein
Hydron
Jane
Jason Natural
Kiehl's
Kiss My Face
L'Occitane
L'Oréal
La Mer
La Prairie
Lancôme
Little Forest Baby Care
Lush
M.A.C.
Marcelle
Mary Kay
Maybelline
Mustela
N.V. Perricone, M.D.
Neostrata
Ole Henriksen Skin Care

Ombrelle
Origins
Orlane
Paula Dorf Cosmetics
Paula's Choice &
    Paula's Select
PEDIAM
Phytomer
Prescriptives
Prestige Cosmetics
ProActiv
Ralph Lauren Polo Sport
Revlon
Sense Usana Skin Care
Serious Skin Care
Seventh Generation
Stila
Sue Devitt Studio
    Makeup
Thalgo
The Body Shop
Tony & Tina
Urban Decay
Vichy
Zirh Men's Skin Care

Companies That Continue to Use Animal Testing

Baby Magic
Banana Boat
Calvin Klein
Chubs (Playtex)
Clearasil

Colgate Shaving Care
Cover Girl
Diaparene (Playtex)
Dove
Edge Pro Gel

Eucerin
Gillette
Huggies (Kimberly-
    Clark)
Lac-Hydrin

Max Factor
MetroGel,
  MetroLotion, and
  MetroCream
Moisturel
Nivea Visage

Noxzema
Olay
Old Spice
Pampers (Procter &
  Gamble)
Pond's

Sea Breeze
Shiseido
Skin Bracer by Mennen
Suave
Wet Ones (Playtex)

Companies with Unknown Animal Testing Status

Acne-Statin
Adrien Arpel's
  Signature Club A
Ahava
Alexandra de Markoff
Aloette
Alpha Hydrox
Anna Sui Cosmetics
Annemarie Borlind
Anthony Logistics
Aqua Velva
Artistry by Amway
Aveeno Facial Care
Awake
B. Kamins Skin Care
Bain de Soleil
bare escentuals
Basis
BioMedic
Black Opal
BlissLabs
Blistex
Body & Soul
Bonne Bell
Borghese
California North Men's
  Skin Care
CamoCare
CARGO

Caudalie
Cellex-C
Cetaphil
Chantal Ethocyn
Chantecaille
Cle de Peau Beaute
Clean & Clear (Johnson
  & Johnson)
Clientele
Clinac
Club Monaco
Complex 15
Coppertone
Corn Silk
Crabtree & Evelyn
Darphin
Dermablend
Desitin (Pfizer)
Diane Young
Doctor's Dermatologic
  Formula (DDF)
Dr. Dennis Gross, M.D.
Dr. Jeannette Graf,
  M.D.
Dr. LeWinn's Private
  Formula
Dr. Mary Lupo Skin
  Care System
Elizabeth Grant

Ella Bache
Ellen Lange Skin Care
English Ideas and Lip
  Last
Epicuren
ERA Face Foundation
Erno Laszlo
Esoterica
FACE Stockholm
Fashion Fair
Flori Roberts
Gatineau
Gerber
Givenchy
Glymed Plus
G.M. Collin
Gold Bond (Chattem)
Guerlain
Guinot
Hard Candy
IGIA
Illuminare
Iman
I-Iman
Jafra
Jan Marini Skin
  Research
Jane Iredale
Joey New York

Johnson & Johnson
Jurlique International
Karin Herzog Skin Care
Kinerase
Kiss Me Mascara
La Roche-Posay
Lancaster
Laura Mercier
Linda Sy
Lip Ink
Liz Earle Naturally
   Active Skin Care
Lorac
Lubriderm
M.D. Formulations
M.D. Forte
Make Up For Ever
Marilyn Miglin
Mario Badescu
Mederma
Merle Norman
Morgen Schick
Murad
Nad's Gel Hair
   Removal
NARS
Natura Bisse
Neutrogena
Neways Skin Care
Noevir
Nu Skin
Nutrifirm Isomers
N.Y.C.

Obagi Nu-Derm
Ocean Potion
Osmotics
Oxy Balance
PanOxyl
Parthena
Peter Thomas Roth
Pevonia
Pharmagel
philosophy
pHisoDerm
Physician's Choice
Physicians Formula
Pola
Porcelana
Posner
Prada
Principal Secret
PropapH
Purpose
Quo Cosmetics
Rachel Perry
Re Vive
Rejuveness
Rejuvenique
Remede
Reversa
Rimmel
RoC
Sage Skin Care
Sephora
Shaklee
Shu Uemura

Sisley
SkinCeuticals
smashbox
Sonia Kashuk
Sothys Paris
St. Ives
Stri-Dex
T. Le Clerc
Tend Skin
Three Custom Color
Tri-Luma
Trish McEvoy
Trucco
Ultima II
University Medical Skin
   Care
Uvavita
Vaniqa
Versace
Victoria Jackson
   Cosmetics
Victoria's Secret
   Cosmetics
Vincent Longo
Wet 'n' Wild
Yon-Ka Paris
Youngblood
Yves St. Laurent
Z. Bigatti Skin Care
ZAPZYT
Zia Natural Skin Care